D1316346

MAGNETIC RESONANCE IMAGING

AND

COMPUTED TOMOGRAPHY

OF THE

HEAD and SPINE

MAGNETIC RESONANCE IMAGING

AND

COMPUTED TOMOGRAPHY

OF THE

HEAD and SPINE

C. BARRIE GROSSMAN, M.D.

Neuroradiologist
Methodist Hospital of Indiana

Clinical Assistant Professor of Radiology
Indiana University School of Medicine
Indianapolis, Indiana

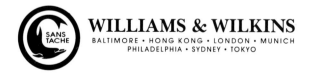

WILLIAMS & WILKINS
BALTIMORE · HONG KONG · LONDON · MUNICH
PHILADELPHIA · SYDNEY · TOKYO

Editor: Timothy H. Grayson
Associate Editor: Carol Eckhart
Project Editor: Shelley Potler
Designer: Norman W. Och
Illustration Planner: Wayne Hubbel
Production Coordinator: Anne G. Seitz

Copyright © 1990
Williams & Wilkins
428 East Preston Street
Baltimore, Maryland 21202, USA

All rights reserved. This book is protected by copyright. No part of this book may be reproduced in any form or by any means, including photocopying, or utilized by any information storage and retrieval system without written permission from the copyright owner.

Accurate indications, adverse reactions, and dosage schedules for drugs are provided in this book, but it is possible that they may change. The reader is urged to review the package information data of the manufacturers of the medications mentioned.

Printed in the United States of America

Library of Congress Cataloging-in-Publication Data

Grossman, C. Barrie, 1938–
  Magnetic resonance imaging and computed tomography of the head and
spine / C. Barrie Grossman.
    p. cm.
  Includes index.
  ISBN 0-683-03768-4
  1. Brain—Tomography. 2. Brain—Magnetic resonance imaging.
3. Spine—Tomography. 4. Spine—Magnetic resonance imaging.
5. Head—Imaging. I. Title.
  [DNLM: 1. Head—radiography. 2. Magnetic Resonance Imaging.
3. Spine—radiography. 4. Tomography, X-Ray Computed. WE 705
G8785m]
RC386.6.T64G76 1990
617'.51'07572—dc19
DNLM/DLD
for Library of Congress   89-5552
                                                                                         CIP

                                                                                       91 92
                                                                             3 4 5 6 7 8 9 10

*To the patients afflicted with
these disorders. May our accurate
diagnoses help to alleviate their suffering.*

FOREWORD

Until computed tomography was developed in 1972, the diagnosis of abnormalities of the brain and spinal cord depended mainly on studies that displayed the subarachnoid spaces, ventricles, and blood vessels—pneumoencephalography, ventriculography, myelography, and angiography. Unless the abnormality being investigated by these methods contained abnormal vessels, the lesion was localized by indirect evidence such as displacement of normal anatomical structures away from a mass. Often an extensive abnormality of the brain or cord was impossible to diagnose by imaging methods then available unless it was associated with edema causing a recognizable mass effect.

The central nervous system presented an unusual, perhaps even unique, challenge for the diagnostician. Very small lesions could cause distinctive neurological symptoms or signs and patients could have subtle abnormalities at the time when they were referred for imaging studies. The neuroradiologist, therefore, was forced to refine the available techniques to meet this diagnostic challenge. Fortunately the brain and spinal cord are almost stationary organs and the normal brain and cord, their blood vessels, and cerebrospinal fluid spaces have a predictable anatomy that has been described in great detail. In order to display these structures to diagnose small and subtle abnormalities it was necessary to have high detail images and the appropriate projections to display or exclude the suspected abnormality. A rigorous, systematic, and detailed analysis of the films was necessary to make some of the more challenging diagnoses.

CT and MR imaging have greatly increased the safety and reduced the discomfort associated with the older imaging methods used for neurological diagnosis. They also demonstrate the brain and spinal cord tissue, thus making it possible to diagnose many abnormalities that could not be shown by older imaging methods.

CT and MR imaging are now the most important techniques for neurological diagnosis. In most cases one or both of these studies will give all the information that is needed in order to proceed with effective treatment of the patient. Modern MR scanners have now been available in many hospitals throughout the world for several years and there are thousands of articles in the medical literature that describe the applications of this technique in detail. We have therefore reached a point in the evolution of this method where it is appropriate to describe it in detail in a hard-cover book.

Dr. Grossman brings to this subject a wealth of personal experience as well as considerable knowledge of the world literature. He also brings to these new modalities the meticulous approach of a neuroradiologist with a detailed knowledge of neuroanatomy and neuropathology gained from experience in the application of the older imaging methods. Just as knowledge of angiography, air studies, and myelography were an asset for the radiologist who was starting to use CT, so also a knowledge of CT is of considerable vlaue for those starting to use MR imaging. The approach of this book—the detailed analysis of CT and MR images of the same patient is clearly an excellent educational method for all students of modern neurological imaging and the very complete discussions of the diagnostic possibilities will make this a valuable text for trainees in radiology, neurology, and neurosurgery. Even experienced neuroradiologists are likely to find the level of discussion and the approach of this book useful.

Finally, at the personal level, it is a special pleasure and satisfaction to see one of my own neuroradiology fellows of some years ago make a significant contribution to the science of modern neuroradiology.

D. Gordon Potts, M.D.
Professor and Chairman
Department of Radiology
University of Toronto

ACKNOWLEDGMENTS

I am grateful to the many people who helped me with this book. Most of all, I want to thank my wife, Sybil, for her constant support and inspiration. She has always encouraged me in my endeavors.

My partner, Richard L. Gilmor, M.D., generously reviewed each chapter in preliminary and final stages for which I am particularly grateful. Many others were consultants and reviewed various chapters in their field of expertise:

Robert J. Alonso, M.D., Methodist Hospital of Indiana, Indianapolis; degenerative diseases

Robert T. Anger, M.S., Methodist Hospital of Indiana, Indianapolis; physics

Jose M. Bonnin, M.D., Methodist Hospital of Indiana, Indianapolis; neuropathology

Malcolm B. Carpenter, M.D., Uniformed Services University of the Health Sciences, Bethesda, Maryland; anatomy

Henry Feuer, M.D., Methodist Hospital of Indiana, Indianapolis; diseases of the spine

Julius M. Goodman, M.D., Methodist Hospital of Indiana, Indianapolis; neoplasms, the pituitary region

Terry G. Horner, M.D., Methodist Hospital of Indiana, Indianapolis; vascular diseases

Benjamin Kuzma, M.D., Methodist Hospital of Indiana, Indianapolis; MR technique

Anthony A. Mancuso, M.D., University of Florida College of Medicine, Gainesville, Florida; ENT diseases

Robert D. McQuiston, M.D., Methodist Hospital of Indiana, Indianapolis; ENT diseases

Valerie A. Purvin, M.D., Methodist Hospital of Indiana, Indianapolis; neuro-ophthalmology

Michael S. Turner, M.D., Methodist Hospital of Indiana, Indianapolis; congenital anomalies of the head and spine, and head trauma

Heun Y. Yune, M.D., Indiana University Medical Center, Indianapolis; petrous temporal bone abnormalities

All of these consultants have been most generous and kind to critique this work, taking time from their busy schedules to help me.

Special thanks to my mentor, D. Gordon Potts, M.D., for starting my career in neuroradiology, training me, reviewing this material and writing the Foreword. His world-famous collaboration with Dr. T. H. Newton serves as the standard for clarity, accuracy, and organization for all authors in neuroradiology. I know that his influence has had a positive effect upon this work.

Thank you, Drs. Mary K. Edwards, Heun Y. Yune, Solomon Batnitzky, and Richard R. Smith for generously donating your excellent case studies. Two Methodist Hospital radiology residents, Robert E. Mehl, Ph.D., M.D., and Jeffrey R. Bessette, M.D., have been particularly helpful to me in reviewing the neuroanatomy and physics material, respectively. Three Methodist Hospital technologists, Michael W. Duncan, R.T., Brenda K. Tabor, R.T., and John R. Dickey, R.T., were most helpful in producing the excellent images throughout this text and in helping with special techniques and technical problems.

Profound thanks to Fran Shaul, radiology secretary, whose cheery optimism, encouragement, consummate skill and dedication has kept this large, ever-changing document in excellent, organized, retrievable order on her magic word processor.

Thanks to Phil and Craig Wilson, artists and photographers, for their excellent, prompt, and efficient work. Many thanks, too, to the Methodist Hospital technical and file room staff for their cooperation and understanding.

Finally, but not least, thanks to the Williams & Wilkins staff: Tim Grayson, medical editor, Carol Eckhart, associate editor, Anne Seitz, production sponsor, Wayne Hubbel, illustration planner, and Shelley Potler, copy editor. It has been a pleasure to work with them.

The joy of completing this text has been tempered by the recent deaths of my mother, Eve Rae Grossman, and my colleague and friend, Dr. J. Michael Gilson—both avid readers and intellectuals. How much I would have wanted them to see this book.

PREFACE

The sudden preeminence of MR imaging for investigation of many head and spine conditions has established a need for one single text to demonstrate state-of-the-art MR and CT investigation and to compare MR and CT imaging indications, techniques, and results. *Magnetic Resonance Imaging and Computed Tomography of the Head and Spine* describes anatomy and pathology, demonstrates MR and CT methods and techniques, and compares MR and CT imaging of normal and abnormal conditions of adults and children. The text is unique because of its prospective side-by-side correlation and comparison, and because of the extensive use of gamuts for lesion identification and differential diagnosis.

Magnetic Resonance Imaging and Computed Tomography of the Head and Spine will hopefully become a handy imaging department reference. It is written particularly for specialists and residents in radiology and the neurosciences. It should also be useful to practitioners and residents in ophthalmology and orthopaedic surgery. The book is divided into four sections.

1. BASIC TECHNICAL CONSIDERATIONS

This section describes, as simply and graphically as possible, the physics and applications of the MR and CT methods. The goal is to provide an easily read basic understanding of fundamental principles. Great effort has been spent creating appropriate illustrations to clarify difficult concepts of physics and applications. The goal of this section is to make topics, that are usually considered tedious and difficult, interesting and easy.

2. THE BRAIN

The inclusion of an extensive MR and CT anatomical atlas is unique to Chapter 4. The anatomical atlas includes side-by-side adult and infant MR and CT anatomy in orthogonal planes with reference to the section level and important landmarks provided by specially prepared line diagram mannequins. Vascular anatomy and neurological clinical correlation are also included. Supplemental anatomical atlas sections of more detailed territorial anatomy such as the sella, temporal bone, face, orbit, and spine appear at the beginning of the appropriate chapters. Other chapters of this section describe intracranial tumors, cerebrovascular disorders, intracranial trauma, infections and inflammatory disease, congenital anomalies, and hydrocephalus and degenerative disease. An extensive gamut section in Chapter 5 (tumors) is included.

3. THE SKULL BASE, SKULL, AND FACE

This section contains chapters on the sella region, temporal region, and the skull and face. Each of these chapters includes an antomical atlas and an illustrated descriptive text. A large gamut section is included in Chapters 11 and 12. The orbit chapter, also in this section, includes an anatomical atlas, an illustrated descriptive text, and a gamut section. In addition, there is a brief applications section.

4. THE SPINE

This is clearly the largest chapter in this text. It also follows the anatomy atlas/illustrated text/gamut organization and includes a brief applications section. Major effort here, as elsewhere in the text, has been directed toward comparison and relative value of the MR and CT methods. The complementary role of CT to MR for both teaching and clinical purposes is particularly striking in this chapter.

A major effort was made to strive for accuracy, clarity, and simplicity in this approach. Stated facts are documented bibliographically. Most importantly, a panel of expert consultants has reviewed this work and, to them, I am humbly grateful and appreciative. Hopefully this expert-reviewed, single-authored, correlative text—which is lavishly illustrated and chock full of gamuts—will simply, usefully, and accurately show the stuff of MR and CT of the head and spine.

C. Barrie Grossman

CONTENTS

SECTION ONE

Part One. Physical Principles of CT Scanning/ Overview/ System Configurations/ Detectors/ Localizer/ X-ray Attenuation Measurement/ Matrix, CT Volumes/ Section Thickness and Partial Volume Effect/ Section Level/ Data Processing/ Multiplanar Display/ Window Level/ Window Width/ Dose/ Artifacts

Part Two. Physical Principles of MR Imaging/ Overview/ Larmor Frequency/ The MR Signal/ Pulse Sequences/ Gradient Fields/ Data Processing and Image Display/ Pixel Size and Field of View/ Flow Effects/ Gating/ Magnetic Field Strength/ Coils/ Spectroscopy/ Artifacts/ MR Contrast Materials

Part One. CT Scanning Technique/ Scan Speed/ Patient Motion and Need for Sedation and Anesthesia/ Patient Positioning/ Section Thickness/ Image Reformation/ Algorithm and Window Level/ Window Width Choice/ Target Scanning/ Rapid Sequence Scanning/ CT Number Evaluation/ Measurement of Lesion Size, Location, and Ventricular Size/ Intravenous Contrast/ Intrathecal Positive Contrast/ Air or Carbon Dioxide Cerebellopontine Angle Cisternography/ Xenon Inhalation Contrast

Part Two. Basic Cranial CT Diagnostic Principles/ Noncontrast Cranial CT Scan/ Normal CT Scan/ High Density Abnormalities/ Mixed Density Abnormalities/ Isodense Abnormalities/ Low Density Abnormalities/ Intravenous Contrast Injection Scan/ Nonenhancement/ Homogeneous Enhancement/ Enhancement of a Solid Tumor Outlining a Cystic or Necrotic Component/ Smooth Ring of Contrast Enhancement Surrounding an Area Lacking Enhancement/ Heterogeneous Contrast Enhancement with Admixed Areas of Nonenhancement/ Multiple Lesions/ Differentiating Tumor and Edema/ Timing Characteristics of Lesion Contrast/ CT Radiotherapy Treatment Planning Program

Part One. MR Scanning Technique/ Introduction/ Scan Speed/ Patient Positioning and Plane of Section/ Pulse Sequence

Choice/ Field of View and Surface Coil Technique/ Section Thickness and Section Spacing/ Location and Measurement/ Intravenous MR Contrast/ Patient Discomfort, Motion, and Need for Sedation/ Patient Monitoring and Ventilatory Assist/ Precautions with the MR System/ Pediatric Considerations

Part Two. Basic Cranial MR Diagnostic Principles/Introduction/ Intensity Interpretation/ Vascular Flow Considerations/ CSF Flow Considerations/ Fundamentals of Diagnostic Technique

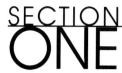

SECTION ONE

Basic Technical Considerations

Physical Principles of Computed Tomography and Magnetic Resonance Imaging

This chapter will briefly describe the physical principles of computed tomography (CT) and magnetic resonance (MR). Both of these diagnostic methods provide remarkable (but selectively different) detail of body parts and of physiological phenomena. Both processes produce sectional images from digital data. Chapters 2 and 3 will discuss applications, techniques, and indications of CT and MR, respectively.

Because of the fundamental physical differences between CT and MR, they will be discussed separately. The introductory section of Chapter 3 briefly compares the two methods of investigation and shows their complementary roles.

PART ONE

Physical Principles of CT Scanning

Overview

CT utilizes x-ray as its imaging source, most often using 120 kVp. The attenuation of the x-ray beam by body parts is measured by detectors and produces the data necessary for image production. Thin x-ray beams traversing the chosen body section at various angles are necessary for the process. Historically, there have been several CT scanner configurations.

Generally, two of these systems (third and fourth generation) are currently in use. An additional scanner configuration (scanning electron beam system) has been introduced and will also be discussed.

System Configurations

Common to all three systems is the gantry. The gantry is the structural frame containing the x-ray source and the detectors. Central to the gantry is the aperture within which the patient lies. The gantry of most third and fourth generation CT systems can tilt up to 20° in either direction. In the standard (third and fourth generation) systems, a thin x-ray fan beam of approximately 40° is generated. The x-ray tube rapidly rotates (usually 360°) in these standard scanner systems. In the third generation system (Fig. 1.1**A**), an array of multiple, small x-ray detectors is affixed opposite the x-ray tube and both rotate as a unit. In the fourth generation system (Fig. 1.1**B**), the detectors are stationary surrounding the walls of the gantry. The fastest head scans from these systems are about 2 sec.

The scanning electron beam system electronically focuses an electron beam generated by a linear accelerator along a stationary tungsten target area to generate the required multitude of x-ray beams. Stationary detectors similar to the fourth generation system then record the x-ray attenuation (Fig. 1.1*C*). The potential for very rapid imaging results. The detectors of all CT systems record x-ray attenuation of the body parts measured at different angles. The fastest scan time for head images on the scanning electron beam system is about 35 msec.

Detectors

The x-ray detectors are made of materials that are sensitive to x-ray attenuation and have the ability to "recover" quickly in order to record the next "reading." The two principal materials used are gas (xenon) or scintillating crystals (such as cesium iodide or bismuth germinate). Gas detectors record x-ray photon intensity due to ionization causing electron excitation; crystal detectors record photon intensity by scintillation. Detector materials vary in efficiency.

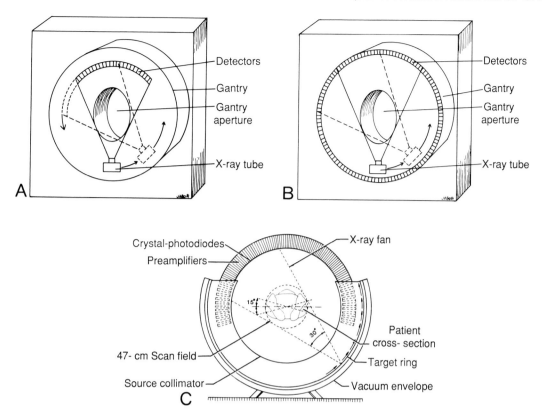

Figure 1.1. The gantry. A, Third generation gantry. Simultaneous rotation of x-ray tube and detector arc around aperture (Courtesy of Churchill Livingstone, Inc.). **B,** Fourth generation gantry. Rotation of x-ray tube only within fixed detector array (Courtesy of Churchill Livingstone, Inc.). **C,** Scanning electron beam CT system. A moving electronically focused high energy electron beam strikes the tungsten target ring at adjacent points producing 30° x-ray fan beams at different angles that course through the object. The fixed detector array (similar to the fourth generation system) records x-ray attenuation (Courtesy of Imatron, Inc.).

Localizer

A digital radiograph (localizer view) is obtained by maintaining the x-ray tube in a stationary vertical or horizontal position while the patient table (couch) is moved an increment per exposure (Fig. 1.2). This digital anteroposterior (AP) or lateral x-ray is then annotated for exact computed slice selection.

X-ray Attenuation Measurement

The x-ray transmission measurements are converted to CT numbers, which are related to the linear x-ray attenuation properties of a particular small volume of the object. X-ray attenuation varies principally with tissue electron density but there is a significant contribution from tissue-effective atomic number. Historically, the energy range that has been used for CT generally has varied from 80–140 kVp. The lower energies have a greater photoelectric effect and the higher energies have a greater Compton effect. The principal advantage of higher energies is the diminution of beam-hardening artifact; another advantage is higher signal-to-noise ratio (S/N). The advantage of lower energy is that the photoelectric effect gives better tissue discrimination. 120 kVp has been almost universally adopted as a compromise.

There is a helpful formula for the understanding of CT x-ray attenuation measurement: $I/I_o = e^{-\mu x}$. (This formula assumes that the x-ray beam is monoenergetic, which it is not.) I_o is the incident x-ray intensity upon an object of thickness x. I is the transmitted intensity through the object, and μ is the linear x-ray attenuation coefficient, which is a constant for a particular substance at a particular energy.[1]

The x-ray attenuation coefficient μ, therefore, can be calculated for each object's small volume and is related directly to a CT number scale called the Hounsfield scale. The Hounsfield scale is based on water having a CT number of zero (0). Air has a CT number of approximately −1000. The upper end of the Hounsfield scale is generally +4000 for most systems. Figure 1.3 demonstrates some characteristic CT number values and the remarkable ability of CT to analyze accurately the x-ray attenuation characteristics within a minute region of the total x-ray spectrum. It is principally this ability of the system to analyze x-ray contrast that has made CT so valuable in diagnosis.[1]

Matrix, CT Volumes

The CT numbers are displayed on a checkerboard-style orderly planar array or grid of squares called a

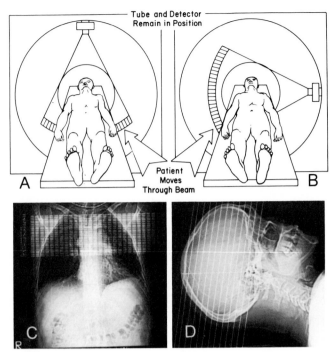

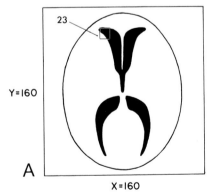

Figure 1.2. The localizer (Fig. 1.2A and B are courtesy of Churchill Livingstone, Inc.). A, AP localizer. The x-ray tube is kept in a fixed overhead position taking exposures coordinated with indexing of the patient couch through the scanner. **B,** Lateral localizer. The x-ray tube is now in a horizontal position. **C,** An AP thoracic localizer image. **D,** A lateral head localizer image.

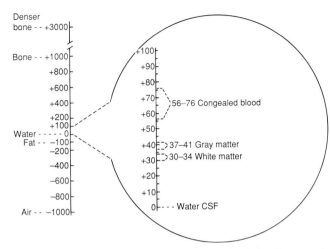

Figure 1.3. The Hounsfield CT number scale. A small segment *(100 H)* of the scale has been expanded to the right side. Only 41 of these 100 units represent normal brain tissue (Courtesy of Churchill Livingstone, Inc.).

matrix (Fig. 1.4A). A single square of the matrix is called a pixel. The pixel represents an object volume called a voxel. The pixel width varies depending on the scanned object field of view (FOV) and the matrix size, i.e.: 256×256, 320×320, or 512×512. That is, a 24×24 cm FOV on a 512×512 matrix has pixel size of 240/512 mm or 0.47 mm. The voxel volume equals pixel area multiplied by the slice thickness.

Section Thickness and Partial Volume Effect

Section thickness is determined by beam collimation. Thinner sections of smaller pixels are obviously most desirable for detail, however, a higher patient dose to maintain the same S/N is required. The thinner section avoids the inclusion (and, therefore, averaging) of undesired body parts within the voxel. An example of this phenomenon is the inclusion of the sella floor on an axial image producing an apparent "dense" pituitary gland. A thin section through the gland would show normal pituitary tissue (Fig. 1.5). The falsely dense gland is an example of the "partial volume effect."[2,3]

Section Level

The level of the body section is determined by the depth of the patient in the scanner because the

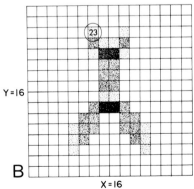

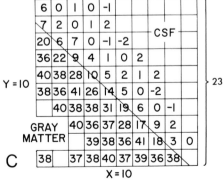

Figure 1.4. The matrix. A, A brain section on a 160×160 matrix at the ventricular level shows good detail. **B,** The same section on a 16 matrix shows a boxy poorly detailed image. A single pixel square shows a Hounsfield number of 23. **C,** Expansion of the pixel *(23 H)* on a 10 matrix demonstrates caudate nucleus (gray matter) from ventricle (CSF) that was visible on **A.** The 10X expansion of the 16-matrix pixel brought each pixel back to 160-matrix geometry and reduced partial volume degradation of detail (Courtesy of Churchill Livingstone, Inc.).

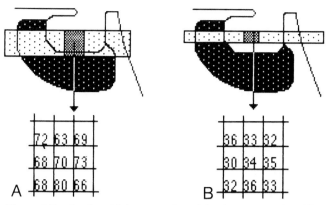

Figure 1.5. Section thickness and partial volume averaging. Midsagittal sella turcica. *Light stipple* = CT section. *Dark area* = sphenoid sinus. *Intermediate area* = volume whose pixels are viewed from above. **A,** Thick section includes sella floor and has abnormally high CT values due to the partial volume effect. **B,** Thin section represents only pituitary gland without sella floor partial volume effect degradation. Note normal CT pituitary Hounsfield numbers.

beam location with respect to the gantry is fixed. The angle of section is determined by the gantry angle and the angle of the body part, such as head flexion and extension (Fig. 1.6).[2,3]

Data Processing

Data computation (the computer system) reconstructs the CT image. The unmanipulated measurements (raw data) are organized in a linear form called profiles, sinograms, and views. These terms are used interchangeably. The profile is the detector readout of all rays that pass through an object at the same common angle. The raw data profile is in analog form and is converted to digital data for processing. This conversion is done by the analog-digital converter. The computer analyzes the x-ray profiles and enters them into a planned sequence of mathematical routines—the algorithm. The algorithm computes attenuation values for all pixels. The method commonly used is filtered back projection. The algorithm may be considered as a two-step system. The first step is the convolution (filter) function, which assigns profile intensity. The second step is back projection of the convoluted profile to each pixel that it crosses. The choice of filter function affects image quality. A smoothing filter function is chosen to examine soft tissue and an edge-enhancement filter is chosen to examine bone (Fig. 1.7).[2,3]

Multiplanar Display

Computer rearrangement of voxels in other planes produces "reformations" (Fig. 1.8). Contiguous or overlapping thin sections are required for this technique. The contiguous slices can also be displayed in a three dimensional (3-D) representation.[4]

Window Level/Window Width

The CT number is imaged as black, white, or a shade of gray (the gray scale). Generally, low CT numbers are displayed as dark shades and high CT numbers are displayed as light shades. The window width (WW) is the range of CT numbers ranging from black to white and can be adjusted to determine object contrast. The window level (WL) is the mean or central CT number that determines the position of the window on the Hounsfield scale (Fig. 1.9). A narrow window would have sharper contrast and a wider window would have greater latitude. The choice of a window is determined by the range of CT numbers to be investigated. For example, investigation of hemorrhage requires a relatively narrow window and the investigation of disease of the middle ear requires a wide window.

Dose

As with any x-ray equipment, dose to the patient must be considered. With respect to head and spine imaging, the most x-ray-sensitive tissues are the lens of the eye and gonads. Avoiding inclusion of these parts when not necessary is important. The dose varies with type of scanner and technique. Scan doses range from 1–10 rads.

Artifacts

Patient motion and beam-hardening artifacts often limit CT quality. Most modern CT scanners can pro-

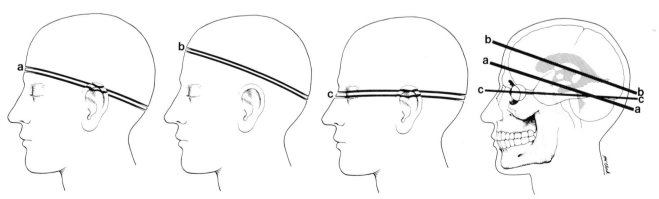

Figure 1.6. Section level and section angle. A, Lower supraorbitomeatal plane section. **B,** Higher supraorbitomeatal plane section. **C,** Infraorbitomeatal plane section. **D,** Diagrammatic representation of **A–C** (Courtesy of Churchill Livingstone, Inc.).

Brain window   Bone window

Soft tissue filter
(smoothing)

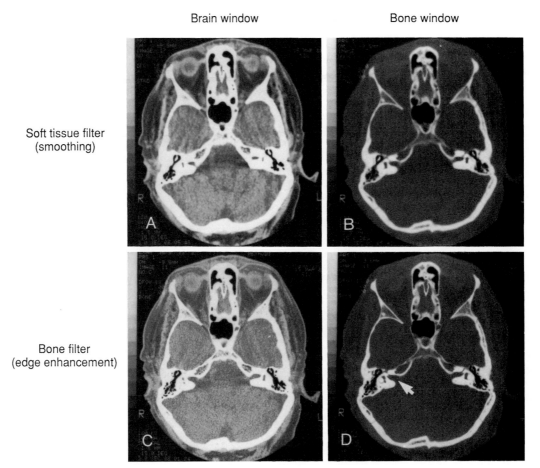

Bone filter
(edge enhancement)

Figure 1.7   Filter functions. A–B, Smooth filter. **A,** and **C,** 38/200 (brain window). **B** and **D,** 38/3000 (bone window). Brain image **(A)** shows good posterior fossa detail but petrous bone detail **(B)** is not sharp. **C–D,** Edge enhancement filter. Brain detail is poor but bone detail is excellent. Note the internal auditory canal and other inner ear structures. **(D,** *arrow).*

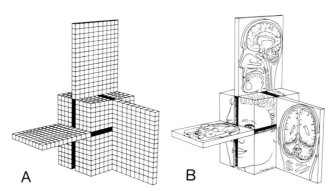

Figure 1.8.   Multiplanar reformation. Layers of voxels from contiguous sections create a "file" from which sections of various planes can be "pulled out." **A,** Digital display. **B,** Analog display (Courtesy of Churchill Livingstone, Inc.).

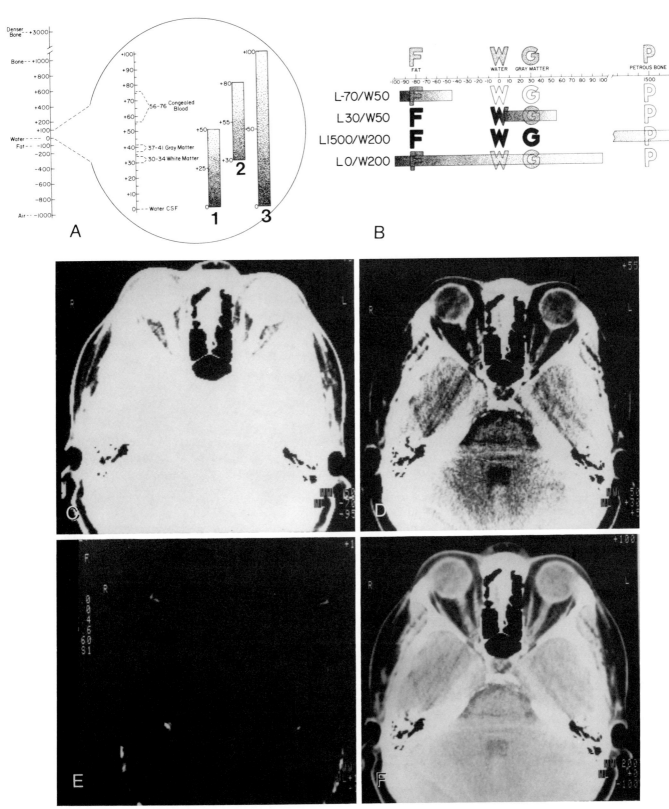

Figure 1.9.   Window level and window width. A, *(1)* L25/W50: CSF, black; gray matter, light gray; *(2)* L55/W50; white matter, black; gray matter, dark gray; *(3)* L50/W100: wide latitude with low contrast of brain structure. **B,** Window level *(L)* and width *(W).* Fat *(F),* water *(W),* gray matter *(G),* and dense bone *(P)* vary in shade depending on the window level *(center of the shaded rectangle)* and window width *(length of the shaded rectangle).* **C,** L70/W50. **D,** L30/W50. **E,** L1500/W200. **F,** L0/W200 (Courtesy of Churchill Livingstone, Inc.).

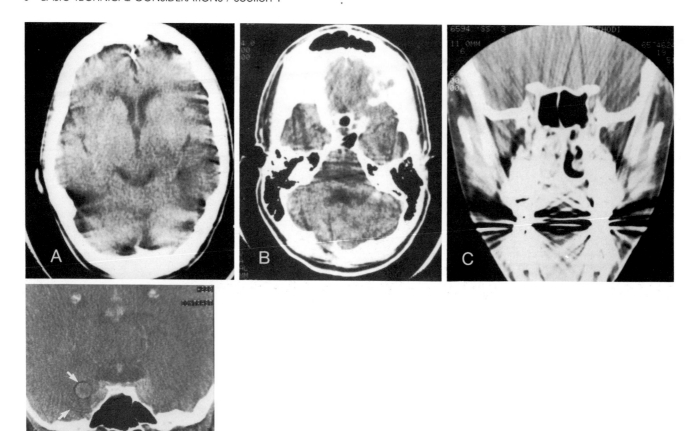

Figure 1.10. CT artifacts. **A,** Motion. **B,** Interpetrous lucency. **C,** Metal. **D,** Ring. Concentric rings *(arrows).*

duce a section in 2 sec, however, these systems still have difficulty with motion artifact when scanning combative patients (Fig. 1.10**A**). Most scanners have a headrest and, often, the use of a Velcro strap of moderate tension helps. Caution is necessary if even mild restraint is used. The scanning beam CT system can produce an image in 35–100 msec that virtually eliminates motion. Beam-hardening artifact (such as the "interpetrous lucency") occurs due to lower energy spectral absorption in areas of high attenuation (Fig. 1.10**B**). Other causes of artifacts are dense foreign bodies such as dental fillings (Fig. 1.10**C**) and detector miscalibration. The latter can produce typical "ring artifacts" on third generation equipment (Fig. 1.10**D**) and a generalized image degradation on fourth generation equipment. Routine maintenance on a regularly scheduled basis limits detector miscalibration problems.

PART TWO

Physical Principles of MR Imaging

The CT technique depends on tissue and contrast media x-ray attenuation that varies with electron density and, to a lesser degree, with atomic number. The routine MR imaging technique depends on the mobile hydrogen concentration of tissue. In addition, MR can identify blood vessels, fluid flow [blood and cerebrospinal fluid (CSF)], and promises to analyze tissue chemistry by spectroscopy. Cortical bone has a very low mobile hydrogen content and is, therefore, essentially signal void. MR lacks the bone-induced artifacts that are so prevalent with CT. CT, however, reveals superior bone detail.

Overview

We have seen with CT that changing filter functions and adjusting windows and levels affect the image. Increasing x-ray tube energy from the standard 120 kVp to 140 kVp can slightly alter the CT number. Dual energy CT scanning has been performed attempting to identify tissue characteristics. By comparison, far more marked changes in image quality, structural identification, and tissue discrimination are obtained with various MR techniques. Present medical MR imaging is more aptly termed nuclear magnetic resonance (NMR) imaging; "nuclear" because the signal detected is generated by the atomic nucleus. At present, we are routinely scanning only hydrogen—the most abundant atom in the body. The hydrogen atom characteristically generates the largest MR signal per nucleus compared to other nuclear species in the body.

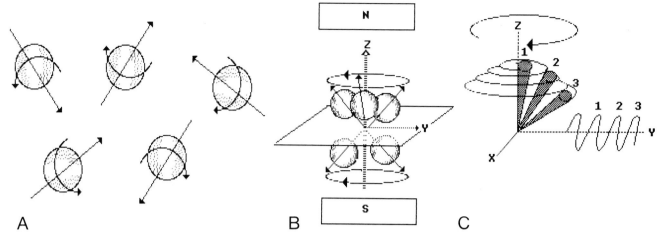

Figure 1.11. Nuclear motion and orientation. A, Random magnetic moment (axis) orientation of rotating nuclei in the absence of a strong external magnetic field. The *straight arrows* indicate nuclear moment (axis) orientation and the *curved arrows* indicate direction of rotation. **B,** Magnetic moments of precessing nuclei distributed randomly about the strong external magnetic field axis forming the surface of a cone. A small surplus of parallel oriented protons forms a net magnetic moment along the longitudinal axis *(arrow Z)*. **C,** The "cone" indicating the locus of nuclear precession in **B** is tilted into the X-Y plane by applied RF. The flip angle and hence the magnitude of the Y axis magnetic moment is proportional to RF duration *(1, 2, 3)*. Under the influence of RF, the motion of the net magnetic moment circumscribes a spiral or "snail shell" 3-D figure.

Each nuclear particle spins about its axis. This spin is an inherent property of individual nuclear particles. A spinning charged particle (or any nucleus with an odd number of protons, neutrons, or both) generates a magnetic moment that has both magnitude and direction along its axis of rotation and will behave as if it is a tiny bar magnet. In the absence of an external field, the nuclear magnetic moments are randomly oriented (Fig. 1.11**A**).

When placed in an external magnetic field, the individual nuclear magnetic moments align themselves along the axis of the external magnetic field, either with the field ("parallel") or against the field ("antiparallel"). The antiparallel energy state is higher than the parallel. There is a small excess of nuclei, usually measured in parts per million (ppm), in the parallel orientation (lower energy state). Application of energy [i.e., radiofrequency (RF)] can raise the proton energy state from parallel to antiparallel. *It is these nuclei that eventually provide the MR imaging signal.*

The individual nuclear magnetic moments do not actually line up in a plane parallel to the axis of the external magnetic field. Instead, the nuclear moments are at an angle to the axis of the field and precess about the axis in a manner similar to a top precessing about the earth's gravitational field. The individual nuclear moments are distributed randomly about the axis of the external magnetic field, forming the surface of a cone. Due to the small excess of nuclei in the parallel direction, a net magnetic moment is generated along the axis of the external magnetic field (Fig. 1.11**B**). The net magnetic moment and the frequency of precession are the basic physical phenomena upon which the MR technique is based.[5,6]

Larmor Frequency

The frequency of precession *(W)* is called the Larmor frequency and is a predictable function of the specific nucleus and the strength *B* of the surrounding magnetic field. This relationship is expressed as $W = \gamma B$. W is expressed in MHz/sec, *B* is expressed in Tesla, and γ is the gyromagnetic ratio of the specific nucleus and is expressed in megahertz/Tesla (MHz/T). The gyromagnetic ratio (γ) for hydrogen is 42.6 MHz/T. At 1.5 T, the Larmor frequency for hydrogen is 63.86 million cycles per sec or 63.86 MHz, the approximate broadcasting frequency of TV channel 3. At 0.6 T, the Larmor frequency for hydrogen is $63.86 \times 0.6/1.5 = 25.54$ MHz, and so on.[6,7] Copper shielding of the MR room prevents outside RF interference.

The precessing nuclei will absorb and induce a signal in RF coils only when the energy is applied at the Larmor frequency. This phenomenon is referred to as *resonance*. All excitation RF pulses are applied perpendicularly to the axis of the external magnetic field. The precessing nuclei absorb energy and the net collective magnetic moment is tipped away from the external field axis. The pulse duration determines the degree of net collective moment deflection. A 90° RF pulse tips the net moment into the X-Y plane perpendicular to the axis of the static field (Fig. 1.11**C**). When the RF excitation pulse is turned off, the individual nuclei begin losing energy as the net magnetic moment begins to return to its original orientation. The excess energy of only those nuclei that are precessing in the X-Y plane induce an alternating current in a detecting RF coil with a RF equal to the precessional or the Larmor frequency. The detecting RF coil is often the same one used to generate the excitation pulse.[6,7]

There are actually two independent exponential processes at work during the de-excitation phase: the recovery of the net magnetic moment along the axis of the static field (Z axis) and the loss of magnetization in the X-Y plane (Fig. 1.12). Immediately after the excitation pulse, the individual nuclei are precessing in phase (all together). During the de-excitation phase the individual nuclei get out of phase, thus dispersing or reducing the magnetic moment in the X-Y plane. *The term "longitudinal relaxation" refers to the net magnetic moment relaxation along the Z axis and "transverse relaxation" refers to phase relaxation.* Loss of magnetization in the X-Y plane is due to the T2 or transverse relaxation, and recovery along the Z axis is due to the T1 or longitudinal relaxation.

The MR Signal

The MR signal is a complex function of the concentration of deflected mobile hydrogen atoms N, T1- and T2-relaxation times, flow or motion within the sample, MR sequence, imaging protocol, and the MR system. N is also called nuclear spin density. It is usually measured in moles/m^3. T1 is the time required for magnetization buildup in the Z axis to reach 63% of its original value. It is also called the spin-lattice relaxation time because energy is lost by the higher energy protons to the environment (lattice) during relaxation from the higher to the lower energy state. Water and other liquids have long T1s. Inhomogeneous and compact molecular environments have shorter T1s. Free "unbound" water has a longer T1 than "bound" water. Bound water is attached to macromolecules and cannot reorient quickly ("tumble") as can free water molecules. T1 increases gradually with increasing field strength. T1 ranges from a few hundred msec to a few sec in different biological tissues.[5,6]

T2 is a measure of the rate of loss of transverse magnetization (in the X-Y plane). It is the time required to reduce the X-Y plane magnetization to 37% of its original value. T2 is also called the spin-spin relaxation time because it results from energy transfer from higher energy nuclei to lower energy nuclei rather than transfer of energy to the lattice as with T1. T2 ranges from a few msec to a few hundred msec. For any specific tissue, T2 is always less than T1.[5,6]

MR signals are stronger from fluid, fats, and soft tissue than from bone (body fluid has a high mobile hydrogen content and bone has a relatively low mobile hydrogen content). Because cortical bone has a low mobile hydrogen content, it is virtually devoid of MR signal. The signal void of bone is also due to the extremely long T1 and extremely short T2 of hydroxyapatite.[8] The signal from muscle is of intermediate strength. Bone marrow, because of its high fat content, has a strong T1 and a moderately strong T2 signal intensity.

Proton relaxation enhancement (PRE) is induced by paramagnetic substances. Paramagnetic substances are characterized by the presence of at least one unpaired electron. Examples of paramagnetic atoms include iron (Fe^{2+} and Fe^{3+}) and gadolinium (Gd^{3+}). When there is free access to water protons in an external magnetic field, paramagnetic substances enhance T1 relaxation by creating local magnetic fields or local magnetic perturbations. There is a lesser PRE effect on T2 that requires greater concentration of the paramagnetic agent. T2 shortening is enhanced preferentially by another mechanism induced by paramagnetic molecules—magnetic susceptibility. If water protons are unable to approximate to within several angstroms of the paramagnetic center, T1 shortening will not occur; if paramagnetic substance concentration is great enough, dephasing of adjacent water protons can occur resulting in selective T2 shortening. Magnetic susceptibility is the ratio of *induced* to applied magnetic fields. These effects increase with increasing magnetic field strength. Such substances as intracellular deoxyhemoglobin and methemoglobin and macrophage-enclosed hemosiderin exert marked susceptibility effects with resultant T2 shortening.[9–13].

Therefore, we see that the effect of paramagnetic substances, in solution, upon T1-weighted images is one of hyperintensity and the effect of paramagnetic substances in high concentration, not in solution, upon T2-weighted images is one of hypointensity.

Pulse Sequences

MR images are obtained by using an appropriate sequence of specific RF pulses, signal (echo)-gathering times (TE), and sequence repetition times (TR).

MR signals (echoes) are measured on a gray scale like CT. Strong signals appear white (hyperintense) and weak signals appear black (hypointense). Figure 1.13 demonstrates TR and TE influences on T1, T2, and proton density (N) effects. The T1 magnetization buildup (T1) curve (Fig. 1.13**A**) plots white matter/gray matter and CSF, and the T2 longitudinal decay curve on the right describes tissue intensities after a 180° RF pulse at TR2000. Because magnetization is related to intensity, T1 white matter is hyperintense to gray matter and gray matter is hyperintense to CSF. This illustration demonstrates TR600 (TR *1*) is at the steep portion of the gray and white matter magnetization curves. A T1-weighted image after the 180°-refocusing RF pulse at TR600 msec results because of optimized gray-white contrast and strong signal (approximately gray and white, 50–60% relaxation).[10] TR2000 (TR *2*) is at the flat part of the curve. Gray matter T1 intensity has already "caught up" to white matter T1 intensity and there is less gray-white contrast.

After the 180°-RF pulse at TR2000, the T2-decay curve (Fig. 1.13**B**) develops. TE20/TR2000 (TE *1*) reveals a T1-weighted image principally because of remaining CSF T1 effects. TE45/TR2000 (TE *2*) is at the CSF-white matter "crossover." At this point, CSF and white matter are distinguishable due to nuclear

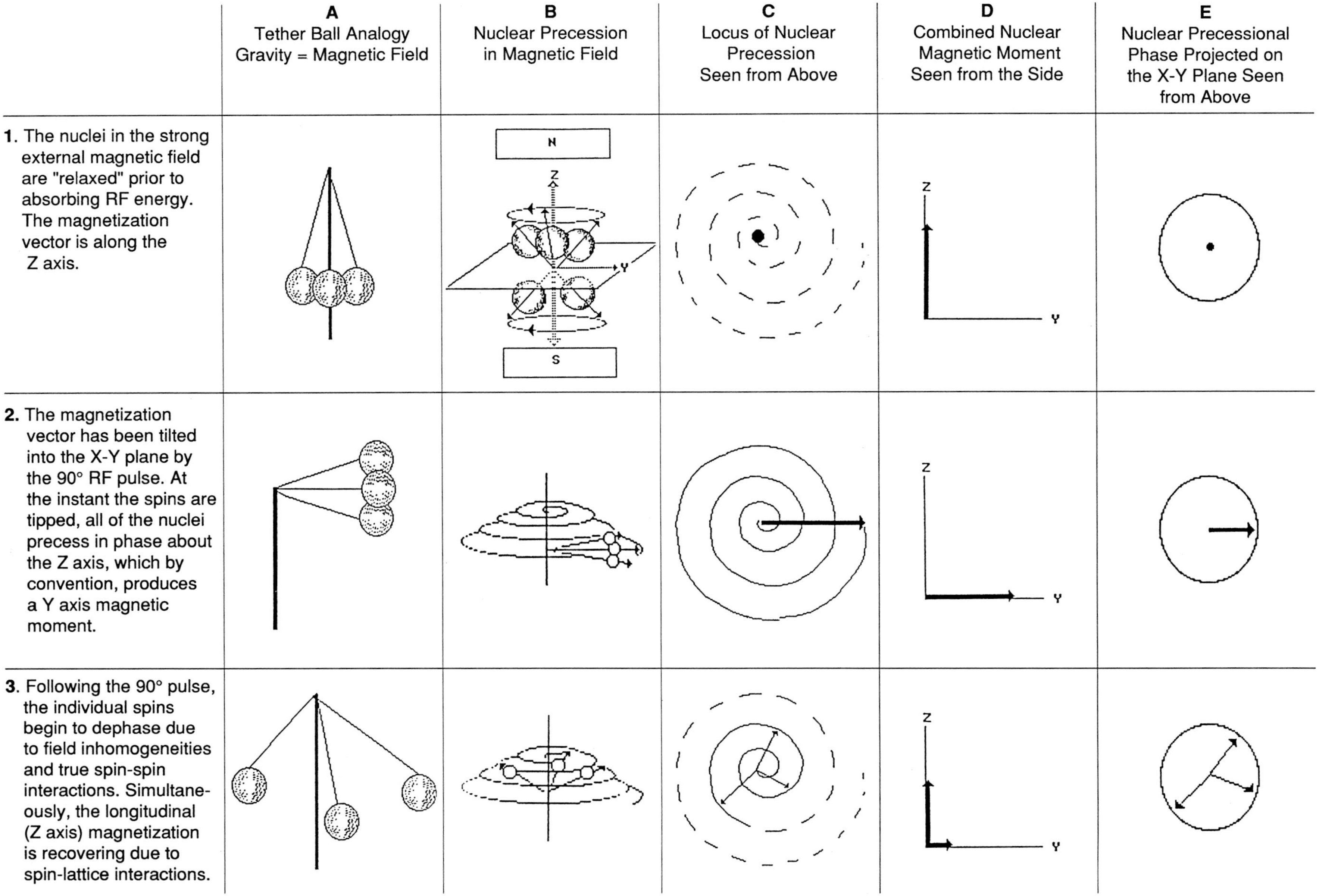

A Tether Ball Analogy Gravity = Magnetic Field	B Nuclear Precession in Magnetic Field	C Locus of Nuclear Precession Seen from Above	D Combined Nuclear Magnetic Moment Seen from the Side	E Nuclear Precessional Phase Projected on the X-Y Plane Seen from Above

1. The nuclei in the strong external magnetic field are "relaxed" prior to absorbing RF energy. The magnetization vector is along the Z axis.

2. The magnetization vector has been tilted into the X-Y plane by the 90° RF pulse. At the instant the spins are tipped, all of the nuclei precess in phase about the Z axis, which by convention, produces a Y axis magnetic moment.

3. Following the 90° pulse, the individual spins begin to dephase due to field inhomogeneities and true spin-spin interactions. Simultaneously, the longitudinal (Z axis) magnetization is recovering due to spin-lattice interactions.

Figure 1.12. **Effect of static magnetic field and RF. A,** Tether ball analogy, gravity, and magnetic field. **B,** 3-D diagram of nuclear precession in a strong external magnetic field. **C,** Locus of nuclear precession seen from above. **D,** Combined nuclear magnetic moment seen from the side. **E,** Nuclear magnetic moment projected on the X-Y plane seen from above.

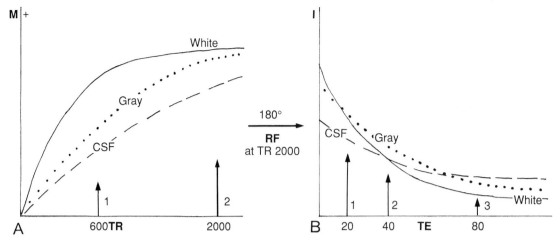

Figure 1.13. TR and TE influences on T1, T2, and proton density (N) effects (after Brant-Zawadzki M[10]). **A,** Z axis magnetization buildup curve. This graph measures Z axis magnetization or relaxation (ordinate) varying with TR (abscissa). TR 1 = TR600 msec results in T1-weighted image after the 180°-RF refocusing pulse due to optimized gray-white matter contrast and strong signal (see Fig. 1.14**A**). TR 2 = TR2000. At TR2000, the gray matter has almost "caught up" to white matter and both are approximately 90% magnetized. There is, therefore, little T1 contrast effect compared to earlier TRs. **B,** After the 180°-RF pulse at TR2000, the T2 decay curve on the right develops. This graph measures intensity (ordinate) varying with TE (abscissa). TE 1 = 20 msec. The 2000/20 image is T1-weighted principally due to persistent CSF T1 effect (see Fig. 1.14**B**). TE 2 = 40 sec. The 2000/40 image reflects proton density (N) due to the signal crossovers with competing and cancelling T1 and T2 signals and low tissue contrast (see Fig. 1.14**C**). TE 3 = 80 msec. The 2000/80 image (see Fig. 1.14**D**) is heavily T2-weighted due to relative absence of T1 effects and water intensity inversion.[10]

spin density effects dominating over low contrast T1 and T2 effects and crossover cancellation of signal by competing T1 and T2 effects. Gray matter, due to its increased free water content, has a proton-density hyperintense signal compared to white matter at the crossover. TE80/TR2000 (TE *3*) produces a T2-weighted signal. T2 contrast is optimized and little T1 effect remains. Note the CSF and the gray-white "inversions" of intensity compared to the T1 effect.[10]

A MR signal detected immediately after a RF pulse is called a free induction decay (FID). A signal occurring sometime after the RF pulse is called an echo. We will not use this technical distinction in this chapter, however, this FID does not contribute to the image.

Different pulse sequences can produce dramatic MR image changes (Fig. 1.14) such as T1 emphasis (T1-weighted), T2 emphasis (T2-weighted), or proton density emphasis. Combined T1, T2, and proton density effects often coexist in the same image, i.e., Figure 1.14**B**. Sequences that are commonly referred to include partial saturation (PS) (often called saturation recovery), inversion recovery (IR), and spin echo (SE).

Ideally, PS images provide a heavily T1-weighted image. It is a relatively fast technique with a high S/N ratio.[3] The PS method is a sequence of 90° pulses separated by pulse repetition time—TR (Fig. 1.15). Data are collected after the second pulse. NEX (number of excitations) is the number of times the pulse sequence is repeated. An increase of NEX improves S/N ratio at the penalty of prolonged scan time. TR is set longer than T2 and shorter than T1 to ensure complete T2 transverse relaxation before the next 90° pulse. Without residual transverse plane mag-

netization, a strongly T1-weighted image results. The signal (echo) is predominantly dependent upon the extent of longitudinal relaxation that has occurred during TR. By changing TR, the image character dramatically changes. If TR is long compared to T1, then total Z axis recovery occurs and the signal is only proportional to spin density (N).[7] We do not currently use the PS sequence.

The IR sequence is a 180° RF pulse followed by a 90° pulse ("flip angle" or "tip angle" of 90°) at an interval called the inversion time—TI (Fig. 1.16). It is a two-pulse sequence. The interval TI is equal to, or less than, T1. The signal is obtained after the second pulse (the 90° pulse). The signal is dependent on the degree of T1 (longitudinal relaxation) occurring between pulses. A large delay is required between pulse sequences due to incomplete longitudinal relaxation.[3] This large delay (greater than $3 \times TI$) makes the technique more time-consuming than PS. The technique has a lower S/N ratio due to its longer TR compared to both PS and SE. Figure 1.17 demonstrates the profound effect of TI variation on the image. Due to the heavy T1-weighting, IR can demonstrate excellent gray-white matter differentiation.[7] We do not currently utilize IR sequences.

SE is a sequence in which a 90° pulse flips the net nuclear moment to the XY axis and the nuclei become phase coherent (Fig. 1.18). After the 90° pulse, loss of phase coherence begins and also the net nuclear moment begins to realign with the Z axis. After a time period (TE/2), a 180° refocusing pulse is applied. TE/2 msec after the 180° pulse, the magnetization partially refocuses to form an echo signal.[6,7]

Both T1 and T2 relaxation times can contribute to SE signal intensity and to contrast. With the SE

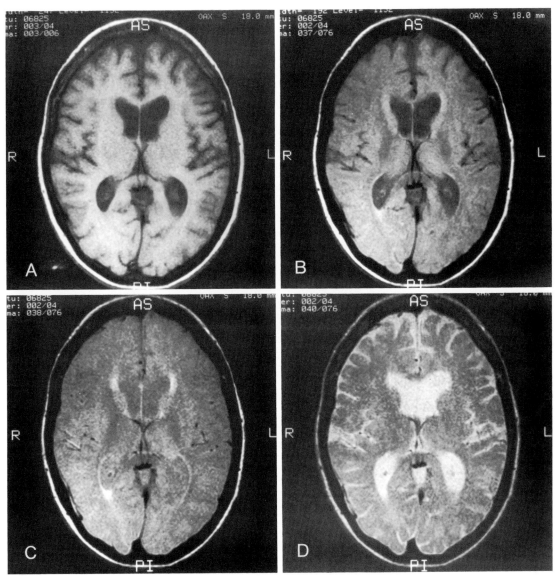

Figure 1.14.   TR and TE influences on brain images. A, SE 600/20 heavily T1-weighted image compares to Figure 1.13A, arrow 1. Gray matter (cortex and basal ganglia) is hypointense to white matter. **B,** SE 2000/20 T1 and proton density-weighted image compares to Figure 1.13B, arrow 1. Note that the gray-white matter crossover point has already occurred. This explains gray matter hyperintensity to white matter on this section. **C,** SE 2000/40. Proton density image. This image compares to Figure 1.13B, arrow 2. The CSF-white matter isointensity is due to the TE (40 msec) at the crossover point for CSF and white matter intensity. **D,** SE 2000/80 T2-weighted image. This image compares to Figure 1.13B, arrow 3. CSF is now hyperintense to both gray and white matter due to the longer TE after the CSF double crossover.

technique and a long TR, the signal intensity becomes relatively independent of T1. If TR is markedly shortened, the signal intensity becomes T1-weighted. SE sequences have become our standard method of obtaining routine T1-weighted images. Figure 1.14**D** illustrates contrast inversion when T2 effects dominate (CSF appears white or "intense"). Because both T1 and T2 effects contribute to SE signal intensity, the T1 and T2 signal contributions can be determined (calculated T1 and T2).[14] We have not found these calculations useful due to difficulty of obtaining values efficiently and accurately.

A major purpose of the SE technique is to obtain T2-weighted images. In order to obtain true T2-weighted images, the effect of magnetic field inhomogeneities must be minimized. This is done by the application of the 180° pulse. This effect is seen in Figure 1.18 where the more rapidly relaxing protons (fast) reverse phase direction ("pancake flip") and "catch up" to the slow protons. T2* is the relaxation time reflecting both true T2 effects and field inhomogeneities. After multiple 180°-refocusing pulses, magnetic field inhomogeneity contributions to T2* are minimized leaving mostly true T2 effects.[10,13]

The conventional SE pulse sequences described have lengthy TRs that approximate T1 water relaxation

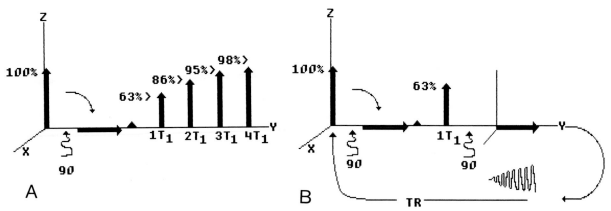

A

B

Figure 1.15. **A 90°-F pulse effect and PS sequence. A,** A 90°-RF excitation pulse deflects net magnetization to the X-Y plane. At time interval $\tau = T1$, 63% of the original net magnetization has recovered along the Z axis. The magnetization recovery is an exponential process approaching 100% after approximately four T1s. **B,** PS se-

quence. One T1 (e.g., T1 gray matter) after an initial 90° pulse, a second 90° pulse is given. After the second pulse, a signal (echo) is obtained. The sequence is then repeated *(long arrow)*. In practice, the TR is greater than T2 and less than T1.

in order to give the image a T2-weighted appearance. These sequences produce high T2 object contrast for pathological conditions in which the water content of tissues is increased. This results in scan

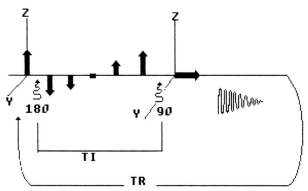

Figure 1.16. **Inversion recovery.** The net magnetization is inverted after the 180° pulse. The recovery of longitudinal (along the Z axis) magnetization grows exponentially. At a time interval (*T1*, inversion time), a 90° pulse is applied and a signal is then produced.

times of approximately 5–15 minutes for a 2-NEX study. Increasing NEX increases signal and increases detail in the absence of motion. Doubling NEX increases signal/noise by $\sqrt{2}$ or by 1.4 ×. (Fig. 1.19).

By using RF excitation pulses of less than 90° (partial flip angles) and substituting gradient reversal for the 180°-refocusing pulse, TRs as short as 10 msec can be used and total scan time can be reduced to less than 3 sec per section.[13] These sequences will be called GRE (gradient recalled echo) techniques. GRE techniques require less RF power deposition (80% less)[15] due to elimination of the 180°-refocusing pulse. Gradient refocusing substitution for the 180°-pulse with short TR/short TE is more sensitive to susceptibility effects. This is due to the lack of the 180°-refocusing pulse. These T2*-weighted images are comparable in appearance to long TR/long TE SE images (T2-weighted images) but with greater susceptibility effect. Heavy T2*-weighting results from smaller flip angles (5–20°).[13,15] Heavily T1-weighted GRE techniques can also be easily obtained. Faster

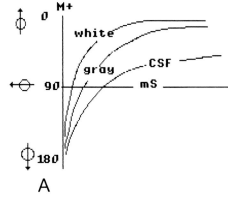

A

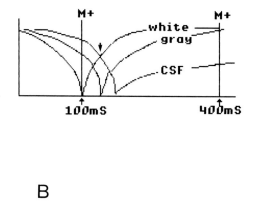

B

Figure 1.17. **Inversion recovery. A,** Longitudinal axis magnetization recovery proceeds from −180° to 0°. At 90°, the Z axis recovery is 0. **B,** The curve can be redrawn this way because the RF coil cannot differentiate between positive and negative Z axis magneti-

zation. Varying TI has a profound effect on tissue intensities. If TI = 100, white matter is hypointense and CSF is hyperintense. At some point, the relationship inverts, for example, at 150 msec *(arrow)*.

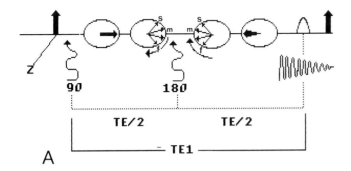

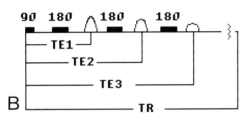

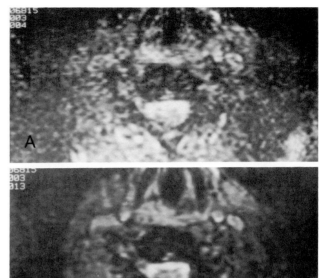

Figure 1.18.   SE sequence. A, One excitation sequence. An initial 90° excitation RF pulse rotates the net magnetization into the X-Y plane *(first oval)*. The *curved arrow* indicates the direction of precession or phase direction. The nuclei are initially phase-coherent in the X-Y plane but quickly become out of phase *(second oval)*. The fast protons *(f)*, those not as slowed by field inhomogeneities, relax ahead of the slow protons *(s)*; *m* = medium rate protons. After a time period of TE/2, a 180° RF pulse is applied which "flips" (or reverses) the axis of the X-Y plane magnetization moment like a pancake. Faster *(f)* protons now trail the slower protons *(s)* thus cancelling out the effects of field inhomogeneities or susceptibility effects. Therefore, phase divergence lost to field inhomogeneities has been converted to phase convergence. This method results in the expression of true T2 relaxation. The lost T2* effect magnetization will not refocus or contribute to the true T2 echo signal. **B,** A variable echo single NEX sequence. Note: diminishing echo intensity.

Figure 1.19.   Effect of increased NEX on spatial resolution. Axial cervical spine. T2-weighted cervical spine images. **A,** 1 NEX. **B,** 4 NEX. Note the improved resolution of the 4 NEX image. No other factors but NEX were changed.

methods are continually being developed and play a role in dynamic scanning (blood flow and perfusion) and 3-D techniques.[13] We currently use the gradient reocusing technique to supplement the SE technique, particularly for spine investigation.[15]

Gradient Fields

So far, we have defined MR, its theory and parameters, and its pulse sequences. We have yet to describe the method of obtaining a sectional image. Let us go back to the formula: $W = \gamma B$, where W is the Larmor frequency and γ is the gyromagnetic ratio. Because resonant frequency W varies with field strength B and γ is a constant for a particular nucleus, small changes of the field strength B slightly alter the resonant frequency W. By applying gradient fields, the magnetic field can be linearly altered during the excitation pulse (Fig. 1.20) and only the atoms in a given section will then be excited by the RF (Fig. 1.21). With a Z-axis gradient (Gz) applied along the long axis of the body, a transverse

(axial) section can be selectively excited by choosing the appropriate frequency for the RF excitation pulse. The thickness of the section depends on the band width of the RF pulse (how many frequencies it contains) and the strength of the gradient field. Stronger gradients and narrower band widths result in thinner sections. Spatial definition within the transverse section is provided by additional gradients in the X (Gx) and Y (Gy) directions. There are three phases of image acquisition: the excitation period, the phase-encoding period, and the readout period (Fig. 1.22). For example, if we are to obtain an axial image, we turn on the Gz during excitation. Now that the body section is defined, it is necessary to define the position of pixels within that section in the X-Y plane. This is done by phase encoding in the Y direction and frequency encoding in the X direction. Gy causes nuclei to precess at frequencies characteristic of their Y-axis location. This introduces phase differences among the nuclei in the Y direction. When Gy is removed, those nuclei all precess at the same frequency but with different phases characteristic of their location; hence phase-encoding of nuclei along the Y direction. During the readout period, the Gx gradient causes the nuclei to precess at frequencies characteristic of their locations in the X direction; hence frequency encoding along the X direction. The order of application of the gradient fields determines the plane of section. If Gx were applied first, the section would be sagittal; if Gy were applied first, the section would be coronal.[7,14]

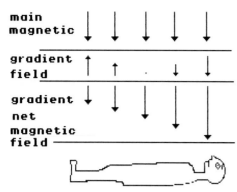

Figure 1.20. Gradient fields. The application of a gradient field (markedly exaggerated) along the X axis linearly alters the main magnetic field during the excitation step of 2DFT.

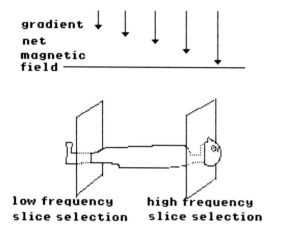

Z-Gradient Defining the Axial Slice

Figure 1.21. Slice selection with the excitation step. Only the nuclei of the selected section can be excited by the RF pulse and, therefore, only the nuclei of the selected section can emit the iso-frequency signal.

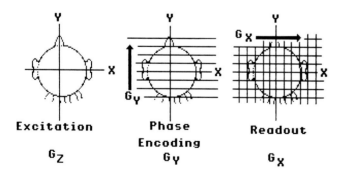

The Three Steps of 2DFT Data Aquisition

Figure 1.22. The three steps of 2DFT data acquisition. During the readout period, the nuclei resonate at characteristic frequencies revealing their location. This is an arbitrary gradient arrangement. GX can become the phase-encoding gradient by operator selection (See Fig. 1.26**E**.)

Data Processing and Image Display

Although each signal contains information from all voxels within the slice, the number of signals necessary to produce an image is the matrix size number, i.e., 128 or 256. The 128 or 256 signals each correspond to a different value of the phase-encoding gradient. Fourier transformation then calculates the intensity values of each pixel: 128^2, 256^2, or 128×256. Therefore, the time required to obtain a single series is $TR \times$ matrix size $(N) \times NEX$. (In the case of a 128×256 matrix, time $= TR \times 128 \times NEX$.) By "interweaving" sequences of different sections, "multisection" imaging can be programmed so that, rather than requiring the multiple of a single section scan time for a complete scan series, the time requirement is lowered 10- to 20-fold.[14] The multisection image data method just described is called the 2DFT method. These sections cannot be reformatted into sections of other planes but rather, sections in other planes including off-axis planes are acquired during a separate series with different gradient selections.

The MR method by which data are simultaneously collected from the entire imaging volume ("slab") is called 3-D. The 3-D method varies considerably in data acquisition as well as image display. Data for 3-D require the RF to be of sufficient band width to include the entire volume. The method provides a higher S/N ratio than the 2-D method at the penalty of increased scan time. It has the advantage of decreased overall scanning time because image reformation in any plane including curved planes (e.g., kyphoscoliosis) is done after the single image acquisition. The technique offers a choice of isotropic and anisotropic data collection. The voxels of isotropic data collection are cubes. Voxels of anisotropic data collection have at least one unequal pixel dimension (Fig. 1.23). Although large volumes can be scanned by the anisotropic method, the highest resolution is obtained in only one plane. The advantage of the isotropic method is the accuracy of images in all planes. Sequences incorporating flip angles of less than 90° make the system more practical with respect to scan time.[5]

Another basic imaging variation is the projection image. This is analogous to the CT scan localizer view and can be used for the same purpose. It is obtained by omitting the slice-selection gradient and using a

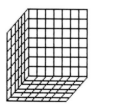
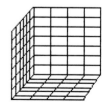

Isotropic   **Anisotropic**

Figure 1.23. 3-D imaging data collection. Isotropic data collection produces less distortions when displayed in other planes.

FOV equal to or greater than the object. It lacks the CT localizer view detail but, in some instances, may be more helpful than the traditional sagittal section MR localizer. To date, we have not used projection imaging at our institution. WL and WW manipulations are used for MR data display. Because MR intensity is not quantitatively specific as are CT numbers, variation in contrast and latitude of the display is the only objective of the WL/WW manipulation rather than intensity quantification.

Pixel Size and Field of View

The choice of FOV determines the pixel size and the resolution. The choice of a small FOV is sometimes referred to as zoom. Increasing gradient strength in the plane of section decreases the FOV and, therefore, increases detail.

Flow Effects

Flow and pulsation influence the MR image. The flow-void phenomenon is the lack of MR signal due to flowing liquid. It is seen in arteries, veins, and CSF. It is due to time-of-flight and first echo-dephasing phenomena.[16,17] The time-of-flight phenomenon occurs when blood flow is too rapid for a pulse to be acquired resulting in lack of signal return. On PS and SE images, complete signal void is seen in ves-

sels of high velocity, such as the carotid arteries. The "flow-related enhancement" phenomenon results from introduction of unsaturated protons resulting in increased signal intensity on the first and last section of the series "entrance sections."[18] Slow flow, such as venous or arterial impeded flow, may produce MR-paradoxical enhancement (Fig. 1.24).[17] This phenomenon can be utilized for blood flow quantitations and blood vessel identification.[16] Flow-related enhancement can be achieved using time-of-flight effects. A flow-related enhancement method utilizing a single section sequence with a short TE (20–25 msec), and a TR varying between 150 and 1000 msec was described in the early literature.[18] A method to eliminate paradoxical flow enhancement perturbs voxels on either side of the slice selection with RF. This method has been called "spatial presaturation."[13]

There is also a CSF signal-void phenomenon in the cerebral aqueduct ("aqueductal signal-void phenomenon") and in the foramina of Monro and Magendie-regions of higher CSF flow rates. This is due more to turbulence than to increased flow.[16,19,20] Physiological CSF pulsation alters the MR proton phase relationship with 2DFT imaging. This can result in signal loss and phase shift (ghost) images.

Even-echo rephasing is another phenomenon that causes slow flow-vessel enhancement on even-echo images of a SE multiecho sequence, such as seen in

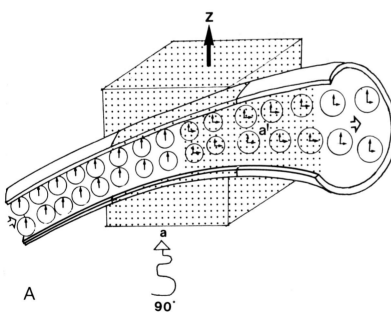
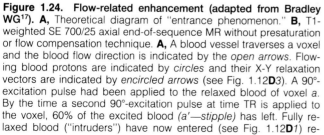
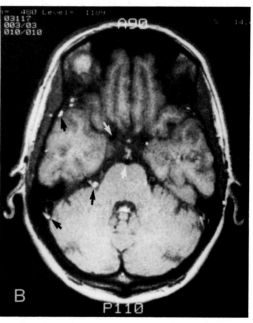

Figure 1.24. Flow-related enhancement (adapted from Bradley WG[17]). A, Theoretical diagram of "entrance phenomenon." **B,** T1-weighted SE 700/25 axial end-of-sequence MR without presaturation or flow compensation technique. **A,** A blood vessel traverses a voxel and the blood flow direction is indicated by the *open arrows.* Flowing blood protons are indicated by *circles* and their X-Y relaxation vectors are indicated by *encircled arrows* (see Fig. 1.12**D**3). A 90°-excitation pulse had been applied to the relaxed blood of voxel a. By the time a second 90°-excitation pulse at time TR is applied to the voxel, 60% of the excited blood (a'—stipple) has left. Fully relaxed blood ("intruders") have now entered (see Fig. 1.12**D**1) re-

placing the energized a' blood. After the second 90° pulse, a 180°-readout pulse to voxel a is applied at which time the echo will falsely demonstrate a shorter T1 relaxation time (contribution from the fully "relaxed intruders"). A bright signal will result. A unit of tissue in a magnetic field that has been equally and simultaneously subjected to a specific pulse sequence is called an "isochromat."[17] The a' *(stippled)* blood is, therefore, an isochromat that has moved due to flow. **B,** Last section of series (number 10 of 10). Paradoxically, contrast-enhanced veins *(black arrows)* signal void of arteries *(white arrows).*

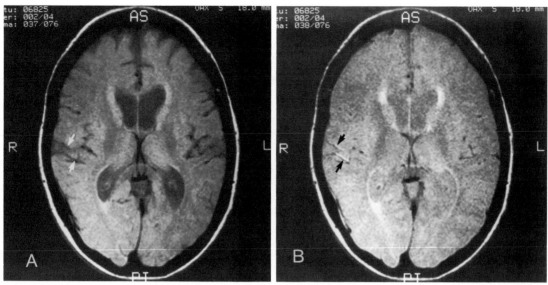

Figure 1.25.   Even-echo rephasing. A, SE 2000/20; **B,** SE 2000/40. Note that blood vessels showing signal void at TE 20 **(A)** are hyperintense at TE 40 **(B).**

Figure 1.14C (Fig. 1.25).[20] Gradient recalled echo techniques with partial flip angles can produce profound arterial, venous, and CSF hyperintensity (Fig. 3.15 p. 50).

Gating (triggering)

Gating serves two goals: the elimination of artifacts and the quantification of blood- or CSF-flow dynamics. Gating is triggered to the pulse or to the cardiac cycle to eliminate flow-related artifacts. Pulse sequence adaptations and complex data manipulation combined with electrocardiographically triggered data acquisition (ECG gating) can produce images with less distortion caused by pulsatile CSF and can result in marked CSF hyperintensity which is useful for spine imaging.[20]

Magnetic Field Strength

The magnetic field strength of the static magnetic field is determined by the type of magnet used. The four common types are resistive, permanent, superconducting, and hybrid resistive/permanent. Resistive magnets require a large power source to maintain the large current demand and continuous water cooling to carry off the heat caused by enormous resistance of the coil windings. This sets a practical limit to field strength of about 2 kilogauss (2 kG) or 0.2 T. The massive frame of a permanent magnet may weigh as much as 100 tons compared to 8 tons for a resistive or superconducting magnet. The field strength of a permanent magnet is limited to about 3 kG (0.3 T). The hybrid resistive/permanent magnets have field strengths of as much as 0.4 T. Superconducting magnets use wires made of superconducting metal alloys that lose their electrical resistance at temperatures approaching absolute zero ($-273°$ or

$0°$ K). Cryogens (liquid helium and liquid nitrogen) are used to maintain this low temperature. New conducting materials are now the subject of intensive research. The coolant requirements for these new materials will be less and may, at least, eliminate the need for liquid helium. Overall operating costs of superconducting systems are the most expensive due to the cryogen requirements. These systems can generate much higher and more stable magnetic fields (15–20 kG or 1.5–2.0 T) but also cannot be readily turned off. Both resistive and superconducting magnets have substantial "fringe fields." These are magnetic lines of force extending outward through their surroundings. Because fringe field extent is proportional to field strength, it is a more serious problem for superconducting magnets. These fringe fields can affect magnetically sensitive devices, i.e., pacemakers, electronic monitoring and recording equipment, and magnetic computer storage media. Conversely, movement of ferrous material within the fringe fields can perturb the uniformity of the magnetic field within the magnet. Permanent magnets do not exhibit such a fringe field and are the least expensive to operate. Hybrid designs also have a small fringe field allowing their use for critical patients with monitoring and life-support devices. In general, the higher magnet field strength produces higher S/N. The S/N rises rapidly up to 0.3 T and then changes more slowly. Neuroanatomical detail appears to be superior with a superconducting system. MR spectroscopy is only practical with superconducting systems of at least 1.5-T field strength. The optimum magnetic field strength for MRI depends on tissue type, body part, imaging sequence, fixed or mobile scanner site, need for chemical shift spectroscopy, etc. For proton MR imaging, the 0.3 to 0.5-MR systems have so far produced satisfactory head, neck, and spine images. The 1- to 2-T systems will likely prove to be the best field strength for multipurpose imaging including 3-D techniques, partial flip-angle sequences, flow, and spectroscopy studies.[21]

Coils

Different body RF coils have been developed to examine different body parts and regions such as head or abdomen. Routine coils are placed under or over the patient. These coils both emit and receive RF signals and are effective at all depths. Specialized coils, called surface coils, have been developed for limited depth penetration of smaller body parts producing increased S/N. These surface coils are designed to approximate the body part closely and some are actually laid on or wrapped around the patient. They have limited depth sensitivity.

Spectroscopy

Utilizing the principle of the Larmor equation (W = γ B), the Larmor frequency W for atoms other than hydrogen (H), such as sodium^{-23}, phosphorus^{-31}, lithium^{-7}, and fluorine^{-19}, can be used and data can be recorded.[23] Weaker MR signals are obtained from these nuclei as compared to hydrogen necessitating high field-strength magnets. Further development of these methods may lead to physiological studies of infarction and ischemia and may help detect early malignancy. At present, we have not found these methods to be practical clinically.

Artifacts

Many types of artifacts degrade the MR image. These can be categorized as artifacts related to extrinsic factors, those related to the MR system, and those related to image processing techniques.[24]

Extrinsic factor artifacts include patient motion and the presence of metallic objects. Patient motion is the most common source of artifactual image degradation (Fig. 1.26**A**). One advantage of the 2DFT method is that it is less susceptible to motion artifact as compared to the CT back projection reconstruction method. Object motion results in typical ghost images in the phase-encoding direction. Metallic artifacts are produced by ferromagnetic as well as other metallic objects (Fig. 1.26**B**). These cause distortions in the main (static) magnetic field and are usually easily recognized. Occasionally, an unusual metallic artifact such as metallic-based eye make-up (Fig. 1.26**C**) or a small paraspinal surgical clip can produce a confusing image distortion.[24]

Artifacts related to the MR system include chemical shift artifacts (Fig. 1.26**D**). This artifact is caused by very slight different rate of proton precession in different tissues and is particularly evident at fat and water interfaces. Because the protons precess at a slower rate in fat than in water, the location will be misinterpreted due to their slightly different precessional frequency. This results in a pixel location shift in the frequency-encoding axis on the matrix. This

artifact is often seen as a hypointense optic nerve margin between the nerve and orbital fat. Chemical shift artifact is more pronounced with high field-strength magnets and increases with narrower band width.[24]

Artifacts related to image processing include phase shift and aliasing artifacts. Pulsating blood and CSF can cause phase shift images ("ghosts") and signal void using the 2DFT method of image reconstruction (Fig. 1.26**E**). This artifact typically obscures anatomical detail of the temporal lobes, brainstem, basal ganglia, and the spinal cord. Peripheral pulse diastolic gating is one method used to reduce this source of image degradation.[25] Another method of reducing pulsation artifact is gradient moment nulling. This method rephases spins that have experienced phase shifts while exposed to magnetic field gradients while moving.[13] Aliasing or "wrap-around" artifacts (Fig. 1.26**F**) occur when the diameter of the object exceeds the FOV. Signal (phase shift) outside the FOV mimics signal from within the FOV from a weak signal location. This type of artifact can produce high intensity signals that can simulate pathology.[24] One method to eliminate this source of artifact is to increase the acquisition FOV to encompass the entire anatomy ("oversampling"). After reconstruction of the raw data, the unwanted portions are discarded.[13]

Truncation or "Gibbs phenomenon" is an artifact characterized by lines paralleling an intensity interface such as brain cortex-bone (rings) and CSF-spine [pseudosyrinx (Fig. 1.26**G**)]. It is related to the data acquisition matrix. Increasing the data collection matrix (192 or 256 pixels) virtually eliminates this artifact.[13]

MR Contrast Materials

Agents (paramagnetic substances) that alter the magnetic environment can shorten T1 and/or T2 resulting in tissue contrast enhancement. The action of contrast enhancement by these agents is indirect (the altered magnetic environment) as compared to the direct effect (x-ray absorption) of x-ray iodinated contrast.[26] Paramagnetic substances have unpaired electrons. Each unpaired electron has a large magnetic field that is more than 650 times larger than the proton-associated magnetic field. Gadolinium (a rare earth element) is one of the most powerful of these substances having seven unpaired electrons per atom. Manganese and iron have five unpaired electrons per atom.[27]

There are three classes of MR contrast-enhancing (magnetic field-altering) agents. These include paramagnetic chelate solutions and superparamagnetic and ferromagnetic particles. Each paramagnetic chelate molecule holds a single paramagnetic atom. These atoms include gadopentetate dimeglumine (Gd-DTPA), iron EDTA, and manganese EDTA. All three chelates decrease both T1 and T2. The superparamagnetic and ferromagnetic particles differ from the chelates in that they are in colloidal suspension and they

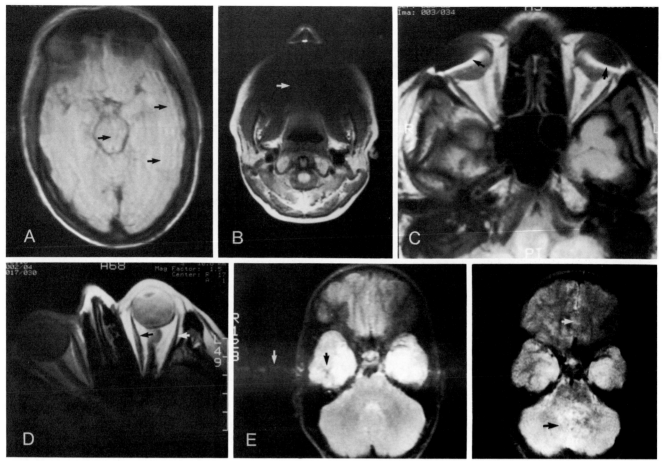

Figure 1.26. MR artifacts. A, Motion artifact. Curvolinear ghost images in the phase-encoding axis *(arrows).* **B,** Metal artifact. Distortion and signal void *(arrow)* due to dental crowns. **C,** Metallic artifact. Ferromagnetic artifact *(arrows)* from metal-containing eye make-up due to magnetic field distortion. **D,** Chemical shift artifact. Hypointense ipsilateral rectus muscle margins *(arrows)* in the frequency-encoding axis of this surface coil SE image. **E,** Pulsation artifact. Left and right SE T2-weighted 2000/80 images, same section and plane.

Left phase-encoding axis is horizontal and *right* phase-encoding axis is vertical. Note the alternating hyperintense reinforcement and hypointense cancellation ghosts *(arrows)* that are *horizontal at left* and *vertical at right* due to the phase-encoding axis shift. The unusual interpeduncular signal void at left is no longer present at *right,* thus documenting it an artifact and not an aneurysm. The cerebellar detail *(right)* is no longer present. On the other hand, temporal lobe detail has returned.

contain 7000–15,000 paramagnetic atoms per particle.

Gd-DTPA is the only approved MR intravenous (i.v.) contrast material to date. Because it enhances relaxation of both T1 and T2, it causes T1 hyperintensity and T2 hypointensity—each effect countering the other. It has been shown that an 80% T1 and T2 reduction results in intense T1 paramagnetic enhancement (see Table 1.1). A dose of 0.1 mmole/kilo body

weight is chosen that satisfies the 80% reduction requirement and heavily T1-weighted pulse sequences are used that emphasize the T1 shortening.

Table 1.1. Effect of Gd-DTPA on T1 and T2 Tissue Relaxation[a,b]

	Without Gd-DTPA		With Gd-DTPA	
	T1 msec	T2 msec	T1 msec	T2 msec
1. Gray	850	75	800	73
2. White	680	65	675	64
3. Extracellular fluid	2500	400	500	80

[a]Note that line 3 demonstrates 80% reduction of both T1 and T2 yet there is ample T1 contrast enhancement.
[b]Data courtesy of Berlex Corporation.

References

1. Phelps ME, Hoffman EJ, Ter-Pogossian MM. Attenuation coefficients of various body tissues, fluids and lesions at photon energies of 18 to 135 KeV. *Radiology* 1975; 117:573–583.
2. Goodenough DJ, Grossman CB. Physics of computed tomography. In Gonzalez CF, Grossman CB, Masdeu JC (Eds). *Head and Spine Imaging.* New York: John Wiley & Sons, 1985;3–41.
3. Goodenough DJ, Grossman CB. Basic radiological principles of computed tomography. In Gonzalez CF, Grossman CB, Masdeu JC (Eds). *Head and Spine Imaging.* New York: John Wiley & Sons, 1985;43–74.
4. Altman NR, Altman DH, Wolfe SA, Morrison G. Three dimensional CT reformation in children. *AJNR* 1986; 7:287–293.
5. Jacobsen HG. Fundamentals of magnetic resonance imaging. *JAMA* 1987; 258:3417–3423.
6. Balter S. An introduction to the physics of magnetic resonance imaging. *Radiographics* 1987; 7:371–383.
7. Harms SE, Morgan TJ, Yamanashi WS, et al. Principles of nuclear magnetic resonance imaging. *Radiographics* 1984; 4:25–47.
8. Oot RF, New PFJ, Pile-Spellman J, et al. The detection of intra-

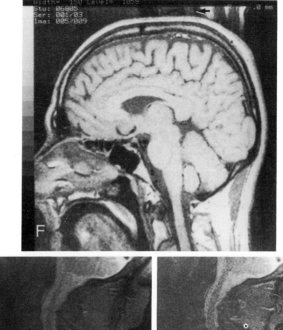

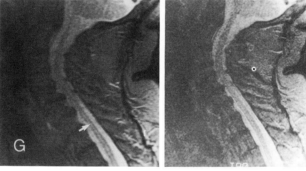

Figure 1.26.F, Wrap-around artifact. Cervical spinal cord *(arrow)* "wrapped" over skull in the phase-encoding direction. **G,** Truncation artifact. "Gibbs phenomenon." *Left:* 256 × 128 matrix. *Right:* 256 × 256 matrix. Note: the centrally located truncation band *(arrow)*. This has been called a "pseudosyrinx" by other authors. *Right:* Same factors but a 256 × 256 matrix. No pseudosyrinx.

cranial calcifications by MR. *Am J Neuro Radiol* 1986; 7:801–809.

9. Bradley WG, Schmidt PG. Effect of methemoglobin formation on the MR appearance of subarachnoid hemorrhage. *Radiology* 1985; 156:99–103.

10. Brant-Zawadzki M. Magnetic resonance imaging principles: The bare necessities. In Brant-Zawadzki M, Norman D (Eds). *Magnetic Resonance Imaging of the Central Nervous System.* New York: Raven Press, 1987; 1–12.

11. Gomori JM, Grossman RI, Goldberg HI. Intracranial hematomas: Imaging by high field MR. *Radiology* 1985; 157:87–93.

12. Drayer B, Burger P, Darwin R. Magnetic resonance imaging of brain iron. *AJNR* 1986; 7:373–380.

13. Wehrli FW. Advanced MR imaging techniques. *GE Publication 7513,* 1987.

14. Wehrli FW, MacFall JR, Newton TH. Parameters determining the appearance of NMR images. *GE Publication 5639,* 1984.

15. Mills TG, Ortendahl DA, Hylton NM, et al. Partial flip angle MR imaging. *Radiology* 1987; 162:531–539.

16. Wehrli FW, Shimakawa A, Gullberg GT, MacFall JR. Time-of-flight MR flow imaging: Selective saturation recovery with gradient refocusing. *Radiology* 1986; 160:781–785.

17. Bradley WG Jr. Pathophysiologic correlates of signal alterations. In Brant-Zawadzki M, Norman D (Eds). *Magnetic Resonance Imaging of the Central Nervous System.* New York: Raven Press, 1987; 23–82.

18. Kucharczyk W, Kelly WM, Davis DO, et al. Intracranial lesions: Flow related enhancement on MR images using time-of-flight effects. *Radiology* 1986; 161:767–772.

19. Citrin CM, Sherman JL, Gangarosa RE, Scanlon D. Physiology of the CSF flow-void sign: Modification by cardiac gating. *AJNR* 1986; 7:1021–1024.

20. Bradley WG Jr. Magnetic resonance appearance of flowing blood and cerebrospinal fluid. In Brant-Zawadzki M, Norman D (Eds). *Magnetic Resonance Imaging of the Central Nervous System.* New York: Raven Press, 1987; 83–96.

21. Bell RA: Magnetic resonance instrumentation. In Brant-Zawadzki M, Norman D (Eds). *Magnetic Resonance Imaging of the Central Nervous System.* New York: Raven Press, 1987;13–22.

22. Koenig H, Lenz M, Sauter R. Temporal bone region: High resolution MR imaging using surface coils. *Radiology* 1986; 159:191–194.

23. Schnall MD, Bolinger L, Renshaw PF, et al. Multinuclear MR imaging: A technique for combined anatomic and physiologic studies. *Radiology* 1987; 162:863–866.

24. Pusey E, Lufkin RB, Brown RKJ, et al. Magnetic resonance imaging artifacts. Mechanism and clinical significance. *Radiographics* 1986; 6:891–911.

25. Enzmann DR, Rubin JB, O'Donohue J, et al. Use of cerebrospinal fluid gating to improve T2-weighted images. Part II. Temporal lobes, basal ganglia and brain stem. *Radiology* 1987; 162:768–773.

26. Runge VM, Wood ML, Kaufman D, Price AC. Gd DTPA future applications with advanced imaging techniques. *Radiographics* 1988; 8:161–179.

27. McNamara MT. Paramagnetic contrast media for magnetic resonance imaging of the central nervous system. In Brant-Zawadzki M, Norman D (Eds). *Magnetic Resonance Imaging of the Central Nervous System.* New York: Raven Press, 1987;97–105.

2 Clinical Computed Tomography Application

PART ONE

CT Scanning Technique

Important variable CT technical parameters include scan speed, mAs, patient positioning, section thickness, planes of section, data manipulation, and rapid sequence scanning.

Scan Speed

Fast scan speeds effectively limit motion artifact and may obviate the need for anesthesia, particularly for children. Some manufacturers offer a rapid sequence scanning package ("dynamic scanning") for the analysis of blood flow, which is described later in this chapter. Scan speeds of less than 5 sec are routine for modern rotate-only third and fourth generation CT systems. The scanning electron beam system can obtain images in approximately 35 msec. Preset programs using function keys are provided for the operator to choose CT scanning technique parameters. Generally speaking, increased scan speed reduces motion artifact and patient dose at the expense of decreased signal-to-noise (S/N) ratio. A longer exposure (increased dose) increases detail (increased S/N) at the expense of increased patient dose and risk of patient motion. X-ray tubes with a high heat-storage capacity are a definite advantage allowing scanning to proceed with virtually all techniques without shutdown periods for tube cooling.

Patient Motion and Need for Sedation and Anesthesia

Rapid scanning of approximately 2 sec decreases the need for sedation or anesthesia. The scanning electron beam system usually obviates the need for anesthesia at our hospital. Light restraint straps are available for most head holders. Use of restraint requires clinical judgment, such as status of the airway, possible aspiration, neck injury, condition of underlying scalp and skull, etc. Gentle care and understanding of the patient cannot be overstressed. Tranquilizing drugs or sedatives can be used to induce somnolence or light sedation. Occasionally, we use chloral hydrate in recommended dosage (see package insert) for infants and children but we prefer to have an anesthesiologist or anestheist administer appropriate light levels of anesthesia. We often use intramuscular or intravenous (i.v.) diazepam in recommended doses (see package insert) for adults. Oral and intramuscular cocktails are often used at other institutions.[1] CT scanning suites should have available oxygen and suction equipment as well as adequate space for hospital beds, anesthesia, and emergency equipment.

Patient Positioning

CT patient positioning technique is used to obtain the appropriate section level and angle of section.

The section level is adjusted by moving the patient couch toward or away from the aperture (see Fig. 1.6). The image localizer (see Fig. 1.2) allows the operator to select the image thickness, levels, and angles before scanning (Fig. 2.1). A laser light reflex is present on most scanners and helps position the patient before the localizer view.

Head extension or flexion and gantry tilt are the methods of adjusting the scanning angle for direct CT scanning. Image reformation (see Fig. 1.7) will be discussed later in this chapter. Section angle for axial intracranial examination varies. Our routine axial brain scan parallels the canthomeatal line (Fig. 2.1A) and our routine spine scan parallels the intervertebral disk space (Fig. 2.1B). A line 0 to −10° to the infraorbitomeatal line (IOML) is recommended for orbital scans[2] and a similar scan angle has also been recommended for evaluation of anter-

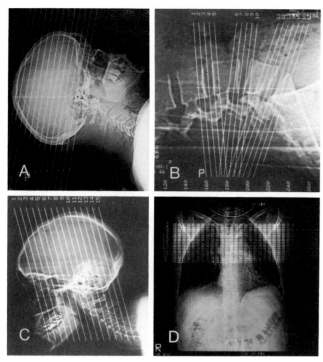

Figure 2.1. Scan plane—scan angle. **A,** Canthomeatal plane head localizer, 1-cm thickness. **B,** L3-S1 localizer paralleling each vertebral interspace, 5-mm thickness. **C,** Direct coronal scan (close to true coronal plane), 1-cm thickness. **D,** AP thoracic spine localizer, 5-mm sections.

omedial temporal lobe structures such as the uncus and amygdaloid nucleus.[3]

Direct coronal CT scanning is performed using the combination of gantry tilt and head hyperextension (Fig. 2.1C). This method usually produces an off-coronal image. The method is particularly helpful for investigation of pituitary, petrous, orbital, and paranasal sinus regions and regions adjacent to axially oriented bones such as the anterior and middle fossa floor. We routinely obtain two thoracic spine localizers. The anteroposterior (AP) thoracic localizer is best for determining the section level (Fig. 2.1D). The lateral thoracic localizer identifies the axial section plane. Direct sagittal cranial images (Fig. 2.2) can be obtained on systems of several manufacturers.[4] The section is off-sagittal and difficult to obtain. We do not find the direct sagittal CT method useful. Cervical spine fractures, severe spondylosis, and subluxation are contraindications to the direct coronal and sagittal methods. Dental fillings often produce severe metallic artifactual streaking. Changing the patient position from supine to prone or vice versa can sometimes help.

Section Thickness

Sections of ten mm are routinely used for head scanning and 5-mm sections for lumbar scanning. Thinner sections, 3 mm, are routinely used for pituitary investigation and 1.5 mm for petrous CT tomography. Thinner sections have less partial volume ef-

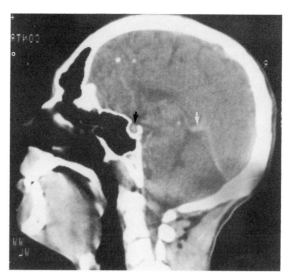

Figure 2.2. Direct sagittal scan. Intravenous contrast 28/300. Sella (black arrow), vein of Galen (white arrow).

fect at the expense of a lower S/N ratio. Increasing scan time (dose) compensates for the lower S/N ratio.

Image Reformation

There are two types of CT image reformations used at our hospital. Both multiplanar and three dimensional (3-D image reformation techniques require multiple thin section images.

Multiplanar reformation can be very useful under certain circumstances, however, initial enthusiasm for reformations has been dampened by clinical experience and the impact of CT-guided stereotaxic biopsy and magnetic resonance imaging (MRI).[5,6] We do not routinely use "reformations" for lumbar disk disease and spondylosis because our diagnostic success with axial sections parallel to intervertebral disk spaces (see Chapter 15). We will obtain reformatted L5-S1 axial images (Fig. 2.3) if the L5-S1 interspace angle cannot be approximated by gantry tilt. The reformatted sagittal image can be helpful for evaluation of lesions in the posterior fossa such as a brainstem tumor (Fig. 2.4) and spine trauma (Fig. 2.5A). Curved plane ("ribbon") reformation for evaluation of scoliosis (Fig. 2.5B) can be useful preoperatively. Image reformation is occasionally useful for brain tumor localization but the direct coronal method is usually sufficient for a complementary planar image display.

Three dimensional (3-D) CT reformation technique has proven useful for pre- and postsurgical evaluation of pediatric craniofacial abnormalities and posttraumatic face and spine deformities (Fig. 2.6). The technique of data accumulation for 3-D reformation is similar to that of multiplanar reformation. It is more useful to surgical planning and postoperative evaluation than to diagnosis. Although its use has been recommended for diagnosis of congenital brain abnormalities, we question the need in most circumstances other than for teaching purposes.[7]

Rapid data accumulation is necessary for these

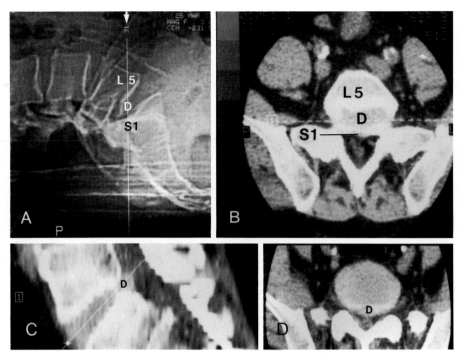

Figure 2.3. Axial lumbosacral spine reformation. A, The lumbosacral angle (37°) far exceeds gantry tilt capacity (20°). L5 and S1 are labeled. L5-S1 disk *(D)*. Unangled section plane *(arrow)*. **B,** Axial section along the section plane labeled by the *arrow* in **A** is part of a "file" of unangled 3-mm sections. Note the L5 bone portion posterior to which is some disk material. The posterior aspect of S1 is next seen dorsal to the disk. **C,** The file is reformatted in the sagittal plane. Note the disk bulge *(D)*. A line cursor selects the axial image L5-S1 disk interspace reformation plane. **D,** Reformatted axial intervertebral plane image demonstrating the disk bulge *(D)*.

Figure 2.4. Multiplanar reformation of pontine glioma. A, Axial 3-mm i.v. contrast scan. Hyperdense mass *(M)*, fourth ventricle *(4)*. **B,** Sagittal reformation. Twinings line (tuberculum to torcular) is divided into two equal parts at the *arrow*. The fourth ventricle lies posterior to the line and is, therefore, displaced, sella *(S)*, torcular *(T)*, anterior *(A)*, posterior *(P)*. **C,** Coronal reformation, fourth ventricle *(4)*, vermis *(V)*, tentorium *(Te)*.

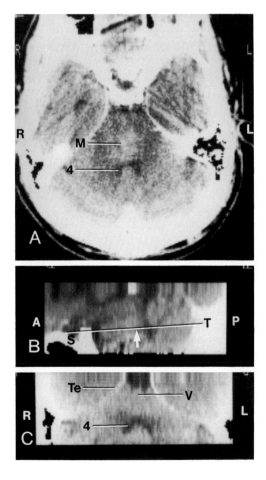

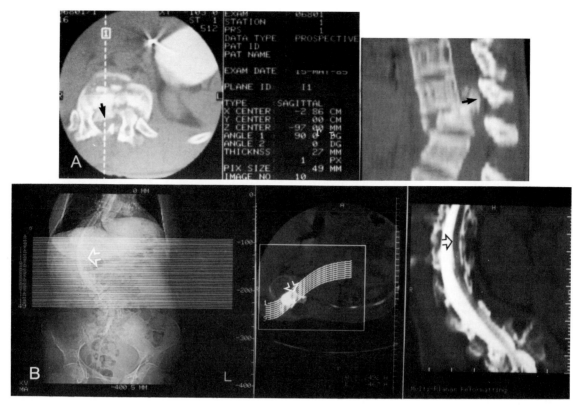

Figure 2.5. Planar reformation. A, Sagittal reformation for spine trauma. T11-T12 fracture dislocation with T12 burst fracture. *Left:* axial T12 5-mm 20/424 image with sagittal cursor line *1.* Sagittal reformation parameters appear in *box at right. Right:* Sagittal section *1.* Note retropulsed frament *(closed arrow)*, T12 burst fracture, wedge compression, and T11-T12 dislocation. **B,** Curved planar ("ribbon") reformation of scoliosis, CT myelogram. *Left:* 49 3-mm axial sections are obtained. *Center:* annotated axial section demonstrating curved coronal planar reformation. *Right:* coronal curved planar reformation. Spinal cord *(open arrow).*

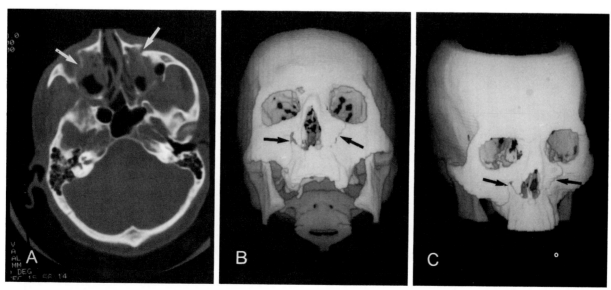

Figure 2.6. A 3-D CT image reformation. Maxillary fractures. **A,** Axial 3-mm thick 200/3000 CT scan. **B,** AP "Waters" and "Towne" oblique. **C,** 3-D-reformatted 49 contiguous 1.5-mm sections. Fractures *(arrows).*

techniques to decrease interval patient motion and to help patient throughput. Fast scanners with high x-ray tube heat capacities are necessary. The unavoidable use of anisotropic voxel collection (Fig. 1.23 and the inability to obtain CT sections thinner than 1.5 mm) produces distortions and inaccuracies with the 3-D CT technique.

Algorithm and Window Level/Window Width Choice

The choice of the appropriate algorithm has already been discussed in Chapter 1 and shown by Figure 1.7. Bone filters (edge-enhancing) are routinely used for petrous pyramid and paranasal sinus imaging. Soft tissue filters (smoothing) are routinely used for brain and spine imaging. The window level (WL) and window width (WW) of the hard copy image varies according to the region investigated and the diagnostic considerations (see Fig. 1.9). Typical "soft tissue" brain and spine WL/WW settings are 35/100 and 30/400, respectively. Bone windows WL/WW (e.g., 350/3000) images are always included on hard copy films of the skull base for brain scans and of all images for spin scans. For lesions that may be obscured by adjacent bone such as a subdural hematoma, an "in-between" setting such as 47/400 is helpful (Fig. 2.7). A "double window" technique is available with some scanning systems. This method simultaneously displays high level/wide window bone and lower level/narrow window brain or spine cord on the same image (Fig. 2.8). We have this latter imaging capability and rarely use it.

Target Scanning

Target scanning is a computer method of processing raw data of a small field of view (FOV) and projecting the small FOV data onto the full matrix. This

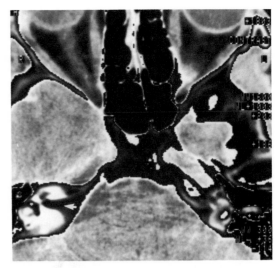

Figure 2.8. Double "window" technique. Simultaneous 1000/1600 and 36/300 axial section demonstrates bone and soft tissue detail. Note brain parenchymal gray tones, orbital and bone detail. The internal auditory canal (arrow).

"expands" the image rather than just "magnifying" it. With the target method, pixels as small as 0.21 mm are obtained (11 cm FOV/512 matrix or 11 mm ÷ 512 = .021).

Rapid Sequence Scanning

Rapid sequence imaging adaptations of present third and fourth generation systems can scan almost twenty sections in less than 30 sec.[8] This method is coordinated with bolus i.v. contrast injection. The change of CT numbers for selected regions can then be plotted on time density curves (histograms). This method has sometimes been called "dynamic scanning." It demonstrates sequential flow images of a particular lesion as well as histographic data (Fig.

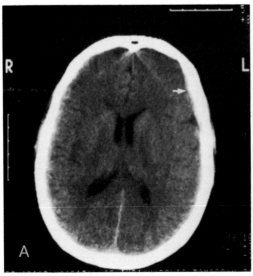

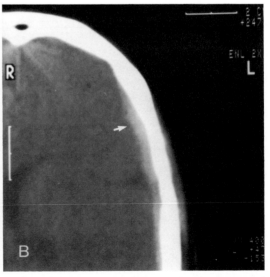

Figure 2.7. "In-between" technique (47/400) for detection of subdural hematoma. A, Noncontrast axial section 33/100 fails to document subdural hematoma. The left frontal bone appears slightly "thicker", however (arrow). **B,** Magnification of the left frontal region of the same section (47/400). Clear evidence of subdural hematoma (arrow).

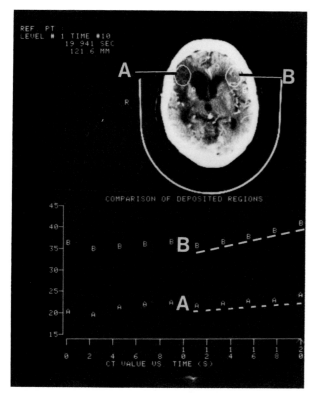

Figure 2.9.   Dynamic CT scan. Remote right middle cerebral artery infarct. Diminished right hemisphere perfusion. Two round cursors *(A and B)* are chosen in corresponding anterior Sylvian regions. A series of 0.6-sec scans at 2-sec intervals at the same level are obtained with a scanning electron beam CT system delayed 5 sec after the i.v. bolus. The CT value (ordinate) vs. time (abscissa) plot shows decreased perfusion and decreased rate of parenchymal contrast increase *(dashed lines)* of the infarcted area *(A)* vs. the normal brain *(B)*. There is slightly delayed circulation time.

Table 2.1.   Classification of CT Numbers

	Hyperdense	Isodense	Hypodense
CT number range (H)	>45	+25 to +45	<25

dense [approimately +40 Hounsfield units (H)]. Clot retraction extrudes serum and increases hemoglobin concentration, thereby increasing the CT number. Recent hemorrhage usually appears homogeneous and usually measures +56 to +76 H.[11,12] Recent clot may be as high as +94 H.[11]

Calcified intracranial regions usually measure higher (or have parts measuring higher) than +80 H. Fat measurements of −100 H are not uncommon.[12]

Lesion CT number values can be hyperdense, isodense, or hypodense with respect to brain tissue and can be homogeneous or heterogeneous with respect to contained CT numbers. Table 2.1 represents a simple (but arbitrary) system for relative density definition.[5]

Methods of CT number measurement are available on all CT systems. The region-of-interest cursor (ROI, Fig. 2.10) is an operator-controlled variable size area enclosure that can be moved to the particular region of interest. Usually the ROI will show the average pixel density and the standard deviation (Fig. 2.10A). Some manufacturers provide a system that displays all the pixel values enclosed within the ROI (Fig. 2.10B). A histogram (Fig. 2.10C) is another method of CT number analysis.

Measurement of Lesion Size, Location, and Ventricular Size

The cursor system of most manufacturers can measure the size of lesions including diameters and area enclosures. Structural shift (e.g., septum pellucidum displacement) can also be measured (Fig. 2.11).

Ventricular size measurements include the ventricular intracranial ratio. This ratio measures the lateral ventricle-frontal horn span divided by the span of the calvarium at the frontal horn level (Fig. 2.12). The average result is approximately 30% between the ages of 15 and 40 years. A slight increase in the ratio (up to 39%) is common in the elderly.[13] We have not found any ventricular size measurements more useful than visual estimates and comparisons.

Lesion localization in a stereotactic neurosurgical apparatus for brain tumor biopsy has been the standard biopsy method at our hospital for over 5 years. The stereotactic apparatus consists of three parts (Fig. 2.13). The base contains pins that affix it to the patient's skull. The CT landmark portion (shown here) is attached to the base. This latter portion is interchangeable with a neurosurgical metal arch portion

2.9). Dynamic scanning, despite its initial promise,[9] has not gained great popularity. Alternatively, more direct means of investigation of vascular malformations and vascular occlusive diseases such as conventional and digital subtraction angiography are favored.

Scanning electron beam CT scanners may renew interest in cerebral vascular perfusion and CT investigation of vascular abnormalities. MR dynamic flow applications are promising but still in the investigative stage at the time of this publication.

CT Number Evaluation

Normal gray matter CT number values of 38.7 ± 2.2 and white matter values of 31.8 ± 2.3 are generally accepted.[10] Younger patients show a smaller gray-white CT number difference than adults. CT tissue numbers may vary with scanning systems and different energies (KV). Investigation of CT gray and white numbers of particular regions can help lead to a diagnosis such as leukodystrophy and generalized cerebral edema or encephalomalacia.

Blood CT number varies linearly with hemoglobin concentration. Flowing blood appears slightly hyper-

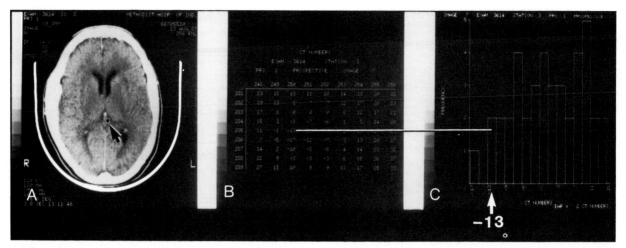

Figure 2.10. Region of interest (ROI) cursor. A, A small rectangular cursor encloses a small hypodense quadrigeminal plate lesion. The average CT density is 2.43 H. **B,** The enclosed pixel CT numbers of the 512 matrix are displayed. **C,** Histogram of the pixel numbers. The histogram column including −13 H has been labeled. The frequency of −12 to −13 is (2) as annotated on the histogram ordinate. A line has been drawn from the −13 H pixel to the histogram column.

The average (mean) density is +2.43. Analysis of the pixel numbers or histogram, however, indicates fat content and, therefore, a diagnosis of lipoma or dermoid tumor seems likely.

that guides the biopsy needle. The CT landmark portion has nine graphite rods (six vertical and three diagonal). By plotting the CT coordinates of the lesion part chosen for biopsy and entering the data into a microprocessor, the angle and depth of the biopsy needle is determined. The CT portion is then removed and the neurosurgical portion is attached to the base. The biopsy needle is then directed through a burr hole according to the microprocessor measurements. A similar type of frame with a nonmetallic landmark portion is used for MR.

Intravenous Contrast

Normal brain tissue demonstrates only slight enhancement with i.v. contrast injection due to the intact blood-brain barrier (BBB).[14] Arteries and veins of the major fissures and cisterns and the choroid plexus of the lateral and fourth ventricles enhance on contrast injection scans. Structures normally lacking a BBB, such as the falx, pituitary gland, and infundibulum also enhance. Each 100 mg of iodine per 100 ml of solution corresponds to 26 H.[14] Using 60% contrast material at 1 ml/kg body weight, the CT number of circulating blood increases 40 H.[15] The distinction between gray and white matter is increased with contrast injection probably because of the more richly vascularized gray matter.[10] Gray matter enhancement of 1.9 H and white matter enhancement of 1.4 H was reported in one series (Fig. 2.14).[10]

The two major methods of i.v. contrast injection are

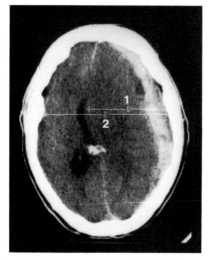

Figure 2.11. Structural shift. Left subdural hematoma with displacement of the septum pellucidum. Axial 37/100 CT scan. Line *2* connecting the skull inner tables measures 11.3 cm. Line *1* from the left inner table to the displaced septum pellucidum measures 6.9 cm. Line *1* minus one-half of line *2* = 1.3-cm displacement to the right side.

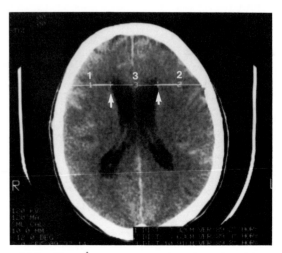

Figure 2.12. The ventricular-intracranial ratio. Axial lateral ventricular level section. A line has been drawn by cursor techniques through the angles of the frontal horns *(arrows)*. The line is divided into three parts. The interventricular span *(3)* divided by the intracranial span *(1 + 2 + 3)* equals 0.37, which is normal for the 63-year-old adult.

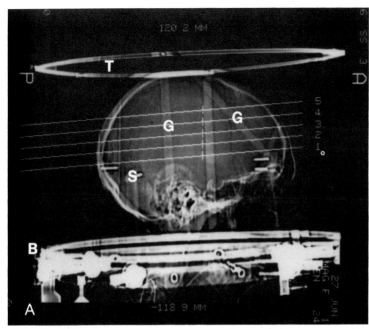

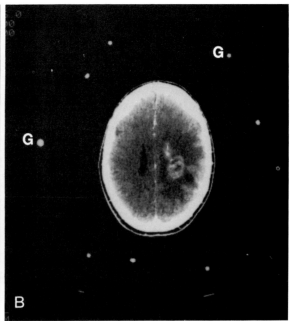

Figure 2.13. Sterotactic neurosurgical apparatus. A, CT landmark portion. The landmark portion is firmly attached to the skull with four screws. Top *(T)* and bottom *(B)* of the frame. Graphite rods *(G)* and screws *(S).* **B,** Axial i.v. contrast CT scan. The nine graphite rods attached to the landmark portion appear as *dots* surrounding the skull. Note the contrast-enhanced left parietal glioma.

bolus and drip. Intravenous drip of 300 ml of 30% solution (approximately 40 g of iodine) for the adult with scanning commencing at half-volume is our routine method. This same dose is occasionally administered for postoperative spine CT differentiation of recurrent herniated lumbar disk versus postoperative scar tissue (Fig. 2.15).[16] Delayed contrast CT

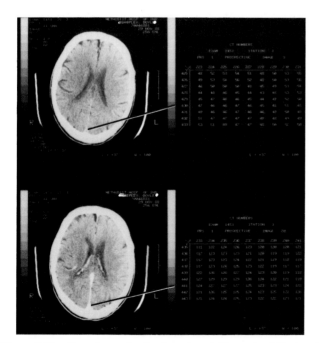

Figure 2.14. Vascular contrast enhancement. Noncontrast *(top)* and i.v. contrast *(bottom)* axial 37/100 lateral ventricle body level CT scans with right-sided pixel display of the posterior superior sagittal sinus. The noncontrast average (46.3 H) has increased to 126.8 H after the i.v. injection of a 42.0-g iodine load.

at 1 hour and 2 hours after the first contrast scan had been initially received with enthusiasm by investigators. It was reported that the delay method was useful for differential diagnosis of some brain tumors.[17] We have not found the delay method to have advantages over the initial routine contrast scan. Our routine for neonates and young children has been 2 ml/kg (approximately 1 ml/lb) of a 30% solution of iothalamate meglumine. Higher pediatric doses have been recommended by others.[18,19] We do not use the sodium salt contrast agents because of probable greater alteration of permeability of the BBB with the sodium salt than with the meglumine salt. No difference of tumor enhancement with these two types of salts is apparent despite the difference in alteration of BBB.[20] Expanded high-dose (double dose) contrast injection has been recommended for improved contrast enhancement of tumors[21] and "isodense" subdural hematomas.[22] We do not use nor recommend the increased dose (80 g iodine load) method. A 3-sec i.v. mechanical injection of 75 ml of 60% contrast injection using a vena cava catheter has been recommended for dynamic scanning. A technique similar to this may be used with the scanning electron beam system.

A preliminary noncontrast scan of the trauma or hemorrhage patient is necessary because contrast enhancement of a lesion and fresh intracerebral clot can be confused. Patient hydration, renal function, and contrast allergy must be carefully considered before injection. Patients with diabetes mellitus and mutliple myeloma are more likely to have compromised renal function after i.v. contrast injection.

There is currently a lot of controversy considering the substitution of ionic i.v. contrast agents with

Figure 2.15. Intrathecal and i.v. contrast-enhanced spine CT scan. Recurrent herniated disk. **A,** Iopamidol CT myelogram L5-S1 level. Left laminectomy *(open arrow).* The contrast-filled thecal sac is overlaid by the *solid arrow* that points to the herniated disk. **B,** Intravenous contrast lumbar CT scan. The margins of the herniated disk contrast enhance.

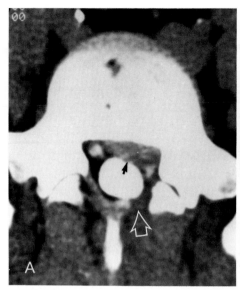 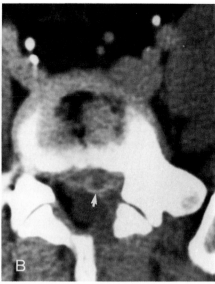

nonionic agents. Iohexol (Omnipaque) and iopamidol (Isovue) are two recently introduced nonionic monomeric contrast agents that have replaced metrizamide as an intrathecal contrast agent. Ioxaglate (Hexabrix) is an ionic dimeric vascular contrast agent also recently introduced in this country. Ioxaglate is often used for arteriography due to lesser induced subjective side effects (pain, heat, metallic taste, and nausea). Intravenous iohexol has even a lower frequency of induced subjective side effects than ioxaglate probably due to its lesser degree of protein binding, decreased liberation of histamines, and lesser inhibition of enzymes. Nonionic agents may have a lesser tendency to cross the BBB, however.[23]

It has yet to be proven that a greater degree of life-threatening i.v. contrast-induced reactions occur with ionics; however, some European reports suggest that there is significantly greater patient safety with the nonionic agents. If such is the case, the cost of i.v. injection examinations will dramatically rise due to the much greater expense of the nonionic contrast agents.

Intrathecal Positive Contrast

We have replaced metrizamide with iopamidol and iohexol at our hospital due to the much fewer and less severe adverse side effects with the newer agents. Contrast density is equal for recommended doses of all three contrast materials.[24–26] We use doses and follow precautions according to the package inserts. One must be aware of contraindications to lumbar puncture such as obstructive hydrocephalus and impending brain herniation. The contrast comes in two intrathecal concentrations. The low concentration is used for lumbar myelography and may be used for lateral cervical puncture and cervical myelography. The high concentration is used for multilevel studies via either the cervical or lumbar approach in order to take advantage of the higher specific gravity bolus before dilution. When we perform CT cisternography

or myelography, it is usually preceded by a conventional myelogram and serves as a complementary study of a specific area for enhanced detail. On the rare occasions that we perform CT-positive contrast cisternography alone, we use reduced doses according to the package insert.

Only approximately 25% of patients receiving myelographic doses of iopamidol or iohexol will have significant adverse side effects. Side effects (headache, nausea, vomiting, and fatigue) are fewer, less severe, and of shorter duration than with metrizamide.[24–26] Although a recent investigation suggests that iohexol is better tolerated than iopamidol,[27] there still remains considerable doubt whether there is significant tolerance difference.

Intrathecal water-soluble contrast material should not be used in patients with seizure disorder. Alternative methods of investigation, such as CT and MRI, should first be performed in seizure patients. Phenothiazine drugs, tricyclic antidepressants, monomine oxidase inhibitors, and other neuroleptic drugs should be withheld 48 hours before examination and 24 hours after it (see package insert).

Because iopamidol and iohexol have a higher specific gravity than cerebral spinal fluid (CSF), the contrast material can be gravitationally distributed with the tilting table until such mixing with CSF has occurred to diminish the specific gravity difference. Scanning can commence immediately. A 2-hour delay CT scan provides equal results and is preferred at many medical centers. Our routine for further CT investigation whether immediate or delayed after lumbar myelography is to roll the patient 360° three times before scanning in order to mix the layered contrast often found in the supine caudal sac (Fig. 2.15). After cervical myelography, the patient is brought to a standing or near-standing position in order to distance the contrast bolus from the brain. A cervical CT myelogram can then be performed (if indicated) immediately or after a delay of 3 hours or

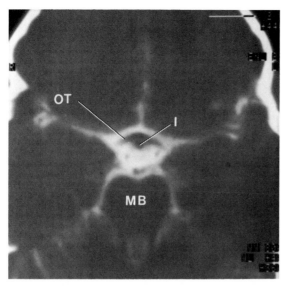

Figure 2.16.   Positive contrast cisternogram. Axial scan at the chiasmatic cistern level. Contrast outlines the midbrain *(MB)*, the optic tracts *(OT)*, and hypophyseal (infundibular) stalk *(I)*.

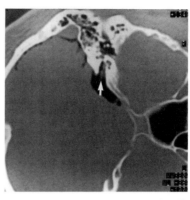

Figure 2.17.   CP air cisternogram, 1.5-mm section. Bone filter (edge enhancement) 3200/−260 lateral decubitus. Air fills the CPA cistern and the internal auditory canal outlining the neurovascular bundle *(arrow)*.

less. Beyond 4 hours, the contrast tends to be too dilute. It is recommended that scanning immediately follow the gravitational mixing of a small intrathecal bolus injected specifically for CT-positive contrast cisternography or CT myelography. Initially, the small bolus of contrast is positioned by table tilt to the area of interest. The cisterns, fissures, and fourth ventricle are almost immediately opacified by table tilt (Fig. 2.16).[28] The direct coronal prone position is used for investigation of CSF rhinorrhea. MR is clearly superior to CT for demonstration of a spinal cord cavity. If CT is used for investigation of a spinal cord cavity, immediate, 6-hour, and 12-hour scans are recommended.

Ventricular shunt injections of 2 ml of low concentration (lumbar concentration) iopamidol or iohexol followed by immediate and delayed scans can demonstrate ventricular pathway obstruction such as aqueductal stenosis.

Air or Carbon Dioxide Cerebellopontine Angle Cisternography

MR with i.v. Gd-DTPA contrast injection is the procedure of choice for investigation of cerebellopontine angle (CPA) tumors. If the CT technique must be used, small quantities of air or carbon dioxide (CO_2) can be introduced easily and safely into the lumbar subarachnoid space and positioned into the CPA. Filtered room air or CO_2, 3–8 ml, is injected into the seated patient with both the head and body tilted 45°. The cranial sagittal plane is then at a horizontal plane parallel to the floor. The petrous pyramid of interest should be the higher (Fig. 2.17). The patient is immediately scanned in the lateral decubitus position with thin section 1.5-mm bone filter wide window technique. If the other CPA requires investigation, the patient can be flipped rapidly to the opposite decubitus position and the head gently tapped in order to position the gas bolus to the now higher CPA.[29]

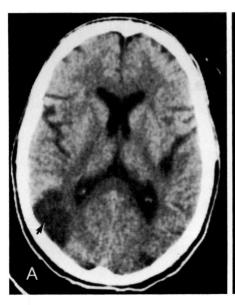

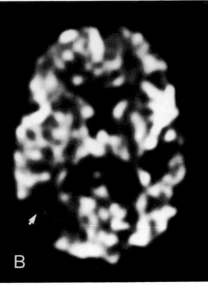

Figure 2.18.   Xenon CT scanning. Acute right middle cerebral artery infarct. **A,** Noncontrast axial 10-mm CT scan. **B,** Xenon CT scan. Note corresponding zone of diminished perfusion of xenon scan that matches the CT infarct *(arrow)* (Courtesy of the General Electric Corp.).

Excellent visualization of the CPA cisterns is demonstrated. Gas enters normal internal auditory canals.

Xenon Inhalation Contrast

Inhaled stable xenon CT dynamic scanning technique quantitates regional cerebral blood flow. Because stable xenon has a high CT attenuation value and freely crosses the BBB, it serves as a method to evaluate cerebral perfusion (Fig. 2.18).[30] A 32% xenon-68% oxygen mixture is breathed by the patient and CT regional enhancement per unit time is mapped. Caution is required because of the anesthetic effects of xenon.[31] (Xenon is a general anesthetic in concentrations over 50%.) We do not use this technique at our hospital.

PART TWO

Basic Cranial CT Diagnostic Principles

The noncontrast axial CT scan is usually the baseline for the choice and order of further CT investigations. In most cases, such as suspected cerebral mestastases, the contrast-only study is sufficient.

Noncontrast Cranial CT Scan

Noncontrast CT scan abnormalities are classified with respect to the density of the lesion and the morphological abnormality. The CT investigation may stop with a normal noncontrast scan or may stop after a clear demonstration of a pathological condition sufficient to institute a therapeutic course. Intravenous or intrathecal contrast injection scanning or imaging in other planes may follow the noncontrast scan. Other neuroradiological procedures such as MR, angiography, or myelography may be necessary for further work-up.

NORMAL CT SCAN

A normal CT scan may be sufficient to eliminate further radiological investigation. A normal scan in a trauma patient or normal ventricular size in a patient with pseudotumor cerebri are good examples.

HIGH DENSITY ABNORMALITIES

A high density abnormality may be diagnostic without requiring injection enhancement such as in extracerebral hematomas and intracerebral hemorrhage. Blood clots usually measure 56–76 H (Fig. 2.19). For many high density abnormalities such as meningioma, i.v. injection is necessary for further definition. Metastases from melanoma, colonic carcinoma, and chorionic carcinoma characteristically are of high density.[32] Calcified lesions are included in the high density category. Some of these lesions with typical-appearing calcifications, such as tuberous sclerosis, toxoplasmosis, and cysticercosis, usually do not require further investigation. Calcified vascular malformations and calcified tumors often require i.v. contrast injection and, possibly, additional coronal

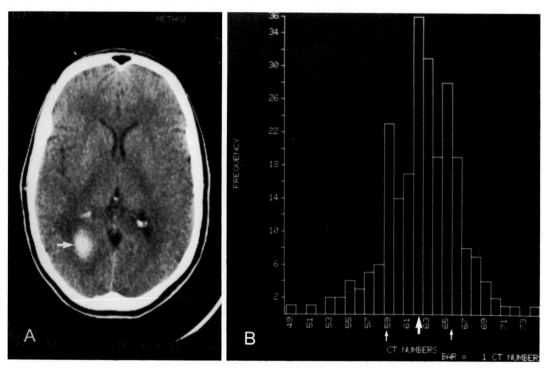

Figure 2.19. Spontaneous right parieto-occipital hemorrhage. Example of homogeneous high density lesion. **A,** A round cursor *arrow* encircles the blood clot. The mean density is 62.5 H and the standard deviation (SD) = 3.6. **B,** Histogram of the encircled pixels in **A.** Mean 62.5 H *(large arrow)*. Notice that most CT attenuation values (68%) are clustered within the first standard deviation *(small arrows)*.

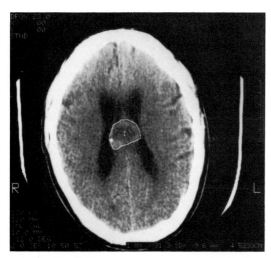

Figure 2.20. **Heterogeneous mixed density lesion.** An irregular cursor encloses a glioma invading the splenium of the corpus callosum. There is peripheral hyperdensity and central hypodensity with a mean density of +31.3 H and a SD of 9.6.

sections. Chondrous and osseous abnormalities are also included in this category.

MIXED DENSITY ABNORMALITIES

Mixed density abnormalities consist of heterogeneous lesions with CT numbers averaging between 25 and 45 H (Fig. 2.20). CT attenuation mean values of mixed density abnormalities have an increased standard deviation. Malignant brain tumors are often found in this category. Intravenous contrast injection is particularly useful for diagnosis of these lesions.

ISODENSE ABNORMALITIES

Isodense abnormalities have CT numbers predominantly ranging from 25–45 H. Isodense subdural hematomas demonstrate these characteristics. Benign tumors and low grade gliomas are often in this category (Fig. 2.21). Intravenous contrast injection is particularly useful for diagnosis of lesions in this category because they are often poorly defined and occasionally not seen on the noncontrast scan.

LOW DENSITY ABNORMALITIES

Low density abnormalities are characterized by having CT numbers below 25 H. Cysts, low grade gliomas (Fig. 2.22), infarcts, cerebritis, leukodystrophies, and abscesses are included in this group.[33,34] Lipid-containing lesions such as cholesteatoma, lipoma, and teratoma are also in this category. Chronic subdural hematomas and white matter degenerative diseases are characterized by low density. Intravenous contrast injection is valuable for investigation of lesions that may show BBB breakdown such as gliomas, infarcts, and infectious disease.

Intravenous Contrast Injection Scan

Certain i.v. contrast injection characteristics help to identify lesions.

NONENHANCEMENT

Nonenhancement indicates a relative lack of BBB breakdown and lack of hypervascularity. Old infarcts and contusions are in this category. Acute infarcts and low grade gliomas often fail to enhance.

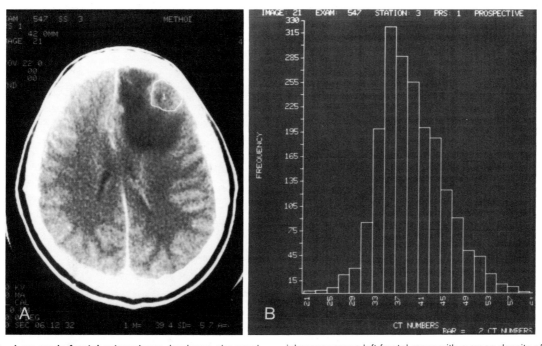

Figure 2.21. **Low grade frontal astrocytoma.** Isodense abnormality. **A,** An i.v. contrast axial scan. Irregular cursor encloses a slightly inhomogeneous left frontal mass with a mean density of 39.4 H, and SD = 5.7. **B,** Histogram of cursor-enclosed region.

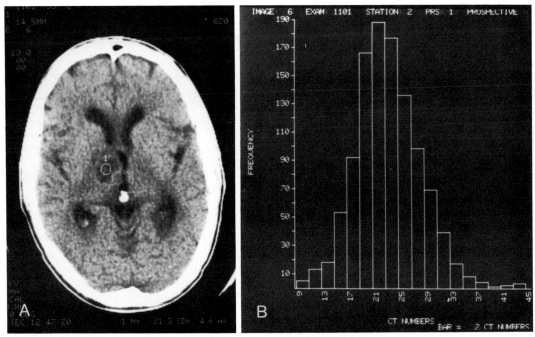

Figure 2.22. **Right thalamic glioma.** Low density lesion. **A,** A round cursor encloses a homogeneous hypodense representative area of the mass. The mean density is 21.3 and a SD = 4.6. **B,** Histogram of cursor-enclosed region.

HOMOGENEOUS ENHANCEMENT

Homogeneous enhancement is commonly seen with meningiomas and can be seen with malignant brain tumors, both primary and metastatic. Smooth margination of a homogeneously enhanced lesion favors benignity (Fig. 2.23).[35,36]

ENHANCEMENT OF A SOLID TUMOR OUTLINING A CYSTIC OR NECROTIC COMPONENT

An irregular zone of contrast enhancement surrounding a nonenhanced central region is often seen with high grade gliomas (Fig. 2.24) and metas-

tases.[37] This pattern can occasionally also be seen in benign tumors, abscesses, infarcts, and contusions.

SMOOTH RING OF CONTRAST ENHANCEMENT SURROUNDING A CENTRAL AREA LACKING ENHANCEMENT

Brain abscesses (Fig. 2.25) commonly appear as a smooth ring surrounding a nonenhanced central area. This pattern is rarely seen with other lesions.

HETEROGENEOUS CONTRAST ENHANCEMENT WITH ADMIXED AREAS OF NONENHANCEMENT

A pattern of heterogeneous contrast enhancement with admixed areas of nonenhancement is seen more

Figure 2.23. **Noncontrast and i.v. contrast meningioma.** Bilateral, right greater than left, falx meningioma. Noncontrast axial 35/100 CT scan demonstrates posteriorly diffusely calcified and anteriorly hyperdense somewhat ill-defined falx mass. After i.v. contrast injection, there is moderately homogeneous contrast enhancement with sharp smooth margination.

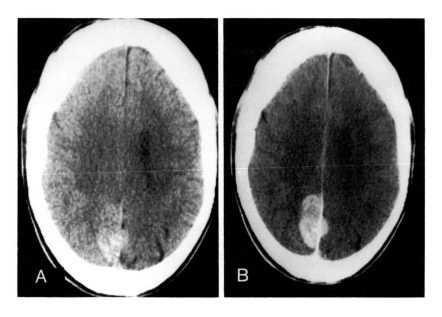

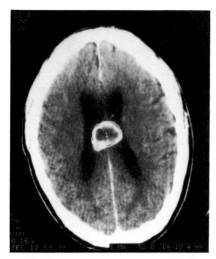

Figure 2.24. Glioma involving the splenium of the corpus calosum, i.v. contrast scan, same case as Figure 2.20. Enhancement of solid tumor surrounding central cystic or necrotic component. A 4.4-cm diameter tumor enclosed within an irregular cursor. Mean density +52, SD = 19.4. The high standard deviation is expected due to the marked heterogeneity.

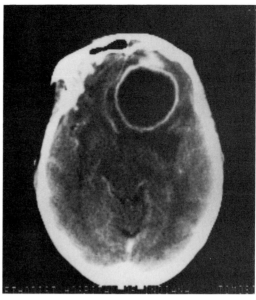

Figure 2.25. Left frontal abscess. Smooth ring of contrast enhancement surrounding a central area lacking enhancement.

commonly with gliomas than with metastases (Fig. 2.26).

MULTIPLE LESIONS

Metasatases (Fig. 2.27) may not be seen clearly without enhancement.[36] Other causes of multiple lesions, such as "multicentric gliomas," multicentric meningiomas, septic emboli, myxomatous emboli, and demyelinating diseases, must also be considered.

DIFFERENTIATING TUMOR AND EDEMA

Metastases, glioblastoma, abscess, and meningioma are often associated with marked edema.[37] Often the tumor component cannot be accurately identified without contrast enhancement. The edema of tumor is confined to white matter and, therefore, is characterized by an interdigitating appearance (Fig. 2.28).

The infarct usually involves a "wedge" of gray and white matter in a vascular distribution and, therefore, lacks the interdigitating appearance (Fig. 2.18A).[38]

CONTRAST ENHANCEMENT OF ENLARGED VEINS

Contrast enhancement of enlarged veins may be seen in vascular malformations and fistulas, strongly suggesting that diagnosis (Fig. 2.29). Enlarged veins may also be seen in association with highly vascular malignant tumors such as glioblastoma.

Timing Characteristics of Lesion Contrast

An infarct usually does not contrast enhance immediately at ictus but is likely to do so 24 hours after ictus. Dynamic scan images with histographic pat-

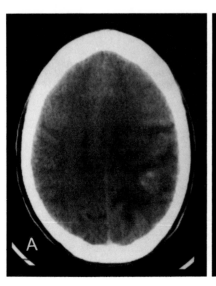

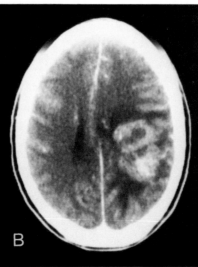

Figure 2.26. Primitive neuroectodermal tumor with heterogeneous contrast enhancement. Axial 10-mm section, 37/100 noncontrast **(A)** and i.v. contrast **(B). A,** Partially calcified heterogeneous density left parietal tumor. **B,** Heterogeneous contrast enhancement.

Figure 2.27. Metastases. Quadrigeminal plate cistern noncontrast **(A)** and i.v. contrast **(B)** 10-mm thickness axial 37/100 CT scans. Note slightly irregular multiple contrast enhancing masses *(1 and 2)*. Calcified choroid plexus *(C)*. Both mass *1* and mass *2* are tissue-density. Mass *1* is not clearly detected before contrast injection. Mass *2* is clearly visible due to the surrounding edema. Note the unexplained edema anterior and lateral to the calcified choroid plexus. Vague contrast enhancement *(arrow)* is noted demonstrating a third metastasis that was confirmed by MR.

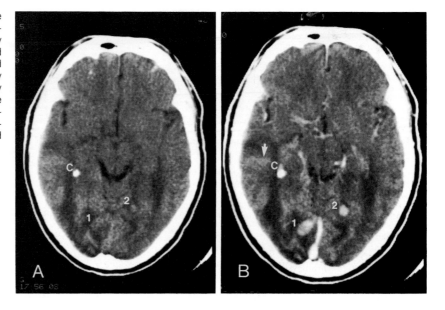

terns can characterize lesions such as infarcts and vascular malformations, however, the technique is rarely used.

CT Radiotherapy Treatment Planning Program

Many manufacturers provide software programs that outline structural contours on the CT image, calculate depth doses, and display isodose contours. These systems assist planning of multiple stationary or rotational fields, wedges, and photon energies.

Multiplanar display of these parameters is provided by some manufacturers to aid in the verification of optimum field size. Annotation of the above treatment parameters produces a permanent hard copy of the treatment plan. The program can be performed at the physician's viewing console or on an independent console.

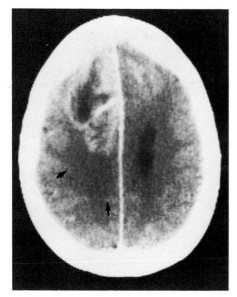

Figure 2.28. Tumor and edema. Right frontal glioblastoma multiforme, i.v. contrast irregular contour and contrast enhancement with surrounding edema *(arrow)*. Note that the edema is interdigitated confined to the white matter as compared to the smooth wedge hypodensity infarct pattern (cellular death and edema) of infarction (Fig. 2.18). The contrast enhancement is of the irregular "ring-type" anteriorly and "sworl-type" posteriorly.

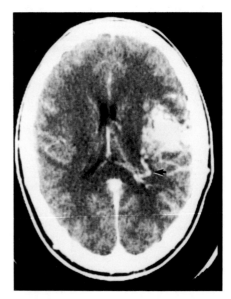

Figure 2.29. Arteriovenous malformation. Axial i.v. contrast 10-mm CT section demonstrating an abnormal tortuous vein *(arrow)* draining the large insular racemose pattern contrast-enhanced malformation.

References

1. Chuang SH, Fitz CR. Computed tomography of head trauma. In Gonzalez CF, Grossman CB, Masdeu JC (Eds). *Head and Spine Imaging*. New York: John Wiley & Sons, 1985; 525.
2. Forbes GS, Earnest F IV, Waller RR. Computed tomography of orbital tumors including late-generation scanning techniques. *Radiology* 1982; 142:387–394.
3. Gammal TE, Adams RJ, King DW. Modified CT techniques in the evaluation of temporal lobe epilepsy prior to lobectomy. *AJNR* 1987; 8:131–134.
4. Osborn AG, Anderson RE. Direct sagittal computed tomographic scans of the face and paranasal sinuses. *Radiology* 1979; 129:81–87.
5. Grossman CB. Basic radiological principles of computed tomography. In Gonzalez CF, Grossman CB, Masdeu JC (Eds). *Head and Spine Imaging*. New York: John Wiley & Sons, 1985; 43–47.
6. Grossman CB, Post MJD. The adult spine. In Gonzalez CF, Grossman CB, Masdeu JC (Eds). *Head and Spine Imaging*. New York: John Wiley & Sons, 1985;781–859.
7. Altman NR, Altman DH, Wolf SA, et al. Three-dimensional CT reformation in children. *AJNR* 1986; 7:287–293.
8. Norman D, Axel L, Berninger WH, et al. Dynamic computed tomography of the brain: Techniques, data analysis and applications. *AJR* 1981; 136:759–770.
9. Dobben GD, Valvassori GE, Mafee MF, et al. Evaluation of brain circulation by rapid rotational computed tomography. *Radiology* 1979; 133:105–111.
10. Arimitsu I, DiChiro G, Brooks RA, et al. White-gray matter differentiation in computed tomography. *J Comput Assist Tomogr* 1977; 1:437–442.
11. New PFJ, Aronow S. Attenuation measurements of whole blood and blood fractions in computed tomography. *Radiology* 1976; 121:635–640.
12. Gado M, Eichling J, Currie M, et al. Quantitative aspects of CT images. In Norman D, Korobkin M, Newton TH (Eds). *Computed Tomography 1977*. St. Louis: CV Mosby Co., 1977; 193–211.
13. Hahn FJY, Rim K. Frontal ventricular dimensions on normal computed tomography. *AJR* 1976; 126:593–596.
14. Gado MH, Phelps ME, Coleman RE. An extravascular component of contrast enhancement in cranial computed tomography. *Radiology* 1975; 117:589–593.
15. Steinhoff H, Lange S. Principles of contrast enhancement in computerized tomography. In Lanksch W, Kazner E (Eds). *Cranial Computerized Tomography*. Berlin: Springer-Verlag, 1976; 60–68.
16. Firooznia H, Kricheff II, Rafii M, Golimbu C. Lumbar spine after surgery: examination with intravenous contrast-enhanced CT. *Radiology* 1987; 163:221–226.
17. Takeda N, Tanaka R, Nakai O, Veki K. Dynamics of contrast enhancement in delayed computed tomography of brain tumors: Tissue-blood ratio and differential diagnosis. *Radiology* 1982; 142:663–668.
18. Kramer RA, Janetos GP, Perlstein G. An approach to contrast enhancement in computed tomography of the brain. *Radiology* 1975; 116:641–647.
19. Harwood-Nash CDF. Congenital craniocerebral abnormalities and computed tomography. *Semin Roentgenol* 1977; 12:39–51.
20. Norman D, Enzmann DR, Newton TH. Comparative efficacy of contrast agents in computed tomography scanning of the brain. *J Comput Assist Tomogr* 1978; 2:319–321.
21. Davis JM, Davis KR, Newhouse J, et al. Expanded high iodine dose in computed cranial tomography: A preliminary report. *Radiology* 1979; 131:373–380.
22. Hayman LA, Evans RA, Hinck VC. Rapid high dose contrast computed tomography of isodense subdural hematoma and cerebral swelling. *Radiology* 1979; 131:381–383.
23. Nakstad PH, Bakke SJ, Kjartansson O, et al. Omnipaque vs. hexabrix in intravenous DSA of the carotid arteries: Randomized double-blind crossover study. *AJNR* 1986; 7:303–304.
24. Kieffer SA, Binet EF, Davis DO, et al. Lumbar myelography with iohexol and metrizamide: A comparative multicenter prospective study. *Radiology* 1984; 151:665–670.
25. Latchaw RE, Hirsh WL Jr, Horton JA, et al. Iohexol vs. metrizamide: Study of efficacy and morbidity in cervical myelography. *AJNR* 1985; 6:931–933.
26. Witwer G, Cacayorin ED, Bernstein AD, et al. Iopamidol and metrizamide for myelography: prospective double blind clinical trial. *AJNR* 1984; 5:403–407.
27. Broadbridge AT, Bayliss SG, Brayshaw CI. The effect of intrathecal iohexol on visual evoked response latency: A comparison including incidence of headache with iopamidol and metrizamide in myeloradiculography. *Clin Radiol* 1987; 38:71–74.
28. Drayer BP, Rosenbaum AE, Kennerdell JS, et al. Computed tomographic diagnosis of suprasellar masses by intrathecal enhancement. *Radiology* 1977; 123:339–344.
29. Krischeff II, Pinto RS, Bergeron RT, et al. Air-CT cisternography and canalography for small acoustic neuromas. *AJNR* 1980; 1:57–63.
30. Yonas H, Good WF, Gur D, et al. Mapping cerebral blood flow by xenon-enhanced computed tomography: Clinical experience. *Radiology* 1984; 152:435–442.
31. Latchaw RE, Yonas H, Pentheny SL, Gur D. Adverse reactions to xenon-enhanced CT cerebral blood flow determination. *Radiology* 1987; 163:251–254.
32. Deck MDF, Messina AV, Sackett JF. Computed tomography in metastatic disease of the brain. *Radiology* 1976; 119:115–120.
33. Osborn AG, Williams RG, Wing SD. Low attenuation lesions in the midline posterior fossa: Differential diagnosis. *CT* 1978; 2:319–328.
34. Williams RG, Osborn AG. Low attenuation lesions in the middle fossa: Differential diagnosis. *CT* 1980; 4:89–97.
35. Near PFJ, Aronow S, Hesselink JR. National Cancer Institute study: Evaluation of computed tomography in the diagnosis of intracranial neoplasms IV meningiomas. *Radiology* 1980; 136:665–675.
36. Davis DO. CT in the diagnosis of supratentorial tumors. *Semin Roentgenol* 1977; 12:97–103.
37. Tchang S, Scotti G, Terbrugge K. Computed tomography as a possible aid to histological grading of supratentorial gliomas. *J Neurosurg* 1977; 46:735–739.
38. Monajati A, Heggeness L. Patterns of edema in tumors and infarcts. *AJNR* 1982; 3:251–255.

CHAPTER

3

Clinical MR Application

PART ONE

MR Scanning Technique

Introduction

We are still in the early stages of the MR era. MR scanning techniques are likely to change markedly and static, dynamic, and spectroscopic imaging and image analysis are likely to improve markedly. The use of MR intravenous (i.v.) contrast agents is in an early phase of development. Because of expectations for rapid changes in MR imaging, it is difficult to write an MR applications chapter beyond generalizations. For this reason, the format of the CT applications chapter (Chapter 2) will be followed but this chapter will be briefer and more limited to fundamentals.

Scan Speed

Choice of MR sequence affects scan time. For example, inversion recovery is considerably slower than certain spin echo (SE) sequences that give comparable results. MR sequences incorporating partial flip "tip" angles and gradient refocusing (gradient recalled echo or GRE) reduce scan time markedly, often without sacrificing image quality. This method reduces repetition times (TRs) by one or two orders of magnitude (2000 msec to 200 msec or 20 msec). Scan speeds of 3 sec per section can be achieved on 1.5T MR scanners.

Other methods are used that proportionately reduce scan time according to the equation $Ts = Ny \cdot TR \cdot NEX$; where Ts = scan time, Ny = lines in the phase-encoding axis, TR = pulse repetition time, and NEX = number of excitations. The number of lines in the phase-encoding axis plane (Ny) are often 256 or 128 for two-dimensional Fourier-transform imaging (2DFT) technique. Ny reduction increases pixel size, reduces resolution for a given field of view (FOV) and increases Gibbs phenomenon (truncation artifact). A compromise using 192 views or lines results in better detail and elimination or diminution of Gibbs artifact. Another method is to acquire only half the number of lines (views). This latter interpolation method is called half-Fourier imaging or, incorrectly, "½ NEX." It reduces scan time by 50%. The drawback to this method is a 1.4X reduction in S/N because only one half of the data is collected. Using a rectangular FOV for regions such as the spine reduces the area imaged, decreases scan time, and maintains signal to noise (S/N) ratio and resolution. Fewer excitations increases scan speed, decreases S/N ratio, and decreases motion artifact.[1] The higher field strength magnets have an increased S/N ratio, thereby requiring fewer excitations (NEX) than a lower strength magnet.[1]

Three-dimensional acquisitions (3DFT) will most likely become a standard technique because only one series will likely suffice for a subject study. Images in any plane and in a variety of thicknesses varying from very thin to thick can be obtained. Imaging time is then reduced to the time of the single 3-D acquisition.[1]

Patient Positioning and Plane of Section

The patient nearly always lies supine in the magnet. A fast T1-weighted multilevel sequence with a relatively large FOV (32 cm) is used as a localizer. From this image, coordinates of the area of interest are determined and smaller FOV images can be obtained with appropriate pulse sequences to produce improved detail.

Software programs are available to annotate images representing the sections to be obtained. Positional coordinates are annotated to each image, which determines the exact 3-D lesion localization.

The multilevel MR plane of section is determined

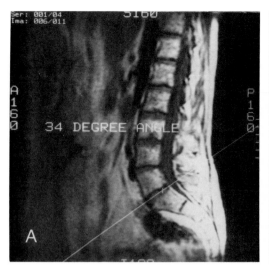

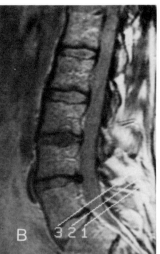

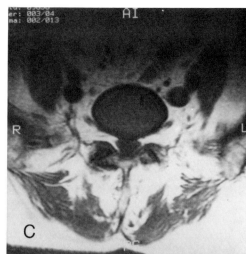

Figure 3.1.   MR section angle selection. Annotated lumbar mid-sagittal SE 600/25 "localizer" **(A)** and SE 2000/20 **(B)** MR scans. Section 2: SE 600/25 **(C)**. The "localizer" section for MR identifies the patient position within the scanner **(A)**. After patient position adjustment inward or outward to the scanner (Z), X and Y axis parameters are determined by adjusting grid slice selection and the de-sired sagittal scan is obtained **(B)**. Slice angle is determined from the localizer (i.e., 34°) and the axial section **(C)** is obtained.

CT is limited to reformation techniques at angles greater than 20° (see Fig. 2.3). MR section angle is not limited by physical factors such as CT gantry tilt.

by the gradient coils and not by changing the patient position as it is with CT direct coronal and sagittal images. At present, the MR multiplanar (2DFT) technique is almost exclusively used so that each pulse sequence produces a series of sections in a single plane only. Because the section angle is not restricted by gantry tilt limitations, the lumbosacral disk can be examined in its exact axial plane (Fig. 3.1). MR 3-D (3DFT) technique is remotely analogous to the CT reformation technique with respect to image reformation in any plane including curved planes. Images such as cervical and lumbar oblique foraminal views can then be conveniently obtained and imaging difficulties with scoliosis and head tilt can be overcome. The axial section is the primary imaging plane for routine cranial MR scans and is necessary for most spine examinations.[1]

As with CT, coronal imaging is helpful for investigation of the pituitary gland (Fig. 3.2), the orbit, petrous pyramids, and regions adjacent to axially oriented bone surfaces such as the skull base and skull vertex. Sagittal imaging is not only used for localization but is very useful for investigation of pituitary, diencephalic, midbrain, pontine vermian, and

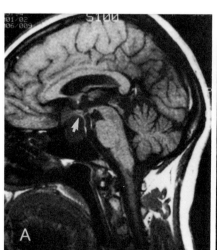

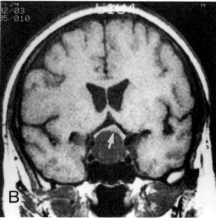

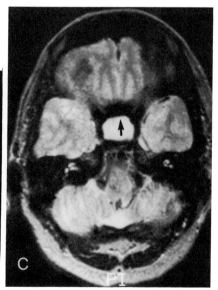

Figure 3.2.   Orthogonal plane imaging. Rathke's cleft cyst. Sagittal **(A)** and coronal **(B)** SE 600/25 heavily T1-weighted images demonstrate a water-slightly hyperintense intra- and suprasellar smoothly marginated mass elevating and deforming the optic chiasm *(arrow)*. Axial SE 2000/80 T2-weighted section **(C)** in the supraorbitomeatal plane demonstrates lesion T2 water isointensity (hyperintense). The optic nerves are seen anterior to the cyst on either side of *arrow*.

spine regions and is of primary importance for investigation of sagittally oriented structures such as the corpus callosum.[1]

Pulse Sequence Choice

Fundamental to the diagnostic value of MR images is spatial and contrast resolution and the comparative intensity of structures with respect to T1- and T2-weighted technique. These T1 and T2 effects vary with the pulse sequence. Spatial resolution is limited by matrix size and FOV for T1, proton density, and T2 effects. Higher S/N is obtained with proton density and T1 techniques than with T2 techniques. Contrast resolution is related to the difference in signal intensity between adjacent structures and S/N. Doubling the number of excitations increases the S/N by $\sqrt{2}$ or by $1.4\times$. As described in Chapter 1, T2*-weighted images are similar to T2 but demonstrate greater magnetic susceptibility effects. The T2* effect is more evident with GRE technique, which demonstrates a markedly hypointense signal for both iron- and calcium-containing tissues.

Present protocols for head and spine examinations will obviously change during these pioneer years of MR imaging. We feel that it is necessary to have at least one very heavily weighted T1 sequence (e.g., 600/25) and one T2-weighted sequence (e.g., 2800/80). Increased signal-to-noise (S/N) and contrast-to-noise (C/N) for spin echo imaging has been achieved with the combined use of pulse triggering and motion compensation techniques. Reducing the band width of the second echo further increases C/N and is currently being successfully used in combination with pulse triggering and MAST.[1a] GRE fast scanning techniques are already routine for spine and 3-D imaging. It is becoming increasingly apparent that MR will play a significant role in CSF and blood flow evaluation in addition to its well-established role in vascular static and dynamic imaging. Fat or water suppression techniques cause signal alteration of fat or water and can be useful for tissue differentiation. Fat suppression can help distinguish fat from paramagnetic contrast-enhanced tissue and from hemorrhage. Short-TI inversion recovery ("STIR") and chemical presaturation are two such techniques[1a] (see page 348).

Field of View and Surface Coil Technique

A relatively large FOV (e.g., 32 cm) is used for the localizer image. From the localizer image, a smaller FOV is usually chosen (e.g., 24 cm). Surface coils study smaller FOVs and accurately receive signals from only surface and shallow structures. The smaller FOV reduces pixel size (e.g., 0.3 mm) by displaying the data on the full matrix analogous to the CT target image. Much improved detail of small structures such as the optic nerve (Fig. 3.3) and the spinal cord results. A significant disadvantage of the technique is the rapid signal drop-off of deeper structures. Smaller FOVs increase wrap-around artifact—a problem that is significant but minor as compared to improved resolution. Software methods have been developed to diminish wrap-around effect.

The surface coil contacts the body surface closest to the object of interest, e.g., a cervical coil wrapped around the neck. Early surface coils served only as receivers of signal. Surface coils have now been developed that both transmit radiofrequency (RF) pulse and receive signal. Another method being developed is the use of separate surface transmitters and receivers functioning in unison.[2]

Section Thickness and Section Spacing

The MR section thickness is determined by gradient strength. Operator-controlled section thickness

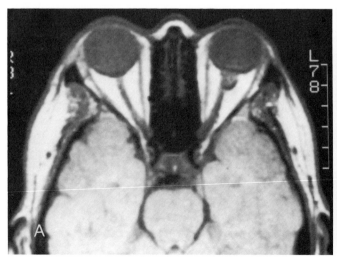
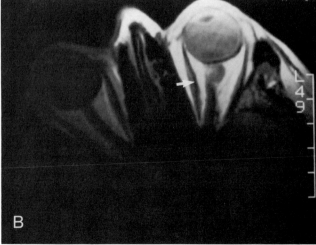

Figure 3.3.   Surface coil technique. Optic nerve meningioma. Note the left optic nerve meningioma in **A** and **B.** SE 600/25 24 cm FOV 1 NEX 1.5 mag **(A)** and SE 600/25 1 NEX surface coil 20 cm FOV 1.5 mag **(B).** Both scans 3 mm thickness and 256×256 matrix. Note the markedly improved globe, rectus muscle, and left ethmoid sinus detail with the surface coil. Since the surface coil has been placed on the left face, there is right-sided signal depletion. Note the chemical shift artifact *(arrow)* along the frequency-encoding axis **(B).** Compare to **(A)** where the chemical shift artifact encircles the posterior globe in the standard Y-axis frequency-encoding direciton.

usually includes 3-, 5-, and 10-mm thick slices. Thinner sections for the same scan time reduce partial volume effect and gives finer detail of small structures with a penalty of decreased S/N ratio. Stronger magnetic fields allow for thin-section increased S/N ratio with shorter scan time.[3] Very thin sections (1–3 mm) are necessary using CT or MR for the study of thin structures such as a cervical disk or facial nerve canal. Partial volume averaging is thus avoided. The very thin section has become an available option for, at least, the high-field strength MR system.

Standard 2DFT pulse sequences produce multiple sections per scan time. Contiguous thin sections can be used for studies of complex regions of thin parts such as the neurovascular bundle of the internal auditory canal, the pituitary gland, the optic nerve, and the cervical spine but the images are often degraded by cross-talk. Cross-talk is the incorrect signal contribution from adjacent sections. It is an entirely different phenomenon than partial volume averaging. In order to avoid cross-talk image degradation, a skip area, usually 20% or greater between sections is used. Another skip area advantage is the ability to scan a larger longitudinal volume with the same number of sections assuming the risk that a very thin lesion confined to the skip area can be missed. Interleaving is a method whereby echoes are received from contiguous sections alternately during a single sequence that produces contiguous sections without cross-talk. Gradient recalled, small flip angle techniques have provided sufficient data for 3-D imaging (3DFT) with 1-mm thick sections and scan times of less than 10 min.[1,3]

Location and Measurement

Lesion location is determined by analysis of spatial coordinates of images of different planes on which the lesion appears. The planes of section can be annotated with system software on the localizer image in order to program an image sequence analogous to the CT localizer.

A MR stereotatic frame for intracranial lesion localization has been developed that is quite similar to the CT device except that the landmark portion is made of nonmetallic material (Fig. 3.4).

Cursor measurement similar to CT technique is a standard operator console function. As yet, no application of intensity quantification has been diagnostically useful. Developments in 3DFT technique will enable volumetric measurements of the ventricles, CSF, brain parenchyma, and masses. Quantitative blood flow measurements are another possible future MR development. MR spectroscopy techniques will hopefully enable physiological and metabolic brain examination. Developments in MR vascular imaging are progressing rapidly. MR investigation of carotid atherosclerotic disease will likely be a practical investigation.

Neonatal ventricle size measurements and estimates of the size of the extracerebral space have been made. Normal values for the ventricular/intracran-

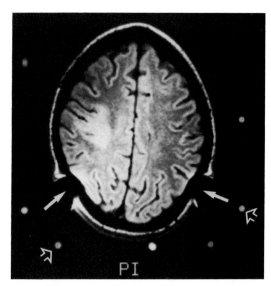

Figure 3.4.   MR stereotactic biopsy device. The nine nonmetallic MR hyperintense rods are similar to those in the CT stereotactic device and appear as hyperintense dots *(open arrows)*. Aluminum screws (plastic screws are optional) are responsible for the artifact *(closed arrows)*. The right parietal hyperintensity proved to be AIDS viral encephalitis.

ial ratio (frontal horn span/intracranial span at the same level) are 0.26–0.34.[4] These values are similar to adult CT values (see Page 27). The same authors measured the size of the neonatal extracerebral space. Although these values are interesting, we have not found them useful.

Intravenous MR Contrast

Presently, only Gd-DTPA (a paramagnetic chelate) is approved for human clinical use as a MR contrast agent in the United States. It is administered in solution of 0.1 mmole/kg with a maximum dose of 10 mmole. Its effect is to increase contrast of abnormal tissues by enhancing relaxation of abnormal extracellular fluid associated with blood-brain barrier (BBB) breakdown. This is similar to the action of x-ray-iodinated contrast material with respect to the extravascular compartment. It should not be administered to patients with hemolytic anemia due to a mild hemolysis effect and may cause delayed headache and nausea within the first 24 hours after the exam. It does not pose nearly the anaphylaxis threat associated with iodinated contrast and, with greater experience, anaphylaxis may not be considered a significant serious use risk. Because it is principally cleared by the kidneys, the drug should be withheld from patients with a creatinine level higher than 2.0 mg/10 ml.[5]

The principal paramagnetic chelate contrast effect is (like that for i.v. x-ray contrast) enhancement of abnormal extracellular tissues associated with BBB breakdown. Unlike CT i.v. contrast effect, is the absence of arterial contrast enhancement due to time-of-flight and rapid dephasing effects. Veins are enhanced, however, due to their slower flow.

MR i.v. contrast technique includes a precontrast, high detail, heavily T1-weighted scan followed immediately after injection by a postcontrast scan with a similar technique. Because T1 hyperintense fat can be confused with paramagnetic contrast enhancement, the precontrast scan provides a baseline in order to exclude a fat-related misdiagnosis. Fat suppression techniques can be concurrently used but they may decrease contrast enhancement. Subacute hemorrhage T1 signal hyperintensity can also be confused with contrast enhancement. Both T1 heavily-weighted SE and T1-weighted GRE techniques are useful MR i.v. contrast techniques.[5]

Basically, the indications for MR i.v. contrast injection are the same as for CT i.v. contrast. They include extra-axial tumors (particularly those at the skull base), intra-axial tumors (particularly metastases), and inflammatory processes. A definite advantage over CT contrast technique is the examination of abnormal tissues adjacent to osseous surfaces. Early results with Gd-DPTA parallel the well-established results of iodinated i.v. x-ray contrast materials.[5,6] For example, low-grade gliomas often fail to enhance, abscesses and central necrotic tumors ring-enhance, and meningiomas and neuromas tend to enhance homogeneously. Gd-DTPA appears to be more sensitive for metastasis. Due to the MR contrast advantage adjacent to cortical surfaces, juxtacortical intracranial and spinal lesions are well suited to MR i.v. contrast investigation (Fig. 3.5). Tumor and edema can be distinguished intracranially and in the spinal canal. The technique helps distinguish recurrent lumbar disk herniation from postoperative scar.

Patient Discomfort, Motion, and Need for Sedation

Claustrophobia is a much greater problem with MR than CT due to the narrow confines of the long mag-netic bore and the isolation of the magnet room. Sedation and anesthesia problems are greater for MR due to the difficulty of having satisfactory monitoring devices and the distance of the patient from personnel administering supportive care. Cardiac monitoring and ventilatory devices are available that can function within a strong magnetic field. Chapter 1 describes the fringe field strength of various types of magnets. The permanent and hybrid types have smaller fringe fields and some configurations allow for relatively unhindered patient support and monitoring.

Patient Monitoring and Ventilatory Assist

The high magnetic field, long bore (aperture), and RF copper-shielded magnet room create unique environmental patient monitoring and ventilatory assist restrictions. MR compatible monitors for body temperature, heart rate, blood pressure, respiratory rate, and ECG waveform are commercially available.[7] We require a nurse or physician present in the magnet room for patients requiring monitoring, ven-

Precautions with the MR System

Patients, personnel, and visitors with cardiac pacemakers, neurostimulators, or monitoring devices are not allowed in the magnet room.[8] Patients with ferromagnetic cerebral aneurysm clips are excluded from study due to the danger of magnetic field torque.[9] Nonferromagnetic aneurysm clips do not deflect or only weakly deflect in the magnetic field. Patients with these MR-compatable aneurysm clips have been scanned at our hospital without complications. Caution is advised, particularly with respect to the documentation of the type of aneurysm clip.[9] Pa-

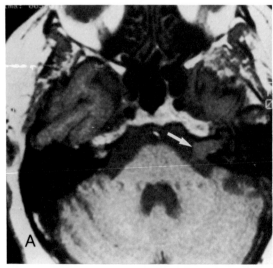
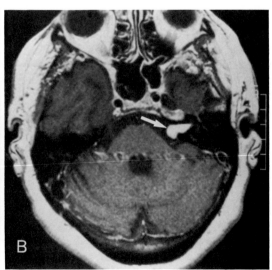

Figure 3.5.   Noncontrast and i.v. contrast Gd-DTPA extra- and intracanalicular acoustic neuroma. Axial internal auditory canal level 3 mm thickness SE 600/25 noncontrast **(A)** and contrast **(B)** MR scans. Note the gray matter isointense **(A)** homogeneously contrast-enhancing **(B)** tumor *(arrow)*.

tients must also be questioned regarding metallic cranial plates, shrapnel injuries, and metallic foreign bodies or devices in the head, heart, spinal canal, ear, or orbit. Ambulatory patients, personnel, and visitors enter the magnet area through an airport security-style metal detector. Ferrous objects such as screwdrivers, scissors, and pens can become lethal missiles in a strong magnetic field. Credit cards, nondigital watches, and paging devices should be removed. ECG leads should be removed from the patient before scanning. Magnetic field-induced currents in coiled or looped wires may heat the wire and injure adjacent tissues. Any wire in the body may carry an induced current in the magnetic field.

Pediatric Considerations

Fetal and neonatal neurosonography is the first order neonatal examination for congenital malformations, hydrocephalus, intracerebral hemorrhage, periventricular cystic changes, tumors, abscess, and meningitis. CT has, before MR, provided a second line method. Although CT probably best confirms acute hemorrhage and adequately investigates all of the above pathological processes, MR better evaluates malformations such as aqueductal stenosis, agenesis of the corpus callosum, and Chiari malformations. Subacute and chronic hemorrhage is also best imaged by MR.

The major technical problem with neonatal MR scanning is anesthesia and monitoring. Neonatal MR scanning requires some form of anesthesia and temperature, cardiac, respiratory, and oxygen saturation monitoring. Insulation is required to prevent loss of body heat.[7,10] An excellent review of these monitoring methods is recommended.[7] As with CT, we prefer to have an anesthesiologist responsible for the anesthetized patient. We do, however, use chloral hydrate and patient monitoring in infants and young children (1–7 years). Under these latter conditions, the patient is monitored by a nurse. The long magnet bore and the magnet room isolation compound the difficulties encountered in CT sedation and anesthesia.

We often utilize "½ NEX" and a 128×256 matrix as a method to reduce scan time in infants. This can result in a variable spin echo sequence of 2.5 minutes still using MAST technique.

PART TWO

Basic Cranial MR Diagnostic Principles

Introduction

MR imaging is more sensitive to many brain and spinal cord abnormalities than is CT. In many ways, MR, as compared to CT, offers a broader choice of technique that markedly influences the imaging result.[11,12] The ability of the MR system to image easily in any plane, including a curved ribbon-like plane

with 3-D technique, is a definite advantage. The MR studies lack specificity of some detected abnormalities, however, in some situations, CT is more specific.[12] For example, CT is highly accurate for diagnosis of acute hemorrhage and is more accurate than MR for calcification.[13] MR, on the other hand, can detect various stages of hemorrhage, multiple sclerosis (MS) plaques, intracanalicular acoustic neuromas, subtle brainstem abnormalities, and spinal cord cavities—all without contrast injection and without artifacts in regions adjacent to dense bones. MR also can detect blood vessels in the normal and abnormal state. Vascular abnormalities such as basilar artery occlusion, venous thrombosis, and atriovenous malformations (AVMs) can be seen without i.v. injection. The normal MR scan excludes brain and spinal cord abnormality with a higher degree of confidence than does CT. However, CT can better characterize certain lesions, such as subarachnoid hemorrhage, types of calcifications, fractures, and other cortical bone and joint abnormalities.[12,13] Some observers feel that noncontrast MR is less sensitive than contrast CT in the detection of benign intracranial tumor.[14] Intravenous contrast MR is more sensitive than i.v. contrast CT for small extra-axial tumors and parenchymal metastases.[5] Although we initially had some difficulty, we now feel that MR is superior to CT for the detection of meningiomas. MR is clearly the method of choice for investigation of MS, pituitary tumors, and acoustic neuromas.

MR Intensity Interpretation

The relative T1 and T2 signal intensities of various substances qualitatively characterize those materials analogous to the way that attenuation values qualitatively and quantitatively characterize substances by CT.

Table 3.1 displays T1 and T2 MR tissue intensity characteristics of a 1.5-T system. Flow void and flow enhancement ("paradoxical enhancement") effects and techniques are not included in this table. We usually obtain a heavily T1-weighted SE image with a short TR and TE (600/25) sequence. Our routine T2-weighted image is usually obtained with a SE with a long TR and TE (2800/80) sequence. Proton density/T1-weighted information is also derived from the later SE sequence with a short TE (2800/30) in addition to the T2 echo. This is why this particular sequence is called a "variable echo sequence." Both T1 and T2* effects can be achieved with GRE partial flip angle sequences. These faster techniques are likely to play an important, if not a commanding, role in the future.

Equally important to a knowledge of the T1 and T2 intensity appearances of Table 3.1 is the analysis of T1 and T2 signal intensity of normal imaged regions. Comparison to normal regions helps to define an abnormal state such as a pituitary cyst (Fig. 3.2). In this case of a Rathke's cleft cyst, not only is there a homogeneous low T1/high T2 intensity pituitary mass, but the intensity within the lesion approxi-

Table 3.1. Biological Tissue and Substance MR T1 and T2 intensities at 1.5 T[a]

substance	++	+/-	--	++	+/-	--
1 water			x	x		
2 white matter		+				-*
3 gray matter		-				+*
4 fat	x					+
5 calcium			x			x
6 ferritin (a,b)		x				x
7 RBC oxyhemog'n		x			x	
8 RBC deoxyhemog'n (b)		x				x
9 RBC methemog'n (b)	x					x
10 free methemog'n	x			x		
11 hemosiderin (b)		x				x
1.5 Tesla	I (T$_1$)			I (T$_2$)		

[a]Symbols used: Hyperintense (++), isointense (+/-), and hypointense (--). Unless otherwise stated, all MR images in this text are generated by a 1.5-T system.
a. High iron concentrations in the globus pallidus, putamen, substantia nigra, red nucleus, thalamus, and temporal subcortical fibers. Approximately 35–50% of this iron is bound in ferritin molecules.[17]
b. T2-marked hypointensity susceptibility effect is seen on conventional SR and SE sequences with high field magnets[15] but may be seen with pulse sequence modifications on midstrength magnets.[16,17] Susceptibility effects are increased with GRE images.
*See Figure 1.13, page 12, for T1/T2 gray/white cortical inversion.

mates that for CSF in the ventricles. The similar analytical technique works well for fat that has a high T1 signal and a slightly high T2 signal. Analysis of Figure 3.6 demonstrates a corpus callosum lipoma by using the same applied principles.

Ferric or ferrous ions alone or within ferritin, methemoglobin, deoxyhemoglobin, and hemosiderin greatly influence the MR signal due to magnetic susceptibility and paramagnetic effects.[15–19] As has been discussed in Chapter 1, magnetic susceptibility effects are more pronounced by GRE techniques than with conventional SE techniques. Shorter TE's diminish the susceptability effect of GRE images. Calcifications with the GRE method also become more hypointense and more clearly detectable, representing an additional clinical application for the technique.[19]

Localized ferritin and ionic iron in the basal ganglia regions are responsible for the T2 signal hypointensity in the adult basal ganglionic regions with high-field strength MR magnets (Fig. 3.7). Protons in the area of the brain with a high ferritin content encounter a local static magnetic field (magnetic susceptibility effect) resulting in decreased T2 signal. This effect is proportional to the square of the magnetic field strength for conventional SE techniques, which explains the difficulty of visualizing normal concentrations of brain iron at lower field strengths with SE sequences.[15,17,18] T2* effects, on the other hand, are linearly related to the applied magnetic field. Low- and midfield strength magnets with GRE technique can take advantage of T2* effects to document iron susceptibility phenomena that could not be documented on these systems with standard T2 SE technique.[19] No detectable iron is present by MR technique in the brain at birth. At six months, the

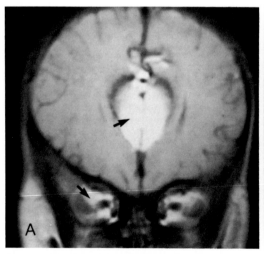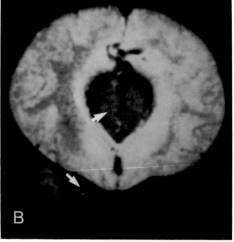

Figure 3.6. Fat signal characteristics and lesion analysis. Corpus callosum lipoma. **A,** SE 2000/20 and **B,** SE 2000/80. Corpus callosum lipoma *(top arrows)* and retrobulbar fat *(bottom arrows)*. Comparison of the signal characteristics of unknown tissues with normal structures helps identify the lesion.

Here, the fat characteristics of T1 hyperintensity and T2 hypointensity are helpful for the diagnosis of lipoma.

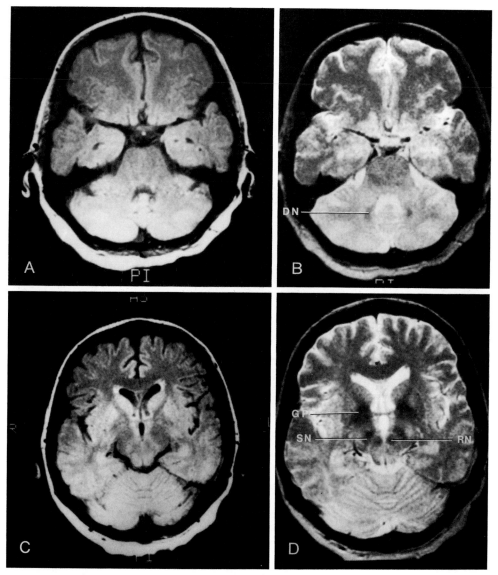

Figure 3.7.   Iron susceptability effects. T1/proton density-weighted 2000/20 supraorbitomeatal fourth ventricle **(A)** and cerebral peduncle **(C)** sections. T2-weighted 2000/80 corresponding images **(B** and **D).** Note T2 iron-induced hypointensity of the dentate nucleus *(DN),* globus pallidus *(GP),* substantia nigra *(SN),* and red nucleus *(RN).*

globus pallidus demonstrates iron content. The substantia nigra, the red nucleus, and the dentate nucleus demonstrate the presence of iron deposits in chronological order over the next 3–7 years. Brain iron is probably independent of hemoglobin metabolism. Iron deposition of hemochromatosis only occurs in brain areas lacking a BBB (e.g., neurohypophysis, pineal, area postrema, choroid plexus, infundibulum, subfornical body).[17]

Table 3.2 demonstrates the stages of intracranial hemorrhage evolution at 1.5 T.[15] The central T2 hypointensity of acute hematomas is most likely caused by deoxyhemoglobin in intact red blood cells (RBCs). Intracellular (RBC) methemoglobin is also markedly T2 hypointense. The T1 and T2 hyperintensity associated with subacute and early chronic hematoma is due to free methemoglobin paramagnetic effects. The

peripheral T1 and T2 hyperintensity effect extending inward in subacute hematomas has been noted at all magnetic field strengths (Fig. 3.8 and 3.9). Hematoma hyperintensity may persist for over a year. The surrounding ring of marked T2 hypointensity is a late development that follows the central hyperintense phase and is probably due to hemosiderin-laden macrophages. This marked T2 peripheral hypointensity is seen using conventional SE sequences with high-field magnets and the T2 hypointensity may persist indefinitely (Fig. 3.10).[15] It may also be seen with T2-weighted MR pulse sequence modifications such as gradient refocusing with midstrength magnets.[16,18,19] By referring to Table 3.1, the MR intensities of hematoma evolution in Table 3.2 can be understood in terms of the state of oxidative denaturation of the hemoglobin molecule and the rela-

Table 3.2. Intracranial Hematoma[a]

Study / Pathology	Acute Day 1	Acute Day 7 / Day 8	Subacute Day 30 / Day 30	Chronic
(P) Pathology RBC oxyhemoglobin (0) oxidized to RBC deoxyhemoglobin (d) and RBC methemoglobin (m). Edema (E). The RBC lysis releases free methemoglobin (m). Perihematoma granulocytes incorporate the (m) biproduct hemosiderin (h).				
(C) CT High hemoglobin (Hb) concentration gives acute high density that decreases with (Hb) breakdown. Hypointense subacute surrounding edema. Subacute rim contrast enhancement may occur. Chronic central hypodense granulation and isodense hemosiderin.				
(T₁) 1.5 T MR I_{T1} Acute (0) isointensity. Surrunding hypointense edema. Subacute central isointense (d) and hyperintense (m). Subacute and chronic hyperintense (m) and isointense hemosiderin in (h). Chronic central hypointense granulation tissue.				
(T₂) 1.5 T MR I_{T2} Acute (0) isointensity. Surrounding hyperintense edema. Subacute (d) and intracellular (m) combined hypointensity later develops extracellular (m) hyperintensity. Subacute and chronic hypointense (h).				
	A	B	C	D	E

[a]The appearance and evolution of intracranial hemorrhage at 1.5 T. This chart (after Gomori et al.[15]) demonstrates the pathological (P), CT (C), T1 and T2 evolution of intracranial hemorrhage along four respective horizontal rows. Time (A–E) progresses left to right from acute (days 1–7) to subacute (days 8–30) to chronic (greater than 30 days). Note that there is some overlap in the early and late acute and in the subacute and chronic appearances.

As already stated in Chapter 1, pulse sequences are chosen that are weighted for particular MR characteristics (i.e., T1, T2, and proton density). Although the chosen characteristic (i.e., T1 effect) is usually predominant on these sequences, substances of high enough concentration and strong enough signal (i.e., deoxyhemoglobin) can produce detectable signals (i.e., T2 effect) usually found on other sequences. This chart is, therefore, an oversimplification.

In order to observe these effects with lower strength magnets, gradient echo techniques are probably necessary.

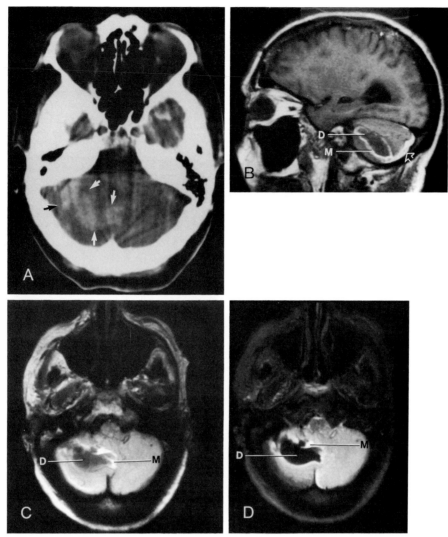

Figure 3.8.   Acute (3 days) cerebellar hemorrhage. A, Axial CT scan 35/200 demonstrates acute hemorrhage hyperdensity *(closed arrows).* **B,** Sagittal T1-weighted 600/25 section demonstrates a hyperintense T1 methemoglobin rim *(M)* surrounding a hypointense deoxyhemoglobin *(D)* center. Subarachnoid and subdural hemorrhage component *(open arrow).* **C** and **D,** T1 2000/20 and T2 2000/ 80-weighted axial MR sections: Note the central T2 deoxyhemoglobin hypointense signal *(D)* and peripheral hyperintense free methemoglobin *(M).* There is a moderate degree of central hypointensity of the hemorrhage on the heavily T1-weighted image **(B).** This is probably due to marked T2 shortening despite the T1-weighted technique.

tionship of these denatured products to cells, proteins, and water.[17] At present, there is some controversy concerning the T2 decreased signal caused by deoxyhemoglobin, particularly at low- and midfield strength magnet systems. The increase of clot hemoglobin concentration caused by clot retraction may play an important role in this phenomenon.[16] Subarachnoid hemorrhage, generally, remains undetected by the MR technique. MR may occasionally detect subarachnoid hemorrhage, however (Fig. 3.8).

Often, different chemical states of hemorrhage are detected in the same patient. MR demonstrates marked hypointensity of some calcified structures. Calcium hypointensity is most marked on T2-weighted GRE (T2*) images (Fig. 3.11).[19] Other substances may occur in pathological states that have paramagnetic properties. One of these substances is melanin, which

may give a high T1 and low T2 signal intensity (Fig. 3.12).

Vascular Flow Considerations

"Time of flight" effects refer to the MR study of fluid (blood and CSF) in motion. The MR lack of signal of flowing blood is called the flow-void effect.[20] Flow-void phenomenon is seen with conventional MR sequences including SE, inversion recovery, and saturation recovery. Flow-void effect within arteries and the dural venous sinuses excludes arterial thrombosis and venous sinus thrombosis, however, care must be taken analyzing both the T1- and T2-weighted images not to mistake thrombus deoxyhemoglobin for flow-void effect. Conversely, the lack of flow-void phenomenon leads to the diagnosis of thrombosis (Fig. 3.13).

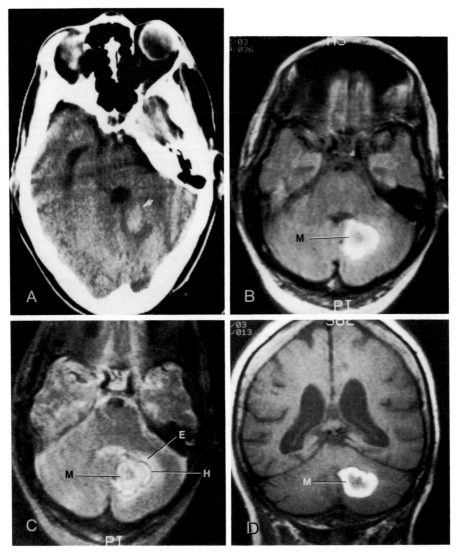

Figure 3.9.   Subacute hemorrhage (2 weeks). A, Axial CT scan 35/ 200 at ictus demonstrates left paramedian clot *(arrow).* **B** and **D,** T1/ proton density-weighted SE 2000/20 axial and coronal sections demonstrate peripheral extracellular methemoglobin *(M).* **C,** T2- weighted SE 2000/80 axial section at same level as **B** demonstrates the extracellular methemoglobin and also demonstrates a thin rim of hypointense hemosiderin *(H)* and hyperintense edema *(E).*

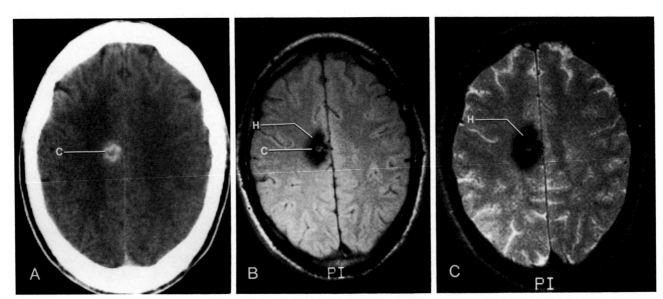

Figure 3.10.   Hemosiderin deposit surrounding occult AVM. A, Axial noncontrast CT scan 35/100. Same level T1-weighted SE 2000/20 **(B)** and T2-weighted SE 2000/80 **(C)** MR scans. Calcification *(C);* hemosiderin *(H);* compare to Table 3.1.

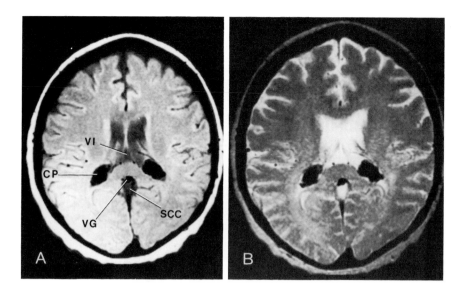

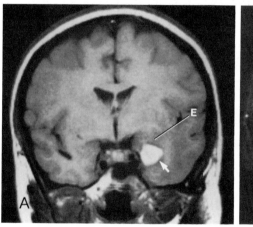

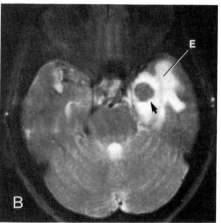

Figure 3.11. Calcific hypointensity. T1- and proton density-weighted 2000/20 **(A)** and T2-weighted 2000/80 **(B)** axial MR scans. Heavily calcified choroid plexus *(CP)* and the vein of Galen *(VG)* have similarly marked hypointensity on both T1- and T2-weighted images. T1 hypointense velum interpositum *(VI)* and supracerebellar cistern *(SCC)* demonstrate T2 hyperintensity.

Figure 3.12. Paramagnetic properties. Metastatic melanoma. **A,** SE 600/25 coronal image T1 hyperintense left temporal mass *(arrow)*. Poorly defined surrounding edema *(E)*. **B,** SE 2000/80 axial image. The mass is now hypointense (T2 white matter-isointense). The surrounding edema is now clearly evident.

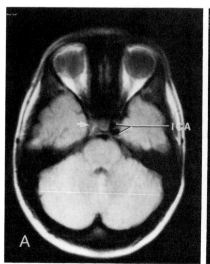

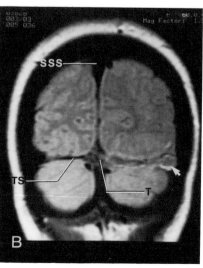

Figure 3.13. Arterial and venous thrombosis (no pulsatile motion artifact suppression technique used). A, T1-weighted SE 2000/20 axial fourth ventricle and cavernous sinus level MR scan. Note signal void (flow-void) of cavernous left internal carotid artery *(ICA)*. Occluded "isointense" right internal carotid artery *(arrow)*. **B,** T1-weighted SE 2000/20 coronal torcular level. Note signal void of the right transverse sinus *(TS)*. Clot in transverse sinus-sigmoid sinus *(arrow)* and torcula *(T)*. Signal void of patent superior sagittal sinus *(SSS)*.

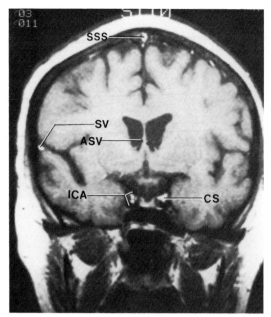

Figure 3.14. Vascular flow-void phenomenon and paradoxical vascular enhancement. No spatial presaturation or MAST technique. Coronal SE 600/25 MR scan without presaturation or flow compensation techniques. Note signal void of internal carotid arteries *(ICA)* and anterior septal veins *(ASV)*. Hyperintensity (paradoxical enhancement) of the superior sagittal sinus *(SSS)*, Sylvian vein *(SV)*, and cavernous sinus *(CS)*.

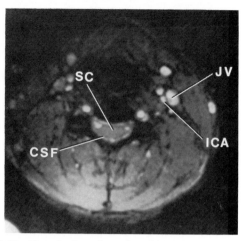

Figure 3.15. Vascular hyperintensity with gradient echo partial flip angle technique. Gradient echo 50/17 20° flip angle 6 NEX 256×256 matrix C4 axial MR section. The internal jugular vein *(JV)* and internal carotid artery *(ICA)* are equally hyperintense. The hyperintense CSF *(CSF)* surrounding the hypointense spinal cord *(SC)* produces a myelographic effect.

Slow flow enhancement (paradoxical enhancement) occurs with short TR/short TE SE sequences (Figs. 1.24 and 3.14). By exciting the "entrance section" tissue with RF, entrance-type enhancement effect is minimized. This latter method is called spatial presaturation. It applies a 90° pulse followed by a dephasing "spoiler pulse" to the sections adjacent to the section of interest. Adjacent slice blood is no longer relaxed and cannot, therefore, contribute to

an increased signal if it should enter the section of interest (Fig. 1.24). GRE techniques with partial flip (tip) angles can produce profound arterial and venous hyperintensity (Fig. 3.15).[21] Motion artifact suppression technique ("MAST") produces enhancement of slow vascular flow.[22] MAST effect enhancement can lead to an erroneous diagnosis of thrombosis when, actually, slow flow is present (Fig. 3.16).

Pulsatile arterial flow is largely responsible for the

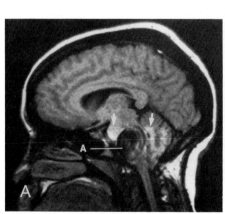
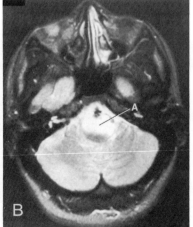
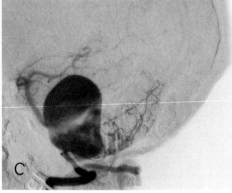

Figure 3.16. Motion artifact suppression technique, "MAST." Application to the arterial flow artifact. Parasagittal SE 600/20, spatial presaturation, no MAST MR scan **(A).** Axial internal auditory canal level SE 2000/80 MAST MR scan **(B).** Lateral left vertebral arterio-gram **(C).** Note the giant left vertebrobasilar junctional aneurysm *(A)* and the flow-induced artifacts *(arrows)* that are not present on the MAST sequence. Note that the aneurysm on the MAST sequence is now hyperintense instead of hypointense-signal void.

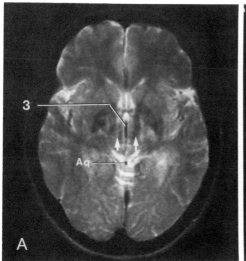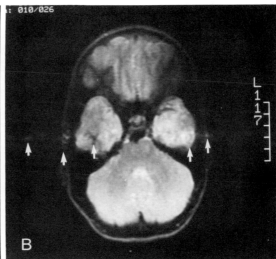

Figure 3.17.   CSF and Arterial flow phenomena. Reinforcement and cancellation. **A,** CSF flow artifact. Axial T2-weighted SE 2000/80 scan. Thrid ventricle level. Markedly hypointense third ventricle *(3)* and cerebral aqueduct *(Aq)* with hyperintense reinforcement and hypointense cancellation signals in the phase-encoding axis *(arrows).*

B, Axial T2-weighted SE 2000/80 scan without flow compensation (MAST). Arterial flow artifact. Sella-carotid siphon level. Horizontal ghost artifact *(arrows).* Hyperintense left temporal lobe (reinforcement) and hypointense right temporal lobe (cancellation).

characteristic "ghosts" occurring in the phase-encoding axis through the perimesencephalic cisterns. "Reinforcement" and "cancellation" phenomena are characteristics of ghost artifacts (Fig. 3.17).[20] Gradient moment nulling is the MAST technique. MAST techniques are also called "flow compensation" techniques. MAST techniques and pulse or cardiac gating markedly reduce ghost artifact (Fig. 3.16). Another method to eliminate ghost artifactual degradation of an area of interest is to change the phase-encoding axis 90° (See Fig. 1.26E). Gradient movement nulling technique is particularly helpful for investigation of parenchymal disorders such as MS, intracranial tumor, brain trauma, or brain or meningeal infection. The technique can be misleading for the investigation of vascular occlusion, aneurysm, or arteriovenous malformation due to flow enhancement (Fig. 3.16).

Much effort is now being directed to developing methods of quantitative blood flow measurements. An example of MR angiography is shown (Fig. 3.18).

CSF Flow Considerations

Turbulent dephasing is the dominant cause of CSF signal loss effects [e.g., signal void of the cerebral aqueduct and third ventricle (Fig. 3.17)] as well as CSF pulsation "ghosts" which particularly degrade cervical spine images.[20,21,23]

CSF signal loss from turbulent dephasing can, however, be useful for diagnosis. For example, without MAST, aqueductal signal void helps establish the diagnosis of communicating hydrocephalus and lack of signal void helps establish the diagnosis of aqueductal stenosis. We use MAST techniques routinely for parenchymal investigation, except for the local-

izer view, due to the markedly improved brain detail obtained.[22] Pulse and cardiac triggering are other methods used to suppress CSF pulsatile motion artifact.[20–23] These methods require synchronization of the pulse wave or ECG wave to the MR sequence. Manufacturers provide the appropriate equipment for pulse and cardiac triggering. Both procedures increase TR and, therefore, scan time. MR methods for

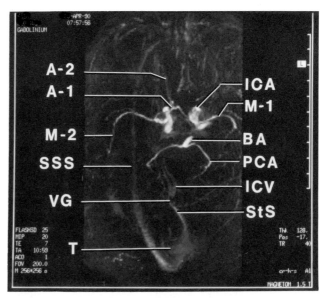

Figure 3.18.   MR Angiogram (MRA). Axial oblique reformation of 3D-FLASH 40/7, 25° i.v. contrast 128 mm slab MRA. Anterior cerebral artery segments (A1, A2). Middle cerebral artery segments (M1, M2). Basilar artery (BA). Posterior cerebral artery (PCA). Superior sagittal sinus (SSS). Internal cerebral vein (ICV). Vein of Galen (VG). Straight sinus (StS). Torcula (T).

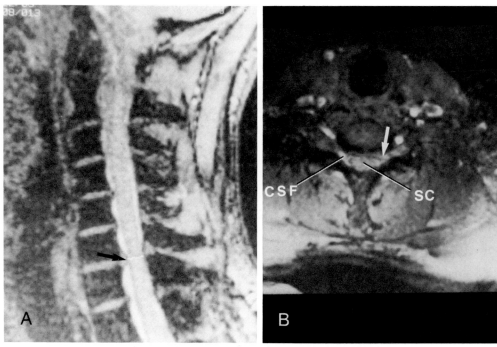

Figure 3.19. GRE spine technique. Midsagittal **(A)** and axial **(B)** C6-7 50/17 flip angle 20° 256 × 256 matrix 6 NEX technique. The C6-7 herniated disk (*arrow* on **A**) causes spinal stenosis (linear cursor = 6.7 mm). It compresses the seventh cervical nerve in the intervertebral neural foramen (*arrow* on **B**). The spinal cord *(SC)* is hypointense compared to the CSF *(CSF)* resulting in a "myelographic effect."

CSF directional flow analysis are now being clinically investigated.

Fundamentals of Diagnostic Techniques

The rapid development of new MR techniques such as GRE 3-D imaging, i.v. MR contrast agents, MR angiography, and artifact suppression methods such as MAST and spatial presaturation has produced frequent protocol changes for MR users. For example, GRE techniques can be used for MR angiography (Fig. 3.18) and for cervical spine "myelographic" effects (Fig. 3.19). It is, therefore, difficult to recommend standard MR pulse sequence techniques similar to those well-established techniques described for CT in Chapter 2. Figure 3.20 is a flow chart of a currently useful method to select the appropriate cranial MR investigative approach. (Spine technique will be discussed in Chapter 15.) A basic rule is that, under most circumstances, a heavily T1-weighted and T2-weighted or T2*-weighted image is necessary to take advantage fully of diagnostic information available by the MR technique. If further information is needed, then MR i.v. contrast technique, surface coil technique, imaging in other planes and MR angiography can be used.

A great problem with MR utilization is the selection of sequences sufficient to make a diagnosis in the least amount of time. As yet, we have no simple solution. For example, if metastases are to be excluded, heavily T1-weighted pre- and postcontrast images can be obtained (Fig. 3.21). Parenchymal disease, such as MS (Fig. 3.22) may be missed, however, without proton density and/or T2-weighted images. T2-weighted intensity characteristics of tumor and edema (Fig. 3.23) complement the T1-weighted exam. Abnormal vessels characteristic of an AVM are often obvious on the T1 localizer image (Fig. 6.39), however, axial and/or coronal T1- and T2-weighted technique will help establish evidence for associated hemorrhage and identify the vascular supply, the arterial nidus, and the draining veins. For the workup of aneurysms or AVMs, MAST technique should be avoided on the localizer view in order to obtain uncompromised spin echo flow effects. MR angiography (MRA) can then be considered (Fig. 3.24). T1 and T2 gray matter isointensity, a broad tumor dural base and a cleft between the tumor and surrounding parenchyma are MR characteristics of meningiomas (Fig. 3.25). Relatively homogeneous i.v. contrast enhancement interrupted by signal void arteries and veins is also typical of meningioma. Tumor multiplicity is characteristic of metastasis and, occasionally, MR i.v. contrast is necessary for diagnosis (Fig. 3.21). Irregular rim contrast enhancement is typical of malignant tumor.

Flowing blood can vary in appearance (hyperintense or hypointense) depending on the MR sequence chosen, the type of scanner, the blood flow velocity and/or the intravenous injection of paramagnetic agents. A presently popular method of MR angiography (MRA) utilizes time-of-flight effects to generate hyperintense signal from flowing blood and suppresses signal from stationary tissue. By using a technique employing 3DFT, short TR and TE and refocussing gradients (GRE), vascular signal is maximized (Fig. 3.18)[24]. Intravenous paramagnetic contrast may be useful, particularly for AVM's.

The 3D volume studied is called a "slab." The individual image "section" in the slice-select plane is called a "partition." Any slice-select plane may be chosen. The individual partitions can be very thin (e.g. 1.4mm in Fig. 3.24B). The 3D data can be reformatted in any plane (e.g. sagittal-oblique, in Fig. 3.18). At present, the images have inferior detail compared to conventional and digital subtraction arteriography[24].

A more recent MRA technique, phase contrast MRA (PC MRA), uses velocity induced phase shifts to distinguish flowing blood from surrounding stationary tissue by subtracting two MRA GRE acquisitions of opposite polarity.

It is superior to time of flight (TOF) MRA for investigation of slow flow and does not require intravenous contrast for venous investigation such as venous sinus thrombosis. Because of its lack of dependence on T1 values, methemoglobin bright signal is not confused with blood flow by PC MRA as it is with TOF MRA. PC MRA can also measure direction and rate of flow. It is our present technique of choice for evaluation of venous sinus thrombosis.

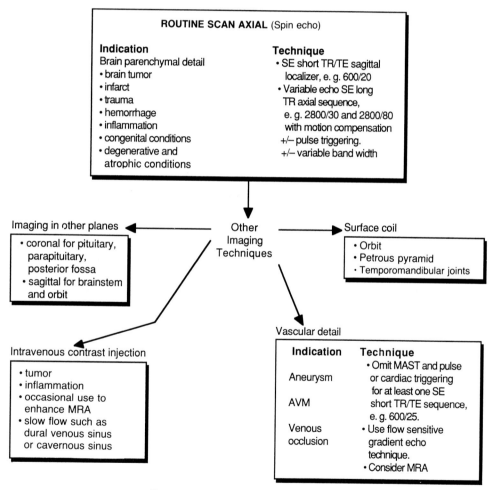

Figure 3.20. Head Scanning Technique.

Figure 3.21. Metastatic bronchogenic carcinoma. Axial fourth ventricle level SE 600/25 noncontrast **(A)** and Gd-DTPA i.v. contrast **(B)** MR scans. Axial subvertex level SE 600/25 noncontrast **(C)** and i.v. contrast **(D)** MR scans. Only the T1-weighted technique was used for this study. Note the irregular ("signet") ring and septated contrast enhancement of the large T1 hypointense cerebellar mass and the fourth ventricle distortion and displacement *(solid arrow).* The sensory cortex (anterior parietal) metastasis *(open arrow)* lacks conspicuity without i.v. contrast.

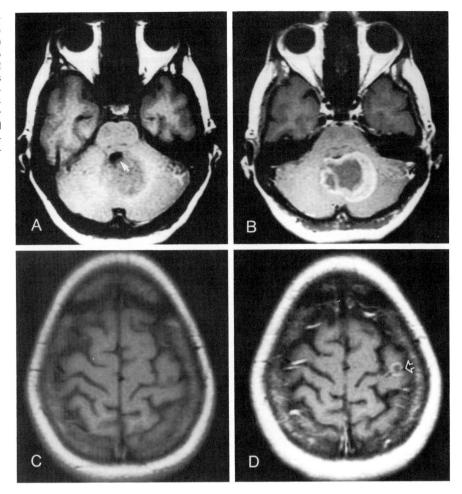

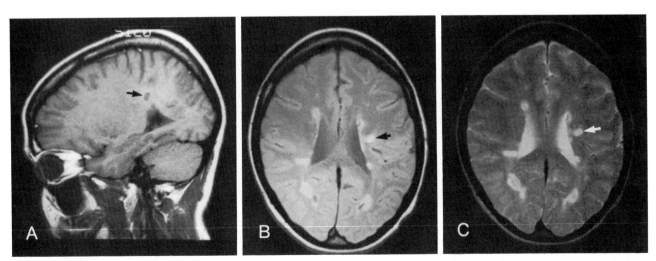

Figure 3.22. **Multiple sclerosis.** Lateral ventricle atrial level sagittal SE 600/25 **(A),** axial SE 2000/20 **(B)** and 2000/80 **(C)** MR scans. Note the T1-gray matter isointense **(A),** proton density and T2 signal hyperintense **(B** and **C)** plaques *(arrows).* Lesion conspicuity is greater with proton density and T2-weighting. The proton density (and T1-) weighted image **(B)** distinguishes between the lateral ventricle and the periventricular plaque. Due to CSF and plaque T2 isointensity, this distinction is lost in **C.** The majority of MS plaques, in our experience, are relatively T1 white matter-isointense and difficult to identify with heavily T1-weighted technique such as SE 600/25.

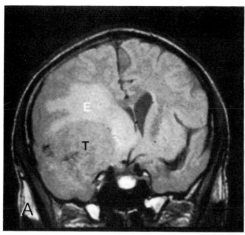

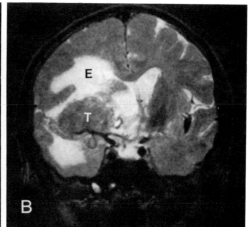

Figure 3.23.   Tumor and edema. T1-weighted SE 2000/20 coronal image **(A).** Same section T2-weighted SE 2000/80 **(B).** Isointense metastatic tumor *(T)* outlined by edema *(E).* The edema is hyperintense to CSF on the T1-proton density image and CSF isointense on the T2-weighted image. More often, tumors are T2 hyperintense and may be difficult to distinguish from edema. In the latter case, Gd-DTPA MR or i.v. contrast CT is necessary.

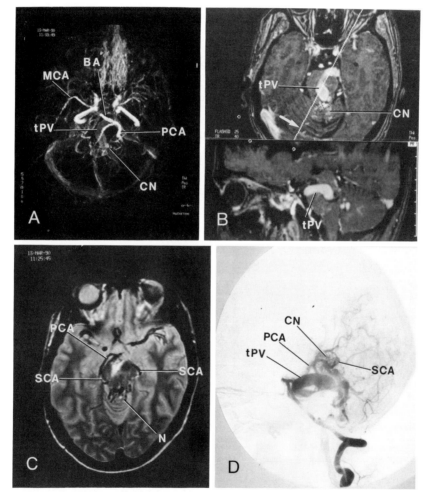

Figure 3.24.   Tectal arteriovenous malformation (AVM) with large transparenchymal midbrain vein—Three-dimensional (3D) time-of-flight MR angiography (MRA). Axial 3D FLASH (Fast Low Angle SHot) 25° flip angle 40/7 84 mm slab 64 partition I.V. Gd-DTPA MR angiogram **(A).** Single partition 1.4 mm thickness section **(B**-top) and oblique sagittal reformation **(B**-bottom) along the annotated line (closed arrow). Axial midbrain-level SE 2745/45 pulse-triggered, MAST MR Scan **(C).** Left vertebral lateral arteriogram **(D).** There is a tectal capillary nidus (CN) arising from both superior cerebellar arteries (SCA) that supplies a large transparenchymal midbrain vein (tPV). The two principal branches of the basilar artery (BA) demonstrated by MRA are probably posterior cerebral arteries (PCA). Right middle cerebral artery (MCA). Note how the oblique sagittal plane optimally demonstrates the abnormal draining vein. Note the GRE flow hyperintensity and the spin echo signal-void hypointensity. The inflow of unsaturated spins into a saturated 3D volume produces optimized hyperintense flow signal against a featureless stationary background. It is very likely that the hyperdynamic flow of the afferent superior cerebellar arteries causes lack of MRA signal due to incomplete rephasing[24]. Signal loss from AVM afferent arteries is a problem with current MRA technique[24]. Hyperdynamic afferent arteries can be demonstrated by conventional spin echo techniques, however **(C).**

Figure 3.25. Tentorial meningioma. Sagittal ventricular atrial level SE 600/25 **(A)** and axial midbrain level SE 2800/80 **(B)** MR scans. Intravenous Gd-DTPA sagittal section identical to Figure **A (C).** Note the characteristic T1 and T2 gray matter-isointense mass *(M)* with an inhomogeneous quality due to prominent blood vessels *(V)* and/or calcifications. The broad dural base *(D)* of the tumor, the relative homogeneous contrast enhancement *(CE)* and the smooth cleft margin *(arrow)* is typical of meningioma. Intravenous contrast injection was probably unnecessary for diagnosis in this case.

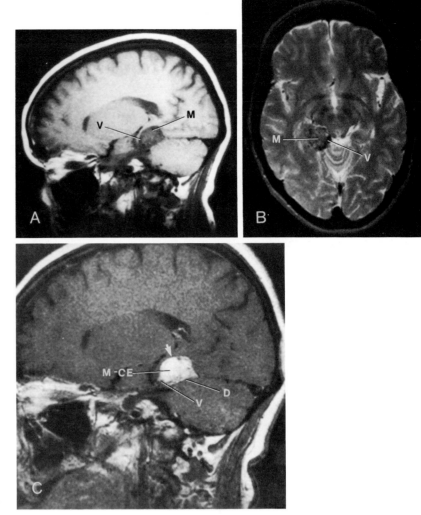

References

1. Spritzer CE, MacFall J. Fast-scan imaging in Pomeranz, SJ. Craniospinal magnetic resonance imaging. Philadelphia, PA, WB Saunders Co, 1989; 71–93.
1a. Enzmann D, Augustyn GT. Improved MR images of the brain with use of a gated, flow-compensated, variable bandwidth pulse sequence. Radiology 1989, 172:777–781.
2. Carlson JW, Arakawa M, Kaufman L, et al. Depth-focused radiofrequency coils for MR imaging. *Radiology* 1987; 165:251–255.
3. Wehrli FW, MacFall JR, Newton TH. Parameters determining the appearance of NMR images. In Newton TH, Potts DG (Eds). *Advanced Imaging Techniques.* San Anselmo, CA: Clavadel Press, 1983; 81–117.
4. McArdle CB, Richardson DJ, Nicholas DA, et al. Developmental features of the neonatal brain. MR imaging. Part II: ventricular size and extracerebral space. *Radiology* 1987; 162:230–234.
5. Brant-Zawadzki M, Berry I, Osaki L, et al. Gd-DTPA in clinical MR of the brain. 2: extra-axial lesions and normal structures. *AJNR* 1986; 7:789–793.
6. Brega RK, Papke RA, Pajunas KW, et al. Benign extra-axial tumors: Contrast enhancement with Gd-DTPA. *Radiology* 1987; 163:427–429.
7. McArdle CB, Nicholas DA, Richardson CJ, Amparo EG. Monitoring of the neonate undergoing MR imaging: Technical considerations—work in progress. *Radiology* 1986; 159:223–226.
8. Pavlicek W, Geisinger M, Castle L, et al. The effects of nuclear magnetic resonance on patients with cardiac pacemakers. *Radiology* 1983; 147:149–153.
9. Becker RL, Norfray JF, Teitlebaum GP, et al. MR imaging in patients with intracranial aneurysm clips. *AJNR* 1988; 9:885–889.
10. McArdle CB, Richardson CJ, Nicholas DA, et al. Developmental features of the neonatal brain. MR imaging. Part 1: gray-white matter differentiation and myelination. *Radiology* 1987; 162:223–229.
11. Runge VM, Wood ML, Kaufman DM, et al. The straight and narrow path to good head and spine MRI. *Radiographics* 1988; 8:507–531.
12. Darwin RH, Drayer BP, Riederer SJ, et al. T2 estimates in healthy and diseased brain tissue: a comparison using various MR pulse sequences. *Radiology* 1986; 160:375–381.
13. Oot RF, New PFJ, Pile-Spellman J, et al. The detection of intracranial calcifications by MR. *AJNR* 1986; 7:801–809.
14. Haughton VM, Rimm AA, Sobocinski KA, et al. A blinded clinical comparison of MR imaging and CT in neuroradiology. *Radiology* 1986; 160:751–755.
15. Gomori JM, Grossman RI, Goldberg HI. Intracranial hematomas: Imaging by high field MR. *Radiology* 1985; 157:87–93.
16. Hayman LA, Taber KH, Ford JJ et al. Effect of clot formation and retraction on spin-echo MR images of blood. An in vitro study. AJNR 1990; 10:1155–1158.
17. Drayer B, Burger P, Darwin R. Magnetic resonance imaging of brain iron. *AJNR* 1986; 6:373–380.
18. Zimmerman RD, Heier LA, Snow RB, et al. Acute intracranial hemorrhage: Intensity changes on sequential MR scans at 0.5 T. *AJNR* 1988; 9:47–57.
19. Atlas SW, Grossman RI, Hackney DB, et al. Calcified intracranial lesions: detection with gradient-echo-acquisition rapid MR imaging. *AJNR* 1988; 9:253–259.
20. Kelly WM. Image artifacts and technical limitations in magnetic resonance imaging of the central nervous system. Brant-Zawadzki M, Normal D (Eds). New York: Raven Press, 1987; 43–82.
21. Porter BA, Hastrup W, Richardson ML, et al. Classification and investigation of artifacts in magnetic resonance imaging. *Radiographics* 1987; 7:271–287.
22. Elster AD. Motion artifact suppression technique (MAST) for cranial MR imaging: superiority over cardiac gating for reducing phase-shift artifacts. *AJNR* 1988; 9:671–674.
23. Enzmann DR, Rubin JB, Wright A. Cervical spine imaging: generating high-signal CSF in sagittal and axial images. *Radiology* 1987; 163:233–238.
24. Marchal G, Bosmans H, Vanfraeyenhoven L, et al. Intracranial vascular lesions: optimization and clinical evaluation of three-dimensional time-of-flight MR angiography. Radiology 1990; 175:443–448.

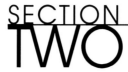

SECTION TWO

The Brain

CHAPTER 4

Normal MR and CT Brain Anatomy

Introduction

The method chosen to present normal MR and CT anatomy begins with a brief introduction to lobar and surface anatomy, and also to functional anatomy. An image atlas presentation then follows. This chapter concludes with a description of the neonatal brain.

Many of the ideas for this chapter are adapted from those of Joseph C. Masdeu, M.D.[1] CT and MR images are shown chosen for anatomical emphasis and, occasionally, to stress a physiological point such as tissue water[2] and iron[3] content.

Sagittal sections are presented first followed by axial and then coronal sections. Before each of these three imaging plane presentations, a group of line diagrams with superimposed image section levels is presented. The canthomeatal axial plane of section has been chosen since it represents a compromise between the supraorbitomeatal and infraorbitomeatal planes. Vascular territories and dural structures will be included in the atlas portion.

Anatomical MR and CT imaging of specific regions are emphasized in different chapters to which the reader is referred: the sella (Chapter 11), the temporal bone (Chapter 12), the skull and face (Chapter 13), the orbit (Chapter 14), and the spine (Chapter 15).

Many excellent brain anatomical references have been used for this chapter and are listed for the reader's convenience.[4-9] Additional excellent references for brain vascular territories are recommended.[1,10-13]

Brain Surface Anatomy

FIGURES 4.1 TO 4.2

Figure 4.1. Lateral convexity (A), medial convexity (B), superior (C), undersurface (D) anatomy.

These figures are presented for correlation with MR and CT sections. They should be helpful for the understanding of the relationship of scan plane angle and anatomical appearances. Because there is considerable individual variation of brain surface anatomy, these surface landmarks should serve as structural approximations. Figure 4.2 illustrates ventricular anatomy related to surface landmarks.

Figure 4.1**A** and 4.1**B** map lateral and medial convexity anatomy, respectively. Figure 4.1**C** maps vertex anatomy and **D** maps the brain undersurface. Lobar landmarks are well defined by the central, parieto-occipital, and lateral sulci and are otherwise estimated between the frontal *(vertical lines)*, the temporal *(horizontal lines)*, parietal *(dots)*, and occipital *(squares)* lobes.

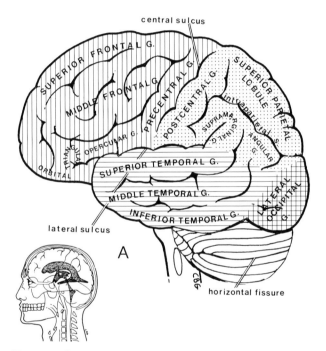

Figure 4.1.A,   Lateral convexity.

The central or "Rolandic" sulcus divides the frontal lobe precentral (motor) gyrus from the parietal lobe postcentral (sensory) gyrus. The lateral sulcus (horizontal portion of the Sylvian fissure) separates the frontal and parietal lobes from the temporal lobe. The lateral sulcus joins the vertical portion of the Sylvian fissure deep to the operculum. The superior lip of the lateral sulcus is formed by opercular portions of the frontal and parietal lobes. Both the frontal and the temporal lobes have three prominent horizontal gyri: superior, middle, and inferior. The inferior frontal gyrus is divided into orbital, triangular, and opercular portions from front to back. The intraparietal sulcus divides the superior parietal lobule from the supramarginal and angular gyri. The inferior parietal lobule is divided into the supramarginal gyrus anteriorly and the angular gyrus posteriorly. Note the small lateral convexity portion of the occipital lobe.

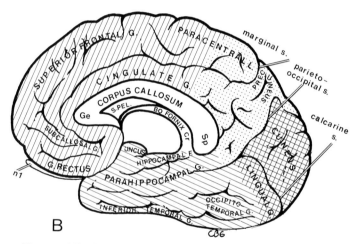

Figure 4.1.B,   Medial convexity surface landmarks (following sagittal division of the corpus callosum and fornix and removal of the diencephalon, midbrain, brainstem, and cerebellum).

The hippocampal formation is artistically demonstrated on this section despite its usually lateral and obscured location to this view. The body *(Bo)* and the crus *(Cr)* of the fornix curve toward the hippocampal formation. The rostrum, genu *(Ge)*, body, and splenium *(Sp)* of the corpus callosum are sectioned through the midline. The cingulate gyrus curves around the corpus callosum and blends with the parahippocampal gyrus. The septum pellucidum *(S. Pel.)* is between the fornix and the corpus callosum. Ge = genu, Sp = splenium of the corpus callosum. Both the cingulate sulcus and the marginal sulcus are reliable anatomical landmarks. The cingulate sulcus demarcates the superior margin of the cingulate gyrus. Posterosuperiorly, it continues as the marginal sulcus that separates the paracentral lobule from the precuneus. Note that the motor cortex is slightly greater than one gyrus width from the marginal sulcus.

The parieto-occipital sulcus is a reliable landmark separating the precuneus (parietal) from the cuneus (occipital). The cuneus is separated from the lingual gyrus by the calcarine sulcus—another reliable landmark.

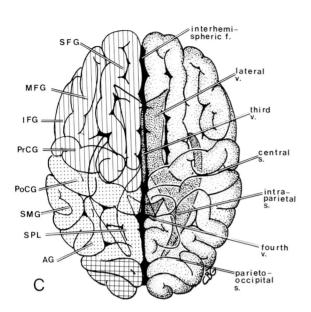

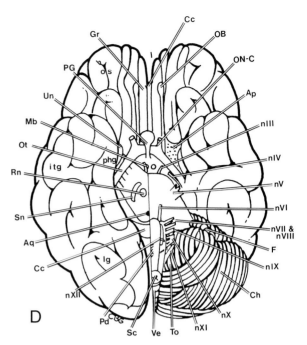

Figure 4.1.C, Brain superior surface anatomy.

On the right side of this diagram, the lateral, third, and fourth ventricles are superimposed over the surface anatomy. The central sulci form a "V" shape because of their slight posteriorly directed course. The interparietal sulcus divides the superior parietal lobule *(SPL)* from the supramarginal *(SMG)* and angular *(AG)* gyri. The parieto-occipital sulcus separates the parietal lobe *(dots)* from the occipital lobe *(squares)*. The central sulcus separates the frontal lobe precentral gyrus *(PrCG)* from the parietal lobe postcentral gyrus *(PoCG)*. Note the frontal lobe superior frontal *(SFG)*, middle frontal *(MFG)*, and inferior frontal *(IFG)* gyri.

Figure 4.1.D, Undersurface of the brain anatomy.

The right side *(reader's left)* of the brainstem has been removed in order to demonstrate the posterior cerebral undersurface. From anterior to posterior, the orbital surface of the inferior frontal gyrus *(os)*, the inferior temporal *(itg)*, parahippocampal *(phg)* gyri, and the lingual gyrus *(lg)* are labeled. The olfactory bulb *(OB)* is the most anterior portion of the olfactory nerve. The optic chiasm *(ON-C)* is anterior to the infundibulum of the pituitary gland *(PG)*. Cranial nerves (nIII–nXII) are also labeled. The genu and splenium of the corpus callosum *(Cc)* are seen through the interhemispheric fissure. The anterior perforated substance *(Ap)* is seen superior and anterior to the optic tract *(Ot)*. The fifth cranial nerve (nV) enters the basilar portion of the pons. The oculomotor nerve (nIII) and the abducens nerve (nVI) arise from the interpeduncular fossa and the medullopontine junction, respectively. The right nIII is superimposed over the mamillary body *(Mb)*. The flocculus *(F)* is seen in the left cerebellopontine angle. The inferior semilunar lobule of the cerebellar hemisphere *(Ch)*, posterior cerebellar vermis *(Ve)*, and the tonsil *(To)* are easily identified. The hypoglossal nerve (nXII) arises from the lateral medullary groove preolivary sulcus and is seen superimposed over the olive. The pyramidal decussation *(Pd)* of the medulla and the central gray matter of the spinal cord *(Sc)* are labeled. The axillary (transverse) section of the midbrain reveals the substantia nigra *(Sn)*, red nucleus *(Rn)*, aqueduct *(Aq)*, and cerebral peduncles. The uncus *(Un)* is continuous with the parahippocampal gyrus. The gyrus rectus *(Gr)* lies medial to the olfactory tract and bulb.

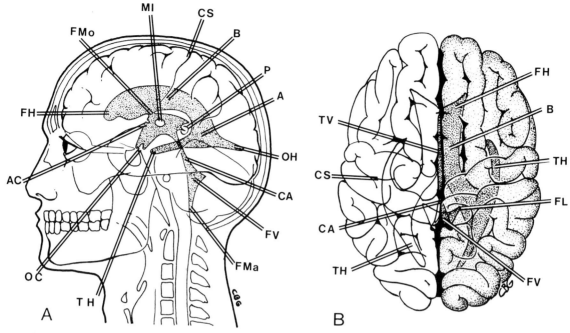

Figure 4.2. The ventricular system
A, Lateral, and **B,** superior diagrams with labeled central sulcus *(CS).* The lateral ventricle frontal horn *(FH),* body *(B),* atrium *(A),* occipital horn *(OH),* and temporal horn *(TH).* The lateral ventricles communicate with the third ventricle *(TV)* via the foramina of Monro *(FMo).* Note the third ventricle massa intermedia *(MI),* the notch for the anterior commissure *(AC),* the optic chiasm *(OC),* and the pineal gland *(P).* Paired anterior and posterior third ventricle recesses are related anteriorly to the optic chiasm and posteriorly to the pineal

gland. The optic recess is anterior and the infundibular recess is posterior to the chiasm producing the characteristic "fish-mouth" appearance. The suprapineal recess is above the pineal gland and the pineal recess projects into the pineal gland. The third ventricle communicates through its caudal outlet, the cerebral aqueduct *(CA),* which in turn, leads to the fourth ventricle *(FV).* The fourth ventricle communicates with the subarachnoid spaces via the midline foramen of Magendie *(FMa)* and bilateral foramina of Luschka *(FL).*

Functional Anatomy

A thorough review of functional anatomy is beyond the purpose of this text. A brief overview of essential functional anatomy is provided, however. For a more thorough functional brain anatomy overview review, the reader is referred to the excellent work by Masdeu.[1]

Four other major regions will only briefly be discussed; these are the internal capsule, the basal ganglia, the brainstem, and the cerebellum. Lesions of the posterior internal capsule usually cause contralateral paresis or paralysis. From front to back, the motor fibers of the posterior limb of the internal capsule are face, arm, and leg. The optic radiations course through the most posterior portion of the internal

capsule. Basal ganglia lesions may produce "extrapyramidal" motor disorders characterized by dyskinesia, bradykinesia, and alterations of muscle tone (i.e., rigidity). Midbrain or pontine tegmental lesions produce eye movement abnormalities and altered consciousness. Bilateral midbrain pontine level corticospinal tract interruption can cause the locked-in state. A midbrain tectal mass may produce Parinaud's syndrome: truncal ataxia, paralysis of upward gaze, and papiledema. Tegmental medullary lesions interfere with respiratory and cardiovascular centers. Ventral or pyramidal brainstem lesions produce contralateral hemiparesis and may also affect the third, sixth, and seventh nerve fibers. Cerebellar lesions produce tremor, ataxia, and asynergic disturbances.

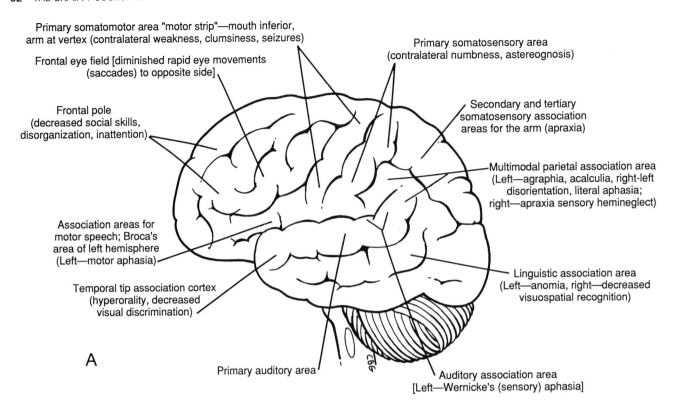

Primary somatomotor area "motor strip"—mouth inferior, arm at vertex (contralateral weakness, clumsiness, seizures)

Frontal eye field [diminished rapid eye movements (saccades) to opposite side]

Frontal pole (decreased social skills, disorganization, inattention)

Association areas for motor speech; Broca's area of left hemisphere (Left—motor aphasia)

Temporal tip association cortex (hyperorality, decreased visual discrimination)

Primary somatosensory area (contralateral numbness, astereognosis)

Secondary and tertiary somatosensory association areas for the arm (apraxia)

Multimodal parietal association area (Left—agraphia, acalculia, right-left disorientation, literal aphasia; right—apraxia sensory hemineglect)

Linguistic association area (Left—anomia, right—decreased visuospatial recognition)

Primary auditory area

Auditory association area [Left—Wernicke's (sensory) aphasia]

A

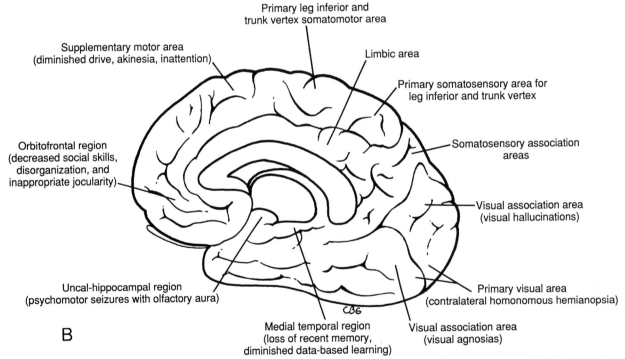

Supplementary motor area (diminished drive, akinesia, inattention)

Primary leg inferior and trunk vertex somatomotor area

Limbic area

Primary somatosensory area for leg inferior and trunk vertex

Orbitofrontal region (decreased social skills, disorganization, and inappropriate jocularity)

Somatosensory association areas

Visual association area (visual hallucinations)

Uncal-hippocampal region (psychomotor seizures with olfactory aura)

Medial temporal region (loss of recent memory, diminished data-based learning)

Primary visual area (contralateral homonomous hemianopsia)

Visual association area (visual agnosias)

B

Figure 4.3. Brain surface functional anatomy. Lateral convexity **(A)**, medial convexity **(B).** Functional anatomical areas are labeled. Beneath each label, in parentheses, are characteristic disorders associated with lesions of the area.

Sectional Anatomy
FIGURES 4.4 TO 4.8

SAGITTAL SECTIONS S1–S4

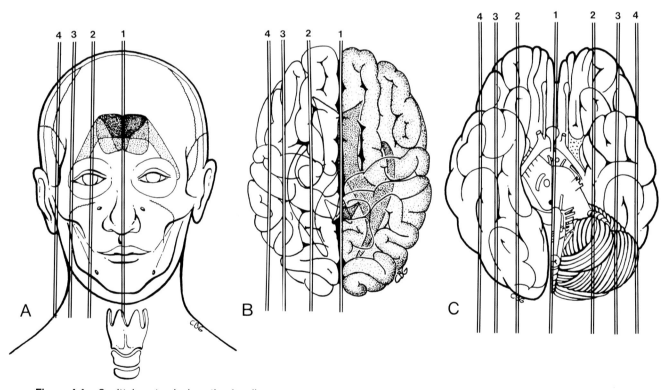

Figure 4.4. Sagittal anatomical section localizers.
Frontal **(A),** superior surface **(B),** and inferior surface of the brain **(C)** localizers demonstrate sagittal sections S1 through S4.

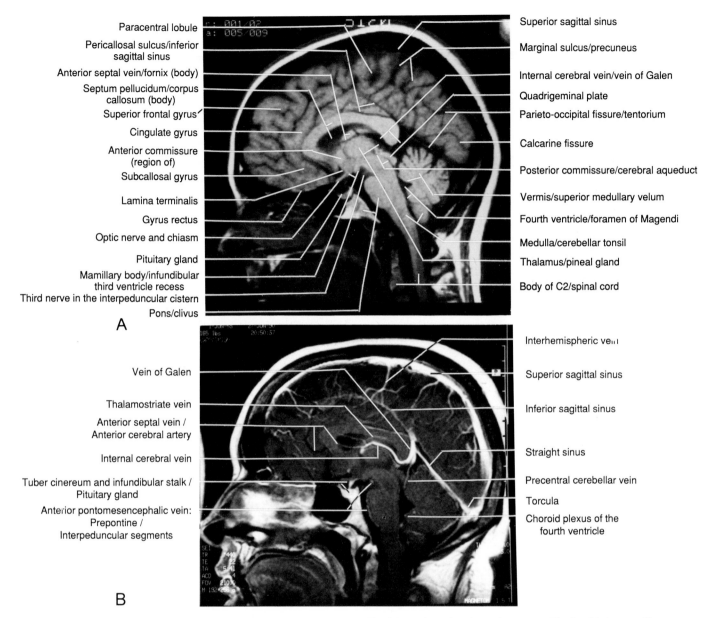

Paracentral lobule
Pericallosal sulcus/inferior sagittal sinus
Anterior septal vein/fornix (body)
Septum pellucidum/corpus callosum (body)
Superior frontal gyrus
Cingulate gyrus
Anterior commissure (region of)
Subcallosal gyrus
Lamina terminalis
Gyrus rectus
Optic nerve and chiasm
Pituitary gland
Mamillary body/infundibular third ventricle recess
Third nerve in the interpeduncular cistern
Pons/clivus

Superior sagittal sinus
Marginal sulcus/precuneus
Internal cerebral vein/vein of Galen
Quadrigeminal plate
Parieto-occipital fissure/tentorium
Calcarine fissure
Posterior commissure/cerebral aqueduct
Vermis/superior medullary velum
Fourth ventricle/foramen of Magendi
Medulla/cerebellar tonsil
Thalamus/pineal gland
Body of C2/spinal cord

A

Vein of Galen
Thalamostriate vein
Anterior septal vein / Anterior cerebral artery
Internal cerebral vein
Tuber cinereum and infundibular stalk / Pituitary gland
Anterior pontomesencephalic vein: Prepontine / Interpeduncular segments

Interhemispheric vein
Superior sagittal sinus
Inferior sagittal sinus
Straight sinus
Precentral cerebellar vein
Torcula
Choroid plexus of the fourth ventricle

B

Figure 4.5. Midsagittal (S1). Short TR/TE T1-weighted MR scans.

A, Noncontrast scan.

Clockwise observations: The cortical gray matter is hypointense compared to white matter. The marginal sulcus separates the paracentral lobule from the precuneus. The internal cerebral vein and vein of Galen course around the splenium of the corpus callosum. The parieto-occipital fissure separates the precuneus from the cuneus. The quadrigeminal plate overlies the cerebral aqueduct. Under the tentorium is the superior cerebellar cistern that is continuous with the quadrigeminal plate cistern. The calcarine sulcus separates the cuneus from the lingual gyrus. The posterior commissure lies anterior-inferior to the pineal gland. The cerebellar vermis overlies the fourth ventricle and rostrally is separated from it by the superior medullary velum. The foramen of Magendi leading to the cistern (vallecula) between the tonsils of the cerebellar hemispheres. The tonsils are at the medullary level and the fourth ventricle is at the pontine level. The thalamus is obscuring the third ventricle water signal.

The interpeduncular cistern is traversed by the third nerve. The pons and clivus between which is the pontine cistern. The mamillary bodies are posterior to the third ventricle infundibular recess. The pituitary gland is slightly deformed by intrasellar extension of the chiasmatic cistern ("partial empty sella"). The optic nerve and chiasm are under the anterior cerebral artery. The lamina terminalis forms the anterior border of the third ventricle optic recess. The gyrus rectus is beneath the subcallosal gyrus. The cingulate gyrus lies over the corpus callosum. The superior frontal gyrus merges with the paracentral lobule. The septum pellucidum lies between the fornix and corpus callosum. The anterior septal vein drains to the internal cerebral vein.

B, Gadolinium DTPA i.v. contrast-enhanced section S1.

Slow flow vascular structures (veins) and structures lacking a blood-brain barrier (pituitary gland and stalk, and choroid plexus) are contrast enhanced. Rapid flow arteries such as the anterior cerebral and basilar arteries are signal-void.

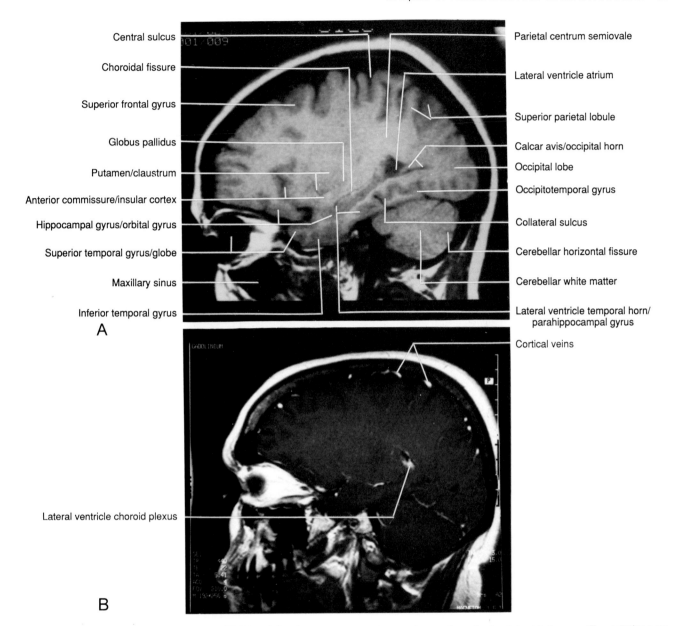

Central sulcus

Choroidal fissure

Superior frontal gyrus

Globus pallidus

Putamen/claustrum

Anterior commissure/insular cortex

Hippocampal gyrus/orbital gyrus

Superior temporal gyrus/globe

Maxillary sinus

Inferior temporal gyrus

A

Parietal centrum semiovale

Lateral ventricle atrium

Superior parietal lobule

Calcar avis/occipital horn

Occipital lobe

Occipitotemporal gyrus

Collateral sulcus

Cerebellar horizontal fissure

Cerebellar white matter

Lateral ventricle temporal horn/
parahippocampal gyrus

Cortical veins

Lateral ventricle choroid plexus

B

Figure 4.6. Sagittal section S2. Short TR/TE T1-weighted MR scans. Hippocampal level.

A, Noncontrast scan.

Clockwise note: The parietal centrum semiovale hyperintensity compared to cortical gray matter. The lateral ventricle atrium and the occipital horn outline the calcar avis. The superior parietal lobule is posterior to the postcentral gyrus. The collateral sulcus is between the occipitotemporal and the parahippocampal gyri. The cerebellar horizontal fissure is shallow at this level. The temporal horn is indented by the hippocampal gyrus. The temporal tip is separated by

the Sylvian fissure from the frontal orbital gyrus. The anterior commissure is beneath the lenticular nucleus (putamen and globus pallidus). The claustrum is anterior to the putamen; the globus pallidus is posterior to the putamen. The anterior insular cortex is sectioned because of its slightly medial location. The choroidal fissure is at the medial aspect of the temporal horn. The central sulcus separates the precentral and postcentral gyri.

B, Gadolinium DTPA i.v. contrast-enhanced section S2. The convexity veins and the lateral ventricle choroid plexus are enhanced.

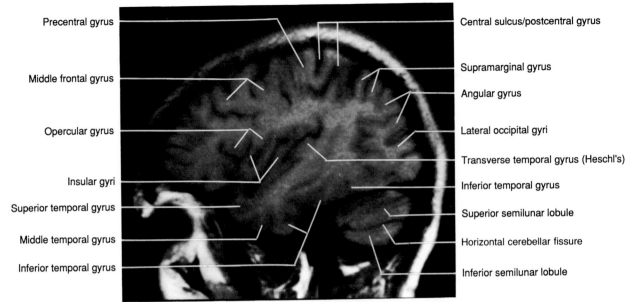

Precentral gyrus
Middle frontal gyrus
Opercular gyrus
Insular gyri
Superior temporal gyrus
Middle temporal gyrus
Inferior temporal gyrus

Central sulcus/postcentral gyrus
Supramarginal gyrus
Angular gyrus
Lateral occipital gyri
Transverse temporal gyrus (Heschl's)
Inferior temporal gyrus
Superior semilunar lobule
Horizontal cerebellar fissure
Inferior semilunar lobule

Figure 4.7. Sagittal section S3. SE 600/25 Insular level.
Clockwise note: The central sulcus separates the pre- and post-central gyri. The supramarginal gyrus is behind the postcentral gyrus and anterior to the angular gyrus. The transverse temporal gyrus is deep within the Sylvian fissure. The cerebellar horizontal fissure is between the superior and inferior semilunar lobules. The insular gyri are below the opercular gyri.

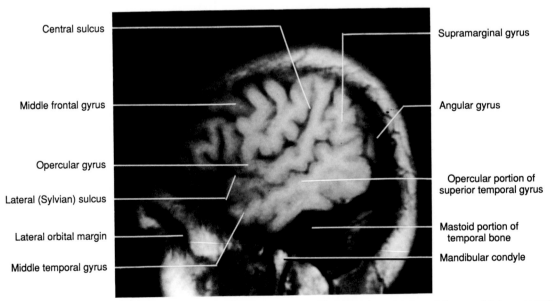

Central sulcus
Middle frontal gyrus
Opercular gyrus
Lateral (Sylvian) sulcus
Lateral orbital margin
Middle temporal gyrus

Supramarginal gyrus
Angular gyrus
Opercular portion of superior temporal gyrus
Mastoid portion of temporal bone
Mandibular condyle

Figure 4.8. Sagittal section S4. SE 600/25 Lateral sulcus fissure level.
Clockwise note: The supramarginal gyrus anterior to the angular gyrus. The frontal, parietal, and temporal lobe opercular portions surround the lateral sulcus. The pre- and postcentral gyri are separated by the central sulcus.

FIGURES 4.9 TO 4.17

AXIAL SECTIONS A1–18

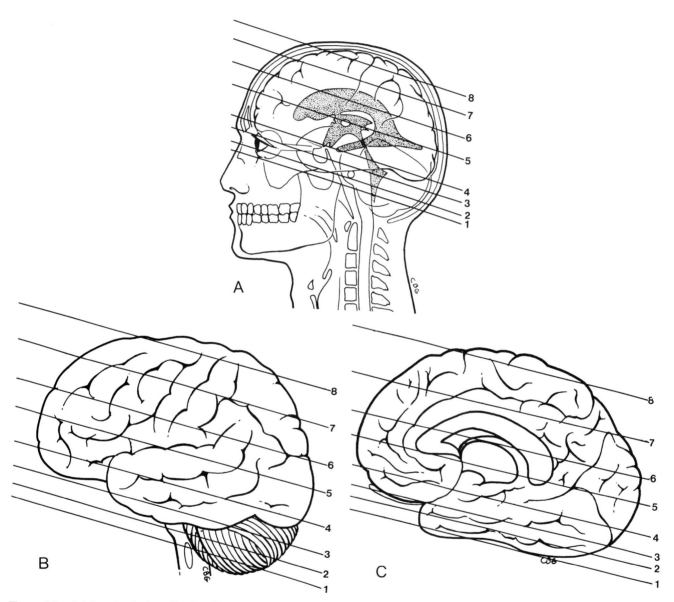

Figure 4.9.   Axial anatomical section localizers.
Lines *1–8* represent the canthomeatal axial planes of section A1–A8. Note how the marginal sulcus is approximately one gyrus width posterior to the central sulcus. The fourth ventricle, the pituitary gland, and the orbit are included together on section A3.

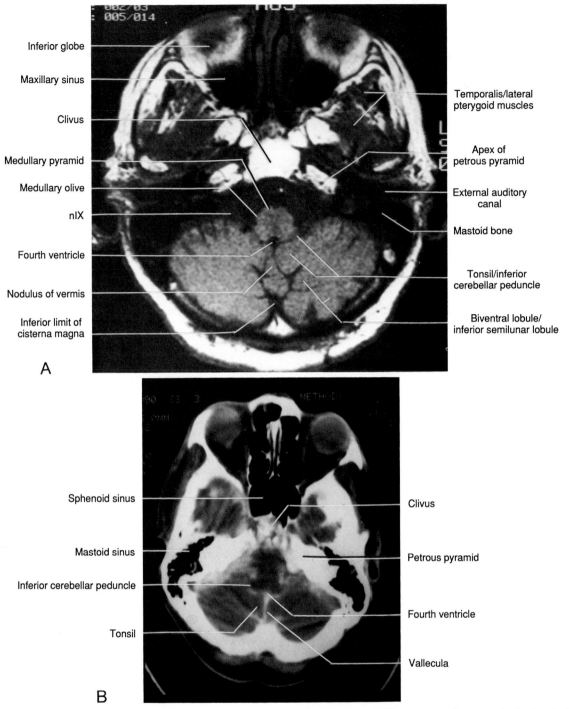

Inferior globe

Maxillary sinus

Clivus

Medullary pyramid

Medullary olive

nIX

Fourth ventricle

Nodulus of vermis

Inferior limit of
cisterna magna

A

Temporalis/lateral
pterygoid muscles

Apex of
petrous pyramid

External auditory
canal

Mastoid bone

Tonsil/inferior
cerebellar peduncle

Biventral lobule/
inferior semilunar lobule

Sphenoid sinus

Mastoid sinus

Inferior cerebellar peduncle

Tonsil

B

Clivus

Petrous pyramid

Fourth ventricle

Vallecula

Figure 4.10.   Axial medullary level section A1.
A. T1-weighted (SE 600/25) 3-mm thickness 16-cm FOV MR. The rectangular shape of the medulla is due to the olivary nuclear complex anterolaterally and the inferior cerebellar peduncles (restiform bodies) posteriorly.[1,5] Note the inferior cerebellar hemisphere lobules and the cerebellar tonsils. **B,** Intrathecal contrast CT cisternogram. The CT cisternogram accurately demonstrates CSF spaces and parenchymal edges. Note the bone detail.

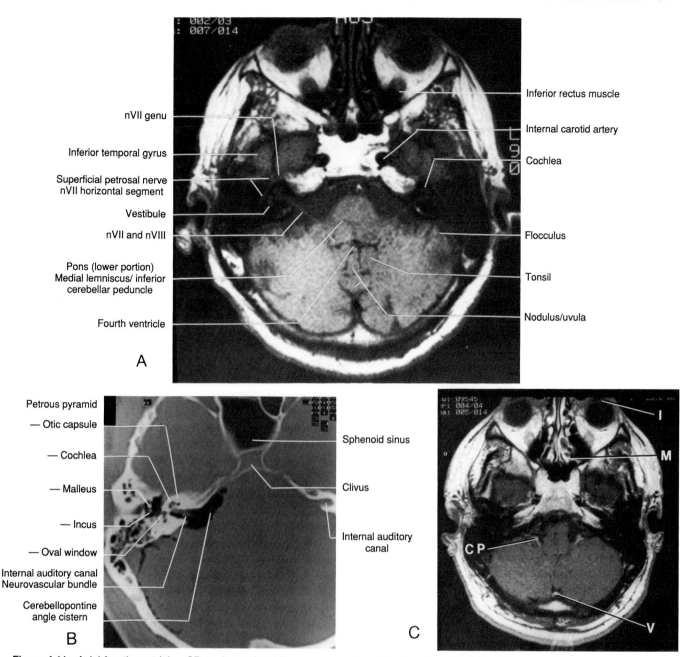

Figure 4.11 Axial fourth ventricle—CP angle section A2.
A, T1-weighted (SE 600/25) MR 3-mm thickness 16-cm FOV section. Note excellent detail of the internal auditory canal neurovascular bundles, the horizontal segment of the facial nerve, and the superficial petrosal nerve. **B,** Cerebellopontine angle air cisternogram (L 200/W 3000). The patient's head is in the left lateral decubitus posi-

tion. Note the air entering the internal auditory canal outlining the neurovascular bundle. **C,** Gd-DTPA i.v. contrast MR SE 600/25 scan. The choroid plexus *(CP)* protruding from the Luschka foramen, a posterior inferior cerebellar vein *(V)*, the occular iris *(I)* and the nasal mucosa *(M)* all prominently contrast enhance.

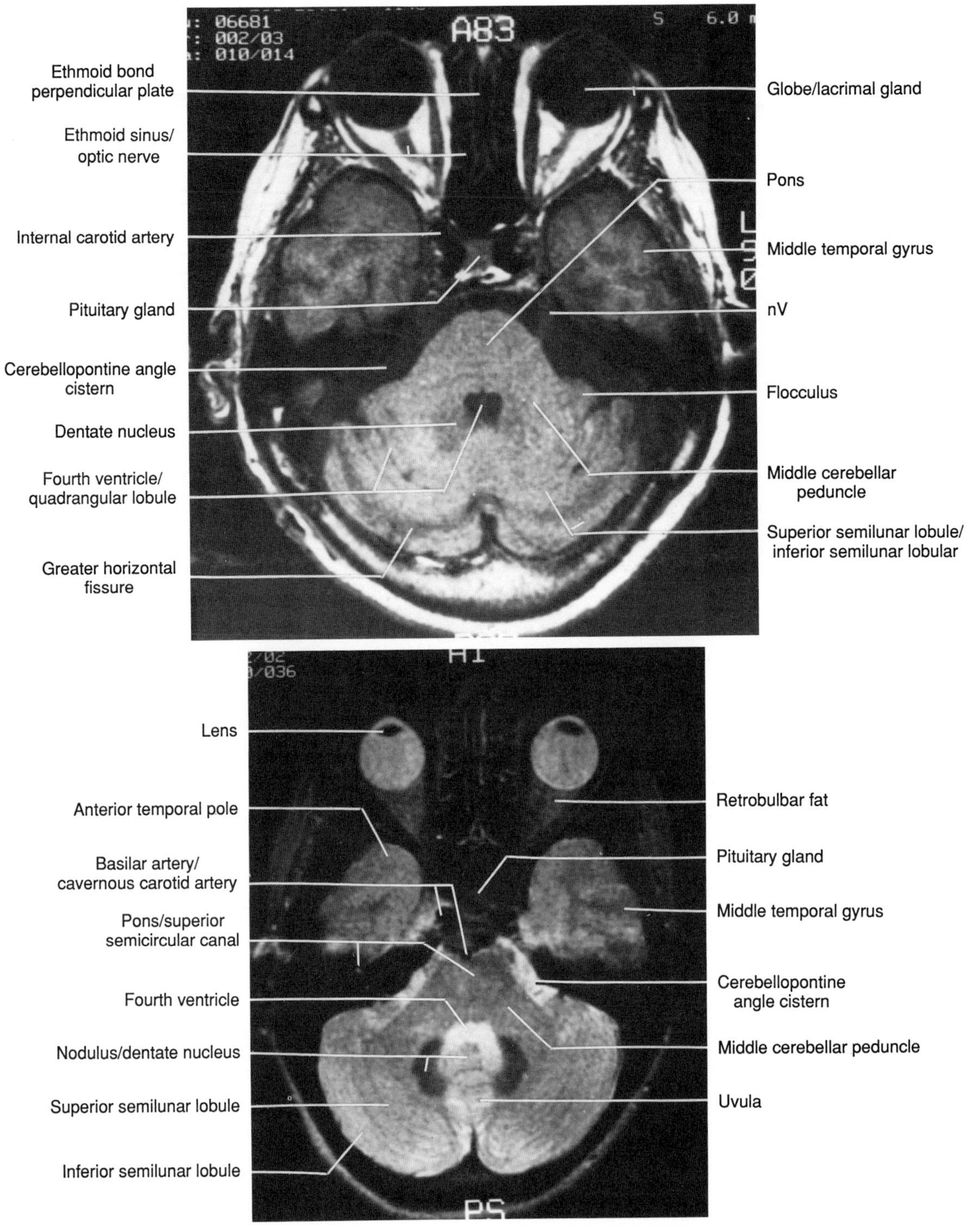

Ethmoid bond
perpendicular plate

Ethmoid sinus/
optic nerve

Internal carotid artery

Pituitary gland

Cerebellopontine angle
cistern

Dentate nucleus

Fourth ventricle/
quadrangular lobule

Greater horizontal
fissure

Globe/lacrimal gland

Pons

Middle temporal gyrus

nV

Flocculus

Middle cerebellar
peduncle

Superior semilunar lobule/
inferior semilunar lobular

Lens

Anterior temporal pole

Basilar artery/
cavernous carotid artery

Pons/superior
semicircular canal

Fourth ventricle

Nodulus/dentate nucleus

Superior semilunar lobule

Inferior semilunar lobule

Retrobulbar fat

Pituitary gland

Middle temporal gyrus

Cerebellopontine
angle cistern

Middle cerebellar peduncle

Uvula

Figure 4.12. Axial fourth ventricle—pituitary section A3.
A, T1-weighted SE (600/25) MR. This section is through the superior part of the fourth ventricle, the pituitary gland, and the midorbit. Carotid artery flow-void phenomenon is seen within the cavernous sinus. Note the high intensity retrobulbar fat. **B,** T2-weighted (SE 2000/90) MR. Note the dentate nucleus T2 iron susceptability effect. Both carotid siphons and cavernous sinus demonstrate flow-void phenomenon. The retrobulbar fat is now only slightly hyperintense. Hypointense lens. Hyperdense orbit aqueous and vitreous humors.

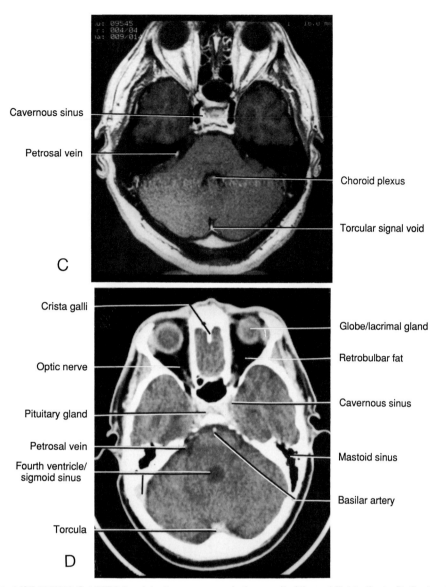

Cavernous sinus

Petrosal vein

Choroid plexus

Torcular signal void

C

Crista galli

Globe/lacrimal gland

Optic nerve

Retrobulbar fat

Pituitary gland

Cavernous sinus

Petrosal vein

Fourth ventricle/
sigmoid sinus

Mastoid sinus

Basilar artery

Torcula

D

Figure 4.12.C, T1-weighted (SE 600/25) Gd-DTPA i.v., injection scan. Note the contrast-enhanced pituitary gland, cavernous sinus, fourth ventricle choroid plexus and petrosal vein. The basilar artery and internal carotid artery signal void and the central torcular signal void is the result of time-of-flight effects. **D,** Contrast (L35/W100) CT. Note contrast within vascular structures and the pituitary gland contrast enhancement. Hypodense retrobulbar fat.

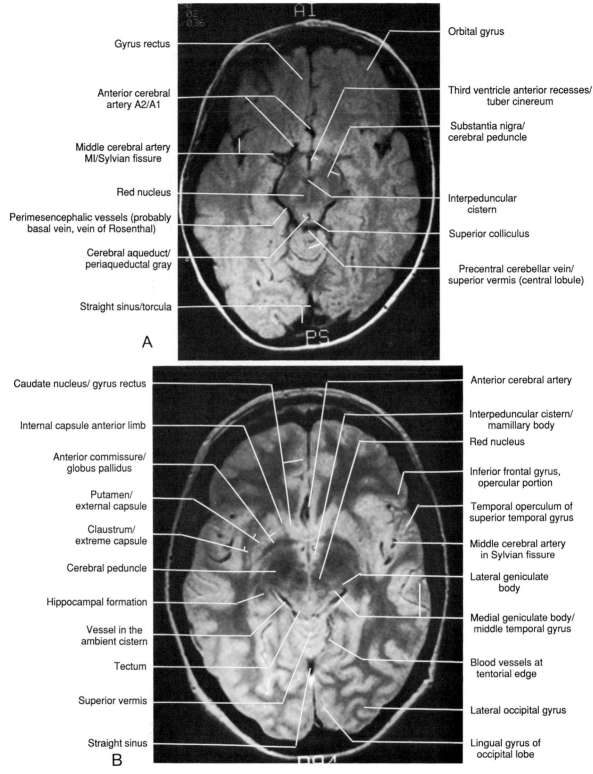

Gyrus rectus

Anterior cerebral
artery A2/A1

Middle cerebral artery
MI/Sylvian fissure

Red nucleus

Perimesencephalic vessels (probably
basal vein, vein of Rosenthal)

Cerebral aqueduct/
periaqueductal gray

Straight sinus/torcula

Orbital gyrus

Third ventricle anterior recesses/
tuber cinereum

Substantia nigra/
cerebral peduncle

Interpeduncular
cistern

Superior colliculus

Precentral cerebellar vein/
superior vermis (central lobule)

A

Caudate nucleus/ gyrus rectus

Internal capsule anterior limb

Anterior commissure/
globus pallidus

Putamen/
external capsule

Claustrum/
extreme capsule

Cerebral peduncle

Hippocampal formation

Vessel in the
ambient cistern

Tectum

Superior vermis

Straight sinus

Anterior cerebral artery

Interpeduncular cistern/
mamillary body

Red nucleus

Inferior frontal gyrus,
opercular portion

Temporal operculum of
superior temporal gyrus

Middle cerebral artery
in Sylvian fissure

Lateral geniculate
body

Medial geniculate body/
middle temporal gyrus

Blood vessels at
tentorial edge

Lateral occipital gyrus

Lingual gyrus of
occipital lobe

B

Figure 4.13. Axial chiasmatic cistern section A4.
A, T1-weighted SE 2000/20 MR scan. The tuber cinereum is seen with the chiasmatic cistern. There are four points of the chiasmatic cistern: posteriorly, the interpeduncular fossa; laterally, the Sylvian fissure; and anteriorly, the interhemispheric fissure. **B,** "Proton density" SE 2800/30 MR scan. Note exceptional gray-white matter contrast with lack of pulsation artifact. The anterior commissure is seen optimally with this technique.

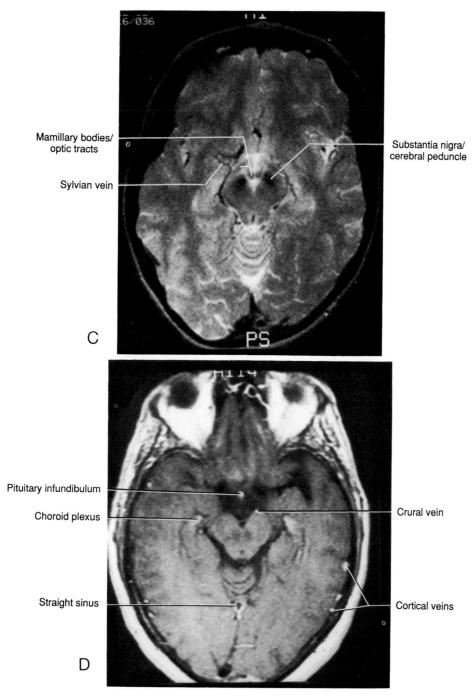

Fiugre 4.13.C, T2-weighted SE (2000/100) MR. Note the hypointensity of the iron-rich substantia nigra. The mamillary bodies and the optic tracts are well seen surrounded by hyperintense chiasmatic cistern CSF. **D,** Gd-DTPA i.v. contrast SE 600/25. There is contrast enhancement of the pituitary infundibulum, choroid plexus, crural vein, and cortical veins. There is partial (central) flow-void within the straight sinus.

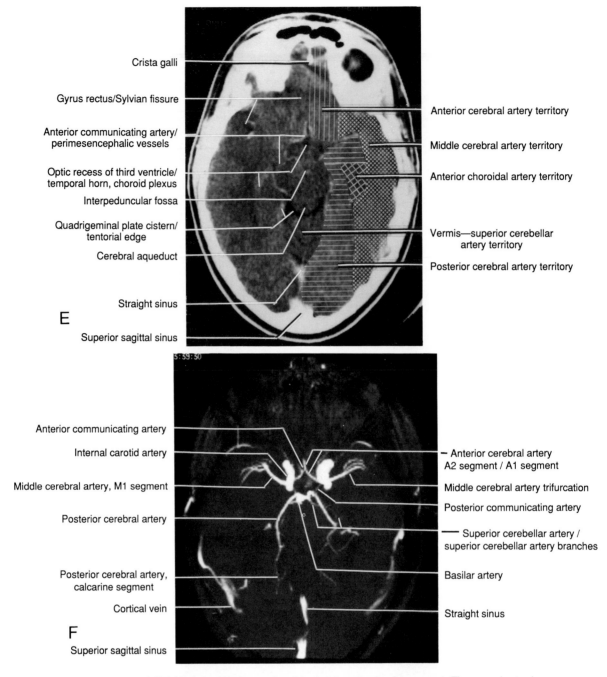

Crista galli

Gyrus rectus/Sylvian fissure

Anterior communicating artery/
perimesencephalic vessels

Optic recess of third ventricle/
temporal horn, choroid plexus

Interpeduncular fossa

Quadrigeminal plate cistern/
tentorial edge

Cerebral aqueduct

Straight sinus

Superior sagittal sinus

Anterior cerebral artery territory

Middle cerebral artery territory

Anterior choroidal artery territory

Vermis—superior cerebellar
artery territory

Posterior cerebral artery territory

E

Anterior communicating artery

Internal carotid artery

Middle cerebral artery, M1 segment

Posterior cerebral artery

Posterior cerebral artery,
calcarine segment

Cortical vein

Superior sagittal sinus

Anterior cerebral artery
A2 segment / A1 segment

Middle cerebral artery trifurcation

Posterior communicating artery

Superior cerebellar artery /
superior cerebellar artery branches

Basilar artery

Straight sinus

F

Figure 4.13.E, Contrast (L35/W100) CT. Note the blood vessel and tentorial contrast enhancement. The vascular territories are labeled on the patient's left side.

Figure 4.13.F,   Circle of Willis MR angiogram. 3-D gradient echo 40/7, 25° flip angle, noncontrast, 32 mm thick slab MRA. Major intracranial arteries and branches are well defined. This 3D volume includes the chiasmatic cistern.

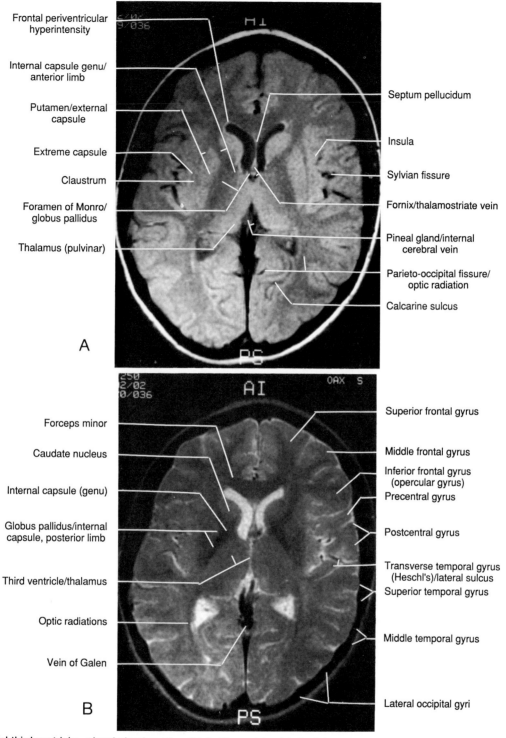

Frontal periventricular hyperintensity

Internal capsule genu/ anterior limb

Putamen/external capsule

Extreme capsule

Claustrum

Foramen of Monro/ globus pallidus

Thalamus (pulvinar)

Septum pellucidum

Insula

Sylvian fissure

Fornix/thalamostriate vein

Pineal gland/internal cerebral vein

Parieto-occipital fissure/ optic radiation

Calcarine sulcus

A

Forceps minor

Caudate nucleus

Internal capsule (genu)

Globus pallidus/internal capsule, posterior limb

Third ventricle/thalamus

Optic radiations

Vein of Galen

B

Superior frontal gyrus

Middle frontal gyrus

Inferior frontal gyrus (opercular gyrus)

Precentral gyrus

Postcentral gyrus

Transverse temporal gyrus (Heschl's)/lateral sulcus

Superior temporal gyrus

Middle temporal gyrus

Lateral occipital gyri

Figure 4.14.   Axial third ventricle—pineal gland section A5. A, T1-weighted (SE 2000/20) MR. The pineal gland hypointensity is probably due to calcification. Gray and white matter structures are clearly identified. Note the punctate high signal intensity just anterior and lateral to both lateral ventricle frontal horns caused by focal diminished myelination and normal regional increased water content.[16] **B,** T2-weighted (SE 2000/100) MR.

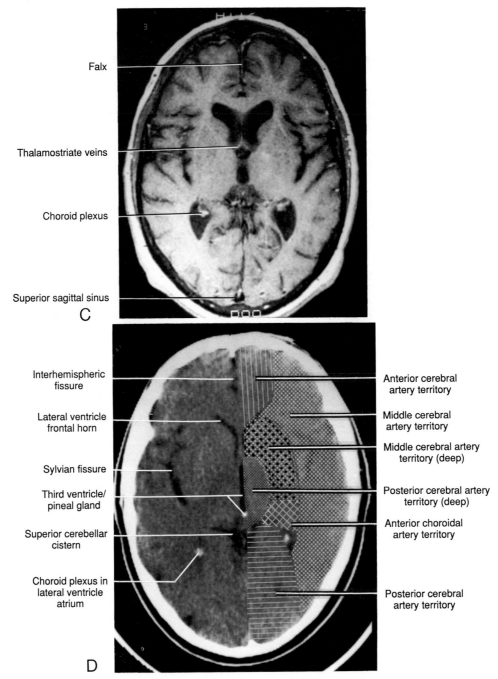

Falx

Thalamostriate veins

Choroid plexus

Superior sagittal sinus

C

Interhemispheric
fissure

Lateral ventricle
frontal horn

Sylvian fissure

Third ventricle/
pineal gland

Superior cerebellar
cistern

Choroid plexus in
lateral ventricle
atrium

Anterior cerebral
artery territory

Middle cerebral
artery territory

Middle cerebral artery
territory (deep)

Posterior cerebral artery
territory (deep)

Anterior choroidal
artery territory

Posterior cerebral
artery territory

D

Figure 4.14.C, Gd-DTPA i.v. contrast SE 600/25 MR scan. Note the contrast-enhanced falx, thalamostriate veins, and lateral ventricle choroid plexus. There is partial signal void of the superior sagittal sinus. **D,** Noncontrast (L35/W100) CT. The pineal gland and choroid plexus are calcified. Vascular territories are mapped on the patient's left side.

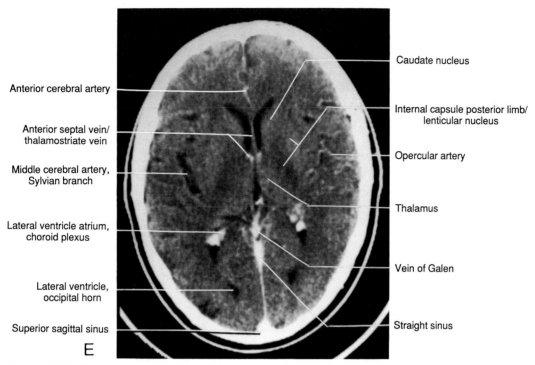

Anterior cerebral artery

Anterior septal vein/
thalamostriate vein

Middle cerebral artery,
Sylvian branch

Lateral ventricle atrium,
choroid plexus

Lateral ventricle,
occipital horn

Superior sagittal sinus

Caudate nucleus

Internal capsule posterior limb/
lenticular nucleus

Opercular artery

Thalamus

Vein of Galen

Straight sinus

E

Figure 4.14.E, Contrast (L35/W100) CT. Note arterial and venous contrast enhancement. The lateral ventricle choroid plexus markedly enhances. Gray-white matter differentiation has improved with i.v. contrast.

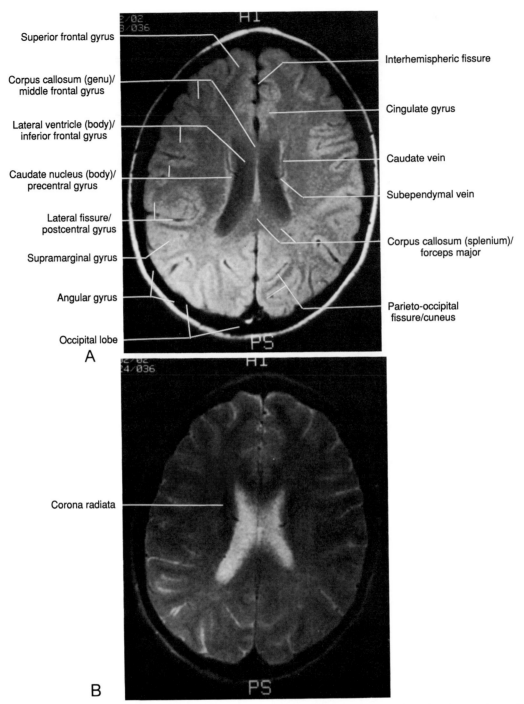

Superior frontal gyrus

Corpus callosum (genu)/
middle frontal gyrus

Lateral ventricle (body)/
inferior frontal gyrus

Caudate nucleus (body)/
precentral gyrus

Lateral fissure/
postcentral gyrus

Supramarginal gyrus

Angular gyrus

Occipital lobe

Interhemispheric fissure

Cingulate gyrus

Caudate vein

Subependymal vein

Corpus callosum (splenium)/
forceps major

Parieto-occipital
fissure/cuneus

A

Corona radiata

B

Figure 4.15. Ventricle body level A6. A, T1-weighted SE (2000/20) MR. The surface anatomy labels match the line diagrams of Figure 4.1 and 4.9. Referencing to these line diagrams will help the reader's understanding of lobar and gyral surface anatomy. Note the caudate body adjacent to the body of the lateral ventricle. **B,** T2-weighted SE (2000/100) MR.

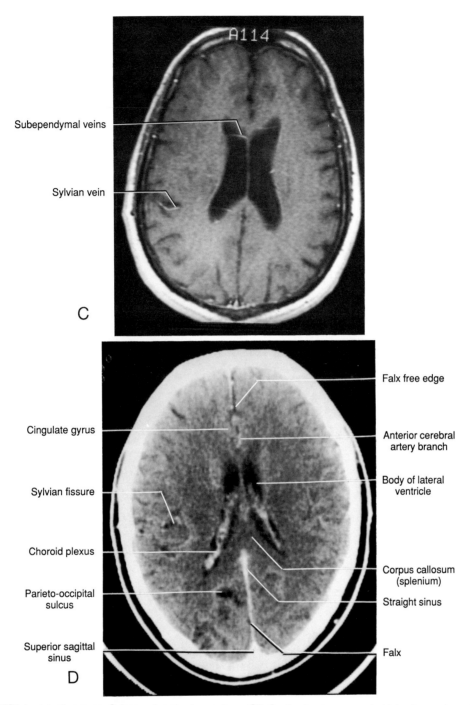

Figure 4.15.C, Gd-DTPA i.v. injection scan. Subependymal veins and a posterior Sylvian vein are well demonstrated. **D,** Contrast (35/100) CT. Contrast enhancement of blood vessels and vascular structures aids structural definition.

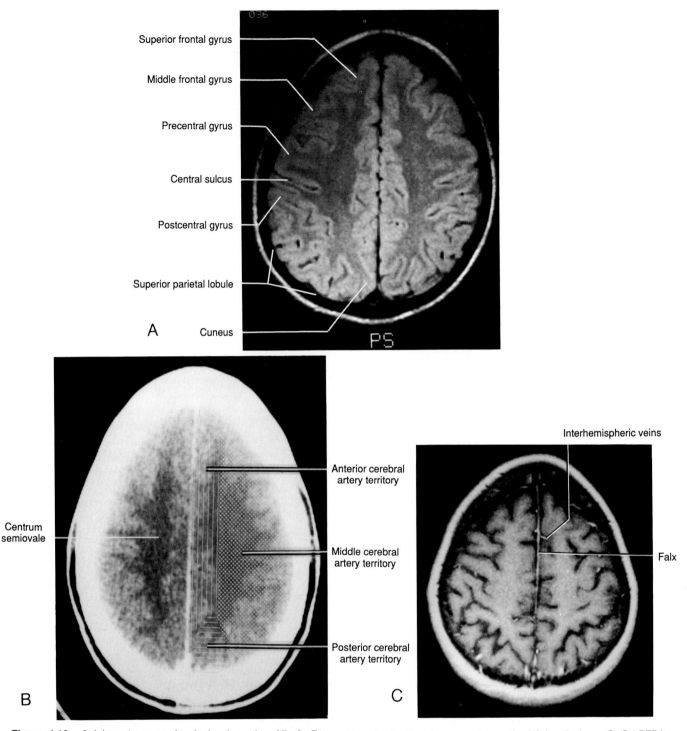

Figure 4.16.   Axial centrum semiovale level section A7. A, T1-weighted (SE 2000/20) MR. Note the lack of exact mirror-image symmetry of the gyral pattern. The gyral labeling represents an accurate estimate and matches Figures 4.1 and 4.9. **B,** Contrast (35/100) CT. Vascular territory is mapped over the left hemisphere. **C,** Gd-DTPA i.v. contrast injection MR scan. The falx and interhemispheric veins cannot be distinguished where they abut. Note that the falx does not contrast enhance as markedly as it does by the CT technique.

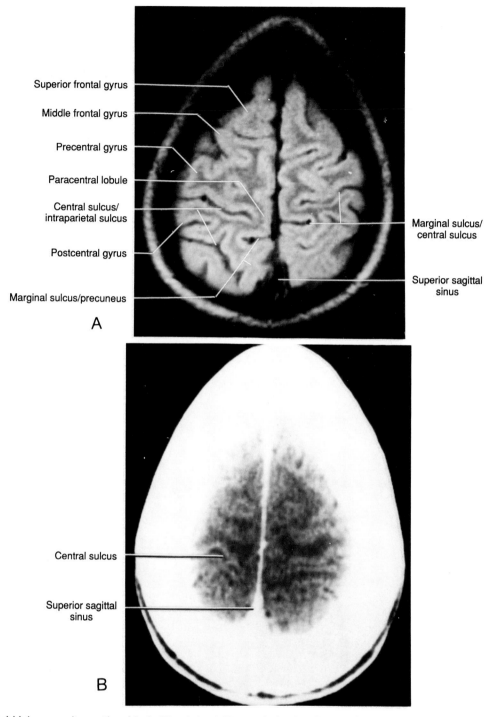

Superior frontal gyrus

Middle frontal gyrus

Precentral gyrus

Paracentral lobule

Central sulcus/
intraparietal sulcus

Postcentral gyrus

Marginal sulcus/precuneus

Marginal sulcus/
central sulcus

Superior sagittal
sinus

A

Central sulcus

Superior sagittal
sinus

B

Figure 4.17.   Axial high convexity section A8. A, T1-weighted SE (2000/20) MR. Labeled gyri should be compared to Figures 4.1 and 4.9. Note the birdwing configuration of the central sulci.[1] The marginal sulcus is posterior by approximately one gyrus width and medial to the central sulcus. **B,** Contrast cranial CT scan (35/100). Part of the central sulcus is identifiable.

FIGURES 4.18 TO 4.24

CORONAL SECTIONS C1–C6

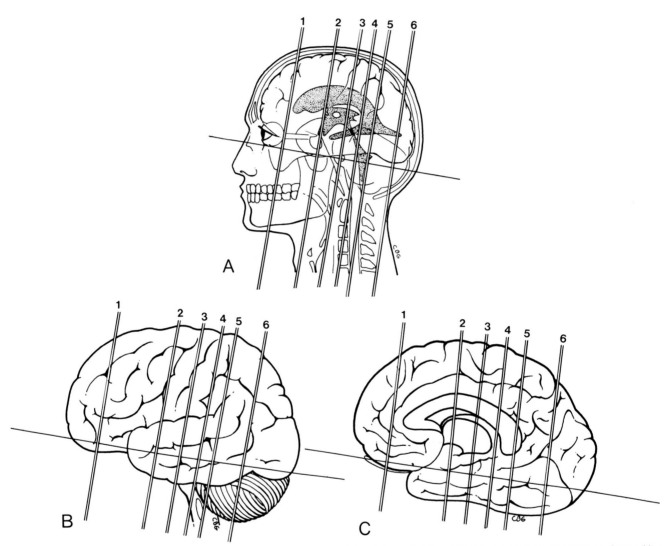

Figure 4.18.   Coronal anatomical section localizers.
    Coronal sections *1* through *6* (C1–C6) are numbered from ante-
rior to posterior *(double black line)* on these three diagrams. The

infraorbitomeatal line *(IOM)* is labeled on all three sections with a
thin black line. The sections are perpendicular to the IOM line.

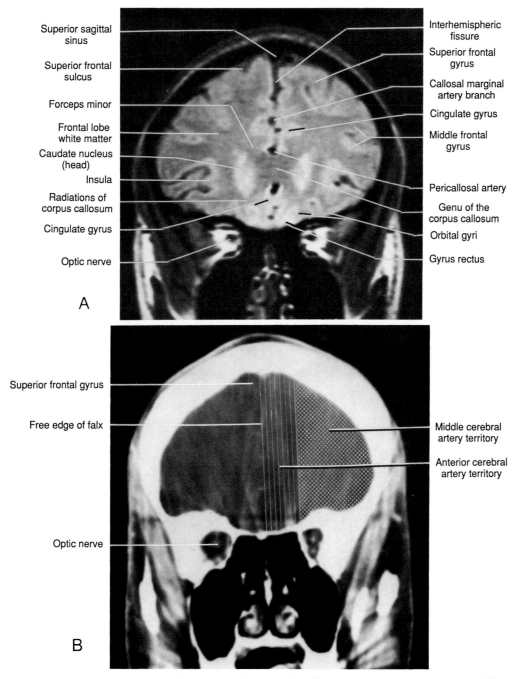

Superior sagittal sinus

Superior frontal sulcus

Forceps minor

Frontal lobe white matter

Caudate nucleus (head)

Insula

Radiations of corpus callosum

Cingulate gyrus

Optic nerve

A

Interhemispheric fissure

Superior frontal gyrus

Callosal marginal artery branch

Cingulate gyrus

Middle frontal gyrus

Pericallosal artery

Genu of the corpus callosum

Orbital gyri

Gyrus rectus

Superior frontal gyrus

Free edge of falx

Optic nerve

Middle cerebral artery territory

Anterior cerebral artery territory

B

Figure 4.19.   Coronal section C1. A, T1-weighted SE 2000/20 MR section. The pericallosal artery and cingulate gyrus are seen closely applied to the genu of the corpus callosum. Compare gyral labeling to Figures 4.1 and 4.18. **B,** Direct coronal i.v. contrast 35/100 CT section. The falx does not reach as deeply at this level as it does on section C4, which explains the arteriographic "round" vs. "square" anterior cerebral artery shift with mass lesions. Note the relatively narrow band of the anterior cerebral artery vascular supply.

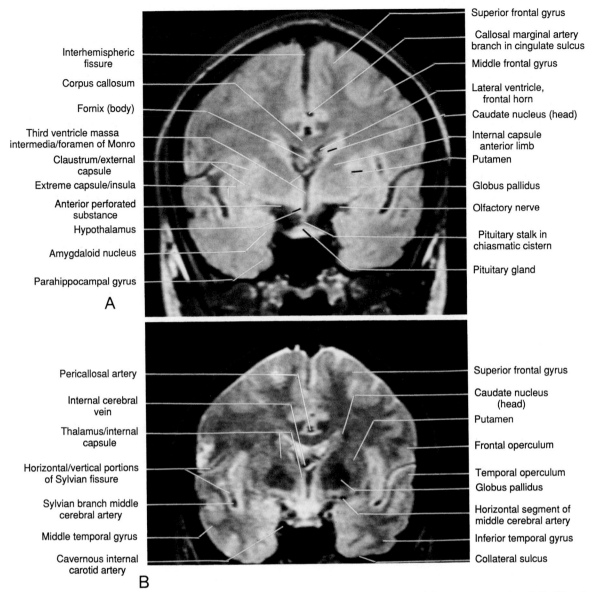

Interhemispheric fissure

Corpus callosum

Fornix (body)

Third ventricle massa intermedia/foramen of Monro

Claustrum/external capsule

Extreme capsule/insula

Anterior perforated substance

Hypothalamus

Amygdaloid nucleus

Parahippocampal gyrus

A

Superior frontal gyrus

Callosal marginal artery branch in cingulate sulcus

Middle frontal gyrus

Lateral ventricle, frontal horn

Caudate nucleus (head)

Internal capsule anterior limb

Putamen

Globus pallidus

Olfactory nerve

Pituitary stalk in chiasmatic cistern

Pituitary gland

Pericallosal artery

Internal cerebral vein

Thalamus/internal capsule

Horizontal/vertical portions of Sylvian fissure

Sylvian branch middle cerebral artery

Middle temporal gyrus

Cavernous internal carotid artery

B

Superior frontal gyrus

Caudate nucleus (head)

Putamen

Frontal operculum

Temporal operculum

Globus pallidus

Horizontal segment of middle cerebral artery

Inferior temporal gyrus

Collateral sulcus

Figure 4.20. Coronal pituitary level section C2. A, T1-weighted (SE 2000/20) MR. Deep structures are well differentiated. The hypophyseal stalk, pituitary gland, and cavernous sinus detail are poor in 10-mm section thickness. (See Chapter 12 for detailed anatomy of the pituitary gland and the cavernous sinus.) **B,** T2-weighted (SE 2000/80) MR image. Note the hypointensity of the iron-rich globus pallidus due to T2 susceptibility effects.

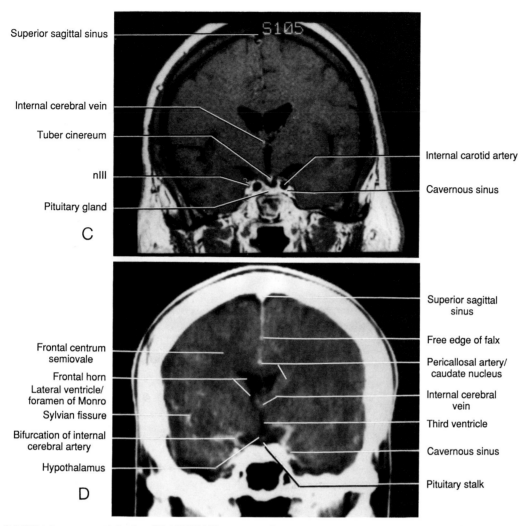

Superior sagittal sinus

Internal cerebral vein

Tuber cinereum

nIII

Pituitary gland

C

Internal carotid artery

Cavernous sinus

Frontal centrum semiovale

Frontal horn
Lateral ventricle/ foramen of Monro

Sylvian fissure

Bifurcation of internal cerebral artery

Hypothalamus

D

Superior sagittal sinus

Free edge of falx

Pericallosal artery/ caudate nucleus

Internal cerebral vein

Third ventricle

Cavernous sinus

Pituitary stalk

Figure 4.20.C, Gd-DTPA i.v. contrast injection SE 600/25 MR scan. Structures lacking a BBB, the pituitary gland and the tuber cinereum, are homogeneously contrast enhanced. There is cavernous sinus contrast enhancement. The *internal carotid* artery flow-void and the occulomotor nerve (n III) cavernous sinus filling defects are well seen. The internal cerebral vein is identified. The superior sagittal sinus demonstrates flow-void on this section. **D,** Contrast (35/100) CT. Note the contrast-enhanced internal carotid, middle, and anterior cerebral arteries.

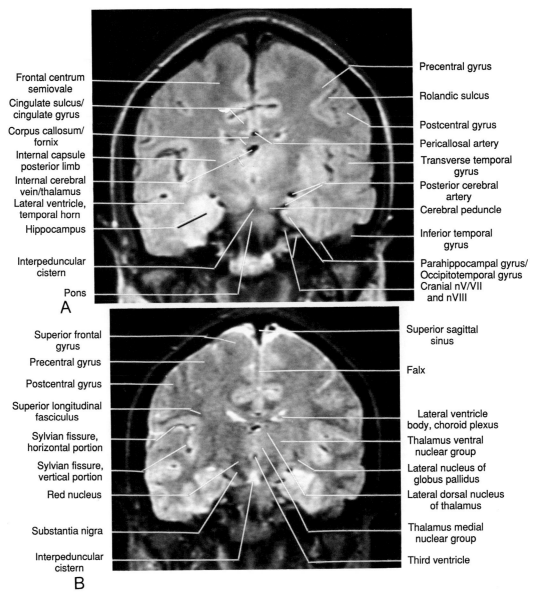

Frontal centrum
semiovale

Cingulate sulcus/
cingulate gyrus

Corpus callosum/
fornix

Internal capsule
posterior limb

Internal cerebral
vein/thalamus

Lateral ventricle,
temporal horn

Hippocampus

Interpeduncular
cistern

Pons

A

Precentral gyrus

Rolandic sulcus

Postcentral gyrus

Pericallosal artery

Transverse temporal
gyrus

Posterior cerebral
artery

Cerebral peduncle

Inferior temporal
gyrus

Parahippocampal gyrus/
Occipitotemporal gyrus

Cranial nV/VII
and nVIII

Superior frontal
gyrus

Precentral gyrus

Postcentral gyrus

Superior longitudinal
fasciculus

Sylvian fissure,
horizontal portion

Sylvian fissure,
vertical portion

Red nucleus

Substantia nigra

Interpeduncular
cistern

B

Superior sagittal
sinus

Falx

Lateral ventricle
body, choroid plexus

Thalamus ventral
nuclear group

Lateral nucleus of
globus pallidus

Lateral dorsal nucleus
of thalamus

Thalamus medial
nuclear group

Third ventricle

Figure 4.21.   Coronal thalamic level C3. A, T1-weighted (SE 2000/ 20) MR. Note the vertical relationship of the fornix, corpus callosum, and cingulate gyrus. The peduncles and pons are both included in this section (refer to Figures 4.18 and 4.5). **B,** T2-weighted (SE 2000/ 80) MR. The substantia nigra and red nucleus are particularly well demonstrated here due to T2 iron susceptibility effects.

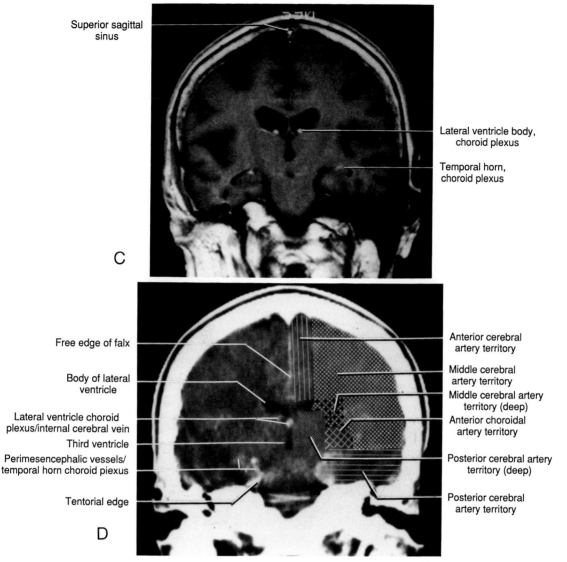

Superior sagittal
sinus

Lateral ventricle body,
choroid plexus

Temporal horn,
choroid plexus

C

Free edge of falx

Body of lateral
ventricle

Lateral ventricle choroid
plexus/internal cerebral vein

Third ventricle

Perimesencephalic vessels/
temporal horn choroid piexus

Tentorial edge

D

Anterior cerebral
artery territory

Middle cerebral
artery territory

Middle cerebral artery
territory (deep)

Anterior choroidal
artery territory

Posterior cerebral artery
territory (deep)

Posterior cerebral
artery territory

Figure 4.21.C, Gd-DTPA i.v. contrast injection SE 600/25 MR scan. The lateral ventricle body and temporal horn choroid plexus are contrast enhanced. The superior sagittal sinus is contrast enhanced on this section. **D,** Contrast (35/100) CT. Note contrast enhancement of the lateral ventricle choroid plexus including that of the temporal horn. The falx free edge reaches the cingulate gyrus. Vascular territory is superimposed over the left hemisphere.

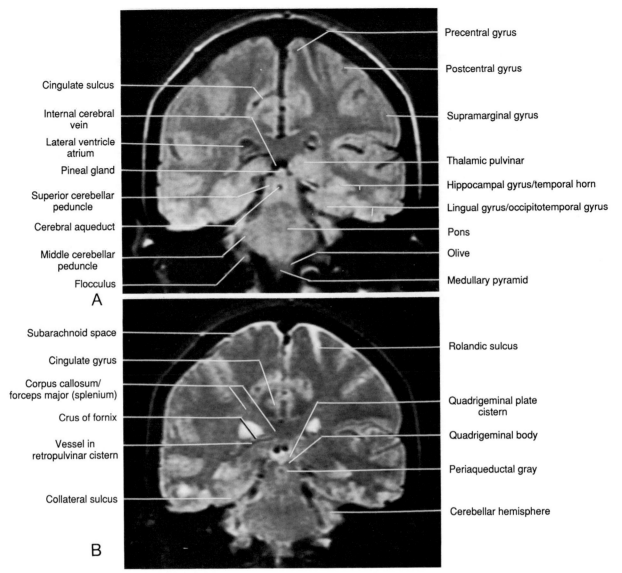

Precentral gyrus

Postcentral gyrus

Supramarginal gyrus

Thalamic pulvinar

Hippocampal gyrus/temporal horn

Lingual gyrus/occipitotemporal gyrus

Pons

Olive

Medullary pyramid

Cingulate sulcus

Internal cerebral vein

Lateral ventricle atrium

Pineal gland

Superior cerebellar peduncle

Cerebral aqueduct

Middle cerebellar peduncle

Flocculus

A

Subarachnoid space

Cingulate gyrus

Corpus callosum/ forceps major (splenium)

Crus of fornix

Vessel in retropulvinar cistern

Collateral sulcus

B

Rolandic sulcus

Quadrigeminal plate cistern

Quadrigeminal body

Periaqueductal gray

Cerebellar hemisphere

Figure 4.22.   Coronal pineal level C4. A, T1-weighted (SE 2000/20) MR. The midbrain and brainstem are well seen without the streak artifact present on the CT image. The pineal gland is superior to the tectum lying between the quadrigeminal bodies. The splenium of the corpus callosum is seen at this level. **B,** T2-weighted (SE 2000/80) MR. Note the periaqueductal gray matter. The crus of the fornix is seen at this level.

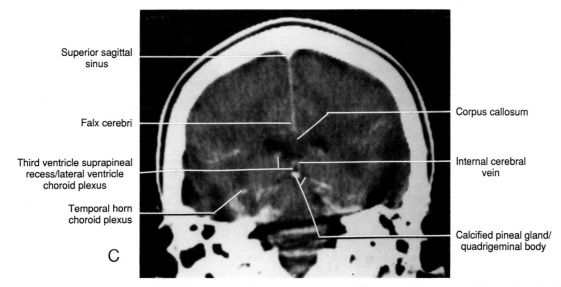

Figure 4.22.C, Contrast (35/100) CT. The contrast-enhanced tentorium and falx are well demonstrated. Note the "deep" free edge of the falx.

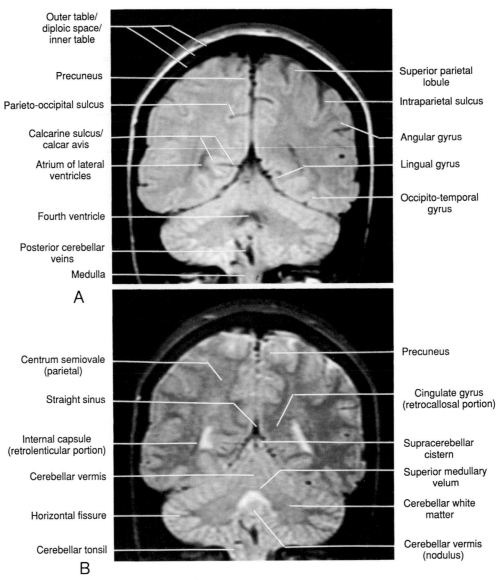

Outer table/
diploic space/
inner table

Precuneus

Parieto-occipital sulcus

Calcarine sulcus/
calcar avis

Atrium of lateral
ventricles

Fourth ventricle

Posterior cerebellar
veins

Medulla

Superior parietal
lobule

Intraparietal sulcus

Angular gyrus

Lingual gyrus

Occipito-temporal
gyrus

A

Centrum semiovale
(parietal)

Straight sinus

Internal capsule
(retrolenticular portion)

Cerebellar vermis

Horizontal fissure

Cerebellar tonsil

Precuneus

Cingulate gyrus
(retrocallosal portion)

Supracerebellar
cistern

Superior medullary
velum

Cerebellar white
matter

Cerebellar vermis
(nodulus)

B

Figure 4.23. Coronal fourth ventricle level C5. A, T1-weighted (SE 2000/20) MR. This section is posterior to the corpus callosum. The intraparietal sulcus separates the superior parietal lobule from the angular gyrus. The right hemisphere "calcar avis" is an indentation of the medial wall of the lateral ventricle caused by the prominent calcarines. The vermis nodulus produces a characteristic imprint upon the fourth ventricle. **B,** T2-weighted (SE 2000/80) MR. The gray-white matter detail is now more prominent.

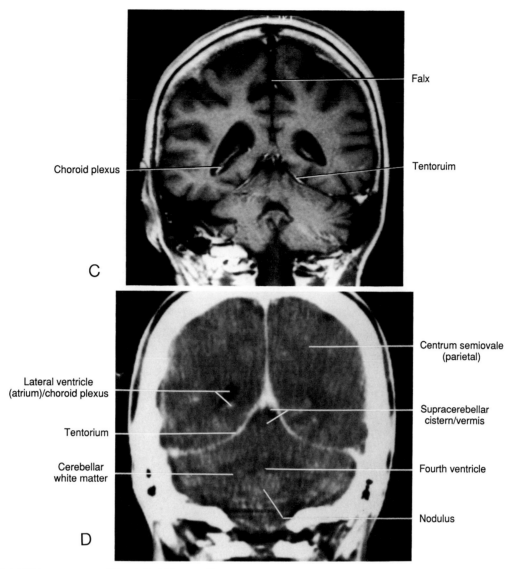

Falx

Tentoruim

Choroid plexus

C

Centrum semiovale
(parietal)

Lateral ventricle
(atrium)/choroid plexus

Supracerebellar
cistern/vermis

Tentorium

Cerebellar
white matter

Fourth ventricle

Nodulus

D

Figure 4.23.C, Gd-DTPA i.v. contrast SE 600/25 MR scan. The lateral ventricle atrium choroid plexus and the tentorium are contrast enhanced. The falx is not contrast enhanced presumably due to relatively rapid flow. **D,** Contrast (35/100) CT. The falx joins the tentorium cerebelli at this level enclosing the straight sinus. The relatively dense nodulus of the cerebellar vermis contrasts with the cerebellar hemisphere white matter creating a commonly misdiagnosed pseudotumor.

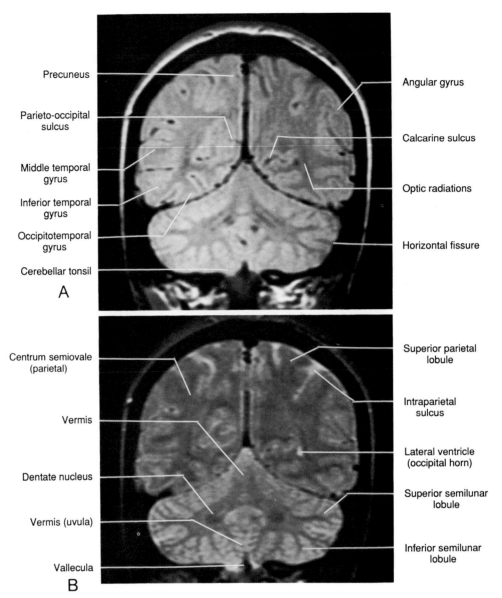

Precuneus

Parieto-occipital sulcus

Middle temporal gyrus

Inferior temporal gyrus

Occipitotemporal gyrus

Cerebellar tonsil

A

Angular gyrus

Calcarine sulcus

Optic radiations

Horizontal fissure

Centrum semiovale (parietal)

Vermis

Dentate nucleus

Vermis (uvula)

Vallecula

B

Superior parietal lobule

Intraparietal sulcus

Lateral ventricle (occipital horn)

Superior semilunar lobule

Inferior semilunar lobule

Figure 4.24.   Coronal dentate nucleus level C6. A, T1-weighted (SE 2000/20) MR. This section is posterior to the splenium. The cerebellar horizontal fissure divides the superior and inferior cerebellar semilunar lobules. The calcarine sulcus is approaching the occipital horn. **B,** T2-weighted (SE 2000/80) MR. The dentate nucleus is lateral and partially posterior to the fourth ventricle (Fig. 4.12). It is well visualized due, in large part, to iron-induced field inhomogeneities. Note the superior parietal lobule (lateral) and the precuneus (medial).

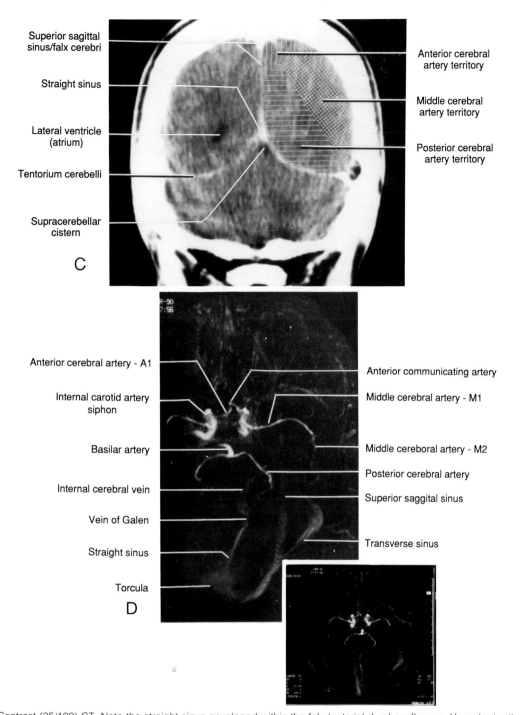

Superior sagittal
sinus/falx cerebri

Straight sinus

Lateral ventricle
(atrium)

Tentorium cerebelli

Supracerebellar
cistern

C

Anterior cerebral
artery territory

Middle cerebral
artery territory

Posterior cerebral
artery territory

Anterior cerebral artery - A1

Internal carotid artery
siphon

Basilar artery

Internal cerebral vein

Vein of Galen

Straight sinus

Torcula

D

Anterior communicating artery

Middle cerebral artery - M1

Middle cereboral artery - M2

Posterior cerebral artery

Superior saggital sinus

Transverse sinus

Figure 4.24.C, Contrast (35/100) CT. Note the straight sinus enveloped within the falx-tentorial dural confluence. Vascular territory is mapped over the left hemisphere.

Figure 4.24D.   Normal vascular anatomy. 3D FLASH axial slice-select 40/7, 25° iv contrast 128mm slab MR angiogram *(inset)* and oblique (head tilt) reformation *(above).* Arteries appear white and veins appear gray against the dark stationary background. The circle of Willis primary and secondary arterial divisions are well demonstrated. The deep veins and dural venous sinuses are also well demonstrated. This is a thick 3D volume which was done for anatomic purposes. Thinner slabs give increased detail with this present system.

Neonatal Brain

The neonatal and pediatric brain on both CT and MR are different in appearance from the adult brain due principally to an increased water content, incomplete myelination, and paucity of iron content. Due to the increased brain water content, the neonatal brain has lower CT attenuation values. The increased water content and incomplete myelinization is responsible for, or at least contributes to, the neonatal diminished CT gray-white distinction (Fig. 4.26D). As the infant matures, brain attenuation values increase and gray and white matter become more distinct.[14]

MR maturation changes of the neonatal brain are more vivid than those of CT. They are due to the decrease of brain water content and to increasing myelination.[2] In addition on T2-weighted images, the lack of brain iron at birth contributes to the T2 basal ganglia, substantia nigra, red nucleus, and dentate nucleus relative hyperintensity compared to the adult.[3] The iron susceptibility effects have already been explained in Chapters 1 and 3 and are particularly evident at high-field strength and with gradient recalled echo (T2*) imaging.

MR neonatal maturation distinctions are best identified on T1-weighted images due to T1 fat (myelin) sensitivity (Figs. 4.25 and 4.26). After 6 months, T2 imaging begins to best identify infantile brain characteristics due to T2 water sensitivity (Fig. 4.27).[2] Myelinated structures have a T1 hyperintensity and T2 relative hypointensity. Brain maturation begins in the brainstem and progresses to the cerebellum and then the cerebrum.

The premature neonate brain demonstrates diminished cortical infolding and immature myelination.

Fetal myelination progresses cephalad from the brainstem at 29 weeks' gestation reaching to the centrum semiovale by 42 weeks' gestation. The corona radiata demonstrates evidence of myelination at 37 weeks' gestation. Whereas cortical infolding approximates that of the adult at full term, myelination appears complete at 18 months after a full-term birth. The normal premature brain must be

Table 4.1. Summary of the MR (1.5 T) Milestones of Normal Brain Myelinization for Neonates of Term Pregnancies[2]

Brain Region	Age (in months) Myelination Detected	
	T1-weighted	T2-weighted
Cerebellar white matter	3	
Corpus callosum		
Splenium	4	6
Genu	6	8
Internal capsule		
Posterior limb	0	
Anterior limb		11
Frontal white matter		14
Adult pattern		18

carefully scrutinized in order to recognize the stage of immature cortical infolding as well as the stage of myelination (Fig. 4.25).[14]

The full-term neonate demonstrates myelination of the middle cerebellar peduncles, cerebellar white matter, and the posterior limb of the internal capsule. At 1 month, optic pathways and paracentral gyri demonstrate myelination. The corpus callosum demonstrates myelination at 7 months, the anterior limb of the internal capsule at 11 months, and the frontal white matter at 18 months. The normal infant brain has an adult pattern at 18 months.[2] A triangular peritrigonal (posterior periatrial) region matures very slowly and produces a round water signal that may persist through young adulthood and should not be misinterpreted as a plaque or infarct (Fig. 4.28).[2,15]

Iron susceptibility effects have been discussed in Chapters 1 and 3. These effects result in T2 hypointensity particularly at high-field magnet strengths and with gradient recalled echo GRE technique. There is no detectable brain iron at birth. At 6 months, iron is detected by laboratory staining methods in the globus pallidus. At 1 year, the substantia nigra, at 2 years, the red nucleus, and at seven years, the dentate nucleus develop iron-staining characteristics. These staining characteristics can be correlated with T2 MR iron susceptability effects.[3]

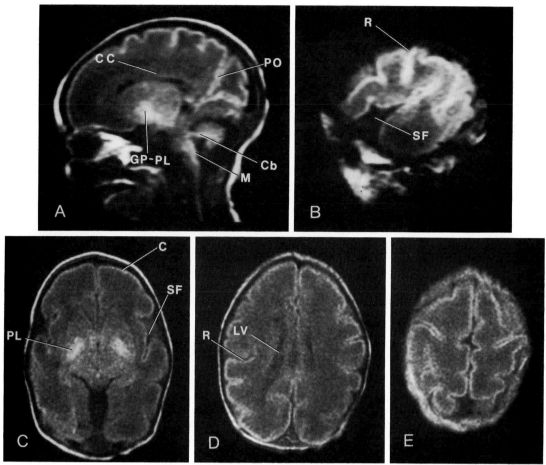

Figure 4.25.   32-week gestation premature infant is shown 6 days postnatally. Sagittal atrial-level **(A)** and lateral convexity-level **(B)** SE 600/25 MR scans. Axial third ventricle-level **(C)**, lateral ventricle body level **(D)**, and centrum semiovale-level **(E)** SE 600/25 MR scans.

The most striking findings on this normal exam are the smooth convexity due to immature shallow and sparse cortical infolding and immature myelination. The Sylvian fossa *(SF)* and major sulci such as the Rolandic *(R)* and the parieto-occipital *(PO)* are identified. The cortical gray matter *(C)* presents as a thin perimeter of hyperintensity enclosing the T1 hypointense white matter. The dorsal medulla *(M)* and pons, the cerebellum *(Cb)*, and the globus pallidus and internal capsule posterior limb *(GP-PL)* show T1 hyperintense myelin.

Figure 4.26. The neonatal brain (2-month-old infant). A, Parasagittal SE T1-weighted 600/25 MR in a 2-month-old. The hyperintense frontal cortical gray matter *(GM-F)* and hypointense white matter *(WM-F)* are the reverse of the adult (compare to Fig. 4.6). The paracentral *(WM-PC)* and the occipital white matter *(WM-O)* demonstrate myelination. Note that the cerebellum is hyperintense compared to frontal white matter. **B,** Axial frontal horn-ganglionic supraorbitomeatal section SE 2000/20. The posterior limb of the internal capsule *(IC-PL)* is faintly detectable. Gray-white matter differentiation is poor. **C,** Same axial frontal horn-ganglionic superorbitomeatal section SE T2-weighted 2000/80 MR. Note the posterior limb internal capsule hypointensity due to myelination *(IC-PL)*. There is lack of identification of the internal capsule anterior limb and lack of globus pallidus *(GP)* iron susceptibility effects. **D,** Noncontrast CT 100/ 35, same case. Frontal *(WM-F)* and temporal *(WM-T)* white matter hypointensity. Relative cerebellar hyperintensity *(Cb)*. Definition of the posterior limb of the internal capsule *(IC-PL)*.

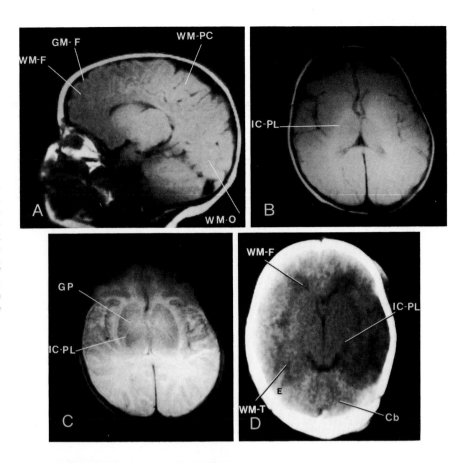

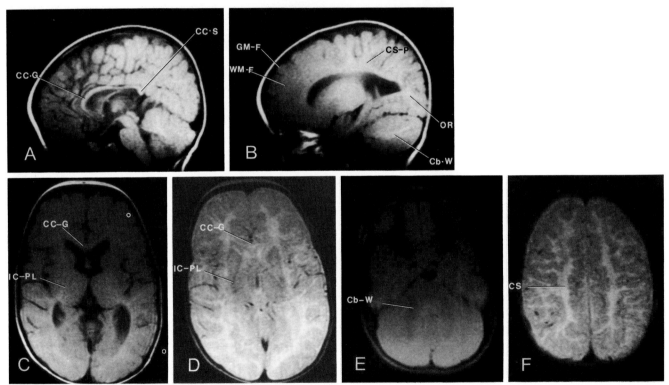

Figure 4.27. Neonatal brain of a seven-month-old infant. Midsagittal **(A)** and atrial level sagittal **(B)** SE 600/25 MR images. Same level, axial third ventricle-level SE 2000/20 **(C)** and 2000/80 **(D)** MR scans. Axial fourth ventricle-level **(E)** and centrum semiovale **(F)** SE 2000/80 MR scans. The lateral ventricles are the upper limit of normal size.

Those structures showing evidence for both T1 and T2 myelinization include the genu of the corpus callosum *(CC-G)*, the posterior limb of the internal capsule *(IC-PL)* and the cerebellar white matter *(Cb-W)*. Those structures showing only T1 evidence for myelinization include the optic radiations *(OR)* and the parietal centrum semiovale *(CS-P)*. Those regions failing to show T1 or T2 evidence for myelinization include the frontal lobe white matter (F-WM) and the anterior limb of the internal capsule. (The splenium of the corpus callosum showed T2 evidence for myelinization on a section not included here.)

Normal Observations and Variants

Foci of hyperintense T2 periventricular signals occur in most patients anterior to the frontal horns[16] and in normal patients through adolescence in the peritrigonal region.[2] The cause of the prefrontal horn T2 hyperintensity is believed to be a combination of low myelin content, gliosis, and increased interstitial fluid.[16] Contributing to the peritrigonal increased T2 signal is delayed myelination (Fig. 4.28).[2]

Normal variants include cyst-like and calcified structures. Among these are cavum septum pellucidum and vergae (Fig. 4.29), cavum velum interpositum (Fig. 4.30), large cisterna magna (Fig. 4.31), cystic pineal gland (Fig. 4.32), and empty sella turcica. Calcified variants include globus pallidus (Fig. 4.33), the choroid plexus (Fig. 4.34) and the habenular commissure (Fig. 4.35).

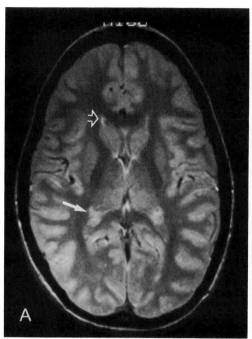
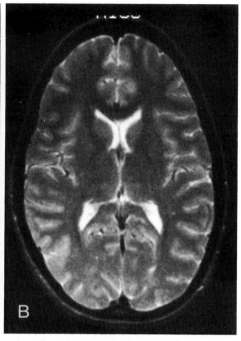

Figure 4.28. Periventricular increased water signal in the normal adolescent.

Axial third ventricle-level SE 2800/30 **(A)** and SE 2800/80 **(B)** MR scans. Note the proton density and T2 hyperintense signals of the deep frontal periventricular region *(open arrow)* and the peritrigonal region *(closed arrow)*. These signals are best seen on the proton-weighted image and tend to be obscured on the T2-weighted image due to the adjacent isointense ventricular CSF.

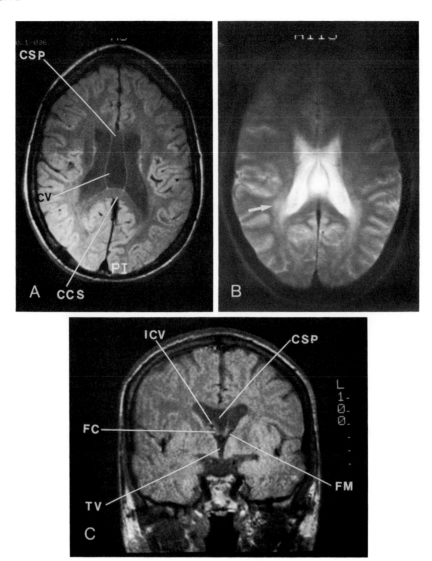

Figure 4.29.   Cavum septum pellucidum and vergae.

The cavum septum pellucidum is a cyst-like collection within the membranes of the septum pellucidum that usually communicates with the lateral ventricle. Its posterior extension (the cavum vergae) abuts the splenium of the corpus callosum and it is located above the fornix. It occurs in more than half of infants born prematurely and in approximately half of the full-term neonates. At 1 month of age, they are often no longer detectable by neurosonography. It is smooth walled, wider posteriorly than anteriorly, and almost always contains CSF-isodense and isointense fluid.

Axial lateral ventricle body level SE 2000/20 **(A)** and 2000/80 **(B)** MR scans. Coronal foramen of Monro level **(C)** and midsagittal

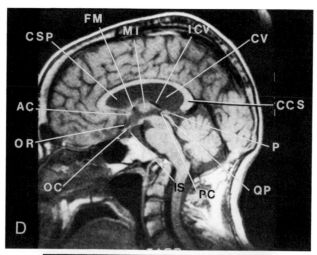

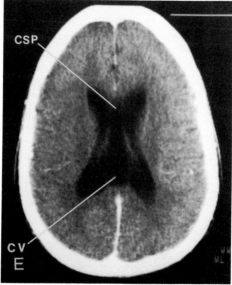

Figure 4.29.(D) SE 600/25 MR scans. Lateral ventricle body-level 37/75 CT scan **(E).**

The cavum septum pellucidum *(CSP)* separates the foramina of Monro *(FM)*, internal cerebral veins *(ICV)*, and columns of the fornix *(FC)*. The fornix lies above the third ventricle *(TV)*. The cavum vergae *(CV)* portion is the widest. It abuts the splenium of the corpus callosum *(CCS)*.

The anterior and posterior recesses of the third ventricle are particularly well seen on the sagittal MR. The optic chiasm *(OC)* is behind the optic recess *(OR)*. The infundibular stalk *(IS)* is emerging below the infundibular recess. The posterior commissure *(PC)* is between the pineal gland *(P)* and the quadrigeminal plate *(QP)*. *MI* = massa intermedia, *AC* = anterior commissure.

Figure 4.30. Cavum velum interpositum.

The cavum velum interpositum is not a true cyst. It communicates with the quadrigeminal plate cistern and is actually a potential subarachnoid space. It is common in infants and uncommon in adults.

Direct coronal **(A)** and axial **(B)** i.v. contrast CT scans. Third ventricle-level **(C)** and midsagittal **(D)** 600/25 MR scans.

It is easy to distinguish from the other cavi. The cavum velum interpositum *(CVI)* displaces the body of the fornix *(FB)* upward, is posterior, and does not involve the septum pellucidum. The lateral ventricular *(LV)* displacement spares the frontal horns. Third ventricle *(TV)*, internal cerebral vein *(ICV)*, corpus callosum *(CC)*.

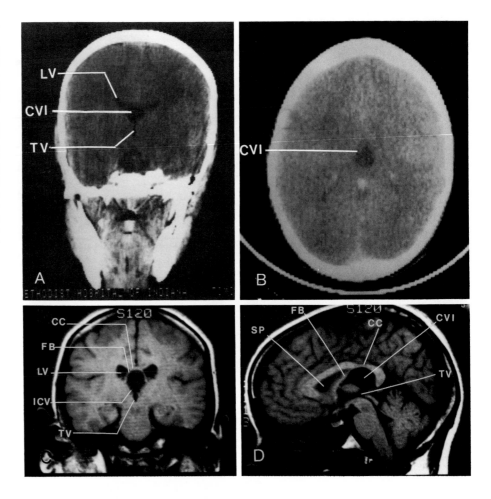

Figure 4.31.

The large cisterna magna can be distinguished from a cyst or cystic tumor by its cisternal shape, symmetry, water signal, lack of structural displacement, or contrast enhancement. Vertical septations (coronal reformation) are characteristic. Positive contrast CT cisternography fills the large cisterna magna.

Large cisterna magna. Contrast CT scans 100/35. *Clockwise:* sagittal and coronal reformations and axial section. Large cisterna magna *(large arrow)*. The fourth ventricle *(small arrow)* is not displaced.

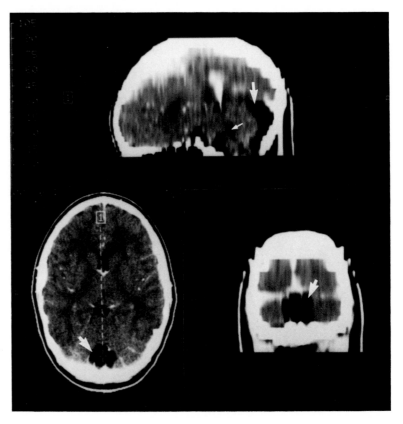

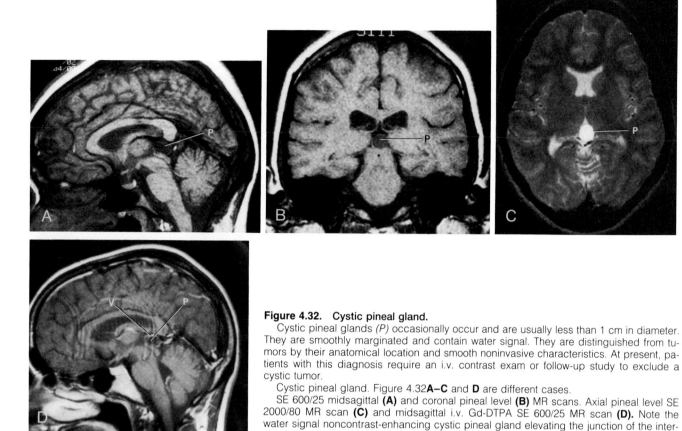

Figure 4.32. Cystic pineal gland.

Cystic pineal glands *(P)* occasionally occur and are usually less than 1 cm in diameter. They are smoothly marginated and contain water signal. They are distinguished from tumors by their anatomical location and smooth noninvasive characteristics. At present, patients with this diagnosis require an i.v. contrast exam or follow-up study to exclude a cystic tumor.

Cystic pineal gland. Figure 4.32**A–C** and **D** are different cases.

SE 600/25 midsagittal **(A)** and coronal pineal level **(B)** MR scans. Axial pineal level SE 2000/80 MR scan **(C)** and midsagittal i.v. Gd-DTPA SE 600/25 MR scan **(D).** Note the water signal noncontrast-enhancing cystic pineal gland elevating the junction of the internal cerebral veins and the vein of Galen *(V)*.

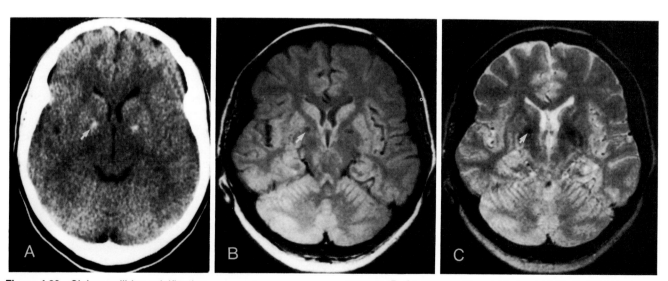

Figure 4.33 Globus pallidus calcification.

Globus calcification is commonly found by the CT technique in normal adults. It can be particularly prominent in hypoparathyroidism and pseudohypoparathyroidism.[1] **A,** 35/100 axial CT without i.v. contrast. **B,** SE 2000/20 T1-weighted axial MR. **C,** SE 2000/80 T2-weighted axial MR. Note that the globus pallidus calcification is obvious by noncontrast CT *(arrow)* is inferred by T1-weighted MR, and is obscured by iron susceptibility effects on the T2 image.

Figure 4.34. Extensive choroid plexus calcification.
Lateral ventricle choroid plexus calcification is almost always seen in adults by the CT technique. Fourth ventricle choroid plexus calcification is uncommon. **A,** Axial 200/35 noncontrast CT scan. Fourth ventricle lateral recess and foramen of Luschka calcification *(arrow).* **B,** 2000/20 SE axial MR scan. Marked hypointensity of the large calcified lateral ventricle choroid plexus glomera *(CP).*

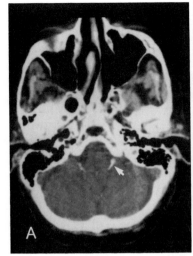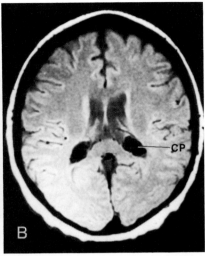

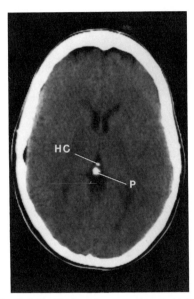

Figure 4.35.   Calcified habenular commissure. Habenular commissure calcification is a frequent normal finding.
Axial pineal level 37/100 CT scan. The calcified habenular commissure *(HC)* is anterior to the calcified pineal gland *(P).* Note lack of lateral ventricle atrial choroid plexus calcification.

References

1. Masdeu JC, Grossman CB. Brain anatomy. In: Gonzalez CF, Grossman CB, Masdeu JC (Eds). *Head and Spine Imaging.* New York: John Wiley & Sons, 1985; 133–222.
2. Barkovich AJ, Kjos BO, Jackson DE, Norman D. Normal matu-
ration of the neonatal and infant brain: MR imaging at 1.5 T. *Radiology* 1988; 166:173–180.
3. Drayer B, Burger P, Darwin R, et al. Magnetic resonance imaging of brain iron. *AJNR* 1986; 7:373–380.
4. Naidich TP, Daniels DL, Haughton VM, et al. Hippocampal formation and related structures of the limbic lobe: Anatomic-MR correlation. Part I. Surface features and coronal sections. *Radiology* 1987; 162:747–754.
5. Naidich TP, Daniels DL, Haughton VM, et al. Hippocampal formation and related structures of the limbic lobe: Anatomic-MR correlation. Part II. Sagital sections. *Radiology* 1987; 162:755–761.
6. Flannigan BD, Bradley WG Jr, Mazziotta JC, et al. Magnetic resonance imaging of the brainstem: Normal structure and basic functional anatomy. *Radiology* 1985; 154:375–383.
7. Carpenter MB. *Core Text of Neuroanatomy,* 5rd Ed. Baltimore: Williams & Wilkins, 1984.
8. Daniels DL, Haughton VM, Naidich TP (Eds). *Cranial and Spinal Magnetic Resonance Imaging: An Atlas and Guide.* New York: Raven Press, 1987.
9. Kilgore DP, Breeger RK, Daniels DL, et al. Cranial tissues: Normal appearance after intravenous injection of gadolinium-DTPA. *Radiology* 1986; 160:757–761.
10. Savoirdo M, Bracchi M, Passerini A, Visciniani A. The vascular territories in the cerebellum and brainstem: CT and MR study. *AJNR* 1987; 8:199–209.
11. Berman SA, Hayman LA, Hinck VC. Correlation of CT cerebral vascular territories with function: I. Anterior cerebral artery. *AJNR* 1980; 1:259–263.
12. Berman SA, Hayman LA, Hinck VC. Correlation of CT cerebral vascular territories with function. III. Middle cerebral artery. *AJR* 1984; 142:1035–1040.
13. Hayman LA, Berman SA, Hinck VC. Correlation of CT cerebral vascular territories with function. II. Posterior cerebral artery. *AJR* 1981; 137:13–19.
14. McArdle CB, Richardson CJ, Nicholas DA, et al. Developmental features of the neonatal brain: MR imaging. Part 1. Gray-white matter differentiation and myelination. *Radiology* 1987; 162:223–229.
15. Williams AL. The neonatal brain. In Williams AL, Haughton VH (Eds): *Cranial Computed Tomography: A Comprehensive Text.* St. Louis: CV Mosby, 1985; 599–625.
16. Sze G, DeArmond SJ, Brant-Zawadzki M, et al. Foci of MRI signal (pseudolesions) anterior to the frontal horns: Histologic correlations of a normal finding. *AJNR* 1986; 7:381–387.

CHAPTER
5
Intracranial Neoplasms and Cysts

Introduction

This chapter will describe MR and CT imaging of adult and pediatric intracranial tumors. The chapter is divided into three parts. Part One concerns MR and CT characteristics and effects of intracranial neoplasms in general. Part Two describes MR and CT imaging of specific tumors and is organized according to histological type. Pediatric brain tumors are not treated as an entirely separate entity but, nevertheless, receive specific attention within the histology-based classification. Brief mention of pertinent clinical characteristics is included. The correlation of imaging findings with the clinical information provided should significantly narrow the list of differential diagnostic possibilities in a given case. Often, a single diagnosis can be reached with a high degree of certainty (i.e., meningioma and glioblastoma). Part Three will briefly discuss the differential diagnosis of brain tumors based on imaging characteristics.

Certain tumors are found only in specific locations. In order to avoid repetition, pituitary tumors and craniopharyngiomas, acoustic neuromas and trigeminal ganglion neuromas, and intracranial tumors arising from bone are principally discussed in Chap-

ters 11, 12, and 13, respectively. The distinction between benign and malignant brain neoplasms is not as clear as it is for other organ system tumors. For example, the so-called benign or low-grade astrocytoma may be slow growing and histologically benign yet may diffusely invade surrounding brain tissue. The low grade gliomas characteristically dedifferentiate to more malignant histological types. The ependymoma may displace rather than infiltrate surrounding brain tissue but does not have a distinct tumor capsule.[1]

Primary central nervous system (CNS) tumors comprise only approximately 10% of total body neoplasms. The majority (85%) of these lesions are intracranial and most of the remaining 15% are intraspinal. Of the primary intracranial tumors, glial origin tumors are the most common (over 40%). The most common clearly benign primary tumors—meningioma, pituitary adenoma, and acoustic neuroma—comprise approximately one-third of intracranial neoplasms (14%, 10%, and 8%, respectively).[1,2]

Whereas most adult primary brain tumors are supratentorial, primary brain tumors of children are frequently located in the posterior fossa. Of these pediatric tumors, astrocytoma, medulloblastoma, and ependymoma are the most common. The majority of pediatric astrocytomas are found in the posterior fossa.[1,2] In a large series of pediatric primary CNS tumors, posterior fossa locations were as common as supratentorial sites. In the same pediatric series, the glial origin tumors constituted approximately 50% of total primary intracranial CNS tumors. The majority (60%) of these glial tumors were located in the posterior fossa (brainstem and cerebellum). Medulloblastoma was the most common cerebellar tumor and represented 17% of total pediatric primary brain tumors.[3]

Metastatic brain tumors account for the largest single group of CNS tumors (40%) in autopsy series.[2] Cerebral metastasis is uncommon in the pediatric group. Subarachnoid spread ("implanting") of certain tumors such as medulloblastoma and germinoma is not uncommon.[4] Some tumors, such as ependymoma, glioblastoma, melanoma, and lymphoma, may invade the ventricular walls.[5] Blood-borne metastasis of a primary brain tumor is a very rare event.[1]

PART ONE

MR and CT Characteristics of Intracranial Neoplasms

Location

Tumor location is important for brain tumor differential diagnosis (Fig. 5.1) and for determining MR and/or CT imaging technique. Extra-axial locations are typical of benign intracranial tumors and parenchymal infiltration is characteristic of malignant brain tumors. Coronal plane imaging of the temporal bones and sella, and MR sagittal imaging of the sella and brainstem are examples of adjusting imaging technique to tumor location.

Multiplicity

Intra-axial tumor multiplicity usually indicates metastatic disease (Fig. 5.2). Multiple primary site gliomas occur rarely. Multiple meningiomas (Fig. 5.3) have characteristic dural surface locations. Multiple sclerosis, emboli, and cerebral abscesses are conditions associated with lesion multiplicity that can mimic multifocal neoplasm. Our new routine for investigation of metastatic brain tumor is a noncontrast and i.v. Gd-DTPA contrast heavily T1-weighted MR scan. Although i.v. contrast CT technique has been relied upon in the past for this investigation, the MR method is more sensitive. Intraventricular (Fig. 5.4) and subarachnoid (Fig. 5.5) tumor spread can be demonstrated by both the MR and CT techniques. Meningeal and ependymal contrast enhancement may occur following craniotomy, intrathecal chemotherapy or shunting in the absence of tumor and therefore, caution is necessary to avoid misdiagnosis.[4]

Intensity and Density

Lesion MR intensity and CT density and degree of homogeniety can be an important clue to tissue type. T1 and T2 are prolonged in almost all brain tumors; however, the degree of prolongation appears shorter in meningiomas. Neuromas, on the other hand, have high T2 intensities—an important distinguishing characteristic for exclusion of meningioma.[6] MR and CT can accurately detect hemorrhage within a tumor.[7,8] The CT detection of calcium within a tumor may suggest a diagnosis such as craniopharyngioma, meningioma, or oligodendroglioma. The presence of fat within a lesion is detected by both MR and CT although the ability of CT to measure fat attenuation directly gives CT the edge in fat detection. A lesion such as a corpus callosum lipoma (Fig. 5.6) is an excellent example.[9] Cystic masses are more accurately evaluated by MR than CT. A water-like low protein pattern of T1 hypointensity and T2 hyperintensity favors arachnoid and postoperative cysts whereas an intermediate pattern of T1 hyperintensity and lower T2 intensity (higher protein) favors

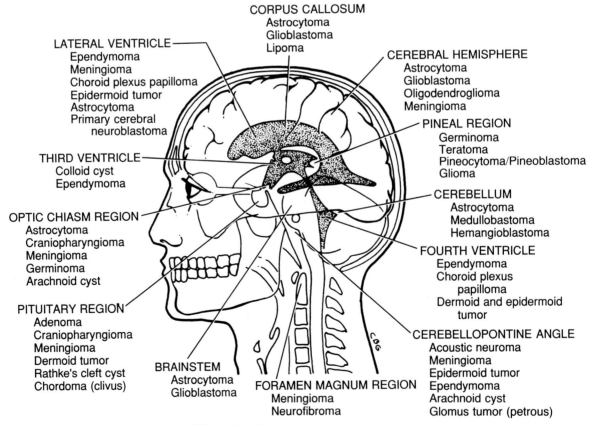

Figure 5.1. Common tumor locations.

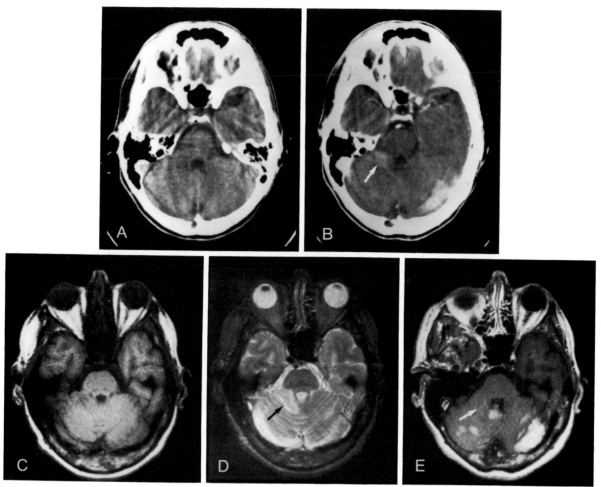

Figure 5.2. Brain metastasis—multiple cerebellar breast metastases. *Noncontrast (A) and contrast (B) axial fourth ventricle-level 35/100 CT scans. SE 600/25 noncontrast (C) and Gd-DTPA contrast (E) MR scans. SE 2800/80 MR scan (D).* The metastases are not identified by noncontrast CT or T1-weighted noncontrast MR. They are well seen by contrast CT, best seen by contrast MR, and moderately well identified by T2-weighted MR. Due to section angulation differences between the CT and MR cases, the metastases on these chosen sections appear somewhat different. Gd-DTPA MR showed far more lesions without artifactual image degradation characteristic of posterior fossa CT. Note the absence of prominent edema. Edema, characteristic of metastases, will be seen in other cases later in this chapter.

nonhemorrhagic tumoral cysts and inflammatory cysts. Both T1 and T2 hyperintensity is characteristic of hemorrhagic cysts and colloid cysts.[10]

Just as important as the intensity and density of tumors is intensity and density homogeneity. For example, an arachnoid cyst (Fig. 5.7) has homogeneous T1 hypointensity, T2 hyperintensity,[10] and water CT attenuation values.[11] It is well known that the imaging characteristics of meningiomas are relatively homogeneous CT hyperdensity or MR isointensity (Fig. 5.8).[1,12] Some degree of signal heterogeneity is a meningioma MR characteristic, however.[8]

MR intensity and CT density quantification, alone, has not been a successful method for tumor histological identification.[1,7]

Margination

Smooth, sharply defined margination favors the diagnosis of benign lesions and irregular, poorly de-

fined margins favor the diagnosis of malignant neoplasm.[1,13] For example, cysts (Fig. 5.7) and meningiomas (Fig. 5.8) have sharply defined and usually smooth margins.[8,10,11,14] A spinal fluid cleft, vascular rim, or dural margin results in an interface between meningiomas and surrounding parenchyma on MR images.[8] A glioblastoma is typically irregularly marginated due to parenchymal infiltration (Fig. 5.9).

Intravenous Contrast Injection

So far, the most clinically tested MR intravenous contrast agent in the United States is gadolinium DTPA (Gd-DTPA). As already mentioned in Chapter 3, MR i.v. contrast will improve sensitivity for small lesions, particularly those close to bone surfaces that would be obscured by CT beam hardening and partial volume artifact (Fig. 5.2). MR i.v. contrast helps characterize lesions and evaluates perfusion and blood-brain barrier (BBB) integrity.[15,16] The well estab-

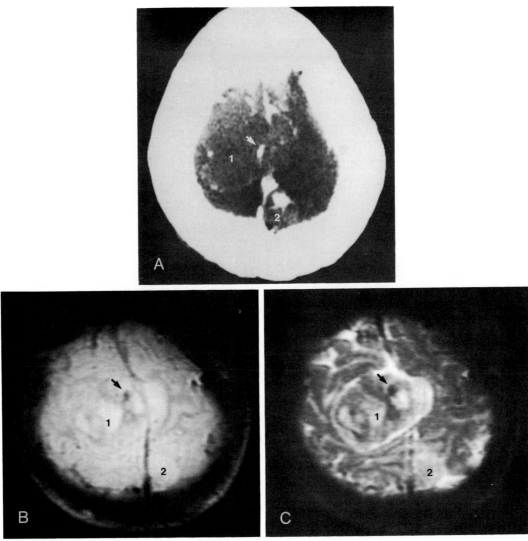

Figure 5.3. Multiple meningiomas. *Noncontrast axial CT 33/100 (**A**), MR SE 2000/20 (**B**), and SE 2000/100 (**C**). The falx (1) and the falx-convexity (2) meningiomas are seen clearly on all images. Calcifi-* cation *(arrows)*. Meningioma contrast enhancement will be discussed later in this chapter.

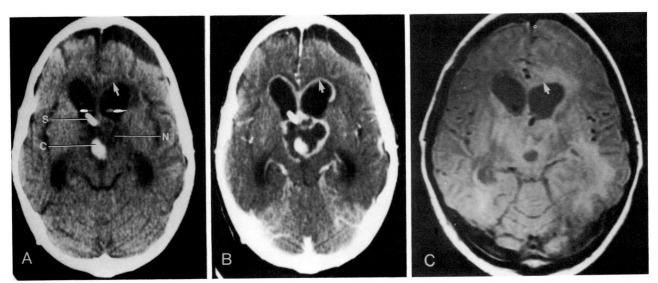

Figure 5.4. Subependymal tumor spread. *A C,* *Hypothalamic glioblastoma multiforme. Axial CT noncontrast (**A**) and i.v. contrast (**B**) sections. Same level SE 2000/20 (**C**) MR section. Note the partially calcified (C) and necrotic (N) tumor. The subependymal tumor* infiltration *(arrows)* is seen on all sections, however, i.v. contrast is necessary to distinguish it from periventricular edema. Note the shunt tube tip at the foramen of Monro (S).

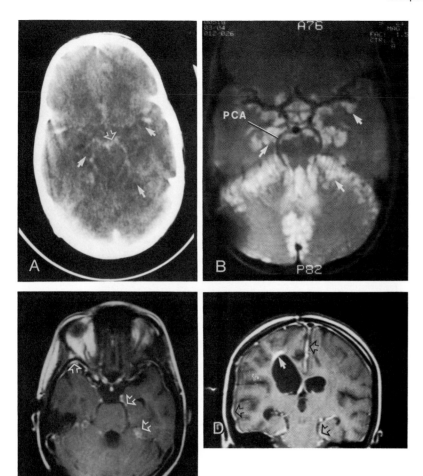

Figure 5.5. Meningeal subarachnoid glioma deposits. *A–B* and *C–D* are different cases. Case A–B demonstrates subarachnoid glioma deposits. Case C–D demonstrates subarachnoid and subependymal tumor deposits. *A–B,* Axial i.v. contrast chiasmatic cistern level CT scan 35/100 *(A)* and SE 2000/80 MR scan *(B)*. CT demonstrates round hypodense lesions *(arrows)* and vascular and/or tumor enhancement *(open arrow)*. MR better demonstrates the T2 hyperintense arachnoid infiltration and demonstrates the signal void of the posterior cerebral artery *(PCA)*. The i.v. contrast CT technique requires very marked perimesencephalic contrast enhancement in order to distinguish subarachnoid tumor enhancement from normal circle of Willis artery and perimesencephalic venous enhancement. *C–D,* SE 600/25 Gd-DTPA i.v. contrast axial fourth ventricle-level *(C)* and coronal posterior third ventricle-level *(D)* MR scans. Right lateral ventricle porencephaly after subtotal glioblastoma resection with adjacent contrast-enhancing tumor *(arrow)*. Note subependymal contrast enhancement of the left lateral ventricle. Meningeal tumor contrast enhancement is quite marked *(open arrows)*. The i.v. Gd-DTPA MR technique is the method of choice for investigation of subarachnoid and intraventricular tumor spread.

Meningeal and ependymal contrast enhancement may occur due to prior surgery and ventricular shunting in the absence of tumor or infection. This is likely due to arachnoid inflammation caused by bleeding at the time of surgery.

*Burke JW, Podrasky AE, Bradley WG Jr. Meninges: benign postoperative enhancement on MR images. Radiology 1990; 174:99–102.

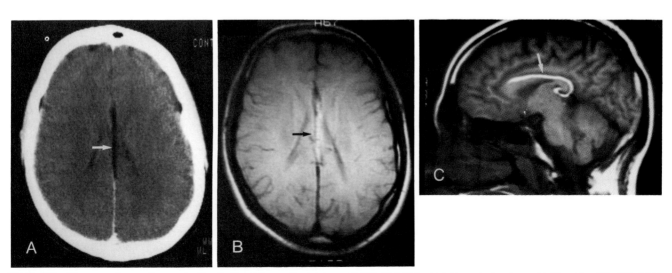

Figure 5.6. Corpus callosum lipoma (or "pericallosal lipoma"). *Axial lateral ventricle body-level 100/35 CT scan *(A)*. Same level SE 2000/20 MR *(B)*. Parasagittal SE 600/25 MR scan *(C)*. Note the CT hypo-dense and T1 hyperintense lesion *(arrows)*. (See also Fig. 3.6, page 44.)

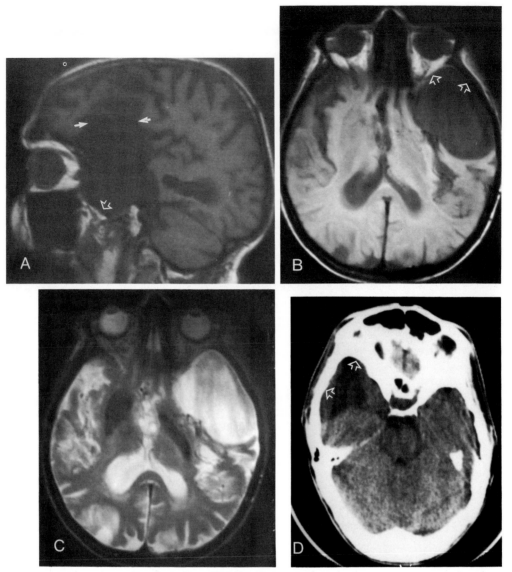

Figure 5.7. Arachnoid cyst. *MR sections (A–C) and CT section (D) are different cases. Sagittal SE 600/25 (A), axial SE 2000/20 (B), and SE 2000/80 (C). Axial sella turcica level noncontrast CT scan (D). Water homogeneous T1 isointensity (A and B) and T2 isointensity* **(C)** smoothy marginated mass expanding the middle fossa *(open arrows)* and continuous with the subarachnoid space *(closed arrows)*. Note the sharp posterior margin.

lished role of CT i.v. contrast is similar to that proposed for MR i.v. contrast use.[17] It is likely, however, that the use of i.v. contrast for MR will be much more selective due to lesion conspicuity without the need for additional study.[6,18,19]

Chapter 2 discussed patterns of CT i.v. contrast enhancement of areas of BBB breakdown and/or hypervascularity as well as of normal vascular structures such as in the cisterns, fissures, and the falx.[1] It is likely, however, that contrast MR examination will routinely follow an initial MR noncontrast scan for work-up of an extra-axial tumor and that the CT method will be relegated to "second best" status.

With specific reference to tumors, homogeneous contrast enhancement favors benign tumor (Fig. 5.8) and inhomogeneous contrast enhancement favors the diagnosis of malignancy (Fig. 5.9). Malignant tumors often demonstrate an irregular rim of contrast enhancement surrounding a necrotic center.[1,20]

Intrathecal or Intraventricular Contrast Injection

The use of intrathecal contrast injection for contrast enhancement has thus far been restricted to CT scanning. For those institutions that have MR scanners, MR has replaced CT cisternography.[21] Positive contrast and gas CT cisternography are virtually no longer used at our hospital.

Positive contrast cisternography or ventriculography has been recommended for dynamic evaluation

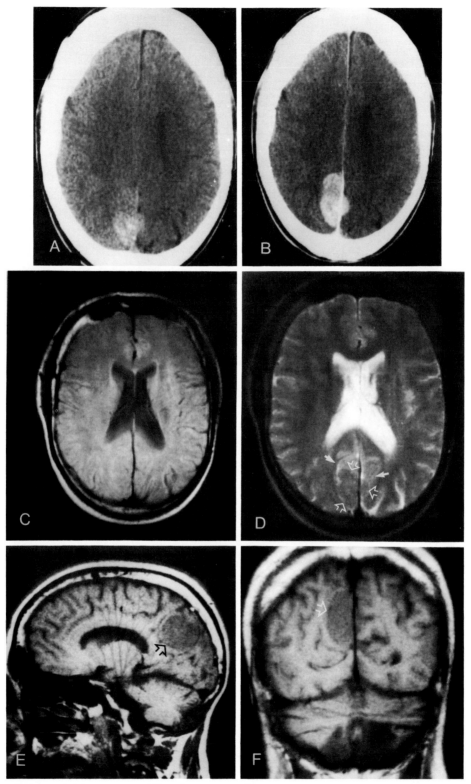

Figure 5.8. Falx meningioma. *Axial noncontrast (A) and contrast (B) CT scans. Axial different angle lateral ventricle-level SE 2000/20 (C) and 2000/80 (D) MR scans. Sagittal SE 600/25 (E) and coronal (F) MR scans. Static artifact is seen on the sagittal scan. The partially calcified falx meningioma is most conspicuous on the i.v. contrast CT scan where the smaller left parasagittal portion is also clearly delineated. The gray matter isointense tumor is virtually undetecta-* ble by MR on **C** and barely detectable on **D** *(open arrows)* where surrounding edema is best demonstrated *(solid arrows)*. It is best detected by MR on heavily T1-weighted images **(E** and **F).** The characteristic capsule and vessels are not demonstrated by this case. MR i.v. contrast enhancement of meningiomas and other MR meningioma features will be illustrated later in this chapter.

Figure 5.9. Glioblastoma multiforme involving the corpus callosum and both frontal lobes—"corpus callosum glioma." *Noncontrast (A) and i.v. contrast (B) axial 37/100 CT scans. Same axial level SE 2000/20 (C) and 2000/80 (D) MR scans.* Markedly irregular contoured centrally necrotic *(N)* tumor with a moderate degree of peripheral edema *(E).* Marked irregular rim contrast enhancement **(B).** Abnormal irregular tumor vessel *(solid arrow).* T2 marginal hemosiderin hypointensity *(open arrow).* Both the CT and MR technique demonstrated here provide sufficient information to reach the correct diagnosis.

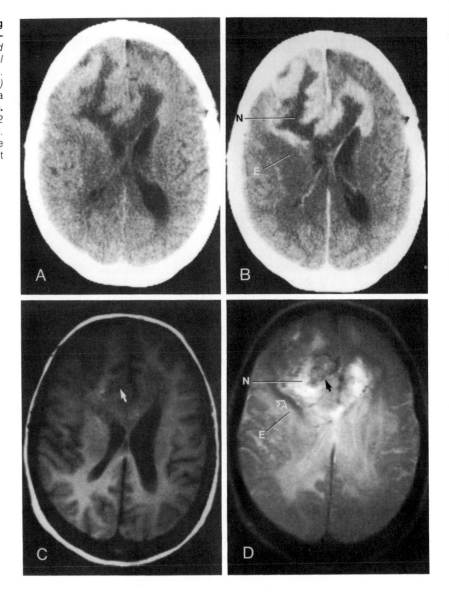

of arachnoid cysts.[11,22,23] Lack of free communication of the cyst and the ventricular system and adverse mass effects of the cyst (e.g., hydrocephalus) requires a direct cyst shunting procedure[23] or open surgery on the cyst.[22] CT ventriculography using 2 ml of io- pamidol or iohexol can be useful for investigation of intraventricular cysts (Fig. 5.10).

For medical institutions without an available MR facility, for patients who also require myelography, or for patients who have contraindications for MR scanning, CT cisternography is still a useful exami- nation for brainstem, midbrain, and for cervicome- dullary imaging (Fig. 5.11).[24,25]

Air cisternography (Fig. 5.12) of the cerebellopon- tine angle (CP angle)[26] for investigation of acoustic neuroma has been replaced as a first choice exami- nation by Gd-DTPA MR scanning.

Vascular Tumor Patterns

MR is superior to contrast CT for the demonstra- tion of enlarged abnormal arteries and veins, arte- rial encasement, and venous sinus occlusion (Fig. 5.13).[8,27] MR, without i.v. contrast, can demonstrate tumor arterial supply (Fig. 5.13).[8] MR techniques are likely to be developed that estimate the rate of blood flow.

Calcification

Tumor calcification is better detected by CT than by MR. Inasmuch as the presence and character of tumor calcification is important to diagnosis, CT has a definite advantage here.[28] For example, the pres- ence of calcium in a suprasellar tumor leads to the diagnosis of craniopharyngioma[3,20] and irregular

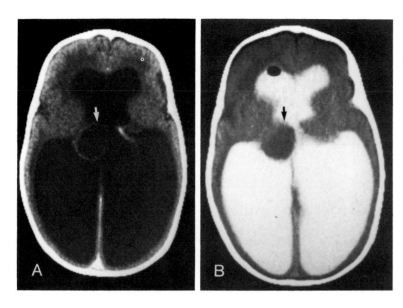

Figure 5.10. Choroid plexus cyst—intraventricular cyst. *Axial noncontrast (A) and ventricular catheter injection contrast (B) CT scans in a hydrocephalic infant. Note the thin-walled cyst (arrows) that does not directly communicate with the lateral ventricles (B). A small air bubble, introduced during ventriculography, is seen in the right frontal horn.*

clumps of tumor calcification suggests the diagnosis of oligodendroglioma (Fig. 5.14).[1,28] A diffusely calcified dural-based mass is most likely a meningioma.[1]

Hemorrhage

Hemorrhage is well detected by both CT and MR as demonstrated by Table 3.2 page 46. A large variety of primary and metastatic, benign and malignant tumors may present with spontaneous parenchymal hemorrhage (Fig. 5.15). The most common tumor in male adults presenting with spontaneous intracerebral hemorrhage is metastatic lung carcinoma. Intratumoral hemorrhage can often be distin-

guished from spontaneous intracerebral hemorrhage by location. Spontaneous intracerebral hemorrhages usually occur in the basal ganglia and are next most often seen in the occipitoparietal location. Intratumoral hemorrhages tend to be peripheral. Perihematoma CT (or MR) contrast enhancement in the early acute state favor the diagnosis of neoplasm.[1]

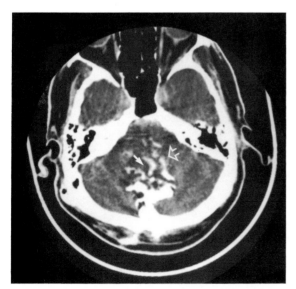

Figure 5.11. CT cisternography of fourth ventricle epidermoid tumor. The tumor has markedly expanded the fourth ventricle. Dense intrathecal contrast *(open arrow)* fills the interstices between the hypodense tumor fronds *(closed arrow)*.

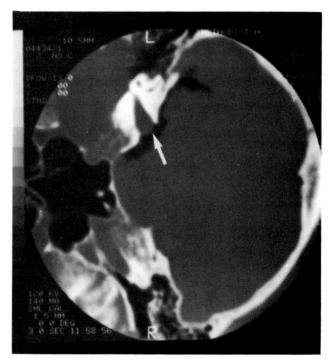

Figure 5.12. Air cisternogram demonstrating acoustic neuroma. *Axial right lateral decubitus 250/4000 left petrous CT air cisternogram, 1.5-mm section. The air-filled left cerebellopontine angle cistern outlines the extracanalicular portion of the acoustic neuroma (arrow). No air enters the internal auditory canal.*

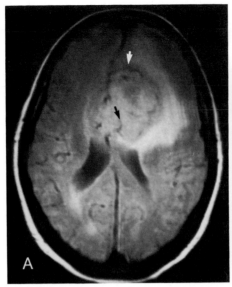

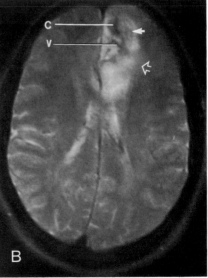

Figure 5.13. Tumor vascular supply. Axial MR SE 2000/20 of falx meningioma **(A)**. Abnormal meningeal artery arising from the anterior falx artery *(white arrow)*. Artery within the tumor *(black arrow)*. Co-

ronal MR SE 600/25 **(B)**. Corpus callosum glioma. Tumor vessel *(black arrow)*.

Edema

Cerebral edema can be classified as cytotoxic, vasogenic, and interstitial (hydrocephalic) types (Table 5.1). Cytotoxic edema results from ischemia with disruption of the cellular ATP-mediated sodium-potassium pump. Pump dysfunction results in sodium entering and potassium leaving the cell. The cellular osmotic gradient increases due to increased intracellular sodium and lactate. Extracellular water then enters and expands the cell producing "cellular edema." Cytotoxic edema, therefore, expands the in-

tracellular space. Cytotoxic edema occurs with cerebral ischemia and is seen in the acute stage of cerebral infarction.[29,30]

Vasogenic edema occurs with BBB breakdown mediated by metabolic and possibly toxic factors that compromise and damage the BBB. This results in the loss of electrolytes, water, and protein from the intravascular compartment and expansion of the extracellular space. Characteristic finger-like imaging pattern of "white matter edema" then develops.

Tumors and abscesses are typically associated with vasogenic or "white matter" edema. Cerebral infarc-

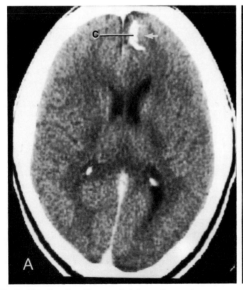

Figure 5.14. Calcified oligodendroglioma. *Axial sections at same frontal anterior pole-level. Intravenous contrast CT 35/100 **(A)** and T2-weighted MR SE 2000/80 **(B)**.* Slight contrast enhancement on CT of noncalcified tumor component *(closed arrow)*. Open arrow **(B)**

represents large edema and/or tumor component not evident by CT. Encased vessel *(V)* seen by MR **(B)**. The calcification *(C)* is CT hyperdense and MR hypointense. It is only clearly diagnostic of calcification by CT.

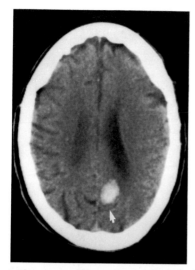

Figure 5.15.   Intratumoral hemorrhage. Metastatic melanoma. Axial 37/100 noncontrast lateral ventricle body-level CT scan. An ovoid well-defined hemorrhagic posterior-medial parietal mass posteriorly displaces and distorts the parieto-occipital sulcus *(arrow).*

tion is initially associated with cytotoxic and then later, after approximately 6 hours, with vasogenic edema. The typical CT gray and white matter distribution infarct hypodensity represents a combination of both cytotoxic and vasogenic edema.[29–31]

Interstitial (hydrocephalic) edema has also been termed transependymal resorption. It occurs when raised intraventricular pressure in the hydrocephalic patient causes transependymal resorption of intraventricular CSF. Periventricular edema can then be detected by CT and MR.[29,30]

CT and MR signal density and intensity is similar in all edema types. The CT signal is hypodense. The MR signal is T1 and proton density slight- to moderate-degree water-hyperintensity and T2 water-isointensity. The T1 and proton water-hyperintensity signal is due to the edema water molecules' approximation to protein molecules.[29]

Malignant tumor peritumoral vasogenic edema oc-

curs due to the greater permeability of the damaged BBB of tumor neovascularity and due to pressure effects upon normal brain. The pressure effect may also result in ischemia and peritumoral infarction adding the additional condition of cytotoxic edema to the already present vasogenic process. Benign tumor pressure effect upon normal displaced brain tissues can cause both cytotoxic and vasogenic edema.[21,29,30]

Meningioma peritumoral edema may be quite marked. It is caused, in part, by pressure effect upon normal brain but the common occurrence of marked degree edema surrounding even small meningiomas is poorly understood.[21] The meningioma peritumoral water signal may be, in part, due to enlarged subarachnoid spaces surrounding the tumor.[32]

It is important to distinguish edema from tumor for purposes of stereotactic biopsy, direct surgical approach, radiation therapy planning, response to therapy, and prognostication. Analysis of CT densities, MR multiecho sequence intensities, contrast enhancement and morphological patterns can usually distinguish tumor from edema (Fig. 5.16). An interesting edema characteristic is the usual tendency of peritumoral edema not to cross the corpus callosum to the contralateral side. Corpus callosal involvement in tumor patients is usually caused by tumor and not, simply, edema (Fig. 5.9).[21]

Cerebral ischemia and infarction are further discussed in Chapter 6.

Displacement and Obstruction

The tumor mass effect results from the tumor mass itself plus edema and possible associated ventricular obstruction. Mass effect may present as a simple shift of midline structures, ventricular compression, or sulcal effacement. Evidence of subfalcial, incisural, or tonsillar herniation may be present (Fig. 5.17). A strategically located small tumor such as a colloid cyst can cause marked hydrocephalus or a lateral ventricular atrial mass may cause lateral ventricular temporal horn entrapment (Fig. 5.18).

Meningioma parenchymal displacement produces

Table 5.1.   Edema[29,30]

	Cytotoxic	Vasogenic	Interstitial (Hydrocephalic)
Clinical setting	Ischemia—infarct	Neoplasms, inflammations, trauma, hemorrhage, infarct after 6 hours	Hydrocephalus
Mechanism	Decreased cellular ATP causes Na-K pump failure	Endothelial tight junction disruption—BBB breakdown	Elevated intraventricular pressure
Substrate	Gray matter and white matter	White matter	Periventricular white matter
Intracellular space	Increases	Decreases	—
Extracellular space	Decreases	Increases	—
Imaging appearance	Sharp margination, water-protein signal[a]	Finger-like white matter, water-protein signal[a]	Periventricular water-protein signal surrounds the lateral, and occasionally, the third ventricles

[a]This term refers to relaxation effects of the water-protein molecular approximation in the edema molecular environment.

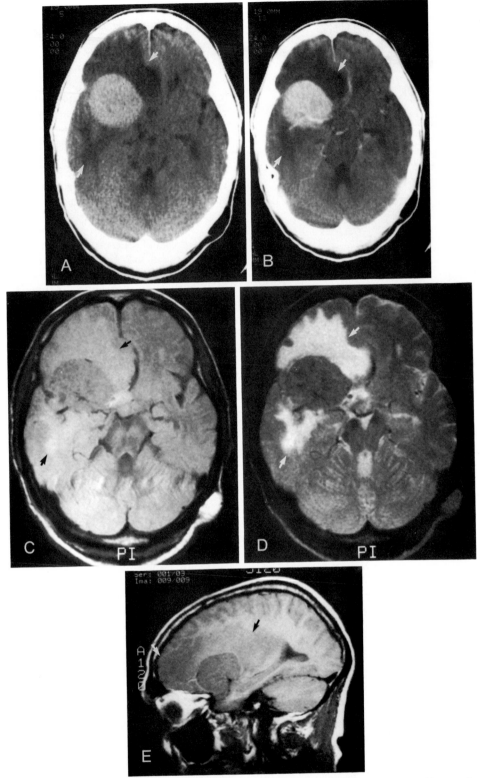

Figure 5.16. Edema. Bronchogenic carcinoma right frontal-basal ganglionic metastasis with marked edema. *Axial noncontrast (A) and i.v. contrast (B) CT scans. Same level axial SE 2000/20 (C) and 2000/80 (D) and sagittal 600/25E MR scans.* CT homogeneous dense and homogeneous contrast-enhancing metastasis with marked surrounding edema *(arrows)* resembles a meningioma. Note the edema relative hyperintensity on the TR 2000 msec images (C and D) and hypointensity on the 600/25 (E) image. MR demonstrates tumor gray matter isointensity similar to a meningioma and fails to document hemorrhage. The lack of CT sphenoid hyperostosis, surrounding cleft, meningeal tumor vessels, and the presence of marginal irregularity in other sections favors the diagnosis of parenchymal tumor.

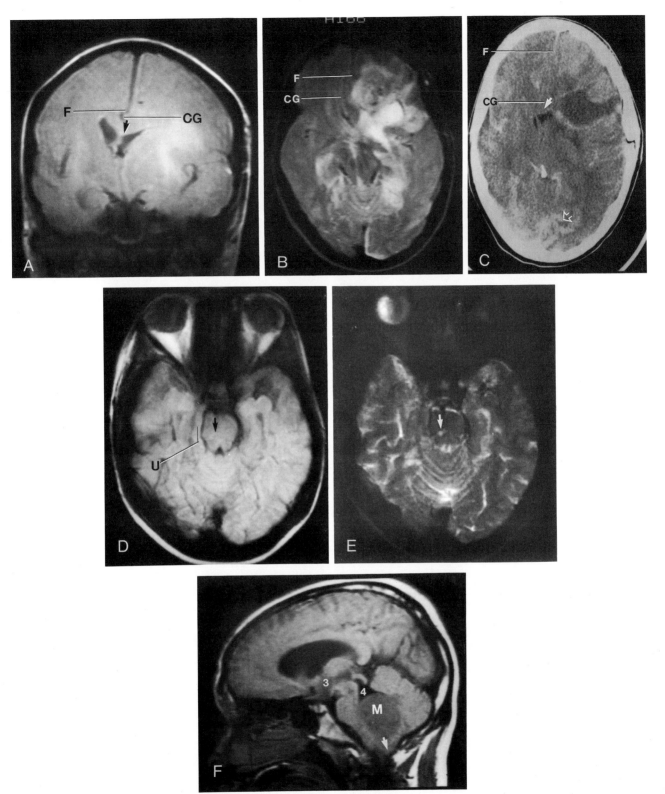

Figure 5.17.   Brain herniations. Subfalcial, tentorial incisural, and cerebellar tonsillar herniations. *A–C; Subfalcial herniation. Left frontal glioblastoma multiforme with marked edema. Coronal MR SE 2000/ 25 (A), axial MR SE 2000/80 (B), and i.v. contrast axial CT 35/100 (C).* The cingulate gyrus *(CG)* is displaced beneath the free edge of the falx *(F)* and the frontal horn of the lateral ventricle is depressed *(arrow)*. There is a contrast-enhancing left posterior cerebral artery infarct *(open arrow)* caused by incisural herniation with arterial compression against the tentorium **(B). *D–E,* Duret's hemorrhage re-** sulting from incisural herniation. Different patient. Axial SE 2000/20 **(D)** and 2000/80 **(E)** MR scans at the midbrain level. The T1 and T2 hyperintense midbrain tegmental hemorrhage *(arrow)*, the right midbrain compression deformity caused by the herniated temporal lobe uncus *(U)* are well seen. **F,** Tonsillar herniation. Different patient. Sagittal MR SE 600/25 of a patient with a vermis medulloblastoma *(M)*. Obstructed dilated fourth ventricle *(4)*, aqueduct, third ventricle *(3)*, and lateral ventricles.

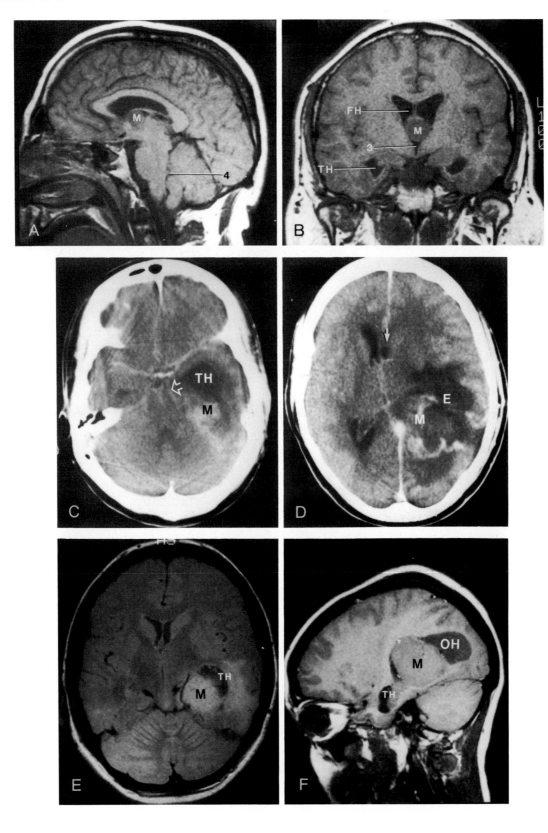

an interface between tumor and brain that is detectable by MR scanning. The interface consists of CSF cleft, vascular rim, and dural margin. MR of large meningiomas may show arcuate convolutional displacement and compression of adjacent gyri analogous to "onion-peel" distortion of the angiographic gyral capillary blush (Fig. 5.8E). Arcuate displacement and compression is absent or uncommon with gliomas probably because of adjacent parenchyma infiltration (Fig. 5.9).[8] The CT equivalent of the meningioma interface and arcuate parenchymal displacement and compression is "white matter buckling." This term refers to the CT preserved but displaced gray-white junction and the compressed or "buckled" adjacent often edematous white matter as seen with extra-axial intracranial masses.[33]

PART TWO

MR and CT of Intracranial Neoplasms and Cysts

Tumors Originating in the Brain and Meninges

GLIAL ORIGIN TUMORS

The glial origin tumor group comprises astrocytomas, "gliomas," oligodendrogliomas, ependymomas, and choroid plexus papillomas.

They are the most common brain tumors of children and the most common primary brain tumors of adults. The tumors in the adult are predominantly supratentorial and, in children, the majority are infratentorial.

Astrocytomas

All astrocytomas are infiltrating to some degree. In the past, they have been histologically graded from I (low grade astrocytoma) to IV (glioblastoma multiforme).

The four-tier Kernohan supratentorial astrocytoma classification has currently been replaced by a new three-tier classification: astrocytoma, anaplastic astrocytoma, and glioblastoma multiforme. Both classifications are based on tumor histology encompassing four major categories: hypercellularity, pleomorphism, vascular proliferation (neovascularity), and necrosis (see Table 5.2). The lesions demonstrate in-

Table 5.2. Supratentorial Astrocytoma Histological Criteria[a]

	Astrocytoma	Anaplastic astrocytoma	Glioblastoma multiforme
Hypercellularity	Slight	Moderate	Moderate to marked
Pleomorphism	Slight	Moderate	Moderate to marked
Necrosis	None	None	Present
Vascular proliferation	None	+/−	+/−
Grade of malignancy	Low	High	High

[a]Adapted from Burger PC, Vogel FS, Green SB, Strike TA. Glioblastoma multiforme and anaplastic astrocytoma. Pathological criteria and prognostic implications. *Cancer* 1985; 56:1106–1111.

creasing malignant histological and imaging characteristics from the astrocytoma through the glioblastoma multiforme. The classification of the astrocytoma series into low and high grade can still be made, however, considering the astrocytoma category as low grade and the anaplastic astrocytoma and the glioblastoma multiforme as high grade. Most adult astrocytomas eventually dedifferentiate into glioblastoma multiforme. Up to 5% of high grade gliomas may arise as a multifocal lesion and thus may mimic metastases.

The CT characteristics of low and high grade astrocytoma series malignancy are generally agreed upon. MR characteristics of these tumors such as margination, necrosis, and contrast enhancement appear to parallel the CT changes with the exception that rapid blood flow produces a spin echo signal void by MR and contrast enhancement by CT. In general, gliomas have an elevated water content that requires careful scrutiny of different CT and MR techniques in order to differentiate tumor tissue from edema for biopsy and/or excision.[1] Intravenous contrast CT and MR can differentiate bulk glial tumor from edema[34] but it should be noted that the surrounding edematous parenchyma is infiltrated to some degree due to the lack of a true tumor capsule.[35] CT contrast technique has long been the procedure of choice after the noncontrast scan. The MR i.v. contrast enhancement technique is clearly superior, however, in regions where CT artifact would obscure detail such as in the posterior fossa. For example, MR contrast techniques can differentiate brainstem tumor and edema in certain cases. The degree of CT

Figure 5.18. Ventricular obstruction by tumor. Figures **A–B, C–D,** and **E–F** are different cases. **A–B,** Lateral ventricle outlet obstruction by a third ventricle colloid cyst. Sagittal **(A)** and coronal **(B)** 600/25 MR scans. There is moderate degree dilatation of the lateral ventricle frontal-horns *(FH)* and temporal horns *(TH)* caused by the cyst *(M)* blocking the foramina of Monro. The third ventricle *(3)* and fourth ventricle *(4)* are collapsed. **C–F,** Temporal and occipital horn entrapment by a mass. **C–D,** Glioblastoma multiforme. *Axial fourth ventricle level **(C)** and lateral ventricle-level **(D)** i.v. contrast CT 35/ 100 scans.* Irregular rim contrast-enhanced tumor *(M)* with marked surrounding vasogenic edema *(E)*. Markedly dilated left temporal horn

(TH). There is marked displacement of the septum pellucidum to the right and there is a characteristic subfalcial cingulate gyrus defect on the left frontal horn *(closed arrow).* This would have the arteriographic pericallosal artery "square shift" effect due to the angular interhemispheric fissure displacement. There is slight dilatation of the right lateral ventricle. Note the uncus incisural herniation *(open arrow).* **E–F,** Intraventricular meningioma. *Axial SE 2000/20 and sagittal SE 600/25 MR scans.* Note the dilated lateral ventricle occipital *(OH)* and temporal *(TH)* horns. There is only slight displacement of the septum pellucidum toward the right without abrupt cingulate gyrus herniation.

(and presumably MR) contrast enhancement is proportional to the degree of malignancy.[34,35] Not all high grade astrocytomas contrast enhance, however.

Supratentorial Low Grade Astrocytomas. CT characteristics of adult supratentorial low grade malignancy astrocytomas include hemispheric white matter location, slight hypodensity, lack of sharp margination, little or no contrast enhancement, occasional calcification, undetectable or minor edema, and minor mass effect.[1,35]

Pediatric supratentorial astrocytomas account for approximately 10% of pediatric brain tumors. The behavior of pediatric supratentorial astrocytomas does not reliably correlate with their imaging appearance. For example, these tumors may markedly contrast enhance.[3] Occasionally, a pediatric cystic astrocytoma will erode the skull inner table (Fig. 5.19).

MR has been found to be generally superior to CT for detection of cystic lesions. This is particularly evident where cysts are located in regions of CT artifact such as the brainstem (interpetrous).[10] MR will usually demonstrate water signal intensities with evidence for an intra-axial position, lack of dural attachment, and lack of sharp margination (Fig. 5.20).

Clinical trial is necessary to determine if lesions failing to contrast enhance by CT will enhance with i.v. MR contrast techniques.

Supratentorial High Grade Astrocytomas. These tumors include anaplastic astrocytoma and glioblastoma multiforme. CT characteristics of high grade adult astrocytomas include heterogeneous density; irregular margination, heterogeneous contrast enhancement often with a central unenhanced portion and an abnormal draining vein, prominent edema, and greater structural displacement (Fig. 5.9). Calcification is rare. Intratumoral hemorrhage is occasionally seen. Periventricular and subarachnoid tumor spread may occur.[1,4] The tumor occasionally occurs multifocally. The MR characteristics of high grade glioma include intra-axial location, heterogeneous T1 hypointensity and T2 hyperintensity, frequent central cyst-like regions, irregular margination, abnormal or encased blood vessels within the mass and enlarged draining veins, possible hemorrhage, edema, and contrast enhancement (Figs. 5.9 and 5.21). Pathologically, areas of necrosis separate anaplastic astrocytoma from glioblastoma multiforme (Table 5.2).[34] Differentiating tumor from edema

Figure 5.19. Supratentorial cystic astrocytoma. *Axial supraorbitomeatal angle lateral ventricle atrial-level i.v. contrast 35/100 **(A)** and 200/3000 **(B)** CT scans. Left sagittal Sylvian level SE 600/25 **(C)** and axial infraorbitomeatal low centrum semiovale SE 2800/80 MR scans **(D)**. Note the fairly sharply marginated homogeneous CT water density and MR T1 water slightly hyperintense and T2 water isointense mass (solid arrows) having eroded the skull inner table.*

Note the frontal gyral "onion skin" displacement (open arrows). There is no detectable edema.

Note: This particular lesion included sections at other levels that had ill-defined margins resembling the case illustrated in Figure 5.20. Onion skin gyral displacement can be occasionally seen in patients with astrocytomas as well as in patients with benign tumors (typically meningioma).

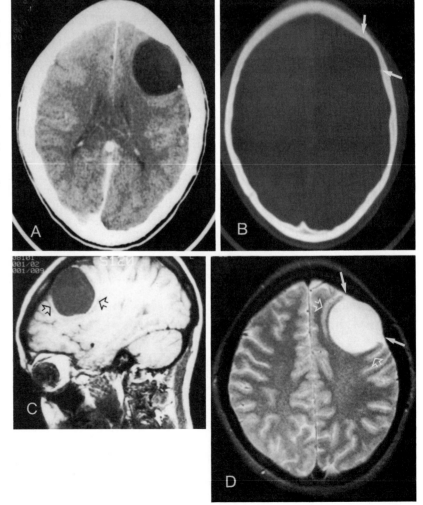

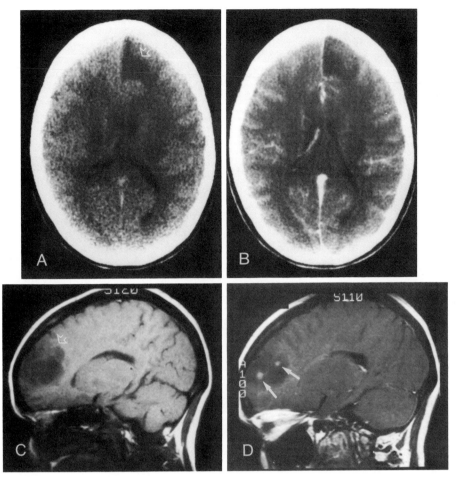

Figure 5.20. Supratentorial low grade astrocytoma. *Axial 35/100 noncontrast* **(A)** *and i.v. contrast* **(B)** *CT scans. Atrial level sagittal SE 600/25 noncontrast* **(C)** *and Gd-DTPA contrast* **(D)** *MR scans. The left frontal CT hypodense MR T1 slight water-hyperintense ill-* defined mass *(open arrows)* does not definitely contrast enhance with iodinated CT contrast but two discrete tumor nodules *(solid arrows)* are enhanced with i.v. Gd-DTPA. No edema was documented by either the CT or T2-weighted (not shown) MR technique.

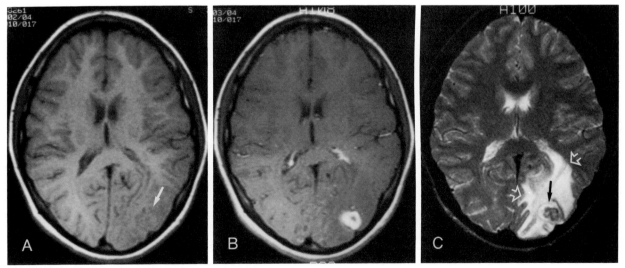

Figure 5.21. High grade glioma. *Axial third ventricle-level SE 600/ 25 without* **(A)** *and with* **(B)** *Gd-DTPA and SE 2800/80* **(C)** *MR scans. The irregularly contoured mixed T2 intensity mass (black arrow on* **C***) is T1 gray matter-isointense* **(A)** *and markedly contrast enhances* **(B).** *The marked surrounding edema (open arrows) is barely identi-* fiable on T1-weighted images. There is a small, irregular, central nonenhanced region within the markedly contrast-enhanced mass presumably representing necrosis.

This case points out the value of obtaining T2-weighted images in addition to the T1 noncontrast and contrast technique.

is often possible by analysis of intensities on different sequences but usually requires MR or CT contrast techniques for greatest accuracy. The orthogonal MR imaging planes are a significant aid to evaluation of structural shift and herniation (Fig. 5.17).

Cerebellar Astrocytomas   This common tumor occurs predominantly in children and young adults. It represents approximately 8% of a series of 164 pediatric brain tumors.[3] The prognosis, compared to that of adult gliomas is very good. Most lesions are larger than 5 cm accounting for the usual moderate to severe hydrocephalus. They are characteristically eccentric involving the midline and one hemisphere. The majority are cystic. The rim that surrounds the cystic portion may be thick and markedly contrast enhanced. Solid portions may, however, predominate. Solid or predominantly solid tumors tend to be smaller and more central.[3]

The CT characteristics of cerebellar astrocytomas include the eccentric location, large size, hypodensity or isodensity, cyst, prominent contrast enhancement of the solid portion, occasional edema, and hydrocephalus. The most common cystic type has a large cyst with a mural nodule that CT contrast enhances. Hemorrhage is not a CT characteristic of these tumors. Solid tumors may calcify.[34] MR imaging demonstrates the solid portion as T1 hypointense and T2 hyperintense with homogeneous lower T1 and higher T2 intensities of the cystic portion. The cyst content is usually water T1 hyperintense and may demonstrate fluid levels.[21]

Brainstem Glioma

In the series by Fitz,[3] brainstem gliomas accounted for approximately 15% of pediatric brain tumors—twice the occurrence rate of cerebellar astrocytomas (8%). Brainstem gliomas may also occur in

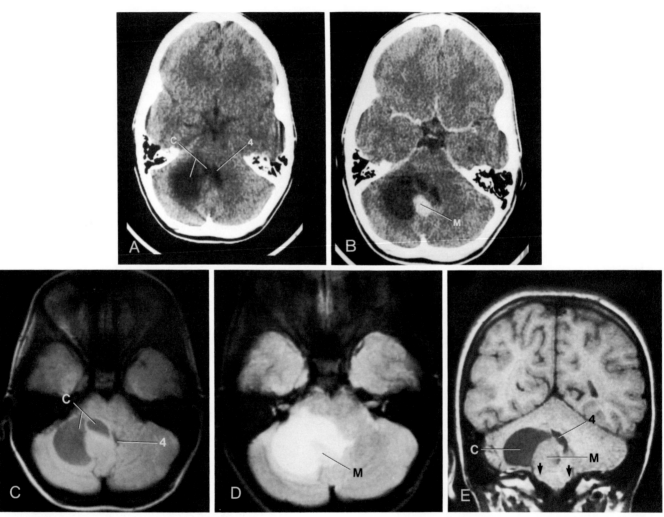

Figure 5.22.   Cerebellar astrocytoma. Axial noncontrast **(A)** and i.v. contrast **(B)** 35/100 CT scans at fourth ventricle-level demonstrating a cystic **(C)** and partially solid *(M)* mass. There is homogeneous contrast enhancement of the round solid portion. Deformed displaced fourth ventricle *(4)*. Axial SE 2000/20 **(C)** and 2000/80 **(D)** MR scans at the fourth ventricle-level. The solid portion is barely discernible and the cystic portion and fourth ventricle cannot be differentiated on the T2-weighted image **(D)**. Note the solid portion and tonsillar herniation *(arrows)* identifiable on the coronal MR section SE 600/25 **(E).**

adults.[36] CT typically demonstrates heterogeneous isodensity or hypodensity within an unsharply marginated mass with heterogeneous contrast enhancement. Cystic portions and hydrocephalus are common.[3] Calcification and hemorrhage may occur. As is so often the case with pediatric astrocytomas, CT characteristics poorly correlate with the histological grade of the tumor. Brainstem gliomas usually begin in the pons. Posterior displacement of the fourth ventricle is the rule (Fig. 5.23). An exophytic tumor may uncommonly displace the fourth ventricle anteriorly. Lateral invasion into the cerebellar peduncles and cerebellar hemisphere may occur.[3,37] Positive con-

trast CT cisternography, before MR, was the most accurate method for investigating brainstem masses.[24,25] This latter procedure is now only rarely performed.

MR is more sensitive than CT for the detection of brainstem gliomas. Although CT cisternography accurately defines the expanded brainstem and adjacent structures, MR also directly visualizes the abnormal signal intensities of tumor tissue and is not compromised by interpetrous artifact. The MR orthogonal plane imaging technique provides a sagittal image that is extremely helpful in brainstem mass evaluation.[36] MR i.v. contrast techniques have become standard for the investigation of these lesions.

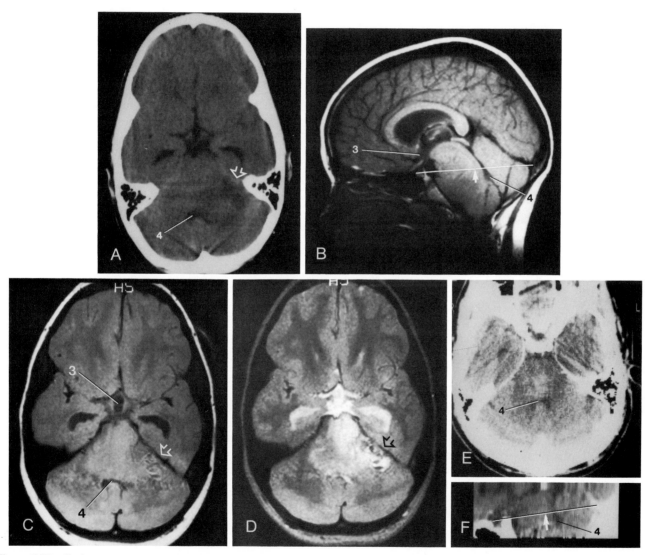

Figure 5.23.   Brainstem tumor—pontine glioma. Figures **A–D** and **E–F** are different cases **A–D,** Noncontrast axial fourth ventricle-level CT scan **(A).** Midsagittal SE 600/25 **(B),** axial fourth ventricle-level SE 2000/20 **(C),** and 2000/80 **(D)** MR scans. Twining line (line of the T's) is drawn from the sella tuberculum to the torcula and is divided into two (closed arrow). The midline should be within the fourth ventricle (4). Note the deformity and posterior displacement of fourth ventricle by the mass. There is a left cerebellar hemisphere area of

low mixed density (open arrows). This latter area demonstrates prominent abnormal vessels best seen on the T2-weighted image. The mass also shows considerable heterogeneous signal intensity in other portions with the T2-weighted technique. **E-F,** Another case. Intravenous contrast axial fourth ventricle level **(E)** and sagittal reformation **(F)** CT scan. Twining line has again been drawn. Note posterior displacement of the fourth ventricle (4) by the contrast-enhanced pontine mass.

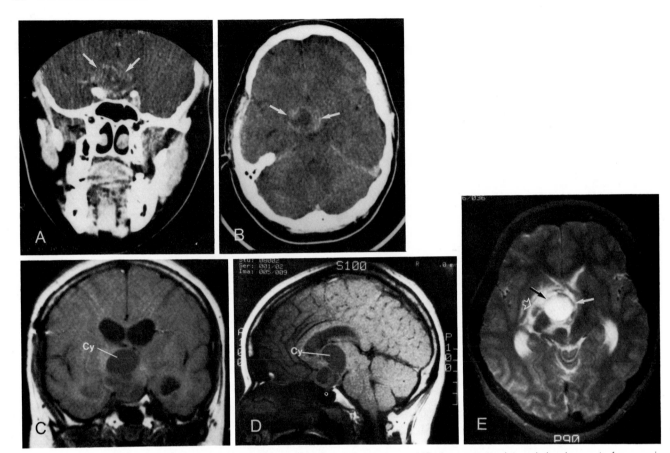

Figure 5.24.   Hypothalamic glioma. Initial CT scan and 3-year MR follow-up. *Coronal sella-level* **(A)** *and axial chiasmatic cistern-level* **(B)** *i.v. contrast CT scans. SE 600/25 coronal sella-level* **(C)** *and midsagittal* **(D)** *and axial 2000/80* **(E)** *MR scans 3 years later.*
    The initial CT demonstrates thick irregular rim contrast enhancement *(closed arrows)* of the suprasellar central hypodense mass.

The follow-up MR demonstrates interval development of a superior cystic portion *(Cy)* that obstructs the foramen of Monro causing hydrocephalus. Note the heterogeneous signal hypointensity of the portion beneath the cyst. There is an irregular T2-hyperintense edematous or infiltrative component peripheral to the cystic portion *(open arrow).*

Hypothalamic Glioma—"Optic Nerve Gliomas"

In Fitz's series of 264 pediatric brain tumors,[3] gliomas involving the optic chiasm and adjacent brain included 14 patients (8%). Of these cases, only four had no optic nerve involvement. One-third (5 patients) of these chiasmatic tumor patients had neurofibromatosis. Hypothalamic gliomas have a relatively benign course.[3] CT characteristics of these primarily hypothalamic tumors include isodensity with prominent contrast enhancement. Calcification is uncommon and cystic areas may occur.[3] The orthogonal plane MR investigation has distinct advantages over CT, especially with the sagittal section (Fig. 5.24). Hypothalamic gliomas are also discussed in Chapter 11 p. 270. Those tumors involving the optic nerve, optic gliomas, are discussed in Chapter 14, p. 355.

Giant Cell Astrocytomas.   Giant cell astrocytomas arise from abnormal astrocytic giant cells in tuberous sclerosis.[38] The presence of a juxtaventricular tumor (particularly at the foramen of Monro) associated with subependymal calcified nodules virtually establishes the diagnosis. They will also be discussed with tuberous sclerosis in Chapter 10.

Oligodendrogliomas

These tumors represents 5–7% of primary intracranial tumors.[38] They usually occur in the adult and are uncommon in young children and the elderly. They commonly involve the centrum semiovale and rarely, the cerebellum. They rarely occur intraventricularly.[39] CT typically demonstrates a calcified unsharply marginated deep location mixed density tumor. The mixed density is due to calcification and cystic degeneration.[20] Prominent clumps of calcium are commonly seen and some form of calcification is seen by CT in up to 90% of oligodendrogliomas.[20] Low grade oligodendrogliomas do not contrast enhance and usually lack edema. The high grade tumors usually contrast enhance and often demonstrate surrounding edema. Ring contrast enhancement, periventricular tumor infiltration, and intratumoral hemorrhage may occur.[1]

MR may demonstrate a mixed and confusing intensity pattern due to the frequent tumor calcification and the occasional hemorrhage.[21,39] For this reason, CT may be more specific for the diagnosis (Fig. 5.25). MR may, however, depict more clearly the in-

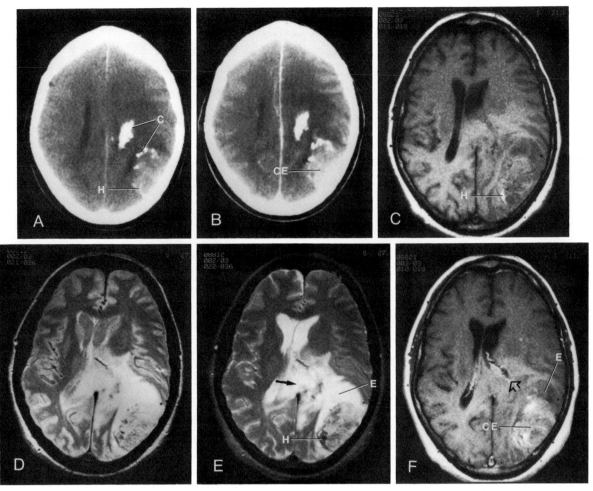

Figure 5.25. Oligodendroglioma with anaplastic astrocytoma portions. *Axial lateral ventricle noncontrast (A) and i.v. contrast (B) 37/100 CT scans. Same level SE 600/25 (C), SE 2800/30 (D), SE 2800/80 (E), and i.v. Gd-DTPA SE 600/25 (F) MR scans.*

The mass displaces and compresses the lateral ventricle atrium *(open arrow)*. Note the particulate and coalesced calcifications *(C)*. Contrast enhancement *(CE)* is seen by both the CT and MR tech-

nique. A small area of probable hemorrhage *(H)* is noted most likely representing intracellular methemoglobin. There is marked surrounding edema *(E)* that shows T1 hypointensity as well as proton density and T2 hyperintensity. Heterogeneous hyperintensity with slight expansion of the corpus callosum splenium *(closed arrow)* is thought to represent tumor invasion.

terface between tumor, edema, and adjacent normal parenchyma.

Ependymoma

This tumor is derived from the ependymal cell and is usually located in or adjacent to ventricles, frequently crossing the ventricle boundary. It represents approximately 6% of all intracranial gliomas. It occurs most frequently in children and young adults. The supratentorial ependymoma tends to occur more frequently in an older age group than does the infratentorial tumor.[3] Sixty percent[2] or greater[40] are located in the posterior fossa usually arising from the fourth ventricle and usually causing hydrocephalus (Fig. 5.26). Supratentorial ependymomas (Fig. 5.27) often cause some degree of hydrocephalus. Ependymomas demonstrate varying grades of malignancy similar to astrocytomas and oligodendro-

gliomas. The higher grade lesions have less distinct margins. Small foci of necrosis commonly occur.

CT demonstrates an isodense to slightly hyperdense, usually contrast-enhancing mass. Calcification is seen by CT in approximately 50% of lesions and tend to be of the multiple small punctate variety. Cystic portions are common in the supratentorial ependymomas and uncommon in the infratentorial locations.[40,41] Edema is usually seen in relation to the extraventricular portion.[1,3,20,40,41] Extension of posterior fossa ependymomas through the fourth ventricle foramina commonly occurs leading to further dissemination into the subarachnoid spaces.[3,20] Intravenous contrast enhancement may document subarachnoid dissemination.

MR orthogonal plane sections are particularly helpful for analysis of the relationship of intraventricular and parenchymal mass components. MR may be less specific for histological diagnosis due to the

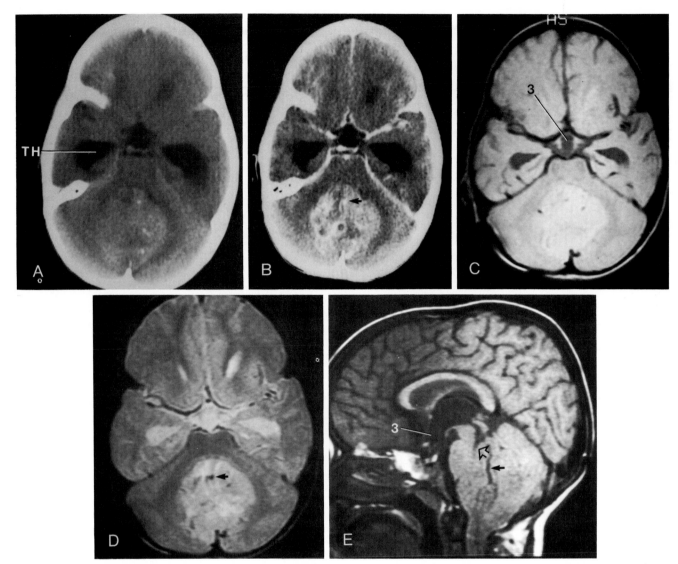

Figure 5.26. Fourth ventricle ependymoma. Axial fourth ventricle level noncontrat **(A)** and i.v. contrast **(B)** CT scans and SE 2000/20 **(C)** and 2000/80 **(D)** MR scans. Midsagittal 600/25 MR scan **(E)**. The large central posterior fossa mass has heterogeneous hyperdensity with calcifications **(A)** that are obscured by heterogeneous contrast enhancement **(B).** Heterogeneous T1 isointensity **(E)** and T2 hyperintensity **(D)** is noted. On the sagittal T1-weighted image, the pons is compressed and displaced anteriorly and tumor margins are unclear. The fourth ventricle *(open arrow)* is compressed and displaced anteriorly and upward. The cerebral aqueduct is dilated. There is signal void from a large abnormal tumor vessel *(arrows)*. Note the dilated lateral ventricle temporal horns *(TH)* and the third ventricle *(3)*.

CT greater specificity for calcium detection. MR i.v. contrast enhancement of subarachnoid dissemination is more accurate than CT contrast enhancement.

Subependymomas are benign, usually solid, slow-growing often asymptomatic subependymal nodular masses that usually extend into the ventricle. The subependymoma may grow quite large and may have identical MR appearances to ependymomas.[40]

Choroid Plexus Papilloma

This rare tumor of infants, children, and young adults arises from the epithelium of the choroid plexus. It occurs in the atrium of the lateral ventricle during the first decade of life and in the fourth ventricle during adolescence and early childhood.

Characteristic CT findings include smooth or irregular frond-like margination, hyperdensity, and marked intravenous contrast enhancement. Calcification is uncommon. Hydrocephalus develops with the lateral ventricle tumor due to presumed CSF overproduction and arachnoid granulation blockage by intermittent hemorrhage (Fig. 5.28A).[1,3,42] The fourth ventricle choroid plexus papilloma produces hydrocephalus by mechanical obstruction (Fig. 5.28B–E).

MR of choroid plexus papillomas may demonstrate the vascular pedicle and choroidal veins as well as the tumor vessels. The orthogonal plane imaging may better establish the choroidal intraventricular origin.

The choroid plexus carcinoma, a very rare tumor, is more aggressive than the papilloma variety. This

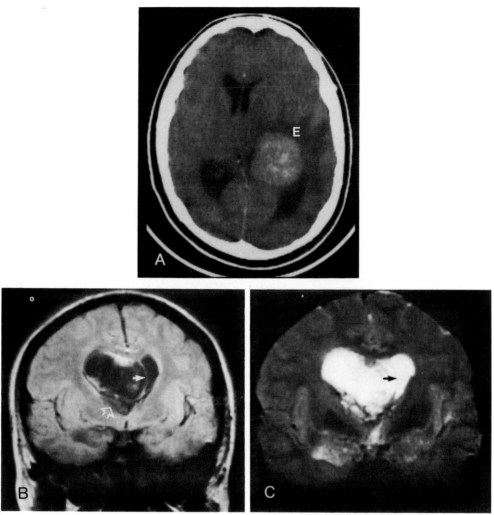

Figure 5.27.   Supratentorial ependymoma. A and **B-C** are different cases. **A,** *Lateral ventricle atrial-level i.v. contrast CT scan.* Heterogeneous enhancing smoothly contoured well-defined left lateral ventricle mass. Note the surrounding edema *(E)* indicating transependymal parenchymal invasion. The septum pellucidum and third ventricle are shifted to the right and there is entrapment of the left occipital horn. **B–C,** *Coronal pituitary-level SE 2000/20* **(B)** *and 2000/* 80 *(C) MR scans.* A large heterogeneous T1 hypointense and T2 hyperintense mass expands the right lateral ventricle and deforms and displaces the frontal horn of the left lateral ventricle *(closed arrows).* Abnormal blood vessels are identified within the tumor inferior portion *(open arrow).* This lower portion appears to have invaded the ependyma and expanded beyond the confines of the lateral ventricle.

latter tumor is more invasive, may be associated with cysts and edema, and has a variable contrast enhancement pattern.[3]

GANGLION CELL ORIGIN TUMORS

Medulloblastoma

Medulloblastoma is included in the ganglion cell section for convenience, even though there is some controversy concerning cell origin.[2] These common highly malignant cerebellar tumors of children and, occasionally, young adults constituted 17% of all pediatric intracranial tumors in Fitz's series.[3] They are characteristically midline tumors often arising in the vermian nodulus location that anteriorly compresses and invades the fourth ventricle. An off-midline location is not uncommon in the adult case. These tumors frequently spread via the subarachnoid space or beneath the ependyma.[4,44]

The lesion is usually fairly well margined by CT with characteristic near-homogeneous high density and near-homogeneous contrast enhancement. Calcification may occur in 25% of cases. Because medulloblastoma is so common, a calcified midline posterior fossa tumor in a child is more likely to be medulloblastoma than cerebellar astrocytoma or ependymoma.[3] The larger tumors are more likely to be cystic and may extend laterally. There is often a small amount of edema. Intratumoral hemorrhage is occasionally seen.[43] Hydrocephalus is common.[1,3] Intravenous contrast injection may demonstrate subarachnoid contrast enhancement of leptomeningeal tumor spread.

MR characteristically demonstrates a homogeneously well-circumscribed T1 hypointense and T2 hyperintense mass.[21] Intravenous gadolinium contrast enhances the tumor and associated leptomeningeal or subependymal tumor deposits, if present. MR orthogonal plane imaging provides sagittal sec-

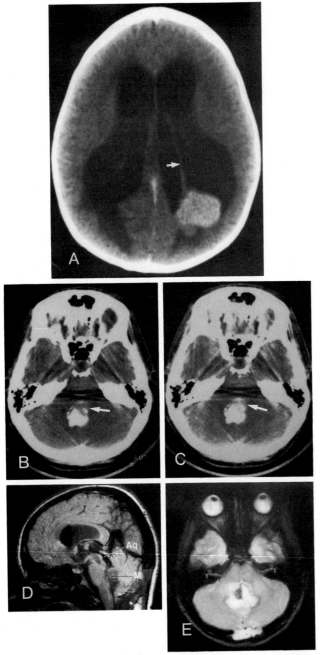

Figure 5.28. Choroid plexus papilloma. A and B–E are different cases. **A,** Axial ventricular-level i.v. contrast CT scan of a hydrocephalic infant. Note the homogeneously contrast-enhanced, sharply marginated, left atrial tumor, the prominent longitudinal vessel *(arrow)*, and the marked hydrocephalus. **B–E,** Calcified fourth ventricle choroid plexus papilloma. *Preoperative fourth ventricle-level axial noncontrast (B) and i.v. contrast (C) CT scans. Midline sagittal SE 2000/20 (D) and axial SE 2000/80 (E) MR scans.* Contrast enhancement of the uncalcified portion is noted *(arrow).* Postbiopsy MR scans demonstrate mixed intensity changes within a large fourth ventricle mass (M), which causes hydrocephalus with cerebral aqueduct dilatation *(Aq).* Note the aqueduct hypointensity compared to the lateral and third ventricles. This "flow-void" phenomenon is due to a combination of transmitted arterial pulsation and flow phenomena. Flow, in this case, is distally obstructed at the fourth ventricle. This case demonstrates that the aqueduct flow-void phenomenon is only a reliable indicator that the aqueduct itself is patent. There is a posterior surgical defect with a small pseudoencephalocele demonstrating T1 and T2 water-intensity. A moderate amount of air is present in the lateral ventricle frontal horns.

tions that are very useful in the posterior fossa (Fig. 5.29).

Primary Cerebral Neuroblastoma

The term "primary cerebral neuroblastoma" is often confused with the term "primitive neuroectodermal tumor." It is most likely a distinct subset of the latter. The primitive neuroectodermal group includes medulloblastoma, medulloepithelioma, neuroblastoma, spongioblastoma, ependymoblastoma and pineoblastoma. Primary cerebral neuroblastomas usually occur in children but may occur in adults. They are usually hemispheric, tend to be deep and may be primarily intraventricular (fig. 5.30)[45]. The tumors are characteristically large (7.4 cm mean diameter in Fitz's series) with an irregular contour. Calcification and cystic portions are very common and there may be hemorrhagic regions. Edema is usually disproportionately small compared to lesion size. Heterogeneous CT density and contrast enhancement of the solid portion is common. MR characteristics vary according to the degree of hemorrhage, cyst formation, vascularity and calcification. Subarachnoid tumor dissemination is common and may occur in 50% of cases. Prognosis is poor due to a tendency for subarachnoid dissemination and local postoperative recurrence[1,3,45].

Ganglioglioma

Intracerebral gangliogliomas are rare benign brain tumors occurring in all age groups but most commonly in children and young adults. In Fitz's series of 264 pediatric tumor cases, ganglioglioma accounted for 3% of tumors.[3] Histologically, they contain both mature ganglion cells and supporting glial origin cells. Malignant change with degeneration into a glioma is unusual. Most gangliogliomas are located in the cerebral hemispheres with the greatest proportion found in the temporal lobes. They may occur in the posterior fossa. CT characteristics are quite variable. Calcification, cystic areas of isodensity or hypodensity, and contrast enhancement are common.[46]

MENINGIOMA

Meningiomas originate from arachnoid cells with the exception of the rare intraventricular meningioma that arises from pia-arachnoid rests. The common extra-axial meningioma represents approximately 15% of all primary intracranial neoplasms. They occur principally in the middle-aged and elderly population and are rarely found in children. They occur in women approximately twice as frequently as in men. In a reported series, 23% of children with meningioma had neurofibromatosis.[47] Multiple meningiomas may occur, particularly in patients with neurofibromatosis. There is considerable controversy concerning the nature of the so-called malignant meningioma. A large angioblastic compo-

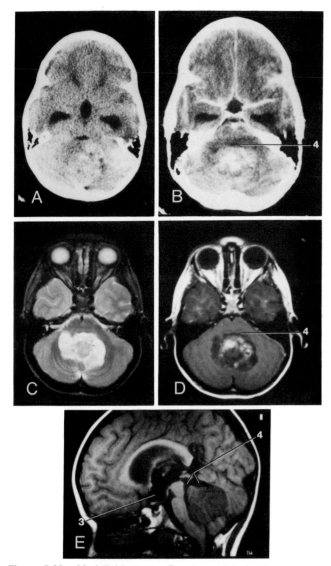

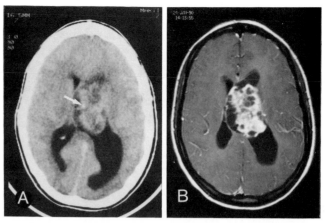

Figure 5.30.   Primary cerebral neuroblastoma. *Axial ventricular level noncontrast **(A)** 35/80 CT scan and i.v. contrast flow compensation SE 800/22 **(B)** MR scan. The predominantly intraventricular multicystic tumor has a small calcification (arrow) and markedly contrast-enhances. There was virtually no detectable edema. The irregular left lateral margination indicates parenchymal infiltration. No intratumoral hemorrhage was detected. The calcification was only detectable on the noncontrast CT scan. It was helpful for suggesting the correct diagnosis.*

Figure 5.29.   Medulloblastoma. *Fourth ventricle level noncontrast **(A)** and i.v. contrast **(B)** CT scans. Same level SE 3008/90 noncontrast pulse-gated **(C)** and 800/22 iv contrast **(D)** mast MR scans. Midsagittal SE 600/15 MR scan **(E)**. A large mixed-density T1 gray matter-hypointense T2 heterogeneous hyperintense contrast-enhancing mass invades, distends, obstructs and markedly displaces the fourth ventricle (4). There is marked brainstem compression and distortion. The third ventricle (3) and aqueduct of Sylvius are markedly dilated.*

nent (including imaging evidence of an abnormal draining vein, heterogeneity of tumor densities or contrast enhancement, irregular tumor margins, and marked surrounding edema) tend to be associated with more aggressive tumors.[27] Rarely (<0.1%) meningiomas may metastasize. Most investigators believe that neither the histological pattern, local aggressiveness, size, nor tumor location are useful characteristics to predict metastatic potential.[2,48] Tumor consistency (hard or soft) may have considerable importance for surgical planning. CT attenuation values over 100 H (Fig. 5.31) suggest "hard" tumor.[12]

The most common locations of the extraventricular lesions are the cerebral convexities both laterally and along the falx (Fig. 5.8), the sphenoid ridge, the juxtasellar region (Fig. 5.32), the posterior fossa (Fig. 5.33), and the olfactory groove. Multiple meningiomas occasionally occur (Fig. 5.3). They occur in unusual locations in the pediatric age group such as intraventricular and optic nerve sheath. The characteristic broad-based dural attachment may become quite large and the adjacent bone may become hyperostotic. The rare intraventricular tumor is usually located in the lateral ventricle (Fig. 5.34).

MR characteristics of meningiomas include a smoothly marginated dural based mass with T1 and T2 gray matter-isointensity. Because of the decreased degree of MR contrast between the meningioma and adjacent normal brain, Gd-DTPA effectively demonstrates detail that may be lacking on the noncontrast MR.[6] Gd-DTPA i.v. contrast enhancement of meningiomas differs from that of i.v. contrast CT due primarily to the tumor arterial signal void. The meningioma characteristically markedly contrast enhances with a mildly heterogeneous pattern. The heterogeneous tumor texture results from tumor vascularity, calcifications, and occasional cystic foci. An interface between meningioma and brain consisting of a CSF cleft and a vascular rim is usually present. Large tumors cause arcuate displacement and compression of adjacent gyri. Edema is usually present and can be differentiated from tumor by both the CT and MR i.v. contrast methods and by analysis of noncontrast CT and MR signals. The meningeal vascular pedicle and other vascular structures can be identified. Venous sinus invasion is better demonstrated by MR than CT.[8] Extra-axial tumors, particularly small tumors, may be difficult to detect by MR

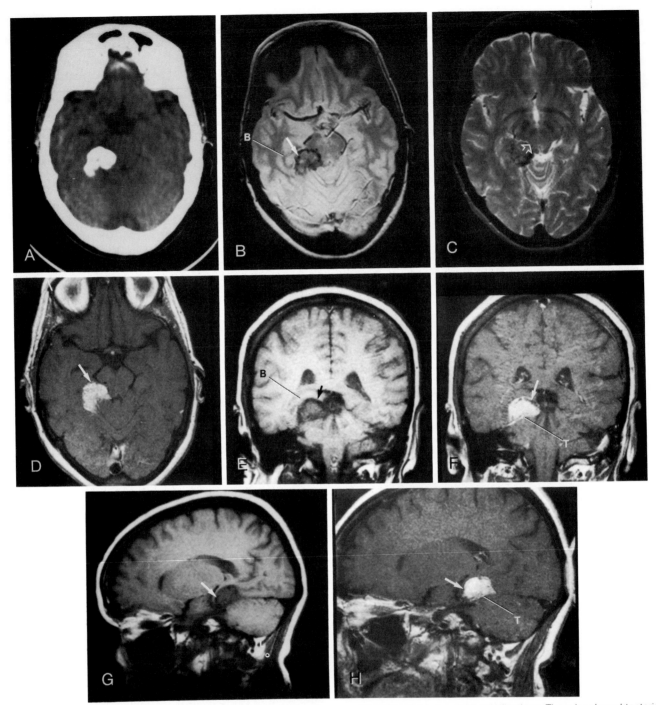

Figure 5.31. Calcified tentorial margin meningioma. *Axial mid-brain-level noncontrast CT Scan **(A)**. Midbrain level SE 2800/30 **(B)**, SE 2800/80 **(C)**, and i.v. Gd-DTPA SE 600/25 injection **(D)** MR scans. Coronal SE 600/25 noncontrast **(E)** and contrast **(F)** MR scans. Sagittal SE 600/25 noncontrast **(G)** and contrast **(H)** MR scans.*

CT demonstrates marked calcification. MR demonstrates T1 **(G)** and T2 **(C)** gray matter-isointensity. Otherwise-homogeneous MR contrast enhancement is interrupted by artery signal void *(closed ar-*

rows) and possibly by small calcifications. There is a broad tentorial tumor base *(T)*. The tumor compresses and deforms the midbrain tegmentum *(open arrow)* and buckles the temporal white matter *(B)*. The tumor "cleft" seen in this case is probably caused by vascular signal void.

Intravenous CT contrast, in this case, failed to demonstrate enhancement. Despite the marked CT calcification, the MR failed to demonstrate calcium signal-void effects.

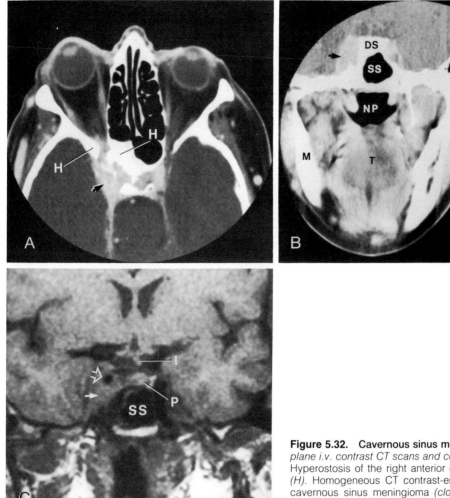

Figure 5.32.   Cavernous sinus meningioma. *Axial **(A)** and coronal **(B)** pituitary plane i.v. contrast CT scans and coronal pituitary plane SE 600/25 MR scan **(C)**.* Hyperostosis of the right anterior clinoid process and the planum sphenoidale *(H).* Homogeneous CT contrast-enhancing and MR T1 gray matter-isointense cavernous sinus meningioma *(closed arrows).* Encased right cavernous segment internal carotid artery *(open arrow).* Displaced infundibular stalk *(I).* Sphenoid sinus *(SS).* Pituitary gland *(P).* Nasopharynx *(NP).*

without i.v. contrast enhancement. These lesions are close to the brain periphery and are subject to partial volume averaging. They are relatively isointense and have varying degrees of vascularity and calcification that can result in unpredictable intensity characteristics.[16,18,49] Gd-DTPA contrast injection is particularly helpful for detection of these small lesions.

CT characteristically demonstrates smooth tumor margination with homogeneous high density and homogeneous contrast enhancement. Low density or cystic meningiomas are uncommon. Calcification is very common ranging from diffuse to punctate to large regions. Punctate and large clump calcification is seen in up to 20% of cases. Peritumoral hypodensity is common and represents edema and, possibly, adjacent subarachnoid space enlargement.[32] Hemorrhage into a meningioma is a rare event. Preservation of the gray-white matter interface and compression of adjacent edematous white matter "buckling" is usually seen.[33] An aggressive meningioma may demon-

strate CT irregularity of contour, heterogeneity of density and contrast enhancement, and abnormal draining veins.

MR i.v. contrast technique has definite advantages compared to i.v. contrast CT technique due to the conspicuity of the hyperintense contrast-enhanced tumor adjacent to signal void bone.

NERVE SHEATH TUMORS

Schwannomas and neurofibromas are nerve sheath tumors which are derived from Schwann cells and from fibroblasts, respectively. The terms schwannoma, neurofibroma, neurolemoma, and neuroma are often used interchangeably despite histological differences. The sensory nerves are usually involved and the vast majority of these tumors affect the eighth cranial nerve. The next most common nerve affected is the fifth cranial nerve. Bilateral eighth nerve tumors as well as tumors of the vagus and glossopharyngeal nerves and of motor roots occur with von Recklinghausen's disease.[2] A full discussion of these

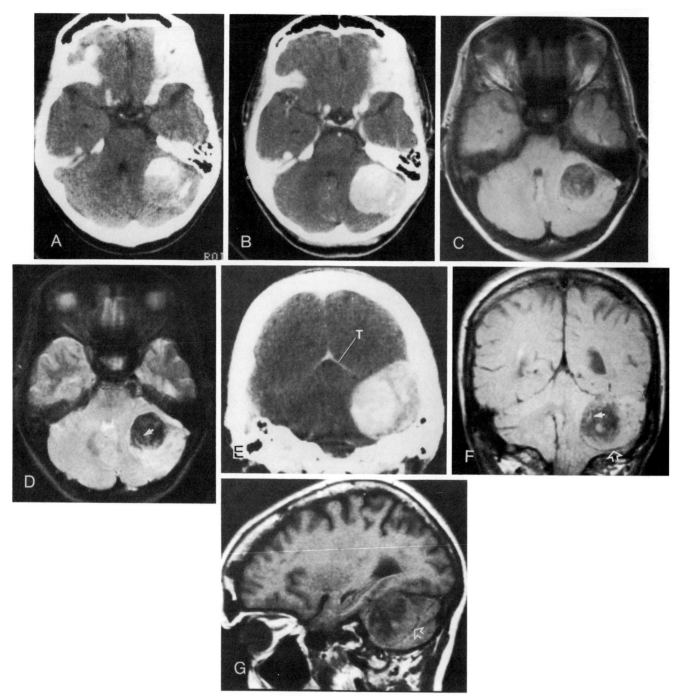

Figure 5.33. Tentorial meningioma. *Axial fourth ventricle-level noncontrast* **(A)** *and i.v. contrast* **(B)** *CT scans compared to SE 2000/ 20* **(C)** *and 2000/80* **(D)** *MR scans. Coronal i.v. contrast CT scan* **(E)** *compared to coronal SE 600/25 MR scan* **(F)**. *Sagittal 600/25 CT scan through the tumor* **(G)**. The heterogeneous density meningioma is more heavily calcified anteriorly and there is marked homogeneous contrast enhancement of less calcified portions **(A–B)**. Note prominent tumor vessels *(closed arrows)*. MR hypointensity appears to correlate with both calcification and vascularity. Note also the marginal tumor vessels producing a ''cleft'' along portions of the tumor perimeter *(open arrows)*. **E** shows the tumor extending through the tentorium *(T)*, a fact not easily appreciated by noncontrast MR **(F–G)**. Note the meningioma broad dural base on multiple images.

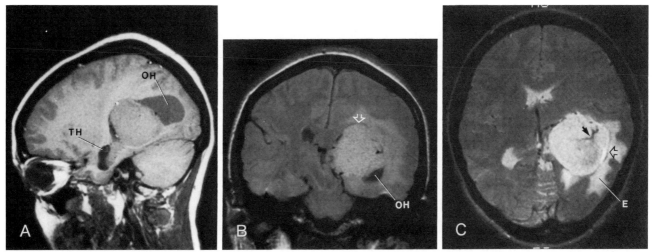

Figure 5.34. Intraventricular meningioma. *Sagittal lateral ventricle atrial-level SE 600/25 **(A)**, coronal SE 2000/20 **(B)**, and axial 2000/80 **(C)** MR scans.* A T1 gray-matter-isointense, large, smoothly marginated, relatively homogeneous intraventricular mass expands the lateral ventricle and obstructs its occipital and temporal horns. Prominent tortuous vessels are seen within the tumor *(closed arrow)*. A partial perimeter "cleft" is noted *(open arrow)*. There is surrounding focal periventricular edema *(E)*. The edema includes ependymoma in the differential diagnosis. Note the trapped left temporal *(TH)* and occipital *(OH)* horns.

tumors is found in Chapter 12. Intracranial malignant schwannomas are very rare destructive lesions that may occur in the petrous area of patients with von Recklinghausen's disease.

PINEAL REGION TUMORS

These tumors are classified into three major groups[2]:

1. Germ cell origin
   Germinoma and embryonal cell carcinoma
   Teratoma
2. Tumors of pineal cell origin
   Pineocytoma
   Pineoblastoma
3. Other tumors

Together, these rare tumors represent 0.4–1.0% of all intracranial tumors. Over 50% are germinomas and less than 25% are of pineal cell origin. Pineal region teratomas and germinomas occur almost exclusively in men. Suprasellar germinomas are more likely to occur in women and they will be discussed in Chapter 11. Pineal cell origin tumors have no sex predominance. Germinomas and embryonal cell carcinomas occur in the 10- to 25-year-old group. Gliomas, meningiomas, and metastases can also be found in this region.[50] Malignant germinal cell and pineal origin tumors have a tendency for subarachnoid metastases. Pineal region tumors often produce hydrocephalus due to compression or invasion of the aqueduct and posterior third ventricle.

CT pineal region tumor characteristics are described in an excellent review of 60 histologically proven cases.[51] CT of germinomas shows characteristically hyperdense areas with tumoral coarse nodular calcification and moderate to marked contrast enhancement. The original pineal gland calcification within germinomas appears to be engulfed by the tumor (Fig. 5.35). These tumors are histologically malignant and invade the third ventricle margins and the subarachnoid space. Contrast enhancement of the tumor "seeding" is characteristic. Benign teratomas are sharply marginated, reveal areas of mixed calcium and fat density, and do not prominently contrast enhance. Intracranial teratomas arising outside of the pineal region are rare. The teratoma may rupture resulting in arachnoid and/or ventricular fatty densities and possible resultant chemical meningitis and/or ventriculitis. Pineocytomas showed hypodense to hyperdense regions with relatively homogeneous contrast enhancement. Pineoblastomas tend to be hyperdense without calcification. They may sometimes be distinguished from the pineocytoma by a low density noncontrast-enhancing center and they are usually invasive. Like the germinoma, they may spread to the ventricles and subarachnoid space. Pineal region gliomas, like those elsewhere, tend to be hypodense or isodense and contrast enhance sometimes producing a ring of enhancement. The glioma tends to displace pineal calcification rather than engulf it. Some of these tumors likely arise from the quadrigeminal plate and the posterior third ventricle. Meningiomas, like those elsewhere demonstrate a tentorial attachment and other meningioma CT characteristics.[51] Marginal irregularity and poor definition of a pineal region tumor favors a malignant lesion.

MR characteristics of germinomas include irregularity of contour, T1 isointensity and T2 hyperintensity relative to gray matter, local mass effect, and hydrocephalus. The sagittal image is particularly

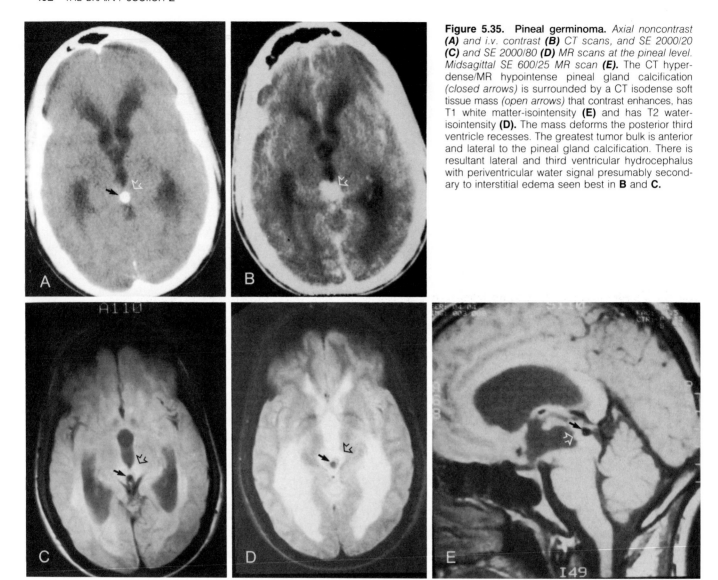

Figure 5.35.   Pineal germinoma. *Axial noncontrast* **(A)** *and i.v. contrast* **(B)** *CT scans, and SE 2000/20* **(C)** *and SE 2000/80* **(D)** *MR scans at the pineal level. Midsagittal SE 600/25 MR scan* **(E).** *The CT hyperdense/MR hypointense pineal gland calcification (closed arrows) is surrounded by a CT isodense soft tissue mass (open arrows) that contrast enhances, has T1 white matter-isointensity* **(E)** *and has T2 water-isointensity* **(D).** *The mass deforms the posterior third ventricle recesses. The greatest tumor bulk is anterior and lateral to the pineal gland calcification. There is resultant lateral and third ventricular hydrocephalus with periventricular water signal presumably secondary to interstitial edema seen best in* **B** *and* **C.**

useful for pineal region examination due to the relationships of the pineal gland, the colliculi, the splenium, third ventricle, and vein of Galen. MR lacks specificity for establishing the etiology of the detected mass as compared to CT due to the accuracy of CT for calcium and fat detection.[52]

Pineal cysts (Fig. 4.32, p. 101) can be confused with pineal tumors. The MR appearance of these cysts includes thin, smooth wall, homogeneous T1 hypointensity and T2 hyperintensity, and possible glandular enlargement (>10 mm). They may produce mass effect and hydrocephalus if they attain sufficient size.[53]

HEMANGIOBLASTOMAS

These tumors usually arise in the cerebellum of young and middle-aged adults. They occur predominantly in men and are the most common primary cerebellar tumors of the adult. Hemangioblastomas are most commonly located in the paramedian cerebellar hemisphere but may have a more lateral or a central location. The tumors are characterized by varying proportions of very vascular solid (often a mural nodule) and cystic components. The tumors extend into the fourth ventricle and hydrocephalus is common. It is a primary feature of Hippel-Lindau syndrome although only a minority of these tumors are associated with the syndrome.[54]

CT of hemangioblastomas shows smooth margination. At least one-half (50%) of the lesions are predominantly cystic. There is usually contrast enhancement that is confined to the capsule and solid portion. Solid tumors are usually of heterogeneous density with homogeneous contrast enhancement. They lack calcification.[44,54]

The several cases that we have seen by MR demonstrate mixed T1 and T2 intensities resulting from combined cystic, highly vascular, and solid components. There is usually sharp margination of a clearly intra-axial tumor and flow-void phenomenon of abnormally dilated vessels (Fig. 5.36).

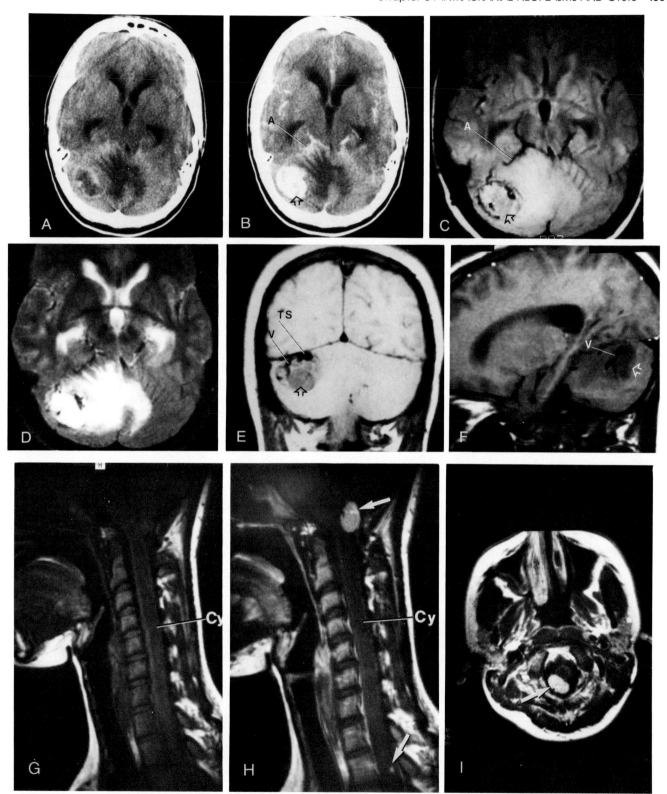

Figure 5.36. Cerebellar and spinal hemangioblastomas. **(A-F)** *Axial quadrigeminal plate-level noncontrast **(A)** and i.v. contrast **(B)** CT scans. Same level axial SE 2000/20 **(C)** and SE 2000/80 **(D)** MR scans. Coronal SE 2000/20 **(E)** and sagittal SE 600/25 **(F)** MR scans.* Note the relatively round, smoothly marginated, right superior cerebellar hemisphere CT hypodense **(A)** contrast-enhancing **(B)** mostly solid and partially cystic *(open arrows)* mass with surrounding feeding arteries arising from the marginal branch of the superior cerebellar artery *(A)*. *Venous (V) drainage **(F)** is to the right transverse sinus (TS). A large amount of surrounding edema is best differentiated from the tumor by contrast CT and "proton density" **(C** and **E)** MR.

Figure 5.36. **(G-I)** *Same patient 3 years later. SE 380/15 noncontrast **(G)** and i.v. contrast **(H)** midsagittal cervical and SE 600/15 axial i.v. contrast foramen magnum level **(I)** MR scans.* There is a large spinal cord cyst (Cy) and uniform contrast enhancement of solid portions (closed arrows).

Tumors Arising from Embryonal Remnants or Structural Duplications

This group of tumors includes arachnoid cysts, epidermoid and dermoid tumors, colloid cysts, lipomas, teratomas, and craniopharyngiomas. Craniopharyngiomas will be discussed in Chapter 11 with sella and juxtasellar lesions. Teratomas have already been discussed in the pineal tumor category of this chapter. The majority of lipomas are in the corpus callosum and will be discussed in Chapter 9 with congenital anomalous conditions.

ARACHNOID CYSTS

These are included here because of their mass effect. They are not neoplasms. They probably originate from duplication or splitting of the arachnoid membrane. They constitute approximately 1% of all intracranial space-occupying lesions. Some arachnoid cysts may develop after trauma or after adhesive arachnoiditis secondary to infection or hemorrhage. They occur in infants, children, and adults. The middle cranial fossa is the most common location and is often expanded (Fig. 5.7). Other locations include the posterior fossa, suprasellar, quadrigeminal (Fig. 5.37), and convexity locations. The posterior fossa cysts occur predominantly behind the cerebellum. Hemorrhage, usually after trauma, may complicate an arachnoid cyst.[1,10]

CT demonstrates sharply marginated homogeneous water-density masses. They lack calcification, contrast enhancement, and fat. The posterior margin of the middle fossa cyst has a characteristic flat margin oriented in the coronal plane (Fig. 5.7). Suprasellar arachnoid cysts cause considerable cisternal expansion and characteristically have marked undulation of contour.[11]

Intrathecal iohexol or iopamidol cisternography may be of assistance for diagnosis as well as surgical planning, e.g., communication of a giant cisterna magna with the fourth ventricle and subarachnoid space without hydrocephalus excludes an obstructing arachnoid cyst. MR intensity analysis may also help in the interpretation of CSF dynamics. For example, signal void may serve as an indicator of flow or communication[11,22,23] and signal hyperintensity may indicate increased protein content due to trapping and lack of communication.

MR of arachnoid cysts demonstrates a typically located smoothly marginated mass with homogeneous T1 and T2 water-isointense signal.[10]

EPENDYMAL CYSTS

These rare lesions occasionally are incidentally discovered by MR (Fig. 5.38). MR can demonstrate the cyst wall separating isointense cystic fluid from ventricular CSF.

EPIDERMOID AND DERMOID TUMORS

These tumors (sometimes called "cysts") are rare intracranially and common when confined to the skull. Occasionally, a lesion of the skull vault extends into the calvarium (Fig. 13.15). Intracranial epidermoid and dermoid tumors account for less that 1% of intracranial tumors. They occur more commonly in men than in women.[1]

The epidermoid tumors occurs with much greater frequency and is more common in the middle-aged adult. The dermoid tumors usually becomes symptomatic in the first decade. The epidermoid tumor is sometimes called a cholesteatoma because of its waxy cellular debris and cholesterol crystals. Dermoid tumors frequently contain calcium and fat. Because of the rarity of the dermoid tumor and the CT similarities of both rare lesions, the two will be discussed together. The CP angle and the parapituitary loca-

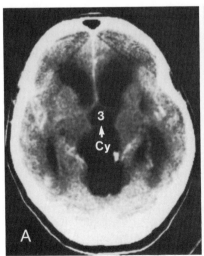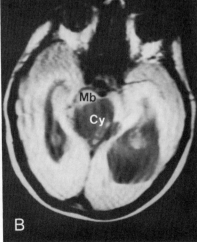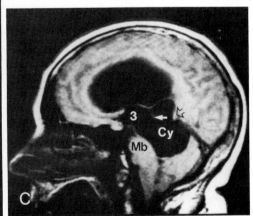

Figure 5.37. Quadrigeminal cistern arachnoid cyst. *Axial CT scan at foramen of Monro level (A). Axial SE 2000/20 MR scan at midbrain level (B). Midsagittal SE 600/25 MR scan (C).* The large posterior fossa cyst *(Cy)* expands the quadrigeminal plate cistern, markedly forward displaces and deforms the midbrain *(Mb)*, anteriorly displaces and deforms *(closed arrow)* the third ventricle *(3)*, and markedly deforms the cerebellum. It extends above the tentorium *(open arrow)*.

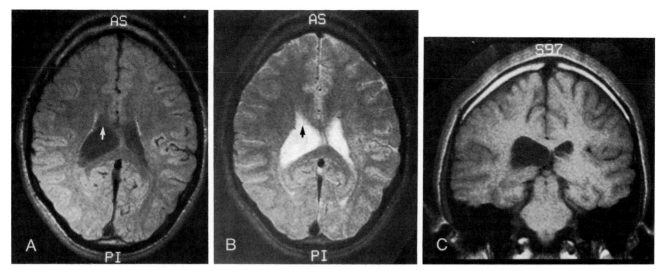

Figure 5.38. Intraventricular cyst (not proven). *Axial ventricular body SE 2000/20* **(A)** *and 2000/80* **(B)**, *and coronal SE 600/25* **(C)** *MR sections.* The water-isodense cyst expands the lateral ventricle atrium and its anterior margin is identified bulging into the ventricle body (arrows).

tions are the most common (Fig. 5.39). These tumors extend along the subarachnoid spaces displacing and encasing structures. Lateral and fourth ventricular locations are rare (Fig. 5.40). There is usually lack of hydrocephalus despite a seemingly strategic tumor location that otherwise might cause ventricular obstruction. They often have frond-like or cauliflower-like contours. The tumor capsule may occasionally rupture reducing the size of the mass and causing "chemical meningitis" (Fig. 5.41).[1,2,9]

CT characteristics of epidermoid tumors include homogeneous water density and smooth or markedly irregular (frond-like) contours which can be demonstrated by positive contrast cisternography (Fig. 5.40). Occasionally, dermoid tumors may demonstrate fat density and calcification. Rarely, the lesion may be hyperdense. These tumors lack hemorrhage, edema, and contrast enhancement. An area (collar) of enlarged subarachnoid space commonly surrounds the tumor.[19]

MR of epidermoid and dermoid lesions has not received the extensive attention in the literature that CT has. In our experience and that of others,[21] epidermoid tumors characteristically demonstrate T1 hypointensity and T2 hyperintensity, irregular contour, and sharp margination. The MR orthogonal plane investigation and high tissue contrast offers particular advantage for investigation of lesions of the fourth ventricle and perimesencephalic cisterns. A lipid-containing dermoid cyst may demonstrate a fat signal (Fig. 5.41).[21]

COLLOID CYSTS

Colloid cysts are probably malformations arising from tissues of the anterior third ventricle-foramen of Monro region. They appear in early adulthood. The smoothly marginated, round, thin-walled, olive-sized mass is filled with gelatinous material. The classic clinical presentation is intermittent headaches, ataxia, fainting spells, and personality changes.[1]

CT of colloid cyst demonstrates a smooth-walled homogeneously hyperdense olive-sized mass at the foramen of Monro with symmetrical widening of the septum pellucidum and hydrocephalus. The hyperdensity is probably caused by a combination of colloid particles within cyst mucin, calcium, and hemosiderin. They may occasionally be hypodense. There is usually a faint degree of diffuse contrast enhancement. Axial and coronal CT images are recommended in order to be certain of the classical appearance in perpendicular planes (Fig. 5.42).[1,55]

MR has been said to be superior to CT for diagnosis of colloid cyst.[10] Since CT is almost pathognomonic for this lesion, we feel that time will tell whether MR is clearly superior. Of course, a sagittal section is quite helpful. These lesions are also smoothly marginated on MR scans. The colloid cyst MR signal tends to be heterogeneous. T1 signal hyperintensity has been reported with high cholesterol concentration within the cyst.[56]

Primary Brain Tumors of Non-neurogenic Origin—Lymphoma

Included in the term "primary lymphoma" is malignant lymphoma, round cell sarcoma, and reticulum cell sarcoma. Primary lymphoma is a rare brain tumor accounting for less than 1% of primary brain tumors but is likely increasing in frequency. Patients with drug-induced immunosuppression are more susceptible to developing this tumor and it also occurs in AIDS patients. The most frequent tumor locations are the basal ganglia, thalamus, and corpus callosum. Multiple lesions are seen in up to 43% of patients. This tumor can also spread along the ventricular margins.

CT characteristics of primary cerebral lymphoma include fairly smooth margination, isodensity to slight

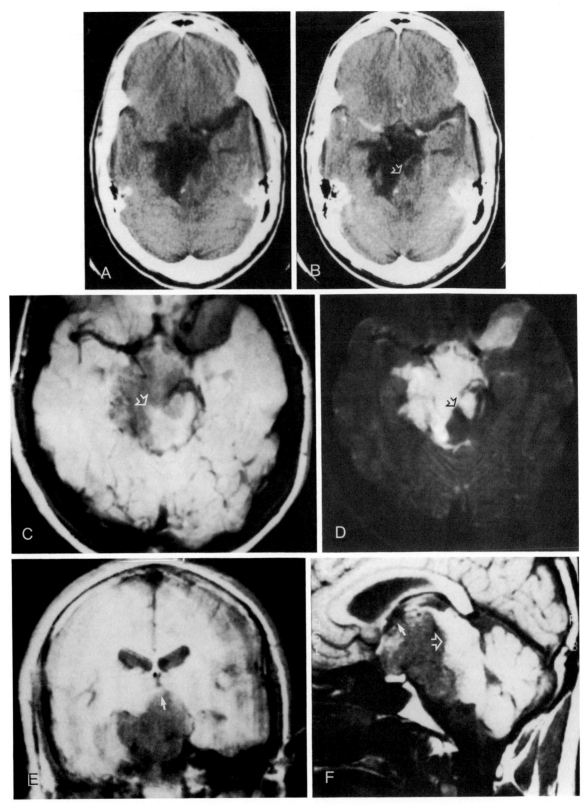

Figure 5.39. Epidermoid tumor. *Midbrain-chiasmatic cistern level noncontrast (A) and i.v. contrast (B) CT sections. Same level SE 2000/ 20 (C) and 2000/80 (D) MR sections. Coronal (E) and midsagittal interpeduncular fossa-level (F) SE 600/25 MR sections. The cauliflower-like mass is CT water-isodense. It is MR slightly T1 water-* hyperintense **(E** and **F)** and T2 water-isointense **(D).** The mass fills the chiasmatic cistern. It compresses, deforms, and posteriorly displaces the midbrain *(open arrows).* There is elevation distortion and compression of the third ventricle *(closed arrows).*

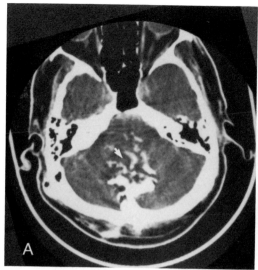

Figure 5.40.   Fourth ventricle epidermoid tumor. *Intrathecal x-ray contrast fourth ventricle-level axial CT cisternogram **(A)**. Chiasmatic cistern level **(B)**.* Between the water-isodense tumor fronds *(solid arrow)* are hyperdense contrast collections. The mass markedly expands the fourth ventricle **(A)** and extends through the fourth ventri-cle into the chiasmatic cistern *(open arrow)* to displace and deform the midbrain tectum anteriorly. Note the contrast-filled dilated lateral ventricle temporal horns, perimesencephalic cisterns, and chiasmatic cistern.

hyperdensity with homogeneous contrast enhancement (Fig. 5.43). Peritumoral edema is common. The lesions lack calcification. Hemorrhage and cavitation or central necrosis are uncommon.[1,21]

Leptomeningeal Infiltration by Non-neurogenic Origin Tumors

The most common form of intracranial involvement by leukemia and lymphoma is leptomeningeal infiltration.[20] Up to 10% of patients with acute leukemia develop CNS involvement, usually in the form of meningeal infiltration.[20] Meningeal lymphoma may present as a mass that is difficult to distinguish from a meningioma by CT technique. Rarely, patients with differing types of leukemia may develop a leukemic parenchymal mass (chloroma).[1] CT of leukemic and lymphomatous meningitis with i.v. contrast injection may demonstrate enhancement of cisterns, fissures, and sulci. MR i.v. Gd-DTPA is a more dependable diagnostic method. Chloromas usually uniformly contrast enhance by the CT technique.[1]

Metastatic Brain Tumors

Hematogenous metastasis to the brain from breast and lung carcinoma and malignant melanoma are the most frequent parenchymal secondary brain tu-

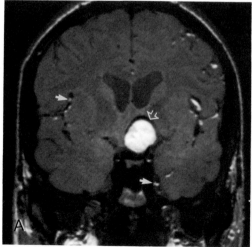
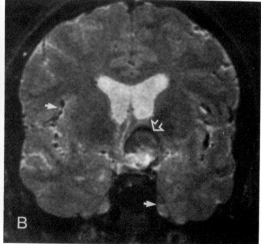

Figure 5.41.   Dermoid cyst rupture (postoperative). *Coronal chiasmatic cistern level SE 2000/20 **(A)** and SE 2000/80 **(B)** MR sections.* The chiasmatic cistern-interpeduncular fossa T1 and T2 fat-isointense mass with a hypointense chemical shift artifact superior rim *(open arrows)* is noted. Also seen are multiple punctate fat T1/T2 isointense subarachnoid deposits *(closed arrows)*. Note: We do not have a CT scan of this case. What is interpreted as chemical shift artifact could represent a superior calcified rim. CT could be helpful in this case due to characteristic attenuation values of fat and calcium.

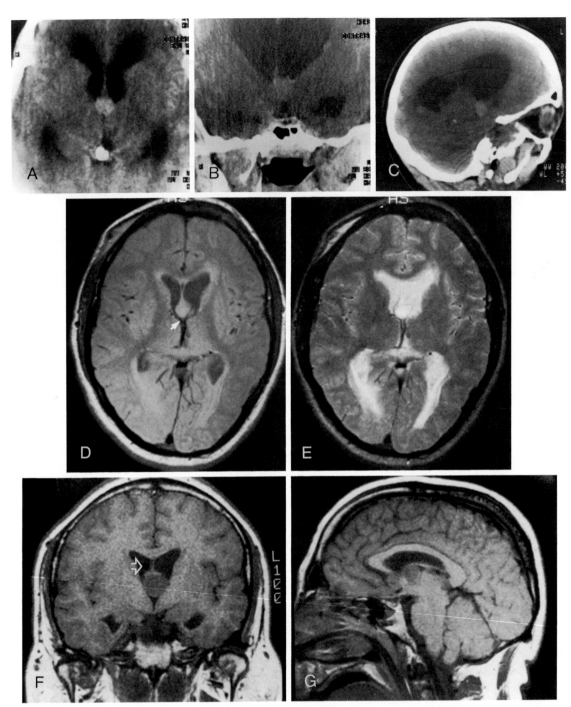

Figure 5.42.   Colloid cyst. *A–C* and *D–G* are different cases. Axial *i.v. contrast 42/75 (A), direct coronal i.v. contrast 42/200 (B), and direct sagittal 51/200 (C) foramen of Monro-level CT sections. Axial SE 2000/20 (D), SE 2000/80 (E), and coronal (F) and sagittal (G) 600/25 foramen of Monro-level MR sections.* The CT homogeneous hyperdense **(A and **B),** MR T1 gray-matter isointense **(F** and **G)** and T2 water-isointense **(E)** mass is midline and separates the foramina of Monro and thalamostriate veins *(closed arrow).* It is round and smoothly marginated. There is hydrocephalus more marked in *case A–C* than in *case D–G.* A ventricular shunt tube is seen on **F** *(open arrow)* explaining lack of marked hydrocephalus. *Note:* there is still evidence of periventricular edema from hydrocephalus before the recent shunt **(D** and **E).**

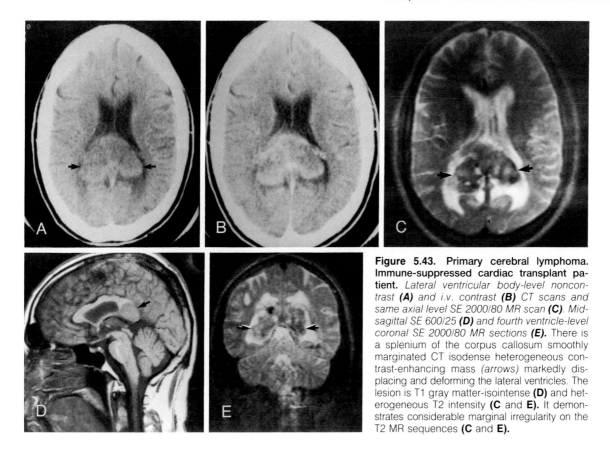

Figure 5.43. Primary cerebral lymphoma. Immune-suppressed cardiac transplant patient. *Lateral ventricular body-level noncontrast (A) and i.v. contrast (B) CT scans and same axial level SE 2000/80 MR scan (C). Midsagittal SE 600/25 (D) and fourth ventricle-level coronal SE 2000/80 MR sections (E).* There is a splenium of the corpus callosum smoothly marginated CT isodense heterogeneous contrast-enhancing mass *(arrows)* markedly displacing and deforming the lateral ventricles. The lesion is T1 gray matter-isointense **(D)** and heterogeneous T2 intensity **(C** and **E)**. It demonstrates considerable marginal irregularity on the T2 MR sequences **(C** and **E)**.

mors. Intra-axial brain metastasis often occurs at the cortical-white matter junction, however, deep metastases are common and parenchyma metastases anywhere in the neural axis occur. The most common intra-axial cerebellar tumor in the adult is a metastasis.

Metastatic tumor growth may simply present as an increase of tumor mass or may infiltrate the periventricular tissues, leptomeninges, or dura. CSF "seeding" of the subarachnoid space produces tumor implants in the cerebral and spinal subarachnoid spaces. Direct tumor growth and infiltration into the ependymal-subependymal and the leptomeningeal-dural tissues is occasionally seen with malignant melanoma, breast, and lung metastasis. Leukemias and lymphomas may infiltrate leptomeningeal and dural tissues. Primary brain tumors such as germinomas and medulloblastomas cause spinal and cerebral subarachnoid implantation "seeding."[1,2,4] These patients may present with symptoms suggestive of meningitis (carcinomatous meningitis).

Multiplicity of lesions, contrast enhancement, and associated edema are well-known CT characteristics of metastases. In our experience, however, single metastases, even of large size, are common. The lesions usually lack sharp margination. Contrast enhancement is usually quite marked and may be ho-

mogeneous, heterogeneous, or ring-like (Figs. 3.21, 5.2, and 5.44). The lesion density before i.v. contrast varies and is usually nonspecific. Malignant melanoma and adenocarcinoma metastases commonly have higher attenuation values (Fig. 5.45). Hemorrhage into brain metastases commonly occurs particularly with melanoma (Fig. 5.15). The intratumoral hemorrhage explains, at least in part, the high CT density of metastatic melanoma.[57] Rarely, a CT hypodense brain tumor may become isointense after contrast injection. Calcification is occasionally seen by CT in brain metastasis particularly those of colonic origin.[1,58]

Contrast CT of dural-leptomeningeal infiltration may demonstrate periventricular, meningeal, cortical, dural, or cisternal enhancement (Figs. 5.4 and 5.5). Hydrocephalus may be the only CT finding in patients with carcinomatous meningitis.[4]

We have found MR very accurate for detecting metastases. MR with i.v. contrast injection has become the imaging method of choice for parenchymal, leptomeningeal-dural, subependymal-ependymal, and cisternal-subarachnoid metastasis. The combined high detectability of paramagnetic contrast agents and bone signal void are the basis for reliance upon the MR imaging technique. Whether protocols for MR contrast investigation of brain tumor will have to in-

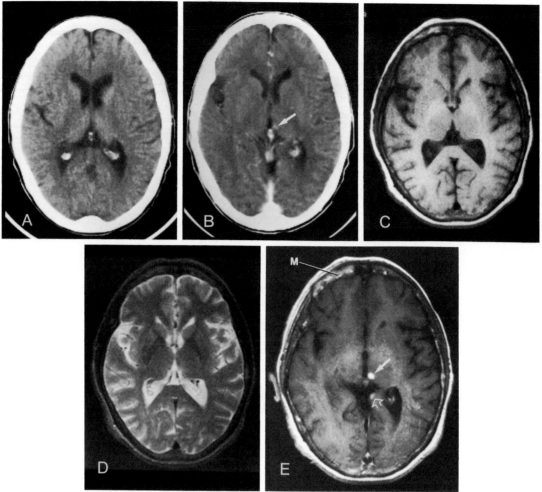

Figure 5.44. Cerebral breast carcinoma metastasis. Use of i.v. CT and MR contrast agents. *Axial noncontrast (A) and i.v. contrast (B) 35/100 CT scans. Axial SE 600/25 (C), SE 2800/80 (D) noncontrast, and i.v. SE 600/25 Gd-DTPA contrast (E) MR scans.* The left pulvinar metastasis *(closed arrow)* is seen only by contrast CT and contrast MR. It is far more conspicuous by i.v. contrast MR. In ad-dition, contrast MR demonstrates an additional deep parietotemporal metastasis *(open arrow)* and skull metastases, which are also seen by T1-weighted MR **(C)** and wide window CT (not included). The skull metastases (hyperintense signals) are far more conspicuous after Gd-DTPA *(M)*.

clude both T1- and T2-weighted sequences will depend upon accumulated clinical experience.

Brain Tumor Treatment

CT AND MR STEREOTACTIC BIOPSY

This method incorporates a three-part neurosurgical apparatus. The frame base has pins that affix to the skull. A CT or MR landmark portion attaches to the frame base and is interchangeable with a neurosurgical metal arch portion that guides the neurosurgical instruments (Figs. 2.13 and 3.4).

RADIATION THERAPY

CT-generated isodose curves and radiotherapy treatment programs have now long been an accepted

practice. Marked tumor regression is often seen. Radiotherapy adverse effects will be discussed in Chapter 10.

PART THREE

Differential Diagnosis of Intracranial Neoplasms and Cysts

Reference is made to Figure 5.1 and generalizations are made regarding differential diagnosis. CT and MR characteristics of tumors within each of the 12 cranial locations identified in Figure 5.1 are discussed in Part Three.

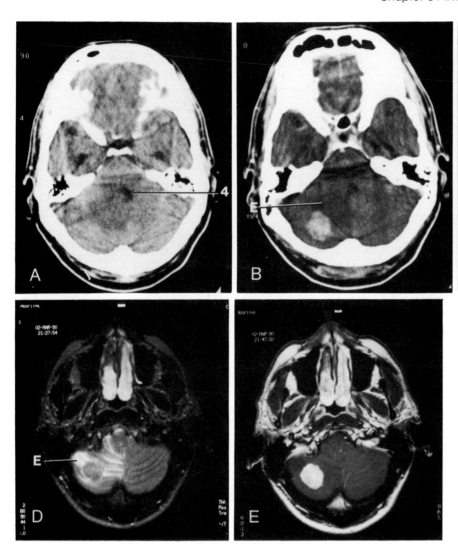

Figure 5.45. Cerebellar melanotic melanoma metastasis. *Noncontrast **(A)** and i.v. contrast **(B)** axial CT scans and SE 600/ 15 **(C)** and 2660/90 pulse-gated **(D)** axial MR scans. Intravenous contrast SE 600/ 22 flow compensated same level axial MR scan **(E)**.* The isodense contrast-enhancing mass is surrounded by edema (E). It is T1 gray matter-hyperintense and T2 gray matter-isointense. It displaces the fourth ventricle (4). The T1 hyperintensity and T2 isointensity is a melanin-induced paramagnetic effect.

Cerebral Hemisphere

Cerebral Hemisphere	Location	Margination	CT Density	Contrast[a]	Calcification	Intensity[b]
Low grade astrocytoma (adult)	Parenchymal	Ill defined	Low	−	−/+	Low T1, high T2
High grade astrocytoma (adult)	Parenchymal	Ill defined	Low, mixed heterogeneous	Heterogeneous ring	−	Mixed T1, high T2
Meningioma	Dural surface	MR = cleft CT = sharp	Iso- or hyperdense homogeneous	MR = homogeneous CT = homogeneous − (CT)	Flecks and clumps, occasional diffuse	Cortex-isointense T1/T2
Oligodendroglioma (low grade)	Parenchymal	Ill defined	Mixed	− (CT)	Clumps	Mixed T1, mixed T2
Metastasis	Parenchymal, frequently multiple	Lacks sharp margination	Varied, may be hyderdense	+ Homogeneous or ring	Unusual	Low T1, high T2
Lymphoma	Deep	Relatively smooth	Iso- or hyperdense	+ Homogeneous or ring	−	Slightly low T1, slightly high T2[c]
Arachnoid cyst	Extra-axial	Sharp	Low	−	−	Low T1, high T2 homogeneous
Primary cerebral neuroblastoma	Parenchymal Deep	Irregular	Varies according to degree of hemorrhage, cyst formation, and calcification	+ Heterogeneous	Common	Varies according to degree of hemorrhage, cyst formation, vascularity and calcification

[a]MR contrast may not enhance arteries and is more sensitive for metastasis.
[b]Varies with calcification, cyst formation, vascularity, and hemorrhage.
[c]From Schwaighofer BW, Hesselink JR, Press GA, et al. Primary intracranial CNS lymphoma. *AJNR* 1989; 10:725–729.

From these several characteristics, meningiomas, arachnoid cyst and metastases are clearly separable. Adjacent hyperostosis is diagnostic of meningioma. Lack or paucity of CT contrast enhancement separates the low grade astrocytoma and oligodendroglioma from the high grade astrocytoma. CT clumps of calcification favor the oligodendroglioma.

Corpus Callosum

Corpus Callosum	Margination	CT Density	CT Contrast	MR Intensity
Low grade astrocytoma	Ill defined	Low	−	Low T1/high T2
High grade astrocytoma	Ill defined	Mixed	+	Mixed T1/high T2
Lipoma (often contains calcium)	Sharp	Fat homogeneous	−	High T1, slightly high T2

The lipoma can easily be separated by its clearly identifiable characteristics. Contrast enhancement tends to separate the high grade from the low grade astrocytoma.

Lateral Ventricle

Lateral Ventricle	Margination	CT Density	Contrast	Calcification	MR Intensity
Astrocytoma	Ill defined	Varies according to degree of malignancy, calcification, and vascularity	+/−	+/−	Varies according to degree of malignancy, calcification, vascularity and hemorrhage
Ependymoma may seed the subarachnoid space	Ill defined	Varies according to degree of malignancy, calcification, and vascularity	+	+/−	Varies according to degree of malignancy, calcification, vascularity and hemorrhage
Choroid plexus papilloma[a]	Smooth or irregular fronds	Isodense or hyperdense	+ Marked	−	Varied signal due to hypervascularity and calcification
Epidermoid/dermoid	Possible foraminal extension, fronds/smooth	Water	−	−	Water
Meningioma	Smooth	Hyperdense homogeneous	+ marked	Clumps or +/− homogeneous	T1/T2 gray matter-isointensity
Primary cerebral neuroblastoma may seed the subarachnoid space	Irregular	Varies according to degree of cyst formation, calcification and hemorrhage	+ Heterogeneous	+	Varies according to degree of hemorrhage, cyst formation, vascularity and calcification

[a] Marked communicating hydrocephalus probably due to overproduction of CSF in the infant.

The fairly clearly identifiable tumors in the lateral ventricle group are the epidermoid tumor, the meningioma, and the choroid plexus papilloma. A giant cell astrocytoma would be identifiable due to other evidence of tuberous sclerosis. The astrocytoma series and the ependymoma share many characteristics.

Third Ventricle

The colloid cyst is easily differentiated from the ependymoma or giant cell astrocytoma by its location, smooth round margination, and homogeneous density. The colloid cyst does not (for practical purposes) contrast enhance as compared to the giant cell astrocytoma, which is likely to enhance detectably, to contain calcium, and to occur in a patient with tuberous sclerosis.

Optic Chiasm

The meningioma can be differentiated from the optic glioma by its dural base, sphenoid hyperostosis, interface on MR, smooth margination, homogeneous high density, homogeneous contrast enhancement, and MR demonstration of dural vascular supply.

Pituitary Lesion

The differential diagnosis of these lesions will be discussed in Chapter 11.

Brainstem

Usually these lesions are gliomas. Rarely, metastasis to the brainstem is seen. Very rarely, a midbrain abscess may occur. Fitz[3] found no CT distinguishing features between low and high grade pediatric brainstem astrocytomas.

Cerebellopontine Angle

The differential diagnosis of these lesions are discussed in Chapter 12.

Foramen Magnum

These tumors are usually meningiomas. Neurofibromas may occur.

Fourth Ventricle

Fourth Ventricle[a]	Location	Margination	CT Density	Contrast	T1/T2 Intensity
Ependymona (may "seed" the subarachnoid space)	4th ventricle	Ill defined	Increased (heterogeneous)	+	Insufficient data
Choroid plexus papilloma (rare)	4th ventricle	Sharp or "frond-like"	Increased	Marked	Varied
Epidermoid/demoid (rare)	4th ventricle	Sharp or "frond-like"	Water/fat	−	Insufficient data
Medulloblastoma (may "seed" the subarachnoid space)	may be hemispheric[b]	Fairly well marginated	Increased (homogeneous)	Marked	−/+

[a]Within or involving the 4th ventricle.
[b]Usually has origin near the vermis nodulus.

Of the fourth ventricle tumors, only the epidermoid and dermoid are clearly separable. Fine punctate calcification, ill-defined margins, and hemorrhagic areas favor ependymoma. Transforaminal extension is characteristic of epidermoid tumor, choroid plexus papilloma, and ependymoma.[44]

Cerebellum

Cerebellum	Location	Margination	CT Density	Contrast	Calcification	Cystic Component	T1/T2 Intensity
Astrocytoma	Favors hemisphere	Irregular	Usually hypodense	+	+25%	+	Varies with degree of hemorrhage, cyst component, vascularity and calcification
Medulloblastoma	Favors vermis, adult, lesion is often hemispheric	Irregular	Hyperdense	+	+25%	May occur	Varies with degree of cyst component, vascularity, and calcification
Hemangioblastoma	Favors hemisphere	Smooth	Varies with degree of cyst component	+	−	+	Varies with degree of cyst component and vascularity

The vermis nodulus location of medulloblastoma in children is an important diagnostic characteristic. The smooth margination of the hemangioblastoma and the feeding artery prominence occurring in the adult is strong evidence for a diagnosis. These tumors can all be distinguished from arachnoid cyst by contrast enhancement and soft tissue signals.

Pineal Region

Pineal Region	Margination	CT Density	Contrast	Calcification	T1/T2 Intensity
Germinoma—often "seed" the subarachnoid space; predominantly found in males	Irregular	Hyperdense	+	+ coarse nodular	T1 water-hyperintense T2 water-isointense
Teratoma—predominantly found in males	Benign-Sharp Malignant-Irregular	Isodense with calcium and fat	−/+	+	Expect fat, calcium, and cystic fluid signal
Glioma	Irregular	Hypodense or isodense	+ Heterogeneous possible ring	−/+	T1 water-hyperintense T2 water-isointense
Pineoblastoma—often "seed" the subarachnoid space	Irregular	Hyperdense	+ Heterogeneous possible ring	−	T1-gray matter iso/hypointense T2-gray matter iso/hyperintense
Pineocytoma	Fairly smooth	Varies	Homogeneous +	+	Insufficient data
Pineal cyst	Sharp	Hypodense	−	+/−	T1/T2 water-isointense

The sharp margination and fat densities of the teratoma make it the most clearly identifiable in this group. The high CT density of the germinoma is a clue but the other tumors of this group tend to share characteristics. The smoothly marginated water isointensity in the noncontrast-enhancing pineal gland cyst is easily distinguished. We have recently found an aneurysm of the quadrigeminal portion of the posterior cerebral artery mimicking a pineal tumor.

References

1. Grossman CB, Masdeu JC, Maravilla KR, Gonzalez CF. Intracranial neoplasms of the adult. In Gonzalez CF, Grossman CB, Masdeu JC (Eds). *Head and Spine Imaging.* New York: John Wiley & Sons, 1985; 225–281.
2. Russell DS, Rubenstein LJ. *Pathology of tumors of the Nervous System,* Ed 4. Baltimore: Williams & Wilkins, 1977.
3. Fitz CR. *Neoplastic Diseases.* In Gonzalez CF, Grossman CB, Masdeu JC (Eds). *Head and Spine Imaging.* New York: John Wiley & Sons, 1985; 483–521.
4. Sze G, Soletsky S, Bronen R, Krol G. MR imaging of the cranial meninges with emphasis on contrast enhancement and meningeal carcinomatosis. AJNR 1989; 10:965–975.
5. McGeachie RE, Gold LHA, Latchaw RE. Periventricular spread of tumor demonstrated by computed tomography. *Radiology* 1977; 125:407–410.
6. Haughton VM, Rimm AA, Czervionke LF, et al. Sensitivity of Gd-DTPA-enhanced MR imaging of benign extraaxial tumors. *Radiology* 1988; 166:829–833.
7. Komiyama M, Yagura H, Baba M, et al. MR Imaging: Possibility of tissue characterization of brain tumors using T1 and T2 values. *AJNR* 1987; 8:65–70.
8. Spagnoli MV, Goldberg HI, Grossman RI. Intracranial meningiomas: High-field MR imaging. *Radiology* 1986; 161:369–375.
9. Zimmerman RA, Bilaniuk LT. Cranial computed tomography of epidermoid and congenital fatty tumors of maldevelopmental origin. *J Comput Tomogr* Vol 3:1, 1979.
10. Kjos BO, Brant-Zawadzki M, Kucharczyk W. Cystic intracranial lesions: Magnetic resonance imaging. *Radiology* 1985; 155:363–369.
11. Gentry LR, Smoker WRK, Turski PA, et al. Suprasellar arachnoid cyst: 1 CT recognition. *AJNR* 1986; 7:79–86.
12. Kendall B, Pullicino P. Comparison of consistency of meningiomas and CT appearances. *Neuroradiology* 1979; 18:173–176.
13. Tchang S, Scotti G. Terbrugge K, et al. Computerized tomography as a possible aid to histological grading of supratentorial gliomas. *J Neurosurg* 1977; 46:735–739.
14. Leo JS, Pinto RS, Hulvat GF. Computed tomography of arachnoid cysts. *Radiology* 1979; 130:675–680.
15. Barkovich AJ, Wippold FJ, Brammer RE. False-negative MR imaging of an acoustic neurinoma (Correspondence). *AJNR* 1986; 7:364.
16. Enzmann DR, O'Donohue J. Optimizing MR imaging for detecting small tumors in the cerebellopontine angle and internal auditory canals. *AJNR* 1987; 8:99–106.
17. Norman D. Stevens EA, Wing SD, et al. Quantitative aspects of contrast enhancement in cranial computed tomography. *Radiology* 1978; 129:683–688.
18. Breger RK, Papke RA, Pojunas KW. Benign extracellular tumors: Contrast enhancement with Gd-DTPA. *Radiology* 1987; 163:427–429.
19. Brant-Zadwadzki M, Berry I, Osaki L. Gd-DTPA in clinical MR of the brain: 1. Intra-axial lesions. *AJNR* 1986; 7:781–788.
20. Williams AL. Tumors. In Williams AL, Haughton VM (Eds): *Cranial Computed Tomography.* St. Louis: CV Mosby Co, 1985; 148–239.
21. Brant-Zawadzki M, Kelly W. Brain tumors. In Brant-Zawadzki M, Norman D (Eds): *Magnetic Resonance Imaging of the Central Nervous System.* New York: Raven Press, 1987.
22. Gentry LR, Menezes AH, Turski PA, et al. Suprasellar arachnoid cysts: 2. Evaluation of CSF dynamics. *AJNR* 1986; 7:87–96.
23. Wolpert SM, Scott RM. The value of metrizamide CT cisternography in the management of cerebral arachnoid cysts. *AJNR* 1981; 2:29–35.
24. Mawad ME, Silver AJ, Hilal SK, Ganti SR. Computed tomography of the brain stem with intrathecal metrizamide. Part I: The normal brain stem. *AJR* 1983; 140:553–563.
25. Mawad ME, Silver AJ, Hilal SK, Ganti SR. Computed tomography of the brain stem with intrathecal metrizamide. Part II: Lesions in and around the brain stem. *AJR* 1983; 140:565–571.
26. Pinto RS, Kricheff II, Bergeron RT. Small acoustic neuromas: Detection by high resolution gas CT cisternography. *AJR* 1982; 139:129–132.
27. Shapir J, Coblentz C, Malenson D, et al. New CT finding in aggressive meningioma. *AJNR* 1985; 6:101–102.
28. Oot RF, New PFJ, Pile-Spellman J, et al. The detection of intracranial calcifications by MR. *AJNR* 1986; 7:801–809.
29. Bradley WG Jr. Pathophysiologic correlates of signal alterations. In Brant-Zawadzki M, Norman D (Eds): *Magnetic Imaging of the Central Nervous System.* New York: Raven Press, 1987; 23–42.
30. McComb JG, Davis RL. Choroid plexus, cerebrospinal fluid, hydrocephalus, cerebral edema, and herniation phenomena. In Davis RL, Robertson DM (Eds): *Textbook of Neuropathology.* Baltimore, Williams & Wilkins, 1985; 147–175.
31. Brant-Zawadzki M, Kucharczyk W. Vascular disease: Ischemia. In Brant-Zawadzki M, Norman D (Eds): *Magnetic Resonance Imaging of the Central Nervous System.* New York: Raven Press, 1987; 221–234.
32. Siegel RM, Messina AV. Computed tomography: The anatomic basis of the zone of diminished density surrounding meningiomas. *AJR* 1976; 127:139–141.
33. George AE, Russell EJ, Kricheff II. White matter buckling: CT sign of extra-axial intracranial mass. *AJR* 1980; 135:1031–1036.
34. Burger PC, Vogel FS, Green SB, Strike TA. Glioblastoma multiforme and anaplastic astrocytoma. Pathological criteria and prognostic implications. *Cancer* 1985; 56:1106–1111.
35. Earnest F, Kelly PJ, Schneithauer BW, et al. Cerebral astrocytomas: Histopathologic correlation of MR and CT contrast enhancement with stereotactic biopsy. *Radiology* 1988; 166:823–827.
36. Lee BCP, Kneeland JB, Walker RW, et al. MR imaging of brain stem tumors. *AJNR* 1985; 6:159–163.
37. Bilaniuk LT, Zimmerman RA, Littman P, et al. Computed tomography of brainstem gliomas in children. *Radiology* 1980; 134:89–95.
38. Rubinstein LJ. Tumors of neuroglial cells. In Firminger HI (Ed): *Atlas of Tumor Pathology, Tumors of the Central Nervous System.* Fascicle 6, Wasington DC: Armed Forces Institute of Pathology, 1972; 257–263.
39. Dolinkas CA, Simeone FA. CT characteristics of intraventricular oligodendrogliomas. *AJNR* 1987; 8:1077–1082.
40. Spoto GP, Press GA, Hesselink JR, Solomon M. Intracranial ependymoma and subependymoma. MR manifestations. AJNR 1990; 11:83–91.
41. Armington WG, Osborne AG, Cubberley DA, et al. Supratentorial ependymoma: CT appearance. *Radiology* 1985; 157:367–372.
42. Hopper KD, Foley LC, Nieves NL, Smirinotopoulos JG. The intraventricular extension of choroid plexus papilloma. *AJNR* 1987; 8:469–472.
43. Weinstein ZR, Downey EF. Spontaneous hemorrhage in medulloblastomas. *AJNR* 1983; 4:986–988.
44. Haughton VM, Daniels DL. The posterior fossa. In Williams AL, Haughton VM (Eds): *Cranial Computed Tomography.* St. Louis: CV Mosby Co 1985; 350–443.
45. Davis PC, Wichman RD, Takei Y, Hoffman JC Jr. Primary cerebral neuroblastoma: CT and MR findings in 12 cases. AJNR 1990; 11:115–120.
46. Dorne HL, O'Gorman AM, Melanson D. Computed tomography of intracranial gangliomas. *AJNR* 1986; 7:281–285.
47. Merten DF, Gooding CA, Newton TH, et al. Meningiomas of childhood and adolescence. *J Pediatr* 1974; 74:696–700.
48. Som PM, Sacher M, Strenger SW. "Benign" metastasizing meningiomas. *AJNR* 1987; 8:127–130.
49. Daniels DL, Millen SJ, Meyer GA, et al. MR detection of tumor in the internal auditory canal. *AJNR* 1987; 8:249–252.
50. Zimmerman RA, Balaniuk LT, Wood JH, et al. Computed tomography of pineal, parapineal and histologically related tumors. *Radiology* 1980; 137:669–677.
51. Ganti SR, Hilal SK, Stein BM. CT of pineal region tumors. *AJNR* 1986; 7:97–104.
52. Tien RD, Barkovich AJ, Edwards MSB. MR imaging of pineal tumors. AJNR 1990; 11:557–565.
53. Mamourian AC, Towfighi J. Pineal cysts: MR imaging. *AJNR* 1986; 7:1081–1086.
54. Naidich TP, Leeds NE, Pudlowski RM, et al. Primary tumors and other masses of the cerebellum and fourth ventricle: Differential diagnosis by computed tomography. *Neuroradiology* 1977; 14:153–174.
55. Ganti SR, Antunes JL, Louis KM, Hilal SK. Computed tomography in the diagnosis of colloid cysts of the third ventricle. *Radiology* 1981; 138:385–391.
56. Maeder PP, Holtås SL, Basibüyük LN et al. Colloid cysts of the third ventricle: correlation of MR and CT findings with histology and chemical analysis. AJNR 1990; 11:575–581.
57. Woodruff WW Jr, Djang WT, McLendon RE. Intracerebral malignant melanoma: high-field strength MR imaging. *Radiology* 1987; 165:209–213.
58. Anand AK, Potts DG. Calcified brain metastases: Demonstration by computed tomography. *AJNR* 1982; 3:527–529.
59. Morrison G, Sobel DF, Kelley WM, Norman D. Intraventricular mass lesions. *Radiology* 1984; 1253:435–442.

CHAPTER 6

Cerebrovascular Disorders

Introduction

The outline of this chapter represents an attempt to organize various cerebrovascular disorders and related conditions into a useful pattern for MR and CT imaging description. The system is primarily chosen to aid diagnosis through imaging findings. Such findings include location, multiplicity, density, intensity, margination, contrast enhancement, vascular pattern, hemorrhage, edema, and mass effect—similar to that in Chapter 5. As much as possible, this order will be kept so that the reader may more easily make comparisons of similar patterns of different etiologies.

Cerebral Infarct, Occlusive Vascular Disease, and Anoxic Brain Damage

ARTERIAL TERRITORY INFARCT

Infarction is caused by ischemia that usually results from atherosclerotic origin emboli. These emboli usually arise from the common carotid artery bifurcation but may be of cardiac origin. Carotid artery occlusions can be responsible for major strokes, however. Major intracranial artery branch primary occlusion is rare.[1] Infarction can also result from severe hypoxia, arterial spasm, and dysmetabolic states.

The size, location, and shape of the infarct help identify the etiology.[2] For example, a middle cerebral artery ascending branch infarct or a middle cerebral artery watershed infarct (distal portion of a vascular territory) are typical of embolic middle cerebral artery branch occlusions. These typical branch occlusion infarcts are small to moderate in size. An infarction involving major portions of both the ipsilateral anterior and middle cerebral artery territory is usually caused by internal carotid artery occlusion. Bilateral globus pallidus infarction suggests asphyxia and/or carbon monoxide poisoning. Ganglionic lacunar infarcts are more common in

hypertensive patients and the majority of these lesions may be primary rather than embolic occlusions.[1,3] It is hoped that the current concepts recognizing embolism as the cause of the majority of cerebral infarcts do not cause the reader confusion. Hemorrhagic infarcts have long been said to be caused by embolic events and nonhemorrhagic infarcts were assumed to be thrombotic.

Hemorrhage develops within an infarct when oxygen deprivation is severe enough to cause necrosis of the capillary endothelial cells which is then followed by re-establishment of blood flow. It is the degree of hemorrhagic component detectable by CT or MR that determines whether we call an infarct "nonhemorrhagic" or "hemorrhagic."[3] A recent review[4] describes four conditions predisposing to hemorrhagic infarction.

1. An embolus lyses after arterial occlusion and the fragments move distally;
2. collateral blood supply develops to the ischemic brain distal to the occlusion;
3. when a hypotensive episode is followed by blood pressure restoration;
4. when there is intermittent compression of the posterior cerebral artery during temporal lobe transtentorial herniation.

Not included in the above categorization is infarction in an anticoagulated patient or a patient with a bleeding diathesis.

Types 1 and 2 imply that watershed zones are particularly susceptible to hemorrhagic cortical infarction. Approximately 20% of all cerebral infarcts are hemorrhagic[4] but smaller petechial hemorrhages may occur in up to 40% of cases.[5] The hemorrhage is almost always confined to the cortex and preferentially involves the deep infolded gyri.[4] Because of MR's greater sensitivity for detecting subacute hemorrhage, the influence of smaller hemorrhages on the decision to anticoagulate the infarct patient may be influenced by data obtained from this newer technique.[5]

Two recent important changes have taken place in imaging of acute cerebral infarcts. The first is high-resolution CT scanning that demonstrates the majority of acute infarcts during the first 24 hours.[6]

Perhaps of even greater importance is the increased sensitivity of MR for acute cerebral infarcts.[1,5]

Chronology of Infarct Imaging

MR intensity and CT density characteristics provide important clues to lesion chronicity. Infarct age will be divided into four periods:

1. Day 1
2. Days 2–7
3. Second Week to 1 Month
4. Older than 1 Month

Day 1 and days 2–7 are considered "acute infarcts." Infarcts from 1 week to 1 month postictus are considered "subacute infarcts" and infarcts older than 1 month are considered "chronic infarcts" (see Table 6.1).

Day 1. The day 1 infarct is usually CT isodense without contrast enhancement during the first 12 hours. The majority of patients with cerebral infarcts demonstrate CT changes of subtle mass effect and/or focal areas of ill-defined decreased density during the first 24 hours. Some of these cases will demonstrate cortical contrast enhancement.[6] In some cases, these early CT changes are seen in the first 3–6 hours after onset of symptoms.[7] Mass effect often manifests as subtle sulcal compression without mid-line shift or ventricular compression (Fig. 6.1).[8] Occasionally, cortical areas of hyperdensity develop. These latter infarcts may have a greater tendency to contrast enhance and also to hemorrhage.

Cytotoxic edema develops within the first 6 hours; then vasogenic edema also develops. MR, because of its increased sensitivity to water detection (edema) compared to CT, can often detect acute infarcts earlier (Fig. 6.2). We expect MR to detect infarction changes routinely 6 hours postictus.[5] MR contrast enhancement of slow flow arteries caused by vascular impedence may occur.

Because day 1 and day 2 hemorrhage detection by MR is dependent on T2 hypointensity of deoxyhemoglobin (see Table 3.2), CT is at least as reliable for hemorrhage detection during the first 24 hours. Another consideration for CT as first method of investigation of early stroke is that some day 1 stroke patients may be too agitated for the MR scan or may need monitoring and respiratory assistance.

Days 2–7. CT hypodensity (from 4–14 H) in a vascular distribution involving both gray and white matter with relatively smooth margins, abnormal contrast enhancement, and mass effect is seen.[3,7] The hypodense region often appears "wedge shaped" conforming to the affected vascular distribution (Fig. 6.3).

Contrast enhancement may be seen and conforms

Table 6.1. Cerebral Infarct Chronology

	Day 1	Day 2–7	2nd week–1 month	Older than 1 month
CT density	Isodense, occasional cortical hyperdensity	Hypodensity	White matter hypodensity; cortical gray isodensity	Gray and white matter-hypodensity
MR intensity	Water (edema) intensity cellular edema for first 6 hours Impedence of arterial flow may be detected by flow-sensitive technique	T1 and T2 water (edema) signal	Varies according to amount of hemorrhage hemosiderin, and edema	Varies—generally T1-weighted, slight water-hyperintensity and proton density/T2-weighted hyperintensity
Mass effect	Subtle	Maximum at this stage; characteristic gray and white matter involvement	Decreases, focal atrophy develops	Ipsilateral atrophy. May develop parenchymal cysts; Wallerian degeneration
CT margination	Ill defined	Relatively smooth	Becomes irregular due to gray matter-isodensity	Sharp
MR margination	Varies	Relatively smooth	Becomes irregular due to cortical isointensity	Less sharp than CT due to cortical isointensity
CT contrast enhancement	Possible cortical enhancement	+ cortical distribution	Cortical distribution maximum at this stage	Usually absent
MR contrast enhancement	May demonstrate contrast enhancement of "slow-flow" arteries	+	+	Insufficient data
Hemorrhage	Occasional	Most likely to appear at this stage; CT hemorrhage signal maximum, particularly if anticoagulated	CT hemorrhage signal decreases; MR hemorrhage signal very sensitive	CT—not seen MR—hemosiderin

to cortical gray matter. Infarction mass effect is greatest at this stage.[5] The mass effect is most often confined to sulcal effacement possibly associated with slight ventricular compression (Fig. 6.3).[3,6] Hemorrhage, if already present, often becomes dense and the hemorrhagic area may enlarge. Hemorrhage not present on day 1 may also appear at this stage.

MR of infarct at days 2–7 will show initially increased gray and white matter edema and mass effect. The influx of protein into the edematous region from breakdown of the blood-brain barrier (BBB) tends to decrease the prolongation of T1 and T2 later in this period resulting in higher T1-weighted and proton density edema signal (Fig. 6.3).[5] MR can distinguish acute hemorrhage from infarct edema by the low T2 signal of deoxyhemoglobin.[4,5] Intracellular and extracellular methemoglobin, is distinguished on heavily T1-weighted images from edema due to T1 methemoglobin hyperintensity and edema T1 hypointensity. T2 and proton density edema signal hyperintensity will obscure T2 extracellular methemoglobin effects. Gd-DPTA contrast enhancement occurs at this stage of developing BBB breakdown.[5]

Second Week to 1 Month. CT of these infarcts demonstrates continued white matter hypodensity, developing irregularity of contour due to cortical gray relative isointensity, decreased mass effect followed by developing focal cerebral atrophy and cortical gray matter contrast enhancement (Fig. 6.4).[3,7,8] Density of hemorrhagic areas will decrease during this period.

MR of second week to 1-month-old infarcts demonstrates decreased mass effect and development of focal cerebral atrophy. Because MR is more sensitive than CT for subacute hemorrhage, cortical hemorrhage methemoglobin is dramatically demonstrated. Infarct intensity may vary at this stage due to interstitial protein molecules, possible foci of hemorrhage (at different stages) or hemosiderin (Fig. 6.4) but generally, the intensity characteristics are T1 hypointense and T2 hyperintense.[5]

Infarcts Older than 1 Month. On CT, after 1 month, both gray and white matter infarct territorial density has decreased. There is now sharp margination of the water-density area. Focal cerebral atrophy occurs and parenchymal cysts may develop (Figs. 6.5 and 6.6). There is usually lack of contrast enhancement but enhancement may last for greater

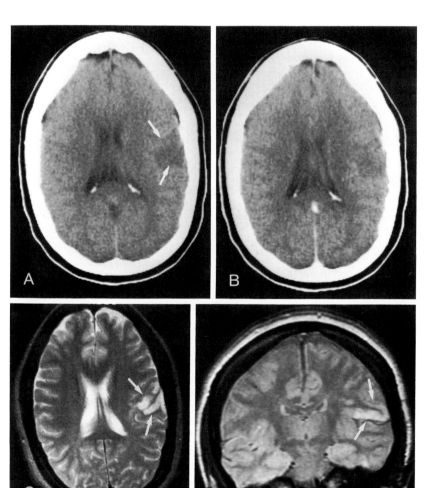

Figure 6.1. Day 1, left middle cerebral artery infarct. **A** and **B,** Day 1. Axial ventricular atrial level 35/100 noncontrast **(A)** and contrast **(B)** CT scans. Note the gray and white matter cortical-based wedge-shaped slightly ill-defined zone of homogeneous slight hypodensity *(arrows)* corresponding to the middle cerebral artery distribution **(A).** The infarct is virtually masked after i.v. contrast indicating slight homogeneous contrast enhancement. **(C)** and **(D)** Day 3. Axial SE 2800/80 **(C)** and and coronal SE 2800/30 **(D)** MR scans. Note the hyperintense perirolandic gyri *(arrows)* more conspicuous on the T2-weighted image probably representing cytotoxic edema. There is slight right-sided displacement of the septum pellucidum.

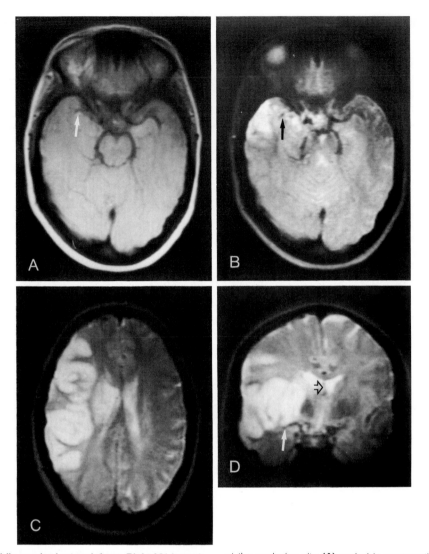

Figure 6.2. Day 1, middle cerebral artery infarct. Right M1 branch embolus and infarct. *Axial midbrain-level SE 2000/20 **(A)** and 2000/ 80 **(B)** MR scans. Axial ventricular body-level **(C)** and coronal pituitary-level **(D)** SE 2000/80 MR scans.* The right middle cerebral artery M1 segment is occluded *(arrow)*. A small hyperintense signal is seen at the occlusion site **(A)** probably representing methemoglobin within clotted blood. Compare to opposite side. There is profound cytotoxic and vasogenic edema, which is poorly seen on the T1-weighted image **(A).** Note the large amount of edema of both gray and white matter and the septum pellucidum shift *(open arrow)*.

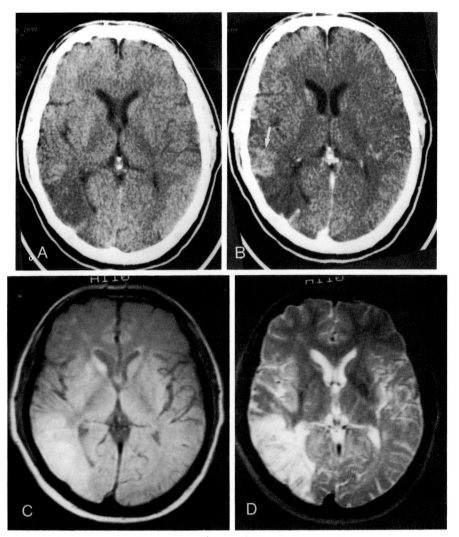

Figure 6.3. Day 2 (CT) and day 6 (MR) acute infarct. **(A)** and **(B):** Day 2. Right middle cerebral artery infarct. **(C)** and **(D):** Day 6. Axial third ventricle-level noncontrast **(A)** and i.v. contrast **(B)** CT scans at day 2. Same level SE 2000/20 **(C)** and 2000/80 **(D)** MR scans at day 6. Note the right middle cerebral artery distribution slightly ill-defined gray and white matter hypodensity associated with sulcal efface- ment and slight occipital horn medial displacement **(A)**. *There is contrast enhancement* (*arrow on* **B**) of the slightly hyperintense ar- terior portion. At day 6, the MR T2 image shows infarct hyperintens- ity **(D).** No hemorrhage was detected on SE 600/25 images (not shown). Note that the proton hyperintensity effects of edema **(C).**

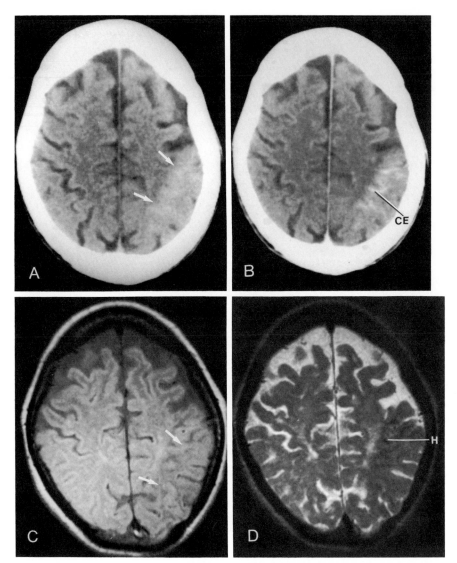

Figure 6.4.   Subacute infarct (chronicity greater than 1 week and less than 4 weeks). Left middle cerebral artery infarct at 11 days (A and B) and 12 days (C and D). *Axial centrum semiovale noncontrast (A) and i.v. contrast (B) 35/100 CT scans. Same level SE 2000/ 20 (C) and 2000/80 (D) MR scans.* There is ill-defined left middle cerebral artery territory hyperdensity and sulcal effacement (*arrows* on **A**) due to hemorrhage and/or hyperemia. There is gyral pattern contrast enhancement *(CE).* The MR T1-weighted image demonstrates vague hypointensity (*arrows* on **C**) and T2-weighted image markedly hypointense bands *(H)* most likely representing deoxyhemoglobin or, less likely, hemosiderin. Although persistent brain swelling is still evidenced by sulcal compression, T2 edema effects are absent.

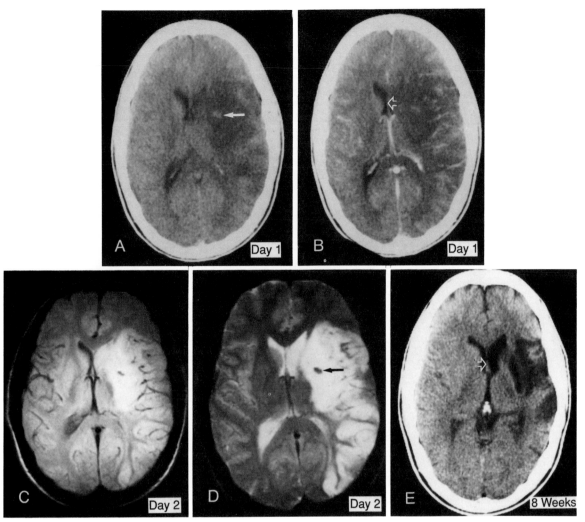

Figure 6.5. Acute to chronic (greater than 1 month old) infarct with day 1 CT (A and B), day 2 MR (C and D) and 8-week follow-up CT (E). *Axial internal cerebral vein-level noncontrast (A) and i.v. contrast (B) 35/100 CT scans. Same level SE 2000/20 (C) and 2000/ 80 (D) MR scans. Eight-week follow-up third ventricle-level noncontrast 35/100 CT scan (E).* Note the large left hemisphere middle cerebral artery territory hypodensity involving both gray and white matter (cytotoxic and vasogenic edema) and the small focal hemorrhage hyperdensity *(closed arrow)*. There is slightly greater contrast en-

hancement of left Sylvian middle cerebral arteries than right possibly indicating luxury perfusion **(A).** The small left lenticular nucleus hemorrhage *(closed arrow)* with T2 hypointensity **(C** and **D)** probably represents deoxyhemoglobin. Note the left hemisphere mass effect *(open arrow* on **B)** and the follow-up left hemiatrophy, encephalomalacia, ipsilateral ventricular dilatation, and septum pellucidum shift *(open arrow* on **E).** The protein influence upon the MR water signal is responsible for the infarct signal hyperintensity on the SE 2000/20 (T1-weighted/proton density) signal.

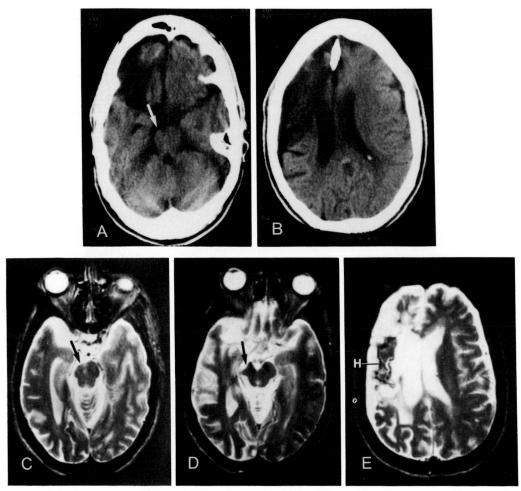

Figure 6.6. Remote ("chronic") middle cerebral artery infarct with Wallerian degeneration. *Noncontrast fourth ventricle-level (A) and lateral ventricle body-level (B) CT scans. Lower midbrain-level (C), upper midbrain-level (D) and lateral ventricle body-level (E) SE 2713/ 90 MAST pulse-triggered MR scans. There is a remote right middle cerebral artery infarct with CT sharply marginated gray and white* matter wedge-shaped hypodense encephalomalacia. A hypointense rim of probable hemosiderin (H) surrounds a T2 isointense "island" within the infarct zone. There is right cerebral peduncle Wallerian atrophy *(arrows)*. The septum pellucidum is slightly displaced toward the involved side and there is right hemispheric gyral atrophy best seen on **(E)**.

than 6 months. In the latter case, the enhancement often is ring-shaped surrounding a central necrotic core. Because some infarcts undergo coagulative necrosis rather than liquefaction, partial calcification may occur.[3,9] Hemorrhage hyperdensity is no longer seen. Wallerian degeneration (distal axonal breakdown after cellular or axonal destruction proximally) can be demonstrated in patients with old large motor cortex infarcts and also in some patients with large capsular infarcts. CT and MR will show ipsilateral cerebral penduncle and pontine atrophy [Wallerian degeneration (Fig. 6.6)].[10,11]

With MR of infarcts greater than 1-month-old, focal cerebral atrophy is also seen. Old infarcts usually show focal areas of cystic change with T1 hypointensity and T2 hyperintensity. Not all infarcts undergo liquefaction, however, so that old infarct intensity can vary but generally will show increased water content.[5] The heavily T1-weighted signal is usually slightly water hyperintense and the proton density and T2-weighted signal is hyperintense. The MR chronic infarct margin is more irregular than the CT margin due to MR cortical isointensity. Hemosiderin deposit in an old hemorrhagic infarct will show characteristically marked hypointensity. MR evidence for hemorrhage may last for months, however. Wallerian degeneration is better demonstrated by MR than CT due to better parenchymal detail of the midbrain and brainstem (Fig. 6.6).[11]

Solitary atherosclerotic embolic infarcts cannot, under most circumstances, be distinguished by CT or MR from embolic infarcts of cardiogenic origin. Some

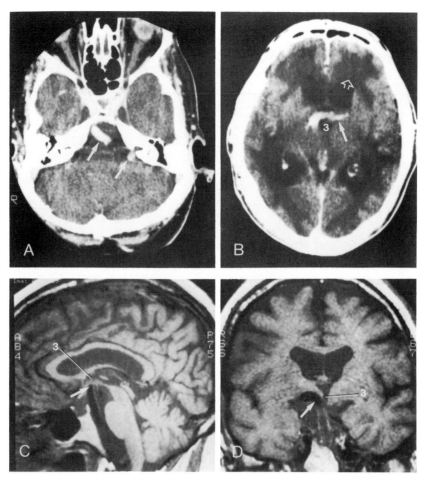

Figure 6.7. Atherosclerotic basilar artery ectasia. *Intravenous contrast axial CT scan at the internal auditory canal level* **(A).** Note the contrast-enhanced tortuous basilar artery vertebrobasilar junction *(right arrow)* and the prepontine-interpeduncular portion *(left arrow)*. The artery is directly opposed to the left internal auditory canal. **B,** Another case. *Axial i.v. contrast injection third ventricle-level CT scan.* The dilated tortuous basilar artery courses from right to left *(arrow)* indenting the undersurface of the third ventricle *(3)*. There is associated hydrocephalus with periventricular edema *(open arrow)*. The hydrocephalus is probably caused by arterial pulsation transmission to the ventricles and compression of the foramina of Monro. **C** and **D,** Another case. *Midsagittal* **(C)** *and coronal anterior third ventricle-level* **(D)** *SE 600/25 MR scans.* Note the elevation and left-sided displacement of the anterior third ventricle by the signal-void dilated and tortuous basilar artery *(arrows)*.

authors believe, however, that the cardiogenic origin infarct has a larger hemorrhagic component.[3]

Table 6.2 (p. 154) lists various causes of brain infarcts.

Atherosclerotic Disease and Infarcts

Direct imaging of the common carotid artery bifurcation with dynamic CT techniques has successfully detected arterial intimal disease.[12] These methods are not generally used, however. MR techniques for examining the common carotid artery bifurcation are being developed.

Vertebrobasilar arterial dolichoectasia is commonly detected by both CT and MR. It can cause compressive cranial nerve deficits and should be included in the imaging report (Fig. 6.7).[13] Carotid artery dolichoectasia is far less common (Fig. 6.8).

Carotid and vertebrobasilar artery occlusions have been diagnosed by both the MR and CT techniques,[14–16] however, we have found only MR accurate for this purpose (Figs. 6.2 and 6.9). We still depend on angiography for confirmatory diagnoses because of its greater accuracy and therapeutic considerations.

Figures 6.1–6.5 demonstrate middle cerebral artery occlusions in various chronological phases. A series of other vascular territory infarcts follows in atlas style: internal carotid artery (Fig. 6.10), anterior cerebral artery (Fig. 6.11), posterior cerebral artery (Fig. 6.12), basilar artery (Fig. 6.13), and posterior inferior cerebellar artery (Fig. 6.14).

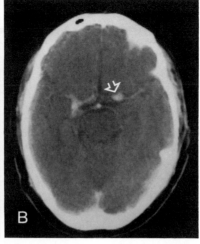

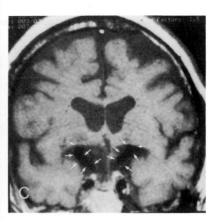

Figure 6.8. Intracranial carotid artery ectasia. *A* and *B,* Axial i.v. contrast cranial CT scans at anteroclinoid level 35/250 *(A)* and chiasmatic cistern level 35/100 *(B).* Note the ectatic partially calcified right internal carotid artery *(closed arrow)* and left internal carotid artery *(open arrow).* **C** (different case), *Coronal pituitary-level SE 600/25 MR scan.* Arrows outline the ectatic supraclinoid internal carotid arteries.

Table 6.2. Causes of Focal (Arterial Territory) Brain Infarct*

1. Atherosclerosis
   Carotid artery origin (embolic)
   Cardiac origin (embolic)
   Primary intracranial artery occlusion
   Vascular dementia (Binswanger's)
2. Hypertension
   Lacunar infarct
3. Emboli of nonatherosclerotic origin
   Bacterial endocarditis
   Cardiac myxoma
4. Arteritis
   Lupus erythematosis
   Polyarteritis nodosa
5. Meningitis
   Granulomatous and fungal (basal) (Fig. 8.9, p. 209)
   Suppurative (convexity) (Fig. 8.5, p. 206)
6. Vasospasm
   Ruptured aneurysm
7. Arterial compression
   Incisural herniation (Figs. 5.17, p. 115; and 7.21, p. 197)
8. Intracranial nonatherosclerotic occlusive disease
   Moyamoya
   Neurofibromatosis
9. Hematological disorders
   Sickle cell disease
   Polycythemia
10. Coagulation disorders
    Disseminated intravascular coagulation (DIC)
11. Drug induced
    Oral contraceptives
    Illicit drug abuse
12. Dissection of intracranial arteries

*This is meant to be a practical rather than an "all-inclusive" list.

Lacunar Infarcts and Other Small Infarcts

Occlusions of deep cerebral vessels such as the lenticulostriate arteries, the anterior choroidal artery, and the thalamoperforating arteries are probably most often caused by thrombus. The small infarcts produced (lacunar infarcts) are associated with arteriolar disease (lipohyalinosis). They commonly occur in hypertensive patients and have a tendency to oc-

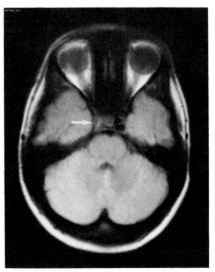

Figure 6.9. Arterial occlusion. Right internal carotid artery occlusion. Axial cavernous sinus level. Note absence of signal void in the right cavernous sinus *(arrow).*

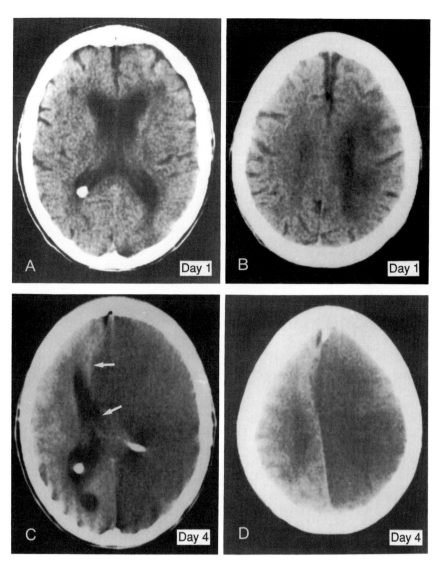

Figure 6.10. Day 1 and day 4 internal carotid artery distribution cerebral infarct. *Noncontrast CT scans. Day 1 (**A** and **B**), day 4 (**C** and **D**). **A** and **C** at lateral ventricle atrial level, and **B** and **D** at centrum semiovale level.* At day 1, abnormal left centrum hypodensity is seen **(B).** At day 4 **(C** and **D),** the entire left hemisphere is hypodense and there is marked subfalx herniation *(arrows).*

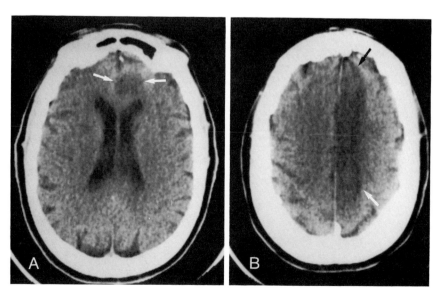

Figure 6.11. Day 2, anterior cerebral artery infarct. Axial noncontrast lateral ventricular body-level **(A)** and centrum semiovale-level **(B)** 37/100 CT scans. Note low density *(arrows)* in the left anterior cerebral artery distribution without detectable mass effect.

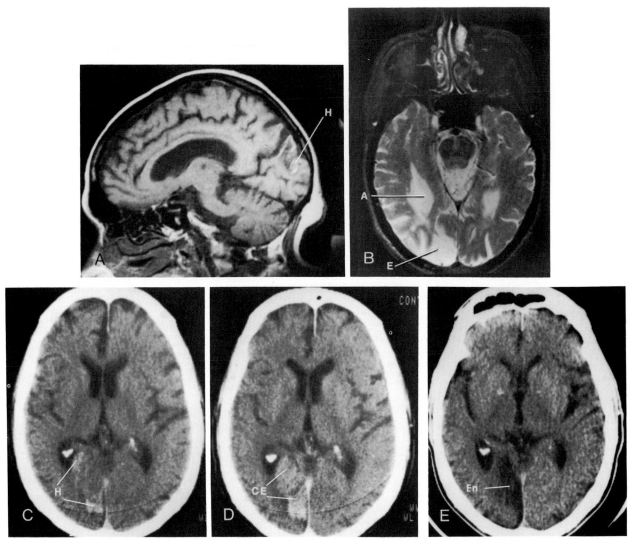

Figure 6.12.   Posterior cerebral artery infarcts (day 3). A–B and **C–E** are different cases. **A–B,** Day 3, right posterior cerebral artery infarct. *Parasagittal 600/25 MR scan (A). Axial 2800/80 MR scan (B).* Note the T1-weighted right occipital rim hyperintensity *(H)* due to methemoglobin effect. Note the right occipitoparietal edema *(E).* Lateral ventricle atrium *(A).* The infarct edema has obscured MR hemorrhage methemoglobin T2-hyperintensity effect **(B). C–E,** Day 3, right posterior cerebral artery infarct **(C** and **D)** and 10-week follow-up **(E).** *Axial third ventricle-level noncontrast (C and E) and i.v. contrast CT scans (D).* Note hyperdense hemorrhagic areas *(H)* and contrast enhancement *(CE)* of the right posterior cerebral artery territory. Note how i.v. contrast has obscured the hemorrhage. There is resulting slightly ill-defined hypointensity at 10 weeks due to encephalomalacia *(En).*

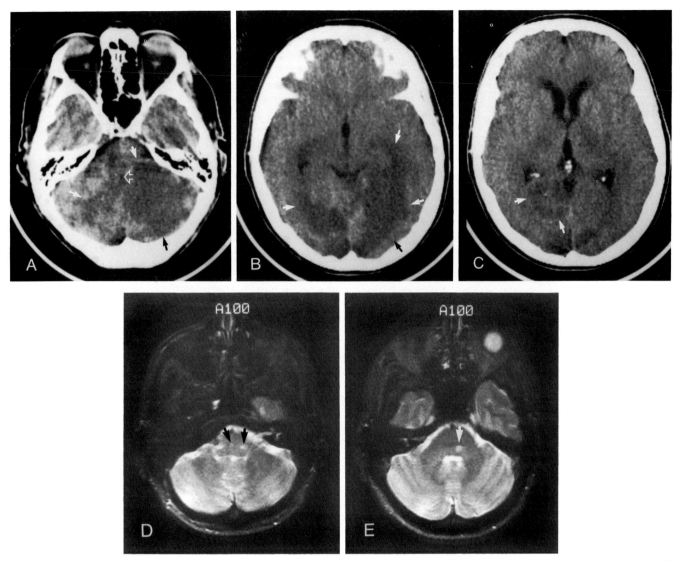

Figure 6.13. Basilar artery infarcts and brainstem infarcts. A–C and **D–E** are different cases. **A–C,** Day 2, basilar artery infarct. *Fourth ventricle-level (A), midbrain-level (B), and third ventricle-level (C) noncontrast axial CT scans.* There is bilateral cerebellar abnormal hypointensity, left greater than right *(closed arrows on **A**).* The fourth ventricle is displaced and deformed *(open arrow).* **B** demonstrates greater left-sided temporoparieto-occipital hypodensity whereas **C** demonstrates greater right-sided involvement. The cerebellar and bilateral hemisphere involvement identifies the basilar artery as the ischemic source. **D–E,** Brainstem infarct, day 2. *Axial brainstem medulla (D) and pons (E) level SE 2800/80 MR scans.* Note the T2 water-isointense bright signals *(arrows).*

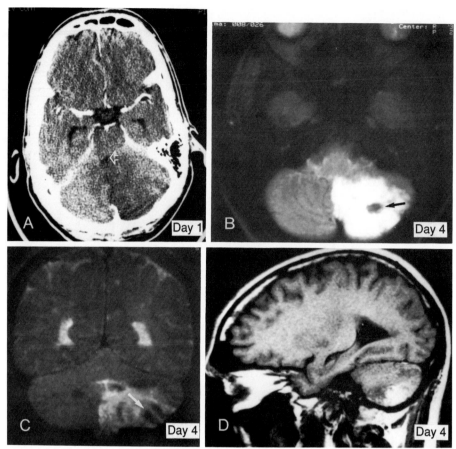

Figure 6.14. Acute posterior inferior cerebellar artery infarct. *Intravenous contrast axial fourth ventricle-level supraorbitomeatal plane CT scan (A) at ictus. Infraorbitomeatal SE 2000/80 MR scan (B). Coronal fourth ventricle-level 2000/80 (C) and left temporal horn-sagittal 600/25 (D) MR scans at day 4.* Note the left inferior cerebellar CT hypodensity and right-sided fourth ventricle displacement *(open arrow).* T1 *(D)* and T2 *(B and C)* hyperintensity indicates a hemor- rhagic component. T2 hypointense foci *(closed arrows)* within the hyperintensity probably indicates deoxyhemoglobin or intracellular methemoglobin. These infarcts often involve the lateral medulla and inferior cerebellar peduncle (the restiform body) producing Wallenberg's syndrome. This case spares the medulla and the restiform body.

cur again at different locations in the same patient.[2,3,17–19]

The MR and CT appearance of lacunar infarcts parallels that of larger infarcts. During the acute stage they are frequently associated with a small amount of surrounding edema and they often contrast enhance in the subacute stage. When acute, the combined infarct and edematous area measures from 1.5–4 cm but later shrinks to less than 1.5 cm in diameter in the "chronic" stage (Fig. 6.15). Small brainstem infarcts that are reliably detected by MR cannot usually be seen by CT due to posterior fossa beam-hardening artifacts (Figs. 6.13**D** and **E**).[15]

Multiple Infarcts

Because the embolic theory of origin of most singular infarcts[1] has been supported in this text, a problem arises in explaining why more singular infarcts are not accompanied by additional infarcts. To counter this argument, why are not more hemorrhagic infarcts (supposedly "embolic" in origin) not accompanied by additional infarcts? Infarcts of different chronicity are commonly seen in the same pa- tient, however (Fig. 6.16). There may be a middle ground in this ongoing argument.[3] Most would agree, at least, that the majority of multiple infarctions are embolic in origin (Fig. 6.17). Cardiac origin emboli occur with myocardial infarction, mural thrombi, arrythmias, subacute bacterial or fungal endocarditis, rheumatic heart disease, and cardiac myxoma.[3] Showers of emboli of the same chronicity are common with bacterial endocarditis and myxoma. Abscesses often develop with endocarditis and pseudoaneurysms often develop with cardiac myxoma and may develop with bacterial and fungal emboli. Patients with severe vasospasm, usually caused by ruptured aneurysm, not uncommonly develop multiple infarcts (Fig. 6.18).

OTHER VASCULAR DISEASES AND CONDITIONS

MR and CT (to a far lesser degree) demonstrate "periventricular" white matter abnormalities in elderly nondemented and demented subjects. MR demonstrates patchy proton density and T2 hyperintense bilaterally symmetrical periventricular and deep

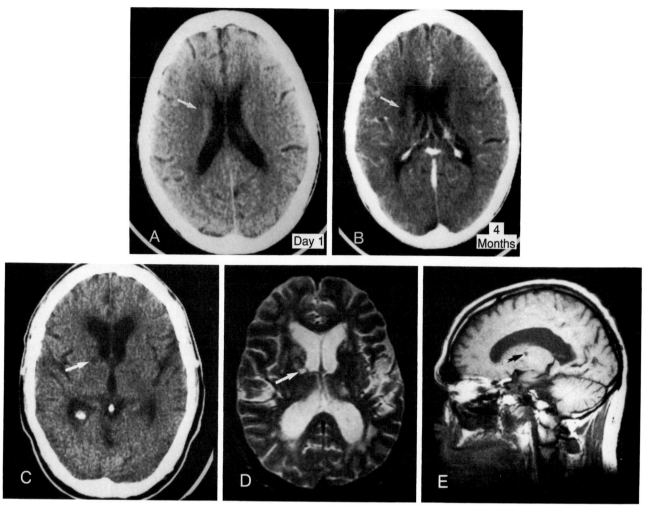

Figure 6.15. Lacunar infarcts. Two different cases. **A–B,** Acute (day 1) and chronic (4 months) lacunar infarct. *Axial lateral ventricle body-level noncontrast CT scan, day 1 (A) and same level i.v. contrast CT scan 4 months later (B).* Note the ill-defined right superior lenticular slightly hypodense infarct **(A),** which is later sharply defined and water-isodense *(arrows)* in the "chronic" state. **C–E,** Remote ("chronic") right globus pallidus lacunar infarct. *Axial foramen of Monro level noncontrast 100/37 CT scan (C) and SE 2800/80 MR scan (D). Sagittal right ganglionic level SE 600/25 MR scan (E).* Water CT density and MR intensity small round globus pallidus lacune *(arrow).* Note smaller similar adjacent lesions seen by both T1- and T2-weighted MR and not by CT.

white matter foci that have slight T1 hypointensity. CT of these lesions often demonstrates slight periventricular and deep white matter patchy hypodensity (Fig. 6.19).[3,20] This appearance, in most cases, is probably caused by atrophic perivascular demyelination[21] although other causes such as subcortical arteriosclerotic encephalopathy (Binswanger's disease)[20,22] may be occasionally responsible. Atrophic perivascular demyelination is a degenerative process resulting from arteriolar wall thickening that is usually unassociated with symptoms.[21] Binswanger's disease is caused by arteriosclerotic and hypertensive vasculopathy, is associated with dementia, and results in multiple infarctions.[21] We have used the term "small vessel disease" to describe the CT and MR appearance because both of the bilateral diffuse conditions, atrophic perivascular demyelination and Binswanger's disease (Fig. 6.20), have similar image appearances and are of vascular origin.

Much less frequent causes of adult diffuse white matter disease are multiple sclerosis, radiation necrosis, methotrexate white matter necrosis, and various leukodystrophies.[20] We have also seen reversible centrum semiovale white matter changes in cases of probable encephalitis and following recent intrathecal methotrexate and brain irradiation.

Cerebral infarction occurs in up to 15% of patients with sickle cell disease. This thrombotic process most frequently involves the carotid system sparing the basilar artery distribution.[23]

Moyamoya disease is a rare condition most often found among patients of Japanese descent. It is a vascular occlusive process of unknown etiology. The main feature of moyamoya is the progressive occlusion of the supraclinoid portion of the internal carotid artery and its branches with the development of extensive parenchymal, leptomeningeal, and

Figure 6.16. Multiple infarcts of different chronicity. Axial foramen of Monro 37/100 i.v. contrast CT scan. Day 1, right internal carotid artery distribution infarct. The entire right middle and posterior cerebral artery territory appears as a homogeneous hypodense mass *(open arrows)* displacing the septum pellucidum and third ventricle to the left. The right posterior cerebral artery arises directly from the right internal carotid artery. Note right anterior medial frontal sparing due to the right anterior cerebral artery supply via the anterior communicating artery. The left frontal lobe more marked hypodensity *(closed arrows),* an enlarged left Sylvian fissure, and ipsilateral left lateral ventricle frontal horn dilatation represent evidence of a remote left middle cerebral artery infarct. There is also left globus pallidus hypodensity representing evidence of additional ganglionic infarction.

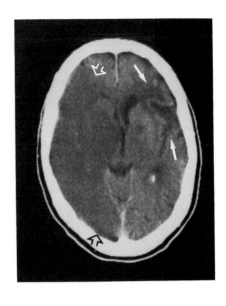

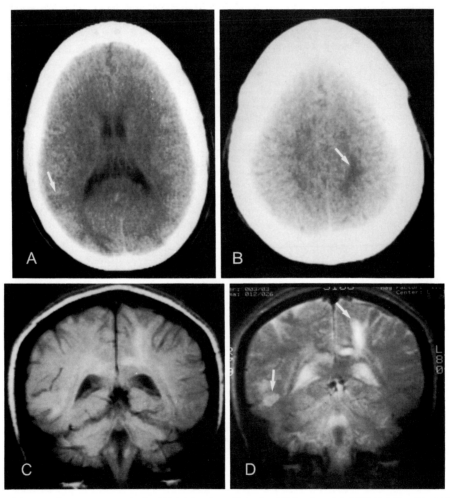

Figure 6.17. Multiple infarcts. Postpartum emboli. Axial lateral ventricle body-level **(A)** and centrum semiovale-level **(B)** CT scans at day 1. Day 2, *coronal atrial level SE 2000/20* **(C)** and 2000/80 **(D).** Note the bilateral parietal CT ill-defined hypodensity **(A** and **B)** and MR T2-weighted hyperintensity *(arrows).* The T2-weighted image lesion conspicuity is much greater than on the T1-weighted image.

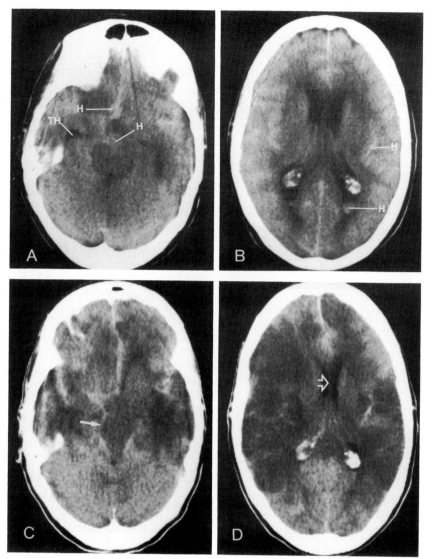

Figure 6.18. Multifocal infarction caused by severe vasospasm. Patient with ruptured anterior communicating artery aneurysm, subarachnoid hemorrhage, resultant vasospasm, infarction and herniation. Axial noncontrast midbrain-level **(A)** and ventricular body-level **(B)** CT scans 5 days after aneurysm rupture. Same level scans, respectively, at 6 days **(C–D)**. Interhemispheric and interpeduncular cistern **(A)** and left Sylvian fissure and intraventricular **(B)** hemorrhage *(H)*. Minimal degree hydrocephalus is evidenced by temporal horn dilatation *(TH)* and there is moderate degree white matter hypodensity at day 5. One day later, there is marked parenchymal hypodensity, downward incisural herniation *(arrow on* **C**), and subfalcine herniation *(open arrow)*. There is now lack of hydrocephalus due to generalized cerebral edema.

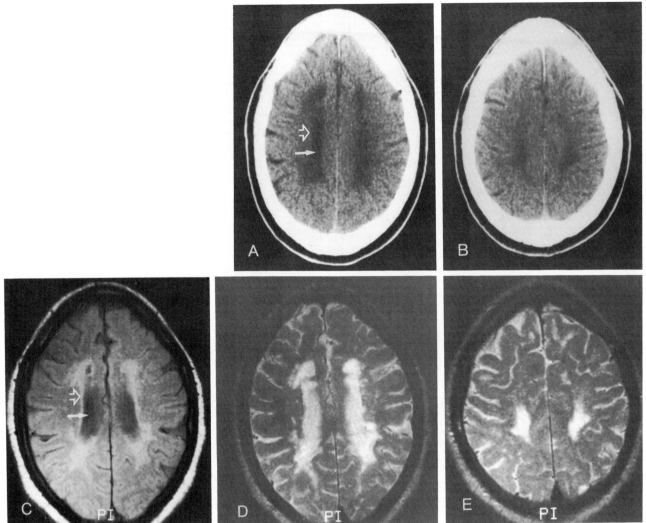

Figure 6.19. Diffuse small vessel disease (perivascular demyelination). *Axial noncontrast superior ventricle body-level CT scan (A) and centrum semiovale scan (B). Same level as scan A, SE 2000/20 (C) and 2000/80 (D) MR scans. Same level as B, SE 2000/80 (E). C best demonstrates the predominantly periventricular water signal of small vessel disease where the ventricular body (closed arrow) is* surrounded by proton signal hyperintensity *(open arrow).* Because the ventricular bodies cannot be adequately distinguished from periventricular hypodensity in **A** or from periventricular T2 hyperintensity in **D**, this relationship is less clear. The T2-weighted images (**D** and **E**) most clearly demonstrate the abnormal signal. Note the smaller, more peripheral "punctate" hyperintense lesions in **D**.

transdural collateral arteries. In childhood, cerebral ischemia is the most common cause of symptoms. Subarachnoid hemorrhage is the most common clinical presentation in the adult. Infarcts also occur. Most symptoms are transient. Intracranial hemorrhage is the usual cause of death. CT demonstrates focal areas of atrophy, subarachnoid hemorrhage and intraparenchymal hemorrhage (Fig. 6.21A and B). Focal areas of hypodensity in the basal ganglia and cortex can be seen. Abnormal CT contrast enhancement is not a characteristic of this disease but tortuous attenuated arteries can be shown with contrast. CT may also demonstrate contrast enhancement of an associated subacute infarct. MR is a better imaging technique for moyamoya. Occlusion or stenosis of the intracranial internal carotid arteries and proximal anterior and middle cerebral artery branches can be

demonstrated by MR. Abnormal basal ganglionic "moyamoya arteries," infarction, and brain atrophy can also be identified.[25] MR may also show hemosiderin deposits with T2-weighted images. We have not seen a case of moyamoya by MR at our hospital yet.[25] Intracranial vascular occlusive disease is an uncommon manifestation of neurofibromatosis.[3] We have studied such a case by MR that demonstrated basal ganglia collateral small caliber arteries (Fig. 6.21C and D).

Systemic lupus erythematosis (SLE) involves the brain in up to 75% of patients. Pathological findings include vasculopathy, infarction and hemorrhage. Both large and microscopic infarctions are common. The most common SLE CT finding is atrophy, which could be caused by steroid therapy.[26] CT can detect small and large infarcts but MR has much greater

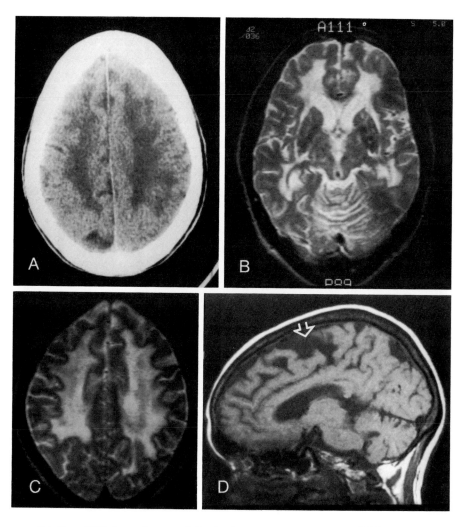

Figure 6.20. Subcortical arteriosclerotic encephalopathy—Binswanger's disease. *Axial noncontrast 37/100 centrum semiovale CT scan (A). Axial SE 2800/80 frontal horn-level (B) and centrum (C) MR scans. Parasagittal SE 600/25 MR scan (D).* Note the florid white matter CT hypodensity and MR T2 hyperintensity. There is marked rolandic and perirolandic atrophy *(open arrow).*

sensitivity. MR has detected both large and small solitary and multifocal infarcts (Fig. 6.22) and has also detected transient T2 hyperintense cortical areas probably representing ischemic areas.[26]

Axial sections using 3-D flow sensative techniques can identify carotid and vertebral artery dissection.

VENOUS OCCLUSIVE DISEASE

Venous sinus thrombosis can be detected by both CT and MR.[27,28] MR, alone, can dependably document deep and superficial venous thrombosis.[28]

Dural venous sinus thrombosis has a variable clinical presentation including headache, behavioral changes, paraparesis, and seizures. Cavernous sinus thrombosis will present typical optic and cranial nerve findings and will be further discussed in Chapter 11. Before the discovery of antibiotics, venous sinus thrombosis was often associated with mastoid sinusitis and facial infections and the transverse sinus was most frequently involved. It is now seen more commonly with altered coagulation states in pregnancy, the puerperium, systemic infection, oral contraceptives, polycythemia, hypercoagulability related to malignancy, thrombotic purpura, neurovascular disseminated intravascular coagulation

(DIC), severe malnutrition, and dehydration. It is also seen with dural invasive tumors such as meningiomas or metastases.[3,27,28]

Hemorrhagic infarction, brain edema, and ventricular compression often occur with dural venous sinus thrombosis. There may be associated deep and cortical vein thrombosis. Deep vein thrombosis is a grave complication, is more frequent in children, causes periventricular infarcts, and is usually lethal. Hemorrhagic infarction is another bad prognostic sign. Isolated cortical vein thrombosis is rare and is prognostically better than the often fatal combined superior sagittal sinus-cortical vein thrombosis.[27]

CT of dural venous sinus thrombosis demonstrates the "delta" or "empty delta" and the "cord" signs (Fig. 6.23). The delta sign is the triangular appearance of the contrast-enhanced margins of the superior sagittal sinus surrounding the lesser density triangular clotted lumen. The outer contrast-enhanced zone is at least partly due to a rich venous collateral network. The delta sign is considered pathognomonic of superior sagittal sinus thrombosis. Care should be taken not to confuse the empty triangle sign with adjacent subdural hematoma, empyema, subarachnoid hemorrhage, or sinus septation.[27] The sign is

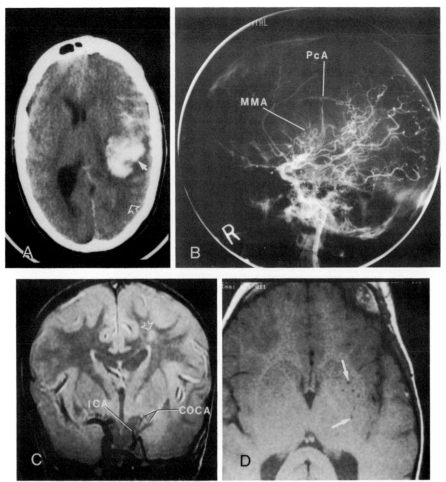

Figure 6.21. Moyamoya (A and B) and vascular occlusive disease of neurofibromatosis (C and D). *A* and *B, Axial lateral ventricle-level noncontrast CT scan (A) and lateral midarterial phase right internal carotid arteriogram (B).* A large left parietal, posterior insular, and ganglionic hemorrhage *(closed arrow)* is surrounded by edema *(open arrow)*. The anterior pericallosal artery *(PcA)* fills retrograde via the posterior pericallosal artery. Note the numerous "moyamoya" small-caliber ganglionic collateral arteries *(MMA)*. **C** and **D,**

Different case. Two-year-old male patient with von Recklinghausen's disease. *Coronal pituitary level. MAST SE 2000/30 (C) and axial basal ganglia-level SE 600/25 MR scans.* Small-caliber stenotic left internal carotid artery *(ICA)*. Abnormal carotid origin collateral arteries *(COCA)*. Note the "moyamoya-like" ganglionic arteries *(closed arrows)*. The left middle cerebral artery Sylvian branch hyperintensity may represent evidence of slow arterial flow. The left frontal forceps minor hyperintensity *(open arrow)* may represent heterotopia or infarct.

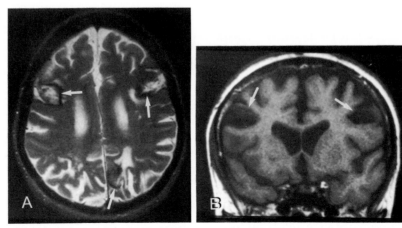

Figure 6.22. Lupus vasculitis. *Axial lateral ventricle body-level SE 2000/80 (A) and coronal SE 600/25 lateral ventricle frontal horn-level (B) MR scans.* Note the T1 water-isointense, T2 mixed heterogeneous hyperintense cortical lesions with peripheral bands of T2 hy-

pointensity *(arrows)*. The CT scan was normal and excluded calcification. The bands probably represent hemosiderin deposits in remote cortical infarcts.

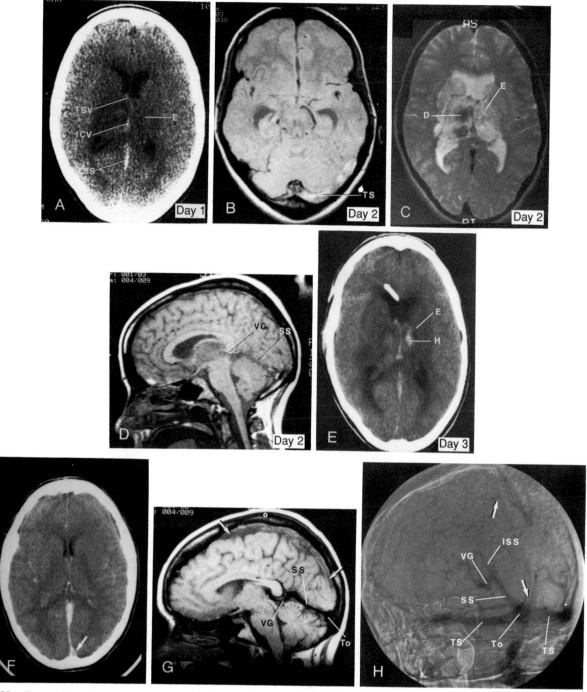

Figure 6.23. **Deep vein and venous sinus thrombosis.** Cases **A–E** and **F–H** are different. **A–E,** *Axial third ventricle-level noncontrast CT* **(A)** *at day 1. All MR scans are at day 2 and no flow-compensation methods were used. Midbrain-level SE 2000/20* **(B),** *axial thalamic-level SE 2000/80* **(C),** *and midsagittal SE 600/25* **(D)** *MR scans. Axial noncontrast CT scan day 3* **(E)** *at same level as* **A** *and* **C.** The CT scans at days 1 and 3 demonstrate hyperdensity ("the cord sign") of the thalamostriate vein *(TSV),* internal cerebral vein *(ICV),* and straight sinus *(SS).* The MR scans demonstrate transverse sinus *(TS),* vein of Galen *(VG),* and straight sinus *(SS)* hyperintensity due to methemoglobin effects. All scans demonstrate thalamic edema *(E)* and thalamic hemorrhage is seen by day 2. Deoxyhemoglobin *(D).* A right lateral ventricle frontal horn drain was placed and CT evi-

dence of thalamic hemorrhage *(H)* is seen at day 3. The delta or "empty delta" sign. Superior sagittal sinus thrombosis. Third ventricle-level axial 35/100 CT scan **(F).** Midsagittal SE 600/25 MR scan **(G),** and digital subtraction oblique cerebral aortography **(H).** No flow-compensation method used. Note the CT contrast-enhanced dural superior sagittal sinus margins outlining the nonenhanced clot *(arrow).* Note that the straight sinus *(SS),* vein of Galen *(VG),* and torcula *(To)* contain signal void. These findings are confirmed angiographically **(H).** Transverse sinus *(TS).* Inferior sagittal sinus *(ISS).* Had flow-compensation methods (MAST) been used, the signal-void effects may have been masked. For this reason, we prefer noncompensated MR technique with emphasis on heavily weighted T1 (600/25).

only detectable in approximately one-third of patients with superior sagittal sinus thrombosis, however.[3,27]

The cord sign is the hyperdensity caused by dural sinus clot (60–80 H). This sign is not as reliable because polycythemic blood also has a high density and knowledge of the patient's hematocrit is necessary for diagnosis. The cord sign can also be seen in cortical veins, the straight sinus, and Galenic system veins with cortical and deep vein thrombosis, respectively (Fig. 6.23A).[3,27] With hematocrits above 60, the dural sinuses, vein of Galen, internal cerebral veins, circle of Willis, and main arterial branches appear "enhanced." In neonates and in patients with diffusely edematous brain parenchyma, the dural sinuses and the blood vessels may appear falsely "dense" by CT compared to brain densities. We recommend measuring CT numbers and comparing them to the patient's hematocrit when this occurs. As stated in Chapter 2, flowing blood at hematocrit of 45 measures 56 H (normal adult HCT = 42–52; normal neonate hematocrit = 37–47). Because the adult gray matter average density is 39, large vessels and the sinuses will appear somewhat dense. Because the normal neonatal brain has slightly lower density than the adult brain, the apparent density of neonatal dural structures is even more pronounced. Despite these diagnostic difficulties, recognition of the dense dural sinus is important because it is a sign of increased blood viscosity. These patients are at high risk for hypoxemic cerebral insult.[3]

MR is superior to CT for diagnosis of dural venous sinus thrombosis because of blood flow time-of-flight effects, accuracy of intensity changes of clotted blood, lack of bone artifact, and orthogonal views including the sagittal (Fig. 6.23).[28] An understanding of MR pulse sequences, time-of-flight phenomena, even echodephasing phenomena, and entrance-exit phenomena, as discussed in Chapters 1 and 3, is essential for interpretation. It is important not to exclusively use flow-compensating sequences if flow effects such as time-of-flight are necessary for the diagnosis.

INFANTILE ISCHEMIA

Infantile ischemia varies from the adult pattern, and because periventricular leukomalacia is unique to the premature neonate, it will be emphasized in this separate section. Infantile ischemia can also result in focal or global infarction. Infarcts in full-term infants characteristically involve the cortical and subcortical regions as compared to the premature periventricular white matter involvement. This difference is due to the premature meningeal collateral cortical perfusion that is lacking in the full-term infant.[29] Intrauterine and perinatal carotid artery infarction may eventually lead to cerebral hemiatrophy or the Dyke-Davidoff-Masson syndrome. In this condition, there is usually atrophy of an entire hemisphere. Compensatory ipsilateral skull thickening, and paranasal and mastoid sinus enlargement develops later in life.[30]

Periventricular leukomalacia results from ischemic periventricular infarction in the premature infant. Subcortical white matter lesions often coexist (Fig. 6.24).[29,30] Periventricular leukomalacia is second only to periventricular and intraventricular hemorrhage as a cause of premature infant cerebral injury. It is rarely fatal but usually results in severe neurological damage. Spastic diplegia or quadriplegia commonly develops with relative preservation of cognitive functions.[31,32] Periventricular white matter coagulation necrosis occurs within a few days after the ischemic insult (stage 1), astrocyte and macrophage proliferation follow at 1–2 weeks (stage 2), and in 3–4 weeks, fluid-filled cavities develop (stage 3).[31] Decreased cyst size and cerebral atrophy follow over the next several months (stage 4). Delayed myelination is characteristic of this condition. There may be coexisting intraparenchymal hemorrhage.[33]

Both CT[33] and MR[31] have been used to image periventricular leukomalacia and, unlike ultrasound, MR can determine the progression of myelination.[29,31] Although CT is of less value in the neonatal period because of the high water content of the immature brain obscuring CT evidence for lack of myelination,[29,33] it is useful in the infant older than 6 months. CT in infants older than 6 months demonstrates periventricular white matter atrophy, particularly at the trigone, periventricular cysts, and enlarged irregularly contoured ventricles.[33] The ventricular contour irregularity is caused by cyst-ventricle porencephaly.[32] MR of periventricular leukomalacia demonstrates the extent of myelination as well as cysts and atrophy.[31]

Focal or hemispheric infarction in the 40-week postconception (full-term) neonate is well demonstrated by CT and MR. Profound focal atrophy may develop.[29] Cerebral hemiatrophy, Dyke-Davidoff-Masson syndrome, has a characteristic CT and MR appearance (Fig. 6.25A and B). There is ipsilateral midline structural shift, ventricular dilatation, and sulcal enlargement. Ipsilateral paranasal sinus and diploic space enlargement is well seen on bone window CT. Adult-acquired cerebral hemiatrophy does not have diploic-paranasal sinus enlargement (Fig. 6.25C–E).[30]

GLOBAL HYPOXIA

Decreased arterial oxygen and/or impaired cerebral perfusion pressure (ischemia) result in global hypoxic brain damage. This is most often caused by cardiorespiratory arrest, severe systemic hypotension, near-drowning, carbon monoxide poisoning, and strangulation.[3,29,34–39] The patients usually exhibit loss of consciousness. The depth and duration of the coma depends on the extent of brain damage and concurrent metabolic factors. Some patients may regain consciousness and relapse into impaired consciousness, spasticity, and hypokinesia due to postanoxic demyelination.[3,37] The basal ganglia and the cortical gray matter are particularly susceptible to anoxia and

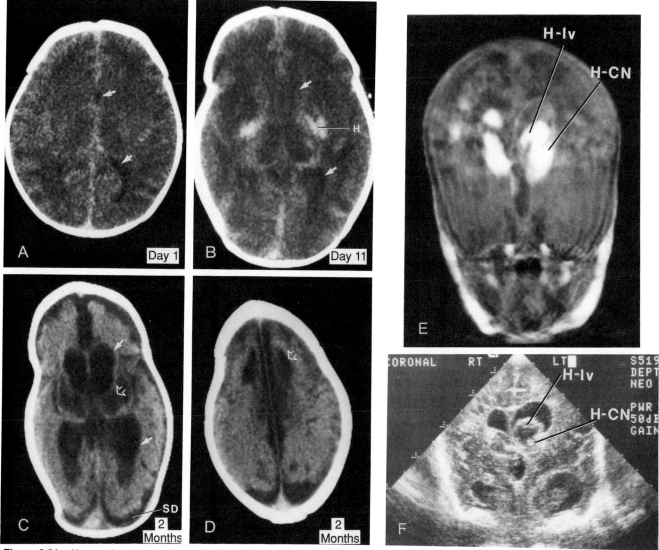

Figure 6.24. **Neonatal asphyxia.** Figures 6.24A-D and 6.24E-F are different cases.

Case 1. **(A-D)** Axial *noncontrast CT scans at birth—day 1* **(A)**, *11 days* **(B)**, *and 2 months* **(C** *and* **D)**. **A–C** are at the same level. At day 1 **(A)**, there is an exaggerated parenchymal hypodensity, relatively "hyperdense" falx and superior sagittal sinus, and "slit-like" lateral ventricles *(solid arrows)*. At day 11, there is bilateral ganglionic hyperdensity from "periventricular" hemorrhage *(H)*. Lateral ventricular expansion has occurred by day 11. The lateral ventricles

are poorly discriminated due to adjacent marked edema. At 2 months, periventricular "cystic" leukomalacia *(open arrows)*, ventricular enlargement *(closed arrows)*, subdural hygromas *(SD)*, and generalized cerebral atrophy has occurred. Note the changing skull configuration. (Courtesy of Mary K. Edwards, M.D., Indianapolis, Indiana.)

Case 2. **(E–F)** *Coronal SE 450/50* MR scan **(E)** and B-sector, ultrasound scan **(F)**. Bilateral caudate nucleus hemorrhage (H·CN) and intraventricular hemorrhage (H·Iv) is seen equally well with both techniques.

ischemia. Basal ganglia infarction frequently occurs. "Laminar necrosis," the term used for preferential necrosis of cortical pyramidal cell layers, may result. Diffuse atrophy is also a common sequella (Fig. 6.26).[3,37]

Early CT findings include diffuse cerebral edema characterized by effacement of fissures, cisterns, and sulci, ventricular compression, lack of gray-white matter distinction and relative hyperdensity of the dura. The cortical involvement is greatest in watershed areas between the anterior, middle, and posterior cerebral artery territories. Gray matter may become hyperdense after several days. Cortical contrast enhancement may develop.[3,39] The CT basal

ganglia low density usually involves the globus pallidus (Fig. 6.27).[3,34,35] Striatal involvement is common, particularly in childhood near-drowning.[38] From 2 weeks to 1 month postictus, generalized atrophy may become quite marked. Hemorrhagic cortical and ganglionic infarction may occur in the subacute stage producing an unusual pattern of serpentine cortical-gray hemorrhage and ganglionic hemorrhage, respectively.[38]

MR of anoxic-ischemic brain insult demonstrates edema, cortical and basal ganglia necrosis, hemorrhage, atrophy, and demyelination with greater tissue contrast and anatomical detail than is demonstrated by CT (Figs. 6.26 and 6.27).[29,35]

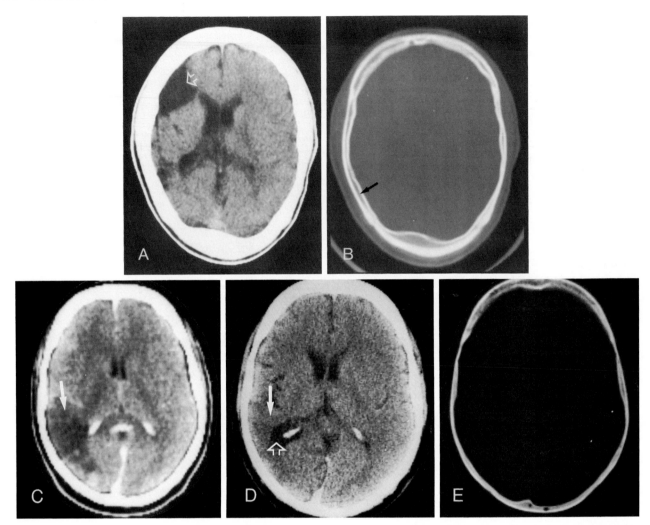

Figure 6.25. Cerebral hemiatrophy. A-B, Dyke-Davidoff-Masson syndrome. *Axial noncontrast ventricle body-level CT scans 35/100 (A) and 30/2000 (B).* Note the triangular water-density right middle cerebral artery infarct *(open arrow)* with ipsilateral right lateral ventricle dilatation and midline structural shift. The right calvarial diploic space is thickened *(closed arrow).* **C-E,** Middle cerebral artery infarct leading to cerebral hemisphere atrophy in an adult. *Axial i.v. contrast third ventricle-level 35/75 160 matrix CT scan (C), 37/100 256 matrix CT scan 3 years later (D), and 37/2000 bone window of D(E).* Note the acute right middle cerebral artery infarct (*closed arrow* on **C**). One and one-half years later **(D),** a persistent "triangle" of hypodensity *(closed arrow)* is associated with ipsilateral ventricular dilatation *(open arrow)* and ipsilateral septum pellucidum and third ventricle shift. Note that there is no diploic widening in **E.**

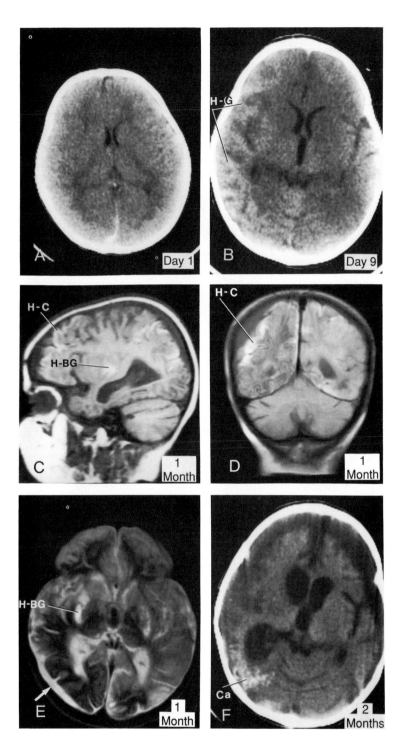

Figure 6.26. Diffuse laminar necrosis and basal ganglia hemorrhage in a 2-year-old after asphyxia. *Axial third ventricular-level, day 1 **(A)** and day 9 **(B)** noncontrast CT scans. MR scans 1 month after hypoxia. Sagittal right lateral ventricular atrial-level SE 600/25 MR scan **(C)**. Atrial-level coronal SE 2000/20 **(D)** and axial third ventricle-level SE 2000/80 **(E)** MR scans. Two-month follow-up atrial-level noncontrast CT scan **(F)**. At day 1, the findings are essentially negative. By day 9 **(B)**, there is gyral hyperdensity (H-G). At 1 month, there is diffuse T1, proton density and T2 gray matter cortical hyperintensity (H-C). The T2 cortical hyperintensity is obscured by the subdural fluid (arrow). There is also profound gyral atrophy. In addition, there is basal ganglia T1 and T2 hyperintensity (H-BG). At 2 months, there is parenchymal calcification (Ca), bilateral subdural hygromas, and profound diffuse atrophy.*

Figure 6.27. Carbon monoxide poisoning. *Axial third ventricle-level i.v. contrast CT scan* **(A).** *Same (approximate) level axial SE 2000/80 MR scan* **(B).** *Coronal third ventricle level SE 2000/20* **(C)** *and 2000/ 80* **(D)** *MR scans.* Note the bilateral globus pallidus CT hypodensity and the MR proton-density weighted and T2-weighted hyperintensity *(arrows).*

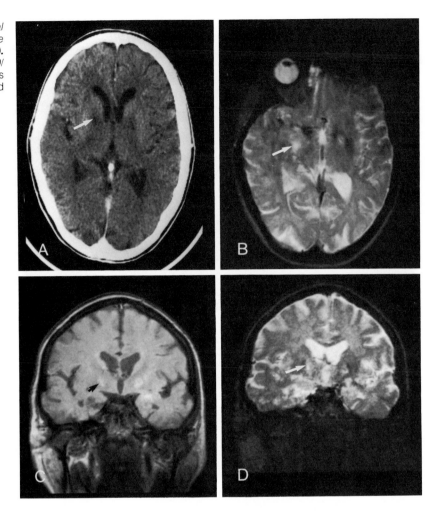

Spontaneous Intracerebral Hemorrhage

PARENCHYMAL

Approximately 70% of spontaneous adult intracerebral hemorrhages occur in hypertensive patients. Hemorrhage occurs in approximately 10% of stroke patients, 70% of whom are hypertensive. Other causes of nontraumatic hemorrhage include ruptured aneurysm or AVM, anticoagulant therapy, hemorrhage into a tumor, bleeding diathesis, amyloid angiopathy,[40] septic emboli, atrial myxoma, Moya Moya, collagen disorders, and venous thrombosis with hemorrhagic infarction.[3] Spontaneous intrancranial hemorrhage also occurs in illegal drug use, i.e., cocaine abuse. Some of these latter conditions will be further discussed in this and other chapters.

The morbidity and prognosis of the spontaneous intracranial hemorrhage is related to its size. Recovery is frequent with small hemorrhage because the hemorrhage dissects primarily between nerve fibers as compared to the neuronal death caused by infarction.[3]

Ninety percent of hypertensive hemorrhages are supratentorial. The putamen, thalamus, head of caudate nucleus, and external capsule ("ganglionic hem-

orrhages") are the most common sites. The most common sites in the posterior fossa are the pons and cerebellar hemispheres. Ganglionic hemorrhages may rupture into the adjacent ventricle. Mass effect is often relatively small with respect to the lesion size.[3]

A recent hemorrhage in an unusual location, such as the cortex, should be investigated for underlying causes, such as brain tumor and AVM.

Noncontrast CT is most accurate for identifying acute stage hemorrhage and is very adequate under most clinical situations. MR has the advantage of identifying subacute and chronic hemorrhage better than does CT; and MR is more accurate for detecting posterior fossa hemorrhage due to lack of streak artifact.[41] Some controversy exists concerning the efficacy of MR during the first few postictal days. This is because of the dependence upon the T2 hypointensity of deoxyhemoglobin for diagnosis. Hemorrhage T1 hyperintensity depends upon methemoglobin, which develops after 2 days.[42]

High-field strength MR of spontaneous parenchymal hemorrhage is characterized by acute, subacute, and chronic phases (Fig. 6.28). The acute phase (<1 week) has T2 central hypointensity. Edema develops in the late acute and early subacute phase. The hy-

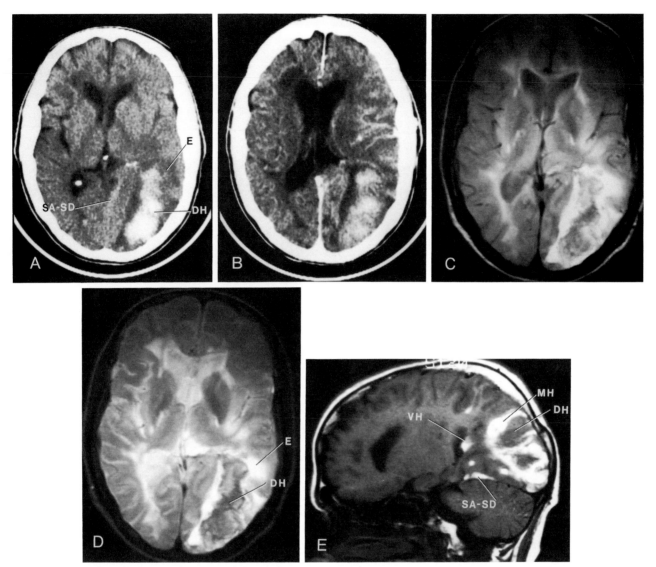

Figure 6.28. Spontaneous parenchymal hemorrhage with subdural and/or subarachnoid hemorrhage in a 53-year-old hypertensive male. Day 1, CT. Day 2, MR. *Axial third ventricle-level noncontrast **(A)** and ventricle body-level i.v. contrast **(B)** CT scans at ictus. Axial SE 2000/20 **(C),** 2000/80 **(D),** and sagittal 600/25 **(E)** MR scans the next day. Deoxyhemoglobin in left occipitoparietal hemorrhage (DH). Subarachnoid and/or subdural supratentorial hemorrhage (SA-SD); edema (E); methyhemoglobin (MH); intraventricular hemor-* rhage *(VH). The CT scan detects the hyperdensity of deoxyhemoglobin, which is MR T2 hypointense and T1 isointense. The heavily T1-weighted MR image distinguishes the methemoglobin portion of the hemorrhage from the surrounding edema which the "proton density" image and the T2-weighted image cannot. Intravenous contrast CT obscures the supratentorial extra-axial hemorrhage. Note anterior displacement of the left lateral ventricle atrium.*

perintense proton density and T2-weighted technique edema can obscure methemoglobin hyperintensity (Fig. 6.12). Subacute hematomas have T1 peripheral hyperintensity followed by T2 peripheral hyperintensity. This hyperintensity fills in the hematoma in the late subacute and early chronic stages. In the late chronic stage, the hematoma center develops water isointensity and the peripheral hemosiderin results in a ring of marked T2 hypointensity.[42] The reader is referred to Chapter 3 for review of MR changes of hematoma progression.[42]

Noncontrast CT of spontaneous parenchymal hemorrhage shows high density clot with slightly ill-defined margins (Fig. 6.29). Extension of hemorrhage

along white matter tracts may occur and produce an irregular contour. There is usually a moderate amount of surrounding edema. Metabolism and phagocytosis of the hemoglobin and an increase of water content leads toward isodensity in the subacute stage. Rim contrast enhancement of the subacute hematoma is common. Focal atrophy also develops during the subacute stage.[3]

SUBARACHNOID HEMORRHAGE

Twelve percent of nontraumatic subarachnoid hemorrhages are sequellae of spontaneous intracerebral hemorrhage. Seventy-five percent are the result of ruptured aneurysms and 10% are due to rup-

Figure 6.29. Basal ganglia hemorrhage. *Axial lateral ventricle body-level 35/100 CT scans day 1 **(A)** and day 2 **(B)**.* Note the small left superior left insular hemorrhage *(closed arrow)* at ictus, which massively increases by day 2 with marked hemorrhage, mass effect, and intraventricular component *(open arrow)*.

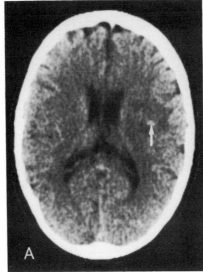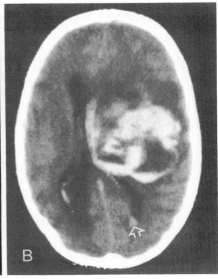

tured AVM. The rest of spontaneous subarachnoid hemorrhages are from other causes and are idiopathic.[3] Noncontrast CT[43] is superior to MR for the detection of subarachnoid hemorrhage probably due to the slower conversion of oxyhemoglobin to methemoglobin of red blood cells in CSF.[44]

CT demonstrates hyperdensity ($\leq$ 80 H) in the perimesencephalic cisterns, Sylvian fissures, interhemispheric fissure, sulci, and juxtatentorial locations (Fig. 6.30).[43] Much has been written of the "pentagonal cistern" (perimesencephalic cistern) and ease of recognition of interpeduncular fossa and chiasmatic cistern subarachnoid hemorrhage. Focality of increased subarachnoid hemorrhage in the an-

terior interhemispheric fissure, in a Sylvian fissure or in the subtentorial compartment, help to localize a ruptured aneurysm to the anterior communicating artery, a middle cerebral artery, or a vertebrobasilar artery, respectively. MR occasionally will demonstrate acute subarachnoid hemorrhage (Fig. 6.28). Subarachnoid hemorrhage develops MR hyperintensity with the passage of time and becomes recognizable 1 week postictus, coincidental with the disappearance of CT hyperdensity due to destruction of the hemoglobin molecule.[44]

Hydrocephalus and spasm commonly complicate subarachnoid hemorrhage. Intraventricular hemorrhage is frequently seen in the occipital horns of the

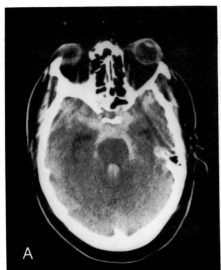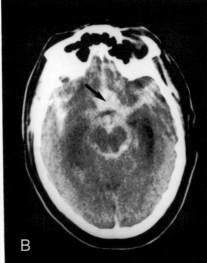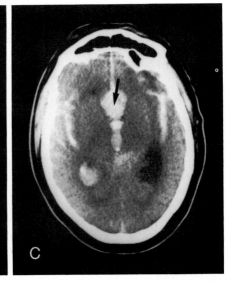

Figure 6.30. Subarachnoid hemorrhage. *Axial 36/100 sella-level **(A)**, chiasmatic cistern-level **(B)** and third ventricle-level **(C)** CT scans.* The massive subarachnoid hemorrhage is caused by the rupture of a small anterior communicating aneurysm. It has dissected into the septum pellucidum *(arrows)*. Hemorrhage is seen in the perimesen-

cephalic cisterns in the Sylvian and interhemispheric fissures and in the third and fourth ventricles.

Occasionally, when only a small amount of subarachnoid hemorrhage is present, it is most conspicuous in the interpeduncular cistern.

lateral ventricles. Those patients with a large amount of subarachnoid hemorrhage tend to have a greater degree of spasm.

NEONATAL INTRACRANIAL HEMORRHAGE

Neonatal intracranial hemorrhage can be classified as extra-axial, intraventricular, and intraparenchymal. Neonatal extra-axial hemorrhage is usually associated with difficult deliveries, particularly those necessitating forceps. These extra-axial hemorrhages are probably due to tearing of superficial cortical veins and/or dural venous sinuses. Neonatal extra-axial hemorrhages are usually subdural but may be epidural or subarachnoid. Neonatal intraventricular and parenchymal hemorrhage is a significant problem in the low birth-weight neonate (Fig. 6.24 and 6.31). Neonatal intracranial morbidity and mortality is roughly proportional to the degree of parenchymal hemorrhage and to the degree of ventriculomegaly.[41,45]

The site of neonatal parenchymal hemorrhage corresponds to the gestational age. Subependymal and intraventricular hemorrhage predominate in premature infants because the subependymal germinal matrix in the premature neonate is particularly susceptible to hypoxic injury. The most common site of subependymal hemorrhage is the caudate nucleus. These hemorrhages often dissect posteriorly along the ependyma adjacent to the lateral ventricle body. Extra-axial and peripheral parenchymal hemorrhage occur more frequently in the full-term infant. These extra-axial hemorrhages are often asymptomatic without long-term clinical consequence. They are found along the lateral convexity, floor of the middle fossa, or falx.[41]

Neonatal hemorrhage sequellae include porencephaly and ventriculomegaly. Porencephalic cysts usually occur in the anterior and midlateral ventricular location but may be peripheral and communicate with the subarachnoid space. They can develop from cavitation of hemorrhage with evacuation into the lateral ventricles or subarachnoid space. Poren-

cephaly may develop as early as the second postnatal week.[41] Posthemorrhagic hydrocephalus may be due to ependymitis. It may also be caused by obstruction of the foramen of Monro, ventricular aqueduct, fourth ventricular outlets, basilar arachnoiditis, or blockage of arachnoid granulations. The lateral ventricular dilatation may be asymmetrical. The presence of neonatal periventricular edema or transependymal absorption is not reliably demonstrated by CT or MR due to the high water content of the immature white matter. The hydrocephalus may require shunting if it does not stabilize.[41,45]

Neonatal neurosonography is still the standard method of examining the neonate for intra-axial hemorrhage. Ultrasound can detect small areas of parenchymal and intraventricular hemorrhage with almost the same accuracy as CT. The ultrasound method cannot distinguish hemorrhage from infarct but this lack of specificity is outweighed by the practicality of the method. Diagnosis of hemorrhage by MR is dependent on T2 hypointensity during the first 2 days and, for this reason, some authors believe it is less accurate during this early period than neurosonography and CT. At 7–10 days, the hemorrhage becomes isodense to CT[45] but the MR hyperintense T1 and T2 signal persists for 2–11 weeks.[41] MR is clearly superior to CT during the late acute and subacute periods for hemorrhage detection, particularly for detection of subacute extra-axial hemorrhages.[41]

In summary, MR and CT (Fig. 6.31) of neonatal intracranial hemorrhage demonstrate the varying progression, maturation, and degree of severity of the hemorrhagic process, and the porencephaly and ventriculomegaly that develops. Neonatal neurosonography remains the standard means of diagnosis and follow-up until 6 months of age.

Intracranial Aneurysms
CONGENITAL "BERRY" ANEURYSMS

Berry aneurysms occur at branches of major intracranial arteries. They probably occur because of a

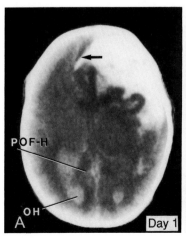
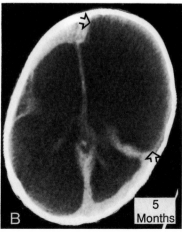

Figure 6.31. Neonatal ICH and sequellae. Premature infant at birth and 5-month follow-up. *Noncontrast axial frontal horn-level, day 1 **(A)**, and 5-month follow-up **(B)** CT scans.* At day 1, there is a large left frontal hemorrhage with a marked shift of the falx *(closed arrow).* The hemorrhage extends laterally to involve the left frontal operculum and insula. There is lateral ventricle occipital horn hemorrhage *(OH)* and subarachnoid hemorrhage in the parieto-occipital fissure *(POF-H).*

Marked left lateral ventricle porencephaly *(open arrows)* and ventricular dilatation has developed at 5 months. Only focal areas of detectable cortical mantle remain.

It seems unlikely that this hemorrhage began in the subependymal-caudate location. The cases currently being examined by CT are complicated; having neurosonographic images that require better definition by CT. We have not scanned the more common subependymal-caudate hemorrhage for a very long time.

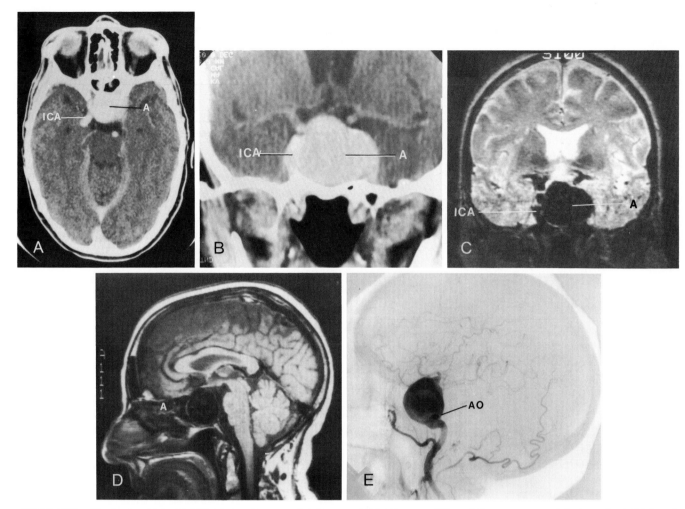

Figure 6.32. Giant cavernous carotid artery aneurysm. *Axial i.v. contrast* **(A)** *and coronal i.v. contrast* **(B)** *CT scans. Coronal SE 2000/ 80* **(C)** *and midsagittal 600/25* **(D)** *MR scans without flow-compensation techniques. Left common carotid arteriogram lateral projection* **(E)**.
Note the right internal carotid artery *(ICA)*, the left cavernous ca-

rotid aneurysm *(A)*, and the aneurysm origin from the left internal carotid artery *(AO)*. There is CT homogeneous contrast enhancement. The MR signal void time-of-flight effect is accompanied by marked bitemporal horizontal flow artifact on the T2-weighted image **(C)**.

congenital arterial wall defect and subsequent degenerative changes associated with aging. Most berry aneurysms are less than 1 cm in diameter. Aneurysms measuring 2.5 cm in diameter or greater are called giant intracranial aneurysms (Figs. 6.32 and 6.33).[46–48] Berry aneurysms are more common in patients with a family history of cerebral aneurysms, longstanding hypertension, and patients with polycystic renal disease. The most common locations are the anterior and posterior communicating arteries and the middle cerebral artery trifurcation. Less common sites include the ophthalmic and anterior choroidal artery origins of the internal carotid artery siphon, the internal carotid artery bifurcation, the distal basilar artery, the anterior and posterior inferior cerebellar arteries, and the pericallosal artery. The most common sites of larger aneurysms are the basilar tip and the cavernous and supraclinoid portions of the internal carotid artery.[3]

Aneurysms usually clinically present when they

rupture producing subarachnoid hemorrhage. Occasionally, they will produce sufficient mass effect to cause neurological symptoms, such as a posterior communicating artery aneurysm causing third nerve palsy. Vasospasm is most common 5–12 days after aneurysm rupture. Spasm is often so marked as to cause cerebral infarction (Fig. 6.18). Patients with a large amount of subarachnoid hemorrhage tend to develop more severe spasm. Anterior cerebral artery infarction, otherwise uncommon, is not an unusual complication of severe spasm after subarachnoid hemorrhage. Communicating hydrocephalus may also develop and can be so severe as to require a ventricular shunt.

Noncontrast CT is the procedure of choice for initial work-up of berry aneurysms due to the usual presentation with subarachnoid hemorrhage. Areas of predominant hemorrhage or areas of associated parenchymal hemorrhage are a strong clue to aneurysm location (Fig. 6.30). A noncontrast CT scan

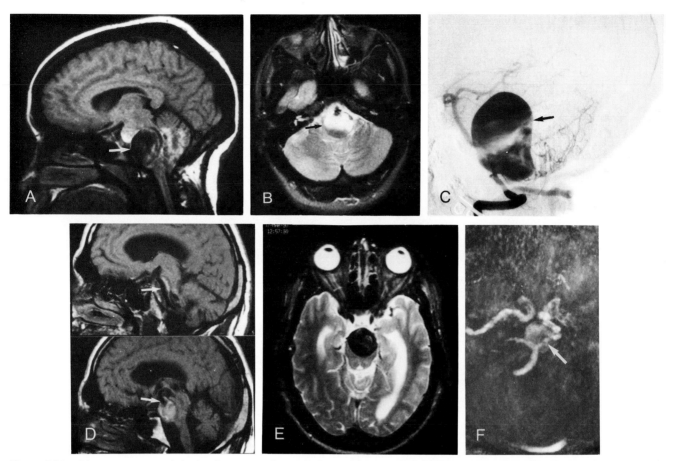

Figure 6.33. Giant aneurysms of the basilar artery. *Cases (A-C) and (D-F) are different patients.*
Case 1 *(A-C)*: *Giant aneurysm at the basilar artery origin. Sagittal SE 600/25 (A) without motion compensation technique (MAST) and axial 2800/80 with MAST (B) MR scans and lateral vertebral arteriogram (C).* Note the non-MAST signal void aneurysm **(A)** appears hyperintense with MAST **(B).** Pulsation artifact in the phase direction in A (closed arrow) is absent in **(B).** Note the hyperintensity of scalp veins **(B).** Arteries in the B sequence were signal-void on other sections. Case 2 *(D-F)*: *Giant aneurysm of the basilar artery tip with small channel within larger clotted portion. Left parasagittal (top) and midsagittal (bottom) SE (600/20 non-MAST noncontrast MR) scans*

(D), *axial 2749/90 pulse triggered, MAST MR scan (E) and MR angiogram 3D FLASH 40/7 20° flip angle (F).* The patent channel within the aneurysm is signal void in **(D)** and hyperintense in **(E)** *(closed arrows).* The different SE sequences on different 1.5T scanners used for Case 1 and Case 2 produce different SE flow effects. Comparing the aneurysm, venous and arterial intensities on different sequences provides clues to the presence of flow and, in Case 1, the presence of slow flow. The flow sensitive GRE (FLASH) technique **(F)** results in hyperintense arteries and veins. The thrombosed portion of the Case 2 aneurysm is T1 hyperintense, T2 hypointense and T2* hyperintense.

should always precede the i.v. contrast scan for investigation of subarachnoid hemorrhage so as not to obscure evidence for hemorrhage or calcification. Aneurysm wall calcification occasionally occurs, is more common in giant aneurysms, and often has a curvolinear shape (Fig. 6.34). The contrast CT scan can demonstrate berry aneurysms greater than 5 mm in diameter (Fig. 6.34) although tortuous arteries can give the false appearance of an aneurysms. Arteriography is necessary for confirmation and detail. Aneurysm wall thrombus is a fairly common occurrence and can be demonstrated by i.v. contrast CT (Fig. 6.35).[46]

MR of berry aneurysms usually fails to demonstrate acute subarachnoid hemorrhage. Even aneurysms as small as 4 mm in diameter may be detected by signal-void effect using spin-echo methods (Fig. 6.34). MR of giant aneurysms demonstrates the pat-

ent lumen by signal-void or flow-enhancement effects and laminated, staged thrombus with intervening layers of hemosiderin and methemoglobin (Figs. 6.32 and 6.33). The methemoglobin tends to have a centripedal distribution in giant aneurysms as compared to the centrifugal distribution in spontaneous parenchymal hemorrhage (Fig. 6.28).[47,48] Contrast MR, due to time-of-flight effects, may fail to enhance aneurysms reliably unless flow is sufficiently slow.

ATHEROSCLEROTIC ANEURYSMS

These aneurysms are fusiform and result from atherosclerotic arterial dilatation and elongation. They predominantly involve the basilar artery (Fig. 6.36). The distinction between atherosclerotic aneurysm and marked atherosclerotic ectasia is not clear. Occasionally, the carotid system is involved (Fig. 6.8). They occur in the older age group, particularly in

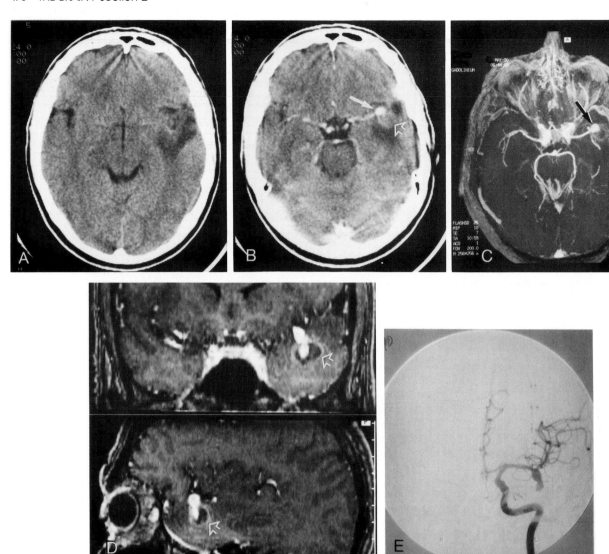

Figure 6.34. Partially clotted left middle cerebral artery aneurysm. *Flow sensitive gradient echo MR technique. Axial chiasmatic cistern-level noncontrast (A) and I.V. contrast (B) CT scans. Same level I.V. contrast 3D FLASH 40/7, 25° 32 mm slab MRA (C) with coronal (D-top) and sagittal (D-bottom) reformations. Left internal carotid arteriogram AP (E).*
There is a CT mixed density partially contrast enhancing aneurysm *(closed arrow)* with surrounding edema. The clotted portion (open arrow) is demonstrated by both the CT and MR methods. The reformations very accurately demonstrate the bilobed character of the aneurysm and compare favorably to the arteriogram. Note the rim contrast-enhanced clotted portion on the MR scans and the clotted portion slight enhancement on the i.v. contrast CT scan.

hypertensive patients. They may cause brainstem and cranial nerve compression. They do not represent a significant risk of rupture and are usually not surgically approached.[49] CT and MR of atherosclerotic aneurysms demonstrate dilatation and tortuosity of the involved artery or arteries. CT demonstrates associated calcification and MR demonstrates flow.

ANEURYSMS OF OTHER ETIOLOGIES

"Mycotic aneurysm" is a term used to define infective aneurysms that occasionally occur in the course of bacterial or fungal endocarditis. They are often mutiple. Septic emboli lodge in a peripheral cerebral artery producing endothelial ischemia. Bacteria invade the arterial wall resulting in aneurysmal dilatation and rupture. These aneurysms may rapidly increase in size and they may also spontaneously disappear. They frequently rupture into the parenchyma and adhesions may prevent the hemorrhage from escaping into the subarachnoid space.[49] Surgical clipping is often necessary to prevent recurrence. CT and MR of mycotic aneurysms may demonstrate multiplicity of peripheral aneurysms, parenchymal or subarachnoid multiple hemorrhagic or nonhemorrhagic infarcts. Abscesses may coexist. Calcification is unlikely.

Trauma-induced cavernous internal carotid aneurysms (Fig. 6.37), as well as caroticocavernous fistulas, occasionally occur.

A rare type of aneurysm results from emboli of

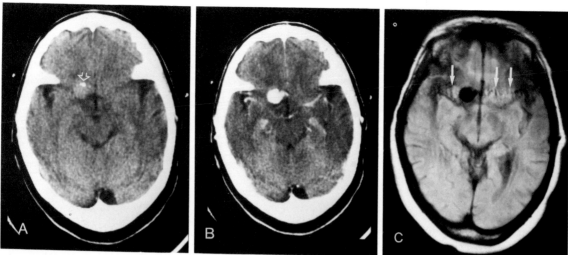

Figure 6.35. Internal carotid artery bifurcation aneurysm-calcification, signal void and flow effect. *Axial noncontrast (A) and i.v. contrast (B) CT scans, and SE 2000/20 non-MAST MR scan (C).* There is a round, smoothly margined, CT hyperdense, homogeneously contrast enhanced paraclinoid lesion that has partial perimeter calcification *(open arrow).* It demonstrates signal void phenomenon and augmentation-cancellation artifact in the phase direction *(closed arrows).*

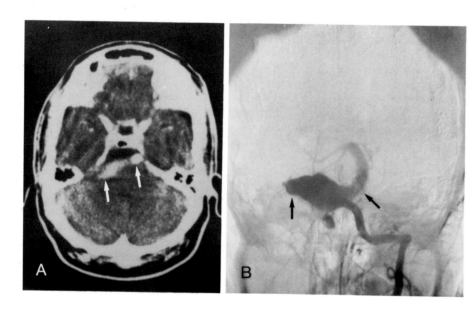

Figure 6.36. Fusiform basilar artery aneurysm. *Axial fourth ventricle-level i.v. contrast CT scan (A). Subtraction left vertebral arteriogram (B).* The fusiform basilar artery aneurysmal dilatation on this CT image extends from the right cerebellopontine angle *(arrows).*

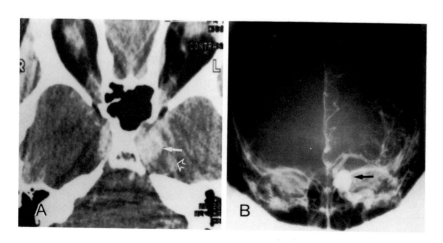

Figure 6.37. Traumatic cavernous carotid artery aneurysm. *Axial sella turcica-level 38/200 i.v. contrast CT scan (A). AP left internal carotid arteriogram (B).* Note the contrast-enhanced aneurysm lumen *(closed arrow)* surrounded by thrombus *(open arrow).* The clivus erosion adjacent to the aneurysm is due to its presence for 6 months.

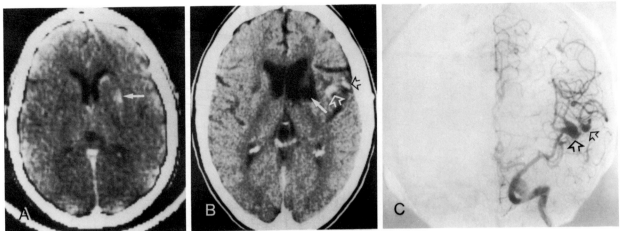

Figure 6.38. Cerebral myxoma. Intracranial hemorrhage, myxomatous aneurysms, and atrophy. *Axial i.v. contrast 160 matrix 35/75 CT scan (A). Same level i.v. contrast 512 matrix 35/100 CT scan 10 years later (B).* Left internal carotid arteriogram at same time as **A(C).**

Note left ganglionic hemorrhage *(A)* progressing to juxtaventricular lacuna (**B,** *closed arrows*). Myxomatous pseudoaneurysms *(open arrows).*

atrial myxoma. Fragments of tumor produce showers of emboli causing arterial occlusions, infarcts, and peripheral pseudoaneurysms within tumor deposits. Different lesion types such as infarct and aneurysm may coexist and since lesions may develop at different times, the multiple infarcts may be at different developmental stages (Fig. 6.38). We only have experience with CT of embolic atrial myxoma at our hospital and have not yet had the opportunity to examine this rare condition with MR. Arteriography is necessary for confirmation and detail of the aneurysm.[3]

ARTERIAL ECTASIA

Dolichoectasia of the distal internal carotid arteries and the proximal cerebral arteries is a rare condition that can occur in the absence of atherosclerosis even in young children. This condition has been implicated in chiasmal and optic nerve syndromes. Both CT and MR will demonstrate the arterial fusiform enlargement and tortuosity (Fig. 6.8). Infarcts may be present presumably secondary to impaired hemodynamics.[50]

Vascular Malformations

ARTERIOVENOUS MALFORMATIONS

AVMs are commonly located in the cerebral and cerebellar hemispheres. They usually clinically present at 20–40 years of age with subarachnoid or parenchymal hemorrhage or seizure. The three types of intracranial AVMs are pure pial, mixed pial dural, and dural.[3,51,52] The former receive arterial supply only from intra-axial arteries. Mixed pial dural malformations receive arterial supply from intra-axial arteries, as well as from dural meningeal branches. Dural AVMs receive arterial supply only from dural arteries. Approximately 75% of AVMs are pure pial, 15% are mixed pial dural, and 10% are dural. Unruptured parenchymal AVMs cause only minor mass

effects as compared to their size.[54] The mass effect can be great with hemorrhage. Edema or gliosis may surround both unruptured and ruptured AVMs and is responsible for T1 hypointensity and T2 hyperintensity effects.[3,51–54]

Both CT and MR are excellent modalities for the investigation of parenchymal AVMs. The CT investigation requires i.v. contrast and the MR technique does not. The adjacent calvarium obscures both CT and MR detail of dural AVMs, however, the MR recognition of serpentine vessels and of flow effects usually is sufficient to identify the lesion. Although CT better detects calcium, MR can detect hemorrhage up to 3 months and better demonstrates blood vessels, particularly in the presence of hemorrhage.[51]

CT of AVMs demonstrates calcification on noncontrast scans or perhaps a subarachnoid or parenchymal hemorrhage. Intravenous contrast enhances the usually large and racemose arteries and veins supplying and draining the AVM but obscures the septae separating vessels within the markedly enhanced nidus (Fig. 6.39). CT often fails to demonstrate dural AVMs due to the adjacent dense skull.[51]

MR of parenchymal AVMs demonstrates clear definition of blood vessels, flow effects, and parenchymal hemorrhage. The blood vessel intensity depends on the velocity of flow and the sequence chosen. As compared to contrast CT, which obscures individual vessels within the nidus, noncontrast MR demonstrates AVM nidus vessels clearly. MR of dural AVMs using flow-enhancement or flow-compensation technique may successfully identify the arterial nidus.[51] Magnetic resonance angiography (MRA) and the individual GRE partitions of 3-D aquisitions show useful detail and are very helpful for therapeutic planning (Fig. 3.24).

Vein of Galen aneurysms are rare lesions that present in the neonatal period usually producing congestive heart failure. They are not true aneu-

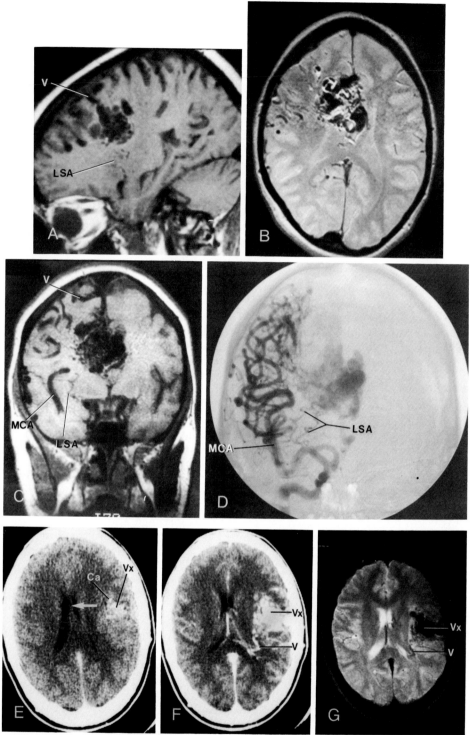

Figure 6.39.   Pial AVMs. Case 1—"Right middle cerebral artery" AVM **(A–D):** *Sagittal orbital-level SE 600/25 **(A)**, axial lateral ventricle-level SE 2800/30 flow compensation (MAST) method **(B)**, and coronal third ventricle-level SE 600/25 **(C)** MR scans. Right carotid arteriogram arterial phase AP **(D)**.* Hypertrophied Sylvian middle cerebral artery branch feeding the malformation *(MCA).* Draining veins *(V).* Hypertrophied lenticulostriate arteries *(LSA)* arising from the M1 segment. Note the large vascular malformation producing signal-void variable caliber vessels on the T1-weighted image and variable flow effect vascular enhancement **(B)** due to flow-compensation (MAST) methods. The confirmation of arterial supply from deep parenchymal vessels (lenticulostriate arteries) has importance for therapeutic embolization consideration and demonstrates the accuracy of MR for demonstrating vascular detail. Case 2—"Left middle cerebral artery" AVM **(E–G):** *Axial lateral ventricle-level 37/100 noncontrast **(E)** and i.v. contrast **(F)** CT scans and SE 2000/80 **(G)** MR scan.* Left insular CT hyperdensity equal to that of the large vein of Galen is mostly due to a large varix *(Vx).* There was no acute hemorrhage despite the slight septum pellucidum shift *(arrow).* A dense anteromedial focus may be calcification *(Ca).* Mass effect is quite unusual in AVM patients lacking acute hemorrhage.

Figure 6.40. Vein of Galen aneurysm. *Axial third ventricle-level noncontrast* ***(A)*** *and i.v. contrast* ***(B)*** *35/100 CT scans. Note the homogeneous slight hyperdensity on the noncontrast scan and the marked homogeneous contrast enhancement after contrast injection of the venous aneurysm (A), the dilated straight sinus (SS), and torcula (T). Other dilated veins are the internal cerebral veins (top arrow) and subependymal veins (bottom arrow).*

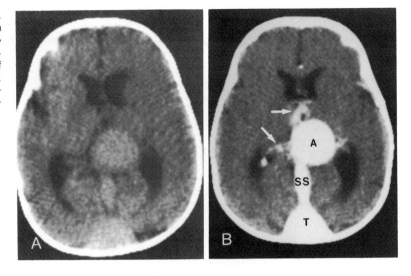

rysms but, actually, are AVMs involving the Galenic venous system.[53] They are associated with a high mortality rate. An initial neurosonography study may suggest the diagnosis (Fig. 6.40) but CT and MR are necessary for confirmation.[55] Arteriography, of course, is the definitive diagnostic examination.

VENOUS ANGIOMAS OR "VENOUS MALFORMATIONS"

Originally thought to be rare, CT and MR are increasingly demonstrating venous angiomas and we categorize their frequency at our hospital as uncommon. The venous angioma consists of a deep cerebral or cerebellar nidus or "body" with a radial distribution of small veins leading to a principal deep medullary or "transcerebral" draining vein. The transcerebral vein leads, in turn, to a superficial cortical vein or dural sinus.[56] No increase in number or caliber of arteries in the nidus area is observed. These malformations are usually smaller and have fewer

vessels than AVMs.[52] In our experience, they usually are discovered by CT and MR as incidental findings unrelated to the patient's presenting complaint. Arteriographic delayed venous phase angiography is the definitive diagnostic procedure. They are usually unassociated with adjacent brain abnormality such as edema, mass effect, or hemorrhage. Hemorrhage may occur, but is far less frequent than with AVMs.[52,57]

CT with i.v. contrast is highly accurate for demonstrating the transcerebral vein. The appearance of the vein on CT images depends upon the plane of section and the orientation of the vein (Fig. 6.41). It may appear as a "dot" of contrast if sectioned perpendicularly or as a straight or curved ribbon of contrast if sectioned longitudinally. There is usually lack of hemorrhage and mass effect and there is always lack of serpentine enlarged arteries and veins characteristic of AVMs. The nidus or body can sometimes

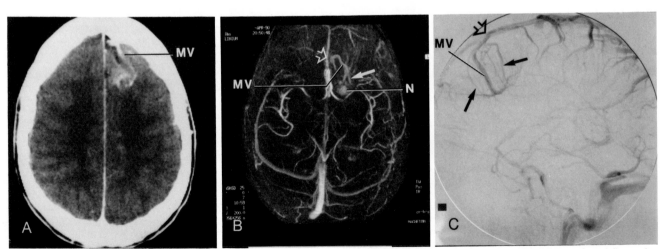

Figure 6.41. Deep venous malformation left frontal lobe. *Axial low centrum-level i.v. contrast CT scan* ***(A).*** *3D-FLASH 40/7, 25° 81 mm slab axial slice-select i.v. contrast MR scan* ***(B).*** *Lateral left carotid arteriogram* ***(C).*** *MRA demonstrates a contrast enhancing deep left frontal vascular nidus (N) with large caliber abnormal medullary veins (closed arrows), the largest of which (MV) leads to the superior sagittal sinus (open arrows). The nidus is demonstrated only by MR in this case.*

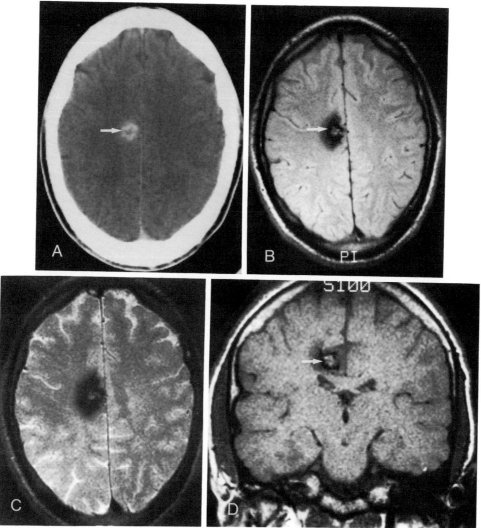

Figure 6.42. Occult vascular malformation. *Axial centrum semiovale-level 35/100 i.v. contrast CT scan* **(A),** *SE 2000/20* **(B),** *and SE 2000/80* **(C)** *MR scan. Coronal third ventricle-level* **(D)** *SE 600/25 MR scans. The cingulate gyrus lesion does not contrast enhance. It is* surrounded by CT hyperdense and MR hypointense calcification *(arrow).* Note the ring of T1 moderate and T2 marked hypointensity of hemosiderin surrounding the calcification on the MR scan. Hemosiderin is not detected on the CT scan.

be seen by CT without contrast due to the intravascular blood content and is usually seen after i.v. contrast.[57]

MR of venous angiomas (Fig. 6.41) demonstrates the enlarged transcerebral draining vein in the vast majority of cases. Spin-echo sequences without flow-compensation will demonstrate the signal-void malformation. In at least one orthogonal plane, the transcerebral vein appears as a curvolinear or straight slow-flow vascular structure. There is usually a lack of parenchymal abnormality other than the radially oriented nidus veins.[52]

ANGIOGRAPHIC CRYPTIC VASCULAR MALFORMATIONS

"Angiographic cryptic" vascular malformations, also called "occult" vascular malformations, are undetectable by angiography and can be demonstrated by both CT and MR (Fig. 6.42). Patients may present with a

parenchymal hemorrhage or seizure; or the lesion may be an incidental finding. These lesions may be AVMs, telangiectasias, and/or cavernous angiomas. They are usually singular but may be multiple and can be found anywhere in the brain including the brainstem. Hemorrhage within these lesions is commonly seen by microscopy. There is usually no mass effect. CT may show slight hyperdensity due to fine calcification and may show faint contrast enhancement. MR may fail to detect the fine calcification. The MR characteristic of occult vascular malformations is a cuff of hemosiderin surrounding a mixed intensity core. Calcification and/or hemosiderin produce central punctate hypointensities. Hyperintensities representing subacute or chronic hemorrhage may be present. MR so far has failed to demonstrate abnormal vessels but may demonstrate faint contrast enhancement. Exclusion of conditions such as infarct might be aided by the presence of calcium on CT.

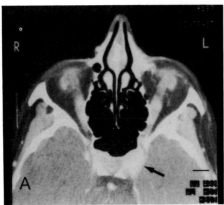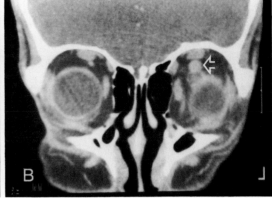

Figure 6.43. Carotid-cavernous fistula. *Axial intravenous contrast pituitary-level **(A)** and coronal cribriform plate-level **(B)** CT scans.* Note the enlarged cavernous sinus *(closed arrow)* and the enlarged superior ophthalmic vein *(open arrow).*

Biopsy can prove dangerous and serial scanning may be a good substitute.[51]

Carotid-Cavernous Fistula

The carotid-cavernous fistula is caused by traumatic cavernous carotid artery rupture or spontaneous rupture of a cavernous carotid artery aneurysm. Symptoms include orbital bruit, chemosis, and pulsatile exophthalmos.

CT demonstrates a prominent cavernous sinus, dilated ophthalmic veins, and proptosis (Fig. 6.43). Dynamic scanning can demonstrate arterialization of the cavernous sinus and superior ophthalmic vein but angiography is necessary for definitive diagnosis and therapeutic planning.[59]

Extracranial Vascular Disease of Neck Vessels

Ultrasound as an initial study and angiography are the principal imaging approaches to neck vessel disease. No doubt the ability of MR to demonstrate blood vessels and estimate blood flow will play an important role in the future and "MR angiography" already shows great promise in the initial investigative phase.[60] Axial sections using 3D time-of-flight techniques can identify carotid and vertebral artery dissection.[61]

References

1. Kricheff II. Arteriosclerotic ischemic cerebrovascular disease. *Radiology* 1987; 162:101–109.
2. Cobb SR, Mehringer CM, Itabashi HH, Pribram H. CT of subinsular infarction and ischemia. *AJNR* 1987; 8:221–227.
3. Masdeu JC, Fine M. Cerebrovascular Disorders. In Gonzalez CF, Grossman CB, Masdeu JC (Eds). *Head and Spine Imaging.* New York: John Wiley & Sons, 1985; 283–356.
4. Hecht-Leavitt C, Gomori JM, Grossman RI. High field MRI of hemorrhagic cortical infarction. *AJNR* 1986; 7:581–585.
5. Brant-Zawadzki M, Weinstein P, Bartkowski H, Moseley M. MR imaging and spectroscopy in clinical and experimental cerebral ischemia: A review. *AJNR* 1987; 8:39–48.
6. Wall SD, Brant-Zawadzki M, Jeffrey RB, Barnes B. High frequency CT findings within 24 hours after cerebral infarction. *AJR* 1982; 138:307–311.
7. Inoue Y, Takemoto K, Miyamoto T, et al. Sequential computed tomography scans in acute cerebral infarction. *Radiology* 1980; 135:655–662.
8. Masdeu JC. Infarct versus neoplasm on CT: Four helpful signs. *AJNR* 1983; 4:522–524.
9. Kapila A. Calcification in cerebral infarction. *Radiology* 1984; 153:685–687.
10. Stovring J, Fernando LT. Wallerian degeneration of the corticospinal tract region of the brain stem: Demonstration by computed tomography. *Radiology* 1983; 149:717–720.
11. Kuhn MA, Johnson KA, Davis KR. Wallerian degeneration: Evaluation with MR imaging. *Radiology* 1988; 168:199–202.
12. Heinz ER, Fuchs J, Osborne D, et al. Examination of the extracranial carotid bifurcation by thin-section dynamic CT: Direct visualization of intimal atheroma in man. *AJNR* 1984; 5:355–366.
13. Smoker WRK, Corbett JJ, Gentry LR, et al. High-resolution computed tomography of the basilar artery: 2. Vertebrobasilar dolichoectasia: Clinical-pathologic correlation and review. *AJNR* 1986; 7:61–72.
14. Vonofakos D, Marcu H, Hacker H. CT diagnosis of basilar artery occlusion. *AJNR* 1983; 4:525–528.
15. Fox AJ, Bogousslavsky J, Carey LS, et al. Magnetic resonance imaging of small medullary infarctions. *AJNR* 1986; 7:229–233.
16. Alvarez O, Edwards JH, Hyman RA. MR recognition of internal carotid artery occlusion. *AJNR* 1986; 7:359–360.
17. Takahashi S, Goto K, Fukasawa H, et al. Computed tomography of cerebral infarction along the distribution of the basal perforating arteries. Part 2: Thalamic arterial group. *Radiology* 1985; 155:119–130.
18. Kashihara M, Matsumoto K. Acute capsular infarction. Location of the lesions and the clinical features. *Neuroradiology* 1985; 27:248–253.
19. Paroni-Sterbini GLP, Mossuto-Agatiello LM, Stocchi A, Solivetti FM. CT of ischemic infarctions in the territory of the anterior choroidal artery: A review of 28 cases. *AJNR* 1987; 8:229–232.
20. Kinkel WR, Jacobs L, Polachini I, et al. Subcortical arteriosclerotic encephalopathy (Binswanger's disease) computed tomographic, nuclear magnetic resonance, and clinical correlations. *Arch Neurol* 1985; 42:951–959.
21. Kirkpatrick JB, Hayman LA. White matter lesions in MR imaging of clinically healthy brains of elderly subjects: possible pathological basis. *Radiology* 1987; 162:509–511.
22. Lotz PR, Ballinger WE Jr, Quisling RG. Subcortical arteriosclerotic encephalopathy: CT spectrum and pathological correlation. *AJNR* 1986; 7:817–822.
23. Gerald B, Sebes JI, Langston JW. Cerebral infarction secondary to sickle cell disease: Arteriographic findings. *AJR* 1980; 134:1209–1212.
24. Fujisawa I, Asato R, Nishimura K, et al. Moyamoya disease: MR imaging. *Radiology* 1987; 164:103–105.
25. Takahashi M, Miyauchi T, Kowada M. Computed tomography of moyamoya disease: Demonstration of occluded arteries and collateral vessels as important diagnostic signs. *Radiology* 1980; 134:671–676.
26. Asien AM, Gabrielson TO, McCane WJ. MR imaging of systemic lupus erythematosus involving the brain. *AJNR* 1985; 6:197–201.
27. Virapongse C, Cazenave C, Quisling R, et al. The empty delta sign:

Frequency and significance in 76 cases of dural sinus thrombosis. *Radiology* 1987; 162:779–785.

28. McMurdo SK Jr, Brant-Zawadzki M, Bradley WG Jr, et al. Dural sinus thrombosis: Study using intermediate field strength MR imaging. *Radiology* 1986; 151:83–86.

29. McArdle CB, Richardson CJ, Hayden CK, et al. Abnormalities of the neonatal brain: MR imaging. (Part II. Hypoxic-ischemic brain injury.) *Radiology* 1987; 163:395–403.

30. Gonzalez CF, Reyes PF. Hydrocephalus, atrophic and degenerative disorders. In Gonzalez CF, Grossman CB, Masdeu JC (Eds). *Head and Spine Imaging.* New York: John Wiley & Sons, 1985; 435–470.

31. Wilson DA, Steiner RE. Periventricular leukomalacia: Evolution with MR imaging. *Radiology* 1986; 160:507–511.

32. Grant EG, Schellinger D, Smith Y, Uscinski RH. Periventricular leukomalacia in combination with intraventricular hemorrhage: Sonographic features and sequellae. *AJNR* 1986; 7:443–447.

33. Flodmark O, Roland EH, Hill A, Whitfield MF. Periventricular leukomalacia: Radiologic diagnosis. *Radiology* 1987; 162:119–124.

34. Miura T, Mitoma M, Kawai R, Harada K. CT of the brain in acute carbon monoxide intoxication: characteristic features and prognosis. *AJNR* 1985; 6:739–742.

35. Horowitz AL, Kaplan R, Sarpel G. Carbon monoxide toxicity: MR imaging in the brain. *Radiology* 1987; 162:787–788.

36. Bird CR, McMahon JR, Gilles FH, et al. Strangulation in child abuse: CT diagnosis. *Radiology* 1987; 163:373–375.

37. Liwnicz BH, Mowradian MD, Ball JB Jr. Intense brain cortical enhancement on CT in laminar necrosis verified by biopsy. *AJNR* 1987; 8:157–159.

38. Fitch SJ, Gerald B, Magill HL, Tonkin ILD. Central nervous system hypoxia in children due to near drowning. *Radiology* 1985; 156:647–650.

39. Taylor SB, Quencer RM, Holzman BH, Naidich TP. Central nervous system anoxic-ischemic insult in children due to near-drowning. *Radiology* 1985; 156:641–646.

40. Wagle WA, Smith TW, Weiner M. Intracerebral hemorrhage caused by cerebral amyloid angiopathy: radiographic-pathologic correlation. *AJNR* 1984; 5:171–176.

41. McArdle CB, Richardson CJ, Hayden CK, et al. Abnormalities of the neonatal brain: MR imaging. Part 1. Intracranial hemorrhage. *Radiology* 1987; 163:387–394.

42. Gomori JM, Grossman RI, Goldberg HI, et al. Intracranial hematomas: Imaging by high-field MR. *Radiology* 1985; 157:87–93.

43. Yeakley JW, Patchall LL, Lee KF. Interpenduncular fossa sign: CT criterion of subarachnoid hemorrhage. *Radiology* 1986; 158:699–700.

44. Bradley WG Jr, Schmidt PG. Effect of methemoglobin formation on the MR appearance of subarachnoid hemorrhage. *Radiology* 1985; 156:99–103.

45. Bowerman RA, Donn SM, Silver TM, Jaffe MH. Natural history of neonatal periventricular/intraventricular hemorrhage and its complications: Sonographic complications. *AJNR* 1984; 5:527–538.

46. Pinto RS, Cohen WA, Kricheff II, et al. Giant aneurysms: Rapid sequential computed tomography. *AJR* 1982; 139:973–977.

47. Olsen WL, Brant-Zawadzki M, Hodes J, et al. Giant intracranial aneurysms: MR imaging. *Radiology* 1987; 163:431–435.

48. Atlas SW, Grossman RI, Goldberg HI. Partially thrombosed giant intracranial aneurysms: correlation of MR and pathologic findings. *Radiology* 1987; 162:111–114.

49. Allcock JM. Aneurysms. In Newton TH, Potts DG (Eds). *Radiology of the Skull and the Brain*, Vol 2, Book 4. St. Louis: C.V. Mosby Co, 1974; 2435–2489.

50. Hinshaw DB Jr, Jordan KR, Hasso AN, Thompson JR. CT cisternography of dolicoectatic arterial compression of the optic chiasm. *AJNR* 1985; 6:837–839.

51. Kucharczyk W, Lemme-Pleghos L, Uske A, et al. Intracranial vascular malformations: MR and CT imaging. *Radiology* 1985; 156:383–389.

52. Lee BCP, Herzberg L, Zimmerman RD, Deck MDF. MR imaging of cerebral vascular malformations. *AJNR* 1985; 6:863–870.

53. Newton TH, Troost BT. Arteriovenous malformations and fistulae. In Newton TH, Potts DG, (Eds). *Radiology of the Skull and the Brain*, Vol 2, Book 4. New York: C.V. Mosby Co, 1974; 2490–2565.

54. Kumar AJ, Vinela F, Fox AJ, Rosenbaum AE. Unruptured intracranial arteriovenous malformations do cause mass efforts. *AJNR* 1985; 6:29–32.

55. Cubberley DA, Jaffe RB, Nixon GW. Sonographic demonstration of galenic arteriovenous malformations in the neonate. *AJNR* 1982; 3:435–439.

56. Augustyn GT, Scott JA, Olson E, et al. Cerebral venous angiomas: MR imaging. *Radiology* 1985; 156:391–395.

57. Olson E, Gilmor RL, Richmond B. Cerebral venous angiomas. *Radiology* 1984; 151:97–104.

58. Norman D. Vascular diseases: Hemorrhage. In Brant-Zawadzki M, Norman D (Eds). *Magnetic Resonance Imaging of the Nervous System.* New York: Raven Press, 1987; 209–220.

59. Williams AL. Trauma. In Williams AL, Haughton VM (Eds). *Cranial Computed Tomography.* St. Louis: C.V. Mosby Co, 1985; 37–87.

60. Goldberg HI, Grossman RI, Gamori JM, et al. Cervical internal carotid artery dissecting hemorrhage: diagnosis using MR. *Radiology* 1986; 158:157–161.

61. Wagle WA, Cousins JP. Magnetic resonance angiography of carotid and vertebral artery dissection. Presented at the American Society of Neuroradiology 28th annual meeting Mar. 19, 1990. To be published in *AJNR*.

CHAPTER

7

Cranial and Intracranial Trauma

Introduction

Serial CT imaging of head trauma has been indispensable at our hospital for over 10 years. CT remains the first procedure of choice for imaging acute cranial trauma due to the ease of obtaining the study and the clear recognition of acute hemorrhage, mass effect, edema, and brain and bone detail. CT has certain weaknesses, however, such as identification of acute nonhemorrhagic contusions, hemorrhages adjacent to bone surfaces which are parallel to the axial plane, brainstem contusions, and "isodense hemorrhages." MR, on the other hand, can demonstrate these abnormalities routinely.[1–5]

MR is the favored imaging method for trauma patients with severe neurological deficits unexplained by CT scan results. MR resolution of neuropathological sequelae is clearly superior to CT in subacute and chronic cases for evaluation of the stage of parenchymal hemorrhage, of CT isodense subdural hematomas, and of parenchymal abnormalities. The difficulty with MR imaging of trauma is management of life-support and monitoring equipment at a distance from the patient within a strong magnetic field and the longer scan time that allows for motion degradation of the images.[3,4] This chapter will demonstrate and compare the results of both CT and MR methods for imaging the common spectrum of trauma-induced cranial and intracranial abnormalities. The reader is referred to Chapters 2 and 3 for technical considerations. In general, however, we recommend noncontrast axial CT scanning with soft tissue and bone windows in the acute stage. After the patient is stabilized, MR scanning in multiple planes utilizing heavily weighted T1, proton density, and T2 techniques are used.

Extracranial Lesions

Neonatal cephalohematomas are usually due to head trauma during labor and delivery. They may be subcutaneous, subaponeurotic, or subperiosteal. Subperiosteal cephalohematomas are confined to suture lines (Fig. 7.1). During the healing stage, shells of bone form over the subperiosteal type. Bone remodeling then develops with a return to normal contours.[1,2]

Fractures

PEDIATRIC CONSIDERATIONS.

Neonatal severe skull fractures with torn dura may rarely become "growing skull fractures" or "leptomeningeal cysts." The meninges herniate through the torn diastatic dura, widening the fracture, and eroding the edges. Brain tissue may be present in the herniated portion.[1,2] CT accurately demonstrates the fracture, meningeal herniation, and the presence or absence of herniated brain (Fig. 7.2).

GENERAL CONSIDERATIONS

The presence or absence of a skull fracture in patients with minor head trauma has little prognostic value for neurological damage.[1,2] Depressed skull fractures are important to document, however, so that

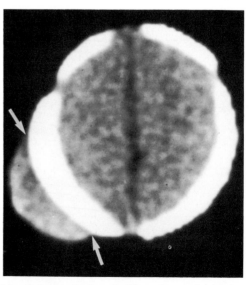

Figure 7.1. Subperiosteal cephalohematoma. *Axial subvertex CT scan.* Note the slightly hyperdense fluid collection confined to the limits of the parietal bone *(arrows).*

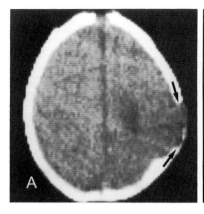
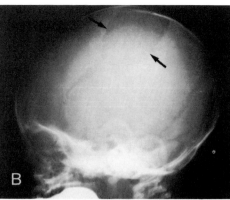

Figure 7.2.   Leptomeningeal cyst. A 2-month-old infant 6 weeks after head injury and a separated linear skull fracture. *Axial 37/100 noncontrast subvertex CT scan* **(A).** *Lateral skull x-ray* **(B).** Note the parietal lobe herniation through the now widely separated fracture and the smooth inner table fracture edge erosion *(arrows).*

a significantly depressed fragment can be surgically elevated or removed (Fig. 7.3). The CT scan and the localizer view in these latter cases usually obviates the need for plain skull x-rays. Detection of cortical bone is far less sensitive with MR.

Extra-axial Hemorrhage
EPIDURAL HEMATOMAS

These hemorrhages develop in the potential space between the skull inner table and periosteum, usually as a result of fracture and meningeal artery tear (Fig. 7.4). Venous epidural hematomas develop from torn diploic veins or venous sinuses and are more common at the skull vertex (Fig. 7.5). The arterial hematoma is usually confined by sutural boundaries due to firm adhesion of the outer dura (periosteum) to the suture line, thus producing a confined lentiform appearance. The majority of epidural hematomas are temporoparietal in location with middle meningeal artery branch hemorrhage. Posterior fossa epidural hematomas are uncommon.[1,6] Those that occur in the posterior fossa are most likely venous in origin due to a dural venous sinus tear.[6] Underlying brain contusion is less likely with epidural hematomas than with acute subdural hematomas.[1,6]

Small (3–5 mm in thickness) epidural hematomas

are frequently seen adjacent to fractures and are usually not significant. Immediate diagnosis and surgery are usually necessary for most larger meningeal artery epidural hematomas. Patients that are surgically treated quickly tend to recover fully. Venous epidural hematomas expand more slowly and symptoms may develop over a period of days. Post-surgical residual collections or reaccumulations are unusual as compared to the subdural hematoma.[1]

CT of acute arterial epidural hematomas demonstrates a biconvex hyperdense collection beneath and adjacent to the calvarium confined to sutural boundaries. There is usually an overlying skull fracture. Most epidural hematomas are small; however, larger hemorrhages with a marked mass effect occur. Acute epidural hematomas may demonstrate a "swirl" of lower density within the dense clot. The swirl represents active bleeding into the clot.[6] There is usually no underlying parenchymal abnormality but when underlying hypodensity is present, it can represent ischemia[6] or a venous or arterial infarct due to compression effects of the hematoma.[1] These homogeneous clots may also be the result of venous hemorrhage.[6] Occasionally, the epidural hematoma patient (particularly the venous type) have only minimal clinical symptoms and surgical evacuation may not be necessary. Chronic venous epidural he-

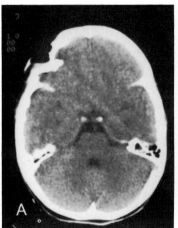
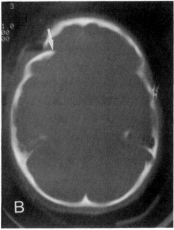

Figure 7.3.   Depressed skull fracture. *Axial chiasmatic cistern-level 37/100* **(A)** *and 650/4000* **(B)** *CT scan.* Note the markedly depressed right frontal bone fragment *(white arrow).* A possible small sphenoid lesser wing subdural hematoma or anterior temporal cortical contusion cannot be excluded.

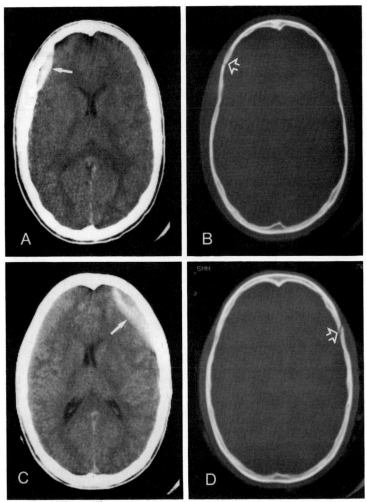

Figure 7.4.   Acute epidural hematoma. A-B and **C-D** are different cases. *Axial lateral ventricle frontal horn-level noncontrast 37/100 (**A** and **C**) and 75/2000 (**B** and **D**) CT scans.* Note the biconvex frontal hyperdensity *(closed arrows)* beneath a linear frontal bone fracture *(open arrows)*. The homogeneous epidural hematoma in **A** is smaller than that of **B.** The heterogeneous (probably active bleeding) epidural hematoma of **C** is associated with moderate degree displacement of the septum pellucidum. These figures do not imply that those epidural hematomas that are actively bleeding are larger.

matomas are predominantly hypodense with contrast-enhancing margins.[6]

MR of acute epidural hematomas is equally accurate as CT, however, as already mentioned, the trauma patient is usually initially evaluated by CT.

If MR is used for initial cerebral trauma evaluation, analysis of T1, proton density, and T2 effects is necessary because of the difficulty of identifying the hematoma lateral margin adjacent to the hypointense skull inner table. MR of subacute epidural hematomas may be more accurate than the CT method due to possible CT isodensity of the lysed clot[6] and to the hyperintense T1 and T2 free methemoglobin. MR has three advantages over CT for the demonstration of venous epidural hematomas. They are: multiple plane imaging, MR accuracy for hemorrhage susceptability effects, and better artifact-free posterior fossa imaging (Fig. 7.5).

SUBDURAL HEMATOMAS

Hemorrhage into the potential space between the dura and the subarachnoid membrane results in a subdural hematoma. The potential subdural space is not confined by sutures as is the potential epidural space and, as a result, the subdural hematoma is free to extend widely over the hemisphere. Recent neuropathological investigations suggest that "acute" and "chronic" subdural hematomas are very different lesions.[1]

The crescentric CT hyperdense collection, which had previously been described as pathognomonic of "acute subdural hematoma," may be the result of severe trauma, trivial trauma, or may result from hemorrhage into a pre-existing chronic subdural hematoma. Those that result from severe trauma behave very differently than those that result from trivial

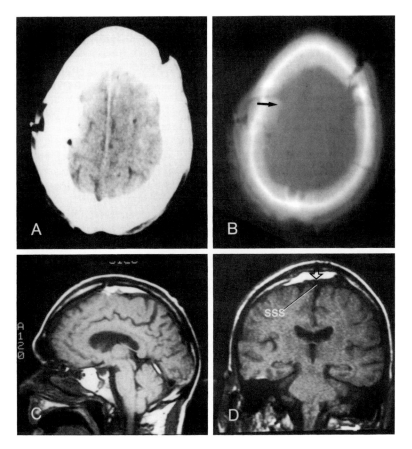

Figure 7.5. Venous epidural hematoma. *Axial sub-vertex 37/100* **(A)** *and 100/2000* **(B)** *CT scans. Midsagittal* **(C)** *and coronal thalamic-level* **(D)** *SE 600/25 MR scans.* CT and MR scans at day 1. Note the CT-demonstrated severe skull fractures with a depressed right frontoparietal portion *(solid arrow).* There is a T1 (shown) and T2 (not shown) hyperintense fluid collection at the vertex *(open arrow)* displacing the superior sagittal sinus *(SSS)* downward. The depressed bone fragment is best demonstrated by CT, however, the epidural hematoma is only demonstrated by MR.

trauma. The severe trauma-type acute subdural hematomas are subdural collections of blood clot or fresh blood that usually result from cortical lacerations or contusions as well as venous tears. Often, this type of acute subdural hematoma is only a secondary manifestation of the underlying parenchymal injury that is primarily responsible for the patient's deteriorating condition (Fig. 7.6). These patients are usu-

ally comatose and have a 30–80% mortality rate. Survivors usually have profound neurological deficits. The subdural collections are often small and often do not require surgical evacuation. The interhemispheric location subdural hematoma is frequently found in battered children and is usually found posteriorly in a unilateral location (Fig. 7.7). There is often associated adjacent parenchymal injury.[1,7]

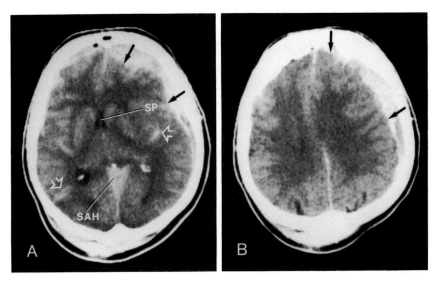

Figure 7.6. Acute (severe trauma-type) subdural hematoma with diffuse axonal injury and subarachnoid hemorrhage. *Axial noncontrast lateral ventricle-level* **(A)** *and centrum semiovale-level* **(B)** *CT scans.* Homogeneous hyperdense partially crescentric subdural hematoma *(closed arrows)* is not confined by sutures. There is a marked right-sided displacement of the septum pellucidum *(SP).* Bilateral deep white matter hyperdense hemorrhagic areas *(open arrows)* of diffuse axonal injury are seen. Subarachnoid hemorrhage is responsible for the superior cerebellar cistern hyperdensity *(SAH).*

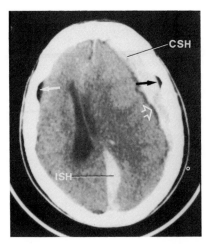

Figure 7.7. Acute severe trauma-type subdural hematoma with interhemispheric fissure component. *Axial lateral ventricle body-level CT scan 37/100, day 1.* Note the crescentric hyperdense convexity *(CSH)* and interhemispheric *(ISH)* subdural hematomas. There is marked compression of the left lateral ventricle with right-sided shift of the septum pellucidum. There are bilateral beam-hardening artifacts *(closed arrows).* The interhemispheric collection is confined to the left side of the falx. Note the hypodense layer beneath the subdural hematoma hyperdense portion *(open arrow).* This may represent plasma extruded from the clot.

The chronic subdural hematoma is usually found in situations where the subarachnoid space is proportionately larger, such as the elderly and cerebral atrophic conditions. It is also not uncommon in the neonate; particularly in the premature infant.[8] They usually result from stretched and torn bridging veins between the cortical surface and the dura.[1] These patients are usually alert, have minor neurological deficits, and have an excellent prognosis despite a tendency to rebleed. A subdural hematoma that develops at the onset of minor injury may have a crescentric homogeneously hyperdense appearance (Fig. 7.8) typical of the severe trauma-type but without associated brain contusion. These patients usually present weeks to months after a trivial traumatic event. This latter type of lesion would be considered by many to fit the "chronic" category better despite the recent hemorrhage.[1]

Most small or moderate-sized severe trauma-type acute subdural hematomas resolve and do not develop into chronic subdural hematomas. For this reason, we will not consider a "subacute" category. Large subdural hematomas and those hematomas causing marked shifts or raised intracranial pressure are almost always surgically evacuated. Ipsilateral atrophy usually develops in these severe trauma patients that survive. The severe trauma-type acute

Figure 7.8. Remote trauma subdural hematoma with recent hemorrhage. Unknown onset with slight left hemiparesis in an elderly patient. Axial noncontrast centrum semiovale-level CT scan *(A).* Axial lateral ventricle body-level SE 2000/20 MR scan *(B).* Coronal third ventricle-level SE 2000/20 *(C).* and 2000/80 *(D)* MR scans. Note the homogeneous crescentric CT moderately hyperdense and T1 and T2 hyperintense subdural hematoma *(arrows).* The septum pellucidum *(SP)* is only moderately left-sided displaced proportionate to the subdural size. There is lack of cerebral contusion. The arachnoid membrane *(AM)* separates the hematoma from subarachnoid CSF. A signal-void cortical vein is seen beneath the arachnoid membrane. Note the incidental small vessel disease *(SVD)* and the signal-void atherosclerotic dilated internal carotid and basilar arteries **(C** and **D).**

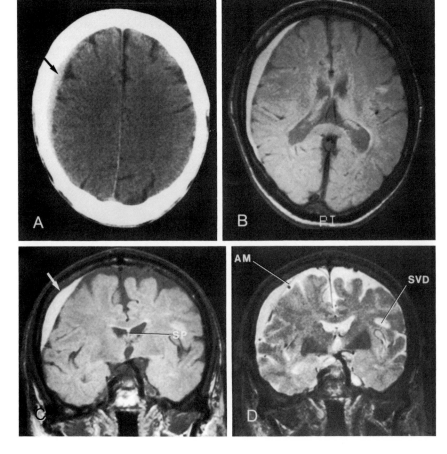

subdural hematoma does not characteristically re-bleed as does the chronic subdural hematoma.

CT of the severe trauma-type of acute subdural hematomas usually demonstrates a homogeneous hyperdense peripheral crescentric mass associated with disproportionately greater structural displacement than would be expected from a mass of that size due to the underlying parenchymal injury (Fig. 7.6). They may have inhomogeneous density and may have a lenticular or irregular shape. The hemorrhage is usually located along the lateral convexities but may occur in subfrontal, subtemporal, or interhemispheric locations. A solitary posterior fossa location is uncommon.[1,10] The subtemporal and subfrontal locations are difficult to identify with axial CT. Coronal CT imaging of these acutely injured patients is not practical and can be dangerous if there is an associated neck injury. Pneumocephalus may result from fracture of an air-filled sinus but it can also develop from vacuum phenomenon within a clot. Occasionally, these acute subdural hematomas may not be present immediately and may develop over the next several days.

Initially, severe trauma-type acute subdural hematomas are uniformly hyperdense unless the patient is anemic (Hb, 8–10 g/dl) in which case the hematoma appears "isodense."[11] Intravenous contrast enhancement may help identify the suspected isodense lesion (Fig. 7.9). We have seen and others have described an isodense acute subdural hematoma in a patient who was overanticoagulated and had a normal hematocrit. Intermediate window settings occasionally identify a subdural hematoma that is not seen with soft tissue window technique (Fig. 7.10). The hyperdense subdural hematomas that are not surgically evacuated become isodense approximately 1–3 weeks postinjury. Most small and moderate-sized severe trauma-type acute subdural hematomas that are not surgically evacuated eventually resolve. Evidence of encephalomalacia is frequently seen on follow-up scans due to the underlying brain injury.[1]

MR scanning of day 1 severe trauma-type acute subdural hematomas is difficult due to patient-life support and monitoring problems. Although the MR oxyhemoglobin signal does not have the marked contrast with brain cortex seen with more oxidized hemoglobin products, the relatively isointense signal within a well-defined crescentric mass can easily be detected on proton-weighted images. MR is superior to CT at day 1 for detection of subtemporal and subfrontal hematomas due to artifact-free multiplanar imaging. We rely on CT for our initial evaluation and use MR several days to 1 week later when the patient is medically stable for evaluation of parenchymal injuries and extra-axial fluid collections. At this stage of post-trauma evolution, T1 and T2 hemorrhage intensity characteristics vividly outline the subdural collections.[3]

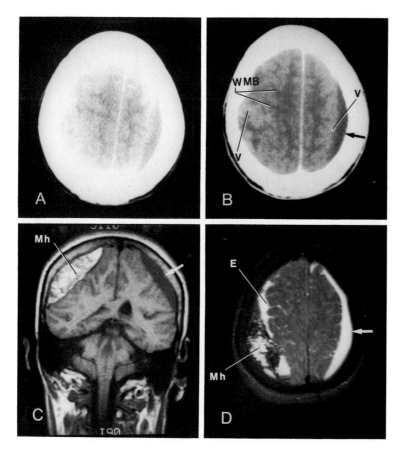

Figure 7.9. Intravenous contrast identifying isodense SDH. Bilateral chronic subdural hematomas with right-sided rebleed. Noncontrast **(A)** and i.v. contrast **(B)** axial centrum semiovale 36/100 CT scans. Coronal lateral ventricle atrial-level SE 600/25 **(C)** and axial centrum-level SE 2800/80 **(D)** MR scans. A biconvex chronic right "isodense" subdural hematoma with inhomogeneous CT densities and MR intensities is seen. There is T1/T2 hyperintense extracellular methemoglobin *(Mh)* and T2 hypointense presumed intracellular methemoglobin (unlabeled). There is adjacent enlargement *(E)* of the subarachnoid space. Intravenous contrast enhancement demonstrates displaced presumed cortical veins *(V)*, which is not as reliable a sign for isodense subdural hematoma as white matter buckling *(WMB)*. The left subdural hematoma *(arrows)* has a homogeneous, slightly greater-than-water CT and T1 signal density/intensity probably due to contained proteins.

Figure 7.10. CT window manipulation to identify thin, acute, severe trauma-type subdural hematoma. *Axial noncontrast lateral ventricle-level CT scan at 38/100 **(A)** and at 47/400 **(B)**.* Note the thin, acute subdural hematoma *(arrow)*. The septum pellucidum is moderately right-sided, displaced which is disproportionate to the thin subdural hematoma and probably caused by a left hemisphere contusion.

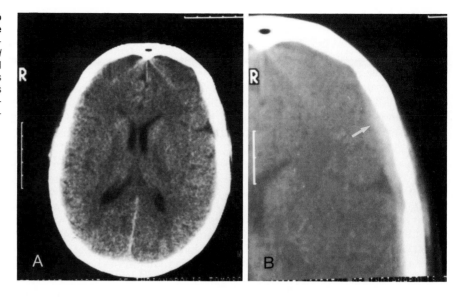

The characteristic CT appearance of the chronic subdural hematoma is a peripheral crescent which is usually homogeneously moderately hypodense. Frequently, there is a clot-fluid level (Fig. 7.11). The lesion may be lentiform in which case it is associated with a capsule that often contrast enhances. There may be more than one subdural hematoma in the same patient and they may be of different chronicity, with different shapes and densities. Isodense subdural hematomas are more difficult to detect but, with high-resolution scanning equipment, they should be seen (Fig. 7.12). Sulcal displacement, "white matter buckling" (Figs. 7.11 and 7.12), a contrast-enhanced capsule, and displaced cortical veins are signs to look for.[1]

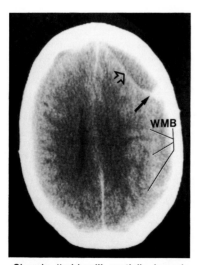

Figure 7.11. Chronic "rebleed" partially hypodense and isodense subdural hematoma. *Axial 37/100 noncontrast ventricle body-level CT scan.* Hypodensity *(open arrow)* and a clot-fluid level *(closed arrow)* are noted. Beneath the hyperdense clot there is isodense subdural hematoma, which is seen indirectly because of white matter buckling *(WMB)*. A thin hypodense right hemisphere subdural collection is also seen.

The subdural hygroma is a subdural location CSF collection without a surrounding membrane presumably caused by a tear in the arachnoid membrane. It is characteristically crescentric and may be smoothly marginated or may appear continuous with the adjacent subarachnoid space producing an interdigitated appearance (Fig. 7.13).[1]

MR of chronic subdural hematomas demonstrate T1 and T2 characteristics of deoxyhemoglobin, methemoglobin, and proteinaceous fluid content of these lesions (Fig. 7.12). Distinct fluid levels are often seen representing evidence of more recent hemorrhage into the chronic fluid collection. Improved detail of the subdural hematoma is noted as compared to CT (Figs. 7.11 and 7.12).[3] We find that CT, in most circumstances, is satisfactory for diagnosis, however.

SUBARACHNOID HEMORRHAGE

The appearance of subarachnoid hemorrhage to both the CT and MR techniques has already been discussed in Chapter 6. It is very common in cerebral injuries but its clinical significance is overshadowed by contusion, parenchymal hemorrhage, and subdural and epidural hematomas (Fig. 7.14). Traumatic subarachnoid hemorrhage usually results from tears of small subarachnoid vessels. The amount of blood in the perimesencephalic cisterns is rarely as great as with ruptured aneurysm. In the vast majority of cases, there are no clinical sequellae from the traumatic subarachnoid hemorrhage itself. Despite the high incidence of traumatic subarachnoid hemorrhage, communicating hydrocephalus is a very uncommon complication.[1] Subarachnoid hemorrhage has often been incorrectly diagnosed by CT in the neonate and young children due to the density of the falx contrasting against either the lower density of the normal neonate brain or the abnormally hypodense edematous brain (Fig. 7.15). Some feel, however, that most vaginal delivery neonates have some degree of subarachnoid hemorrhage. A smooth, thin,

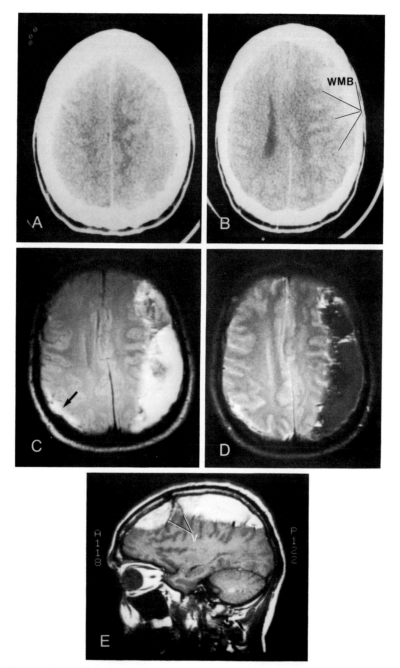

Figure 7.12. Chronic CT-isodense subdural hematoma. *Axial low centrum (A) and lateral ventricle body-level (B) 37/100 CT scans. Low centrum SE 2000/20 (C) and 2000/80 (D) MR scans. Sagittal insular level 600/25 MR scan (E).* Note the CT isodense left hemispheric mass with associated white matter buckling *(WMB).* The subdural hemorrhage is T1 hyperintense **(E)**. It is T2 principally hypointense with small areas of peripheral hyperintensity suggesting central intracellular methemoglobin content. Note an additional small right parietal subdural hematoma *(arrow)*. Cortical veins *(V)* are seen on the sagittal image partially surrounded by hemorrhage.

Figure 7.13. Subdural hygroma. Development over a 10-day period. *Axial lateral ventricle body-level noncontrast 37/100 CT scans at day 1 (A) and day 10 (B).* Note the water-isodense crescentric extra-axial fluid collections that appear continuous with the subarachnoid space *(arrows).*

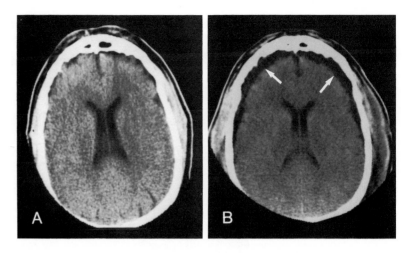

long hyperdense posterior falx which is isodense with the vein of Galen on a nonenhanced CT scan is a normal finding (Fig. 7.15). It is easily confused and often indistinguishable from interhemispheric subdural hematomas (Fig. 7.7) and subarachnoid hemorrhage (Fig. 7.14).[12] Subarachnoid hemorrhage has an interdigitating pattern, however.

INTRAVENTRICULAR HEMORRHAGE

Intraventricular hemorrhage (Fig. 7.16) occurs with both trivial and severe head trauma. Minor amounts of intraventricular hemorrhage in the adult are usually without clinical sequellae. Massive intraventricular hemorrhage may result in marked ventricular dilatation and require drainage. MR and CT establish the diagnosis. MR best excludes associated parenchymal injury.

Neonatal anoxic intraventricular hemorrhage has already been discussed in Chapter 6. Birth and perinatal trauma are responsible for a minority of these cases.

Contusions
MECHANISMS OF INJURY

Direct mechanical injury and secondary pathophysiological changes affect the outcome of head trauma. During the head injury event, different combined stresses are applied to the jelly-like brain substance.[1]

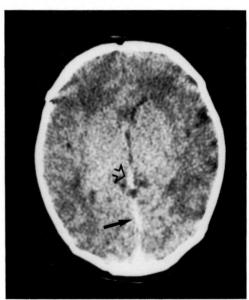

Figure 7.15. Vein of Galen, straight sinus, and torcular prominence ("the false falx sign"). Neonate having had one apneic episode. Note the prominent straight sinus *(closed arrow)* leading to the torcula. The density is similar to that of the vein of Galen *(open arrow).* No cisternal hyperdensity is present on lower sections and no sulcal interdigitated hyperdensity is seen.

In the proper clinical setting, such as a history of trauma or suspected ruptured aneurysm, subarachnoid hemorrhage would have to be considered. The normal flowing blood density contrasts with the normal parenchymal hypodensity of the neonate.

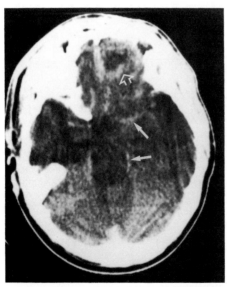

Figure 7.14. Subarachnoid hemorrhage and left frontal cortical contusion. Axial chiasmatic cistern-level noncontrast 37/100 CT scan. Note cistern and fissure hyperdense subarachnoid hemorrhage *(closed arrows)* and left frontal orbital gyrus and gyrus rectus hemorrhage *(open arrow).*

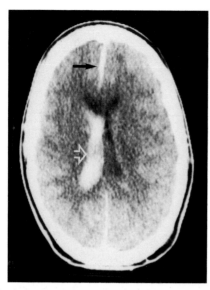

Figure 7.16. Intraventricular hemorrhage, day 1, head trauma. *Axial lateral ventricle body-level noncontrast 37/100 CT scan.* Right lateral ventricle hemorrhagic "cast" *(open arrow).* Interhemispheric subdural hematoma *(closed arrow).*

Table 7.1. Cerebral Contusion

Type	Location	Lesion Size	Hemorrhage Frequency	Frequency of Occurrence
Diffuse axonal injury	White matter	5–15 mm	20%	Most frequent
Cortical contusion	Cerebral cortex	20–40 mm	50%	Second most frequent
Subcortical gray matter injury	Thalamus and basal ganglia			
Primary brain-stem lesion	Midbrain and brain-stem			

Direct mechanical injury is immediately produced by physical forces. A direct blow tends to produce a localized lesion in proportion to the applied force. The applied force (acceleration) causes the brain motion to lag behind skull motion with resultant impact of the brain upon the skull opposite to the blow (deceleration). The result is a contrecoup injury. Contrecoup injuries tend to occur at the dural edges, sphenoid wings, petrous ridges, and orbital roofs. The disproportionate skull-brain motion during impact is further aggravated by rotational forces. Rotational forces are responsible for a contrecoup injury location not directly opposite the impact injury. Rotational acceleration and deceleration forces are also responsible for deep shearing stresses upon central brain structures due to the relative spin of the superficial brain structures twisting around the central brain structures held back by inertial lag. These rotational stresses can be strong enough to tear nerve fibers and even blood vessels.[1,4,13]

There are also secondary physiological changes in response to intracranial injury such as edema and raised intracranial pressure and extracranial pathological changes such as decreased cardiac output, hypotension, decreased peripheral resistance, acid-base imbalance, and arterial hypoxia.

The severity of brain swelling and edema usually increases after the injury and peaks at approximately day 6. This may be due to release of vasoactive substances and toxic byproducts after cellular injury. Blood-brain barrier (BBB) breakdown with increased vascular permeability to serum proteins results in progressive increase in tissue water content producing CT and MR vasogenic edema characteristics. More severe injuries are associated with vascular disruption and hemorrhage.[4,13]

The terms "cerebral contusion," "brain bruises," and "cerebral parenchymal injuries" can be used interchangeably.[1,4] Cerebral contusions can be anatomically classified by imaging appearance into diffuse axonal injury, cortical contusion, subcortical gray matter injury, and primary brainstem injury (Table 7.1).[3,5] Multiple types of lesions within this classification frequently coexist. We use the anatomical nomenclature method to avoid inaccurate pathophysiological diagnoses such as "coup/countrecoup" and "laceration" to describe each lesion.

DIFFUSE AXONAL INJURY

Diffuse axonal injury (also called "diffuse white matter injury") occurs because severe trauma with rotational force produces shear stress on the brain parenchyma. This is the most common type of brain contusion as reported in a recent series.[5] These patients usually have severe impairment of consciousness. Differing physical characteristics of gray and white matter help to explain the common occurrence at gray and white matter interfaces.[4] The corticomedullary junction of the frontal and temporal lobes is most frequently involved. Deeper structures such as the corona radiata, corpus callosum (usually the splenium), and the internal capsule are also commonly affected.[5] Greater severity rotational forces are thought to cause deeper shear stress injuries.[13] Most patients present with a multiplicity of these lesions often combined with other forms of contusion and subdural hematoma.

Diffuse axonal injuries are most often nonhemorrhagic (approximately 80%) by CT and MR techniques and therefore MR, due to superior contrast resolution, is more sensitive for detection (Figs. 7.17 and 7.18).[3,5] The hemorrhagic lesions tend to occur more frequently in locations that are more vascular such as the internal capsule and the lobar white matter and with reduced frequency in the less vascular corona radiata.[5] Both CT and MR can detect secondary effects resulting from brain injury such as edema and infarction, brain structural displacement, brain herniation effects, encephalomalacia, subdural

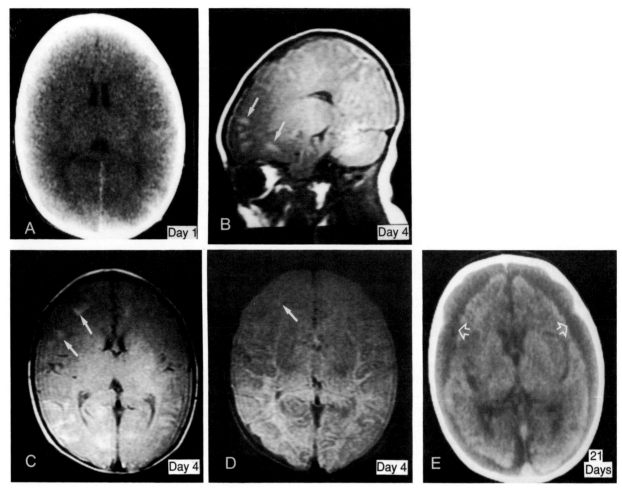

Figure 7.17.   Diffuse axonal injury. *Axial lateral ventricle frontal horn-level noncontrast day 1 CT scan* **(A).** *Sagittal lateral ventricle atrium-level SE 600/25 day 4 MR scan* **(B).** *Axial lateral ventricle frontal horn-level SE 2000/20* **(C)** *and 2000/80* **(D)** *day 4 MR scans. Axial same level noncontrast 3-week follow-up CT scan* **(E).** *The day 1 CT scan is normal. The day 4 MR scan demonstrates subcortical white matter ovoid T1 and T2 hyperintense lesions (closed arrows). The 3-week follow-up CT scan demonstrates bilateral chronic subdural hematomas (open arrows) and generalized cerebral atrophy.*

hematomas, porencephaly, atrophy, and hydrocephalus. MR, however, more accurately demonstrates these secondary changes.

CT of acute diffuse axonal injury demonstrates diffuse cerebral swelling with obliteration of the perimesencephalic cisterns, punctate deep white matter hemorrhage and, often, subarachnoid hemorrhage (Figs. 7.17 and 7.18). CT usually cannot identify acute nonhemorrhagic white matter shear stress injuries.[5] The CT-detected diffuse axonal injury foci usually appear smaller than those detected by MR.

MR of diffuse axonal injury demonstrates that most of the lesions are not hemorrhagic and that they are most often multiple. They usually are from 5–15 mm in size and are usually ovoid or elliptical with the long axis parallel to the direction of the axons (Figs. 7.17 and 7.18).[3–5]

CORTICAL CONTUSIONS

The term "cortical contusion" should not be confused with the term "brain contusion." Cortical contusion is a type of brain contusion characterized by primary involvement of the superficial cortex, and relative sparing of the deep white matter. Although they can occur in any lobe or the cerebellum, they are most frequent in the temporal lobes. The frontal lobes are the next most common location. The vast majority of frontal lesions are lateral or inferior. The frontal pole location is unusual.[5] Cortical contusions tend to be multiple and are much larger than diffuse axonal lesions, often measuring 2–4 cm diameter.[3,5] They are more frequently (approximately 50%) associated with significant hemorrhagic components.[5] The hemorrhagic cortical contusions occur most often along the inferolateral surfaces of the frontal and temporal lobes similar to that of the nonhemorrhagic lesions. Cortical contusions frequently coexist with diffuse axonal injury.

The CT findings of cerebral cortical contusion include heterogeneous mixed hyperdense and hypodense cortical regions representing admixed hemorrhage and edema (Fig. 7.19). The mass effect is

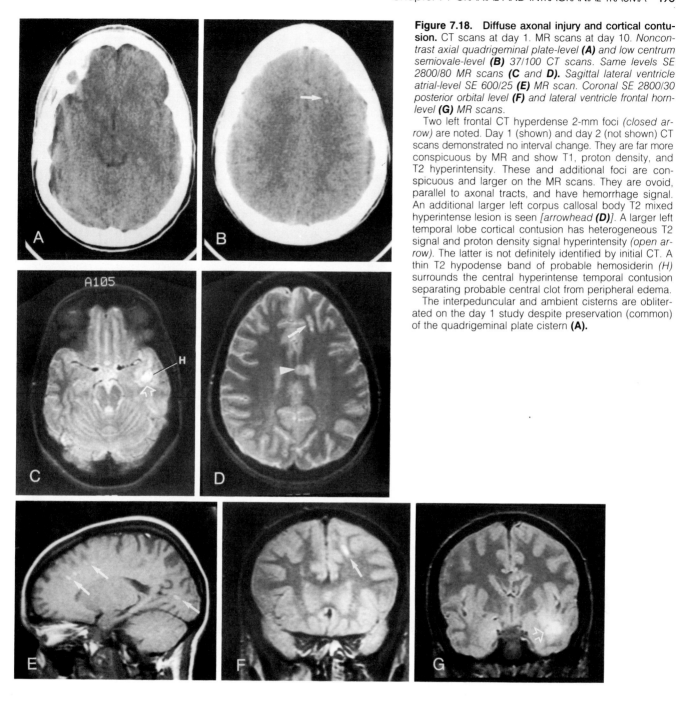

Figure 7.18.   Diffuse axonal injury and cortical contusion. CT scans at day 1. MR scans at day 10. *Noncontrast axial quadrigeminal plate-level **(A)** and low centrum semiovale-level **(B)** 37/100 CT scans. Same levels SE 2800/80 MR scans **(C** and **D)**. Sagittal lateral ventricle atrial-level SE 600/25 **(E)** MR scan. Coronal SE 2800/30 posterior orbital level **(F)** and lateral ventricle frontal horn-level **(G)** MR scans.*

Two left frontal CT hyperdense 2-mm foci *(closed arrow)* are noted. Day 1 (shown) and day 2 (not shown) CT scans demonstrated no interval change. They are far more conspicuous by MR and show T1, proton density, and T2 hyperintensity. These and additional foci are conspicuous and larger on the MR scans. They are ovoid, parallel to axonal tracts, and have hemorrhage signal. An additional larger left corpus callosal body T2 mixed hyperintense lesion is seen *[arrowhead **(D)**]*. A larger left temporal lobe cortical contusion has heterogeneous T2 signal and proton density signal hyperintensity *(open arrow)*. The latter is not definitely identified by initial CT. A thin T2 hypodense band of probable hemosiderin *(H)* surrounds the central hyperintense temporal contusion separating probable central clot from peripheral edema.

The interpeduncular and ambient cisterns are obliterated on the day 1 study despite preservation (common) of the quadrigeminal plate cistern **(A)**.

proportional to the size of the injury. The appearance of diffuse cerebral bihemispheric edema with hypodensity and obliteration or compression of the peri-mesencephalic cisterns may be the dominant CT findings despite the presence of a focal area of cortical hemorrhage and edema (Fig. 7.20). The focal mass effect becomes maximum at approximately 5 days and then starts to diminish. Small areas of hemorrhage may be initially evident but often become more prominent during the first few postictus days (Fig. 7.21). The CT hemorrhagic hyperdensity dissipates in a few days to weeks depending on the hemorrhage

size.[4] A nonhemorrhagic contusion most often appears hypodense acutely and becomes isodense usually from 2–3 weeks due to decreased edema and vascular proliferation. The contusion often contrast enhances at this stage but may contrast enhance even in early stages.[2] CT usually underestimates cortical contusion sizes.[3] Secondary effects such as encephalomalacia and hydrocephalus are well demonstrated.

We rely on the MR cortical contusion proton density image for anatomical localization and T1- and T2-weighted images for tissue identification such as edema and hemorrhage (Fig. 7.18). The lesion size is

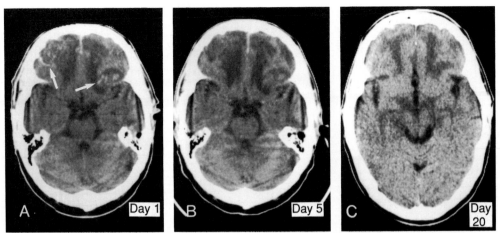

Figure 7.19.   Bifrontal cortical contusions. *Axial inferior frontal lobe-level noncontrast CT scans at day 1 (A), day 5 (B), and day 20 (C).* Bifrontal partially hemorrhagic *(arrows)* mixed density contusions are present at day 1. The hemorrhagic component is no longer detected by day 5 and the regions of abnormal hypodensity are smaller by day 20.

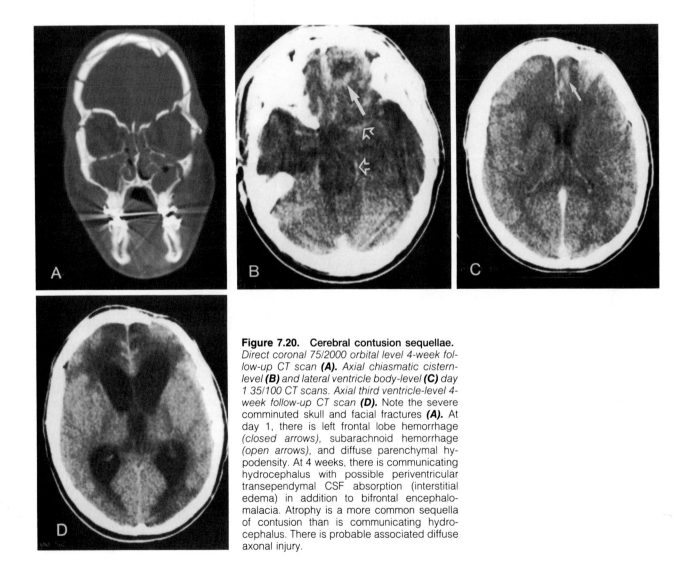

Figure 7.20.   Cerebral contusion sequellae. *Direct coronal 75/2000 orbital level 4-week follow-up CT scan (A). Axial chiasmatic cistern-level (B) and lateral ventricle body-level (C) day 1 35/100 CT scans. Axial third ventricle-level 4-week follow-up CT scan (D).* Note the severe comminuted skull and facial fractures *(A).* At day 1, there is left frontal lobe hemorrhage *(closed arrows),* subarachnoid hemorrhage *(open arrows),* and diffuse parenchymal hypodensity. At 4 weeks, there is communicating hydrocephalus with possible periventricular transependymal CSF absorption (interstitial edema) in addition to bifrontal encephalomalacia. Atrophy is a more common sequella of contusion than is communicating hydrocephalus. There is probable associated diffuse axonal injury.

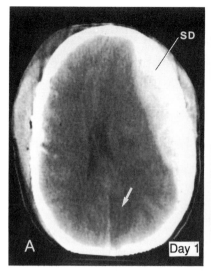
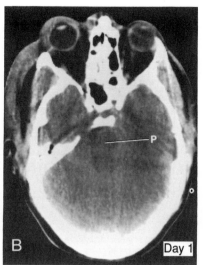
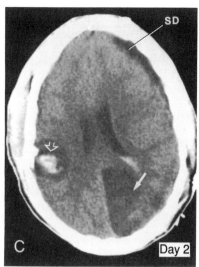

Figure 7.21. Delayed hemorrhagic component of a contusion. Coexistent large acute subdural hematoma and posterior cerebral artery infarct due to incisural artery compression. *Day 1 noncontrast axial lateral ventricular body-level* **(A)** *and upper pons-level* **(B)** *CT scans. Day 2 atrial level* **(C)** *noncontrast CT scan.* Note the day 1 large left acute subdural hematoma *(SD)*, an acute left posterior ce-

rebral artery infarct *(closed arrow)*, and the lack of perimesencephalic cisterns surrounding the upper pons *(P)*. The subdural hematoma was surgically evacuated and, on day 2, only a small hypodense collection of fluid is present *(SD)*. A hemorrhagic cortical contusion *(open arrow)* is now conspicuous in the right temporoparietal location. The infarct hypodensity has enlarged.

more accurately assessed by MR than CT and MR is far more specific for nonhemorrhagic contusions. MR also accurately identifies lesions at the skull base and the less common cerebellar cortical contusions, whereas CT scans are limited by beam-hardening artifacts in these locations. Chronological evolution

changes such as lesion size and intensity differences and secondary effects are easily identified (Fig. 7.22).[3,5]

SUBCORTICAL GRAY MATTER LESIONS

These lesions often occur together with other forms of contusion such as diffuse axonal injury and corti-

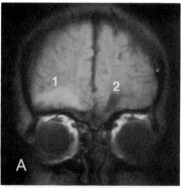
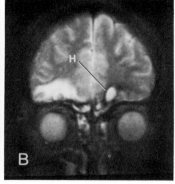
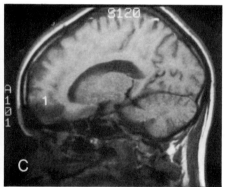
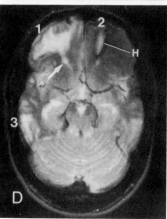

Figure 7.22. Remote changes of cortical contusions. Eighteen-month follow-up. *Coronal anterior orbital level SE 2000/20* **(A)** *and SE 2000/80* **(B)** *MR scans. Sagittal right lateral ventricle body-level SE 600/25* **(C)** *and axial midbrain-level SE 2000/80* **(D)** *MR scans. No flow-compensation methods were used.* There are three principal remote contusions *(1, 2,* and *3)* in typical locations. They all have a cortical location in common. The right inferior frontal lesion *1* demonstrates a broad cortical base. Lesion *2* demonstrates more hemosiderin *(H)* than lesion *1.* Lesion *3* shows only a minor amount of peripheral hemosiderin. Lesion *1* demonstrates a higher proton signal density **(A)** than lesion *2.* Lesion *1* shows white matter involvement *(arrow)* possibly representing Wallerian degeneration greater than that seen for lesions *2* or *3.*

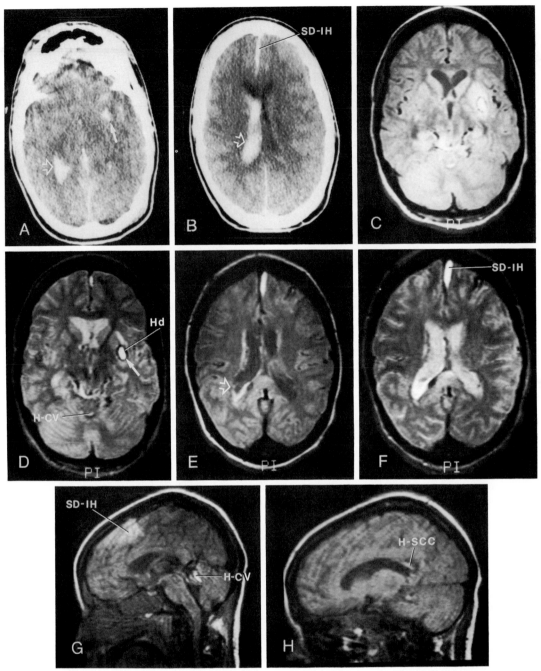

Figure 7.23. Subcortical gray matter contusion with interhemispheric subdural hematoma and corpus callosal and cerebellar vermis diffuse axonal injury. Day 1 CT scans; 3-week follow-up MR scans. *Axial basal ganglionic level (A) and lateral ventricle body-level (B) CT scans. Axial basal ganglionic level SE 2000/20 (C) and 2000/80 (D) MR scans. Axial lateral ventricular body-level SE 2000/20 (E) and 2000/80 (F) MR scans. Midsagittal (G) and right parasagittal (H) SE 600/25 MR scans.* A left putamen hemorrhagic contusion *(closed arrow)* is seen at day 1 by CT and at 3 weeks by MR. The T2 surrounding hypointensity represents hemosiderin *(Hd)*. Both the CT at ictus and the 3-week MR demonstrate interhemispheric subdural hematoma *(SD-IH)*. Intraventricular hemorrhage *(open arrow)* is seen at day 1 and 3 weeks. The MR demonstrates hemorrhagic axonal injuries of the splenium of the corpus callosum *(H-SCC)* and the vermis central lobule *(H-CV)*. The 3-week MR scan demonstrates periventricular hyperintensity the nature of which is not understood.

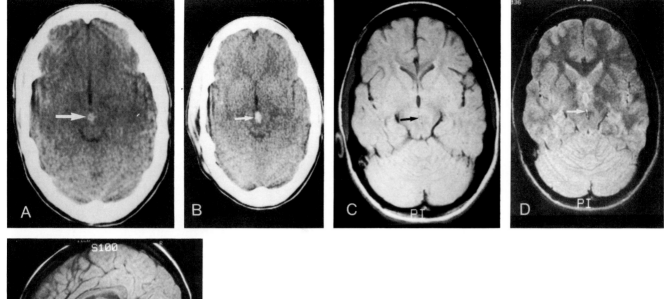

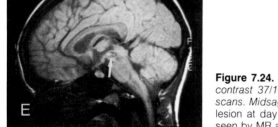

Figure 7.24. **Primary midbrain contusion.** *Axial midbrain-level day 1* **(A)** *and day 2* **(B)** *non-contrast 37/100 CT scans. Axial midbrain-level 3-week SE 2000/20* **(C)** *and 2000/80* **(D)** *MR scans. Midsagittal SE 600/25 MR scan* **(E)** *also at 3 weeks.* A central ovoid hyperdense midbrain lesion at day 1 moderately enlarges by day 2 *(arrows).* The T1 and T2 hyperintense signal is seen by MR at 3 weeks *(arrows).*

cal brain contusion. These patients tend to have severe neurological impairment. Subcortical gray matter lesions are frequently hemorrhagic possibly due to disruption of small perforating blood vessels. Most of these lesions occur in the thalamus.[3–5]

Both CT and MR accurately identify hemorrhagic subcortical gray matter lesions (Fig. 7.23). MR is far more specific for identification of nonhemorrhagic lesions and for frequently associated coexisting other forms of contusion and possible associated extra-axial hemorrhage (Fig. 7.23).[3,5]

PRIMARY BRAINSTEM LESIONS

These lesions probably represent diffuse axonal injury of the brainstem. Primary brainstem lesions are so named because they are caused by the initial trauma. This group of patients is associated with severe impairment of consciousness. These lesions are usually localized to the posterior and lateral midbrain and upper pons.[3–5]

CT is generally less sensitive than MR for detection of brainstem abnormalities due to petrous artifact and superior MR resolution. Only hemorrhagic lesions, above the petrous level, are consistently well seen by CT (Fig. 7.24). Flow-compensation MR methods are particularly helpful. Midbrain and upper pons hemorrhagic and nonhemorrhagic lesions are well demonstrated by the MR technique.[4]

Penetrating Injuries

The most common cause of penetrating head injury is the gunshot wound. Using "bone windows," CT can demonstrate the entrance wound and the exit wound (if present). The bullet, metallic and bone fragments, and the hemorrhagic tract are also identified. Streak artifacts from the dense metallic bullet and/or fragments compromise detail. CT is the study of choice due to the more severe MR metallic artifact image degradation and possible magnetic field effect on the fragments. There is usually subarachnoid hemorrhage and diffuse cerebral edema (Fig. 7.25). Pneumocephalus may be present. Although the prognosis is grave in many or most of these cases, careful attention to the pathological changes are necessary for those cases where surgery may be helpful and for forensic purposes. Other foreign objects may penetrate the skull and attention to brain and bone detail is required for diagnosis.

CSF Rhinorrhea

CSF rhinorrhea can develop spontaneously, as a result of trauma or as a result of surgery. Spontaneous CSF rhinorrhea may be idiopathic or may develop in cases of empty sella turcica and in patients with raised intracranial pressure.[15] This condition has an insidious onset and may continue for years.

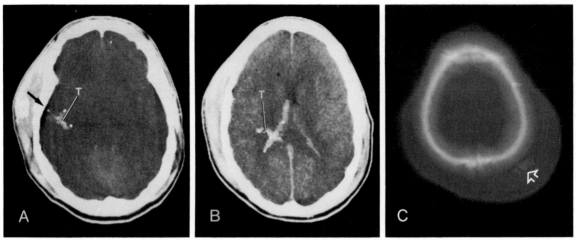

Figure 7.25. Gunshot wound of the brain. *Axial midbrain-level 40/ 100 (A), lateral ventricle body-level 35/100 (B), and subvertex 70/ 2000 (C) CT scans.* Note the entrance *(closed arrow)* and exit *(open arrow)* wounds. The metallic bone fragments and hemorrhagic tract *(T)* are easily identified. A small amount of air is seen in the tract and the right lateral ventricle frontal horn. There is intraventricular hemorrhage. The perimesencephalic cisterns are obliterated and there is generalized parenchymal hypodensity caused by edema. Large subgaleal hematomas are seen. A slight structural shift to the left is noted.

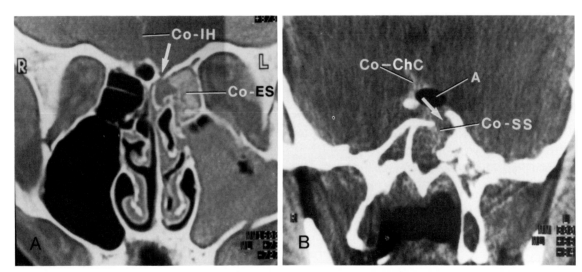

Figure 7.26. Cerebrospinal fluid rhinorrhea caused by a trauma-induced dural tear. A and **B** are different cases. *Direct prone coronal anterior planum sphenoidale 73/1600 (A) CT cisternogram.* Note the interhemispheric fissure *(Co-IH)* and posterior ethmoid sinus *(Co-ES)* contrast. The site of CSF leak is at the medial planum sphenoi- dale *(closed arrow).* The fractured left maxillary sinus is fluid filled. *Direct prone coronal sella turcica level 66/300 (B) CT cisternogram.* Chiasmatic cistern contrast (CoChC) has entered the sphenoid sinus *(Co-SS)* through the lateral sella floor fracture *(arrow).* Air *(A)* has entered the chiasmatic cistern.

Post-traumatic CSF rhinorrhea usually has an abrupt onset within 48 hours of the trauma with spontaneous remission in 70% of patients within 1 week. Up to 50% of those cases that do not remit develop meningitis.[14]

CT cisternography is performed in the prone position during a period of active CSF rhinorrhea in order to document the fistula site (Fig. 7.26). The most common sites are ethmoidal, frontoethmoidal, and sphenoidal.[14] Cisternography for diagnosis of otor- rhea caused by petrous fracture would probably not be successful due to the dense petrous bone and lack of large air spaces in which to identify contrast leak- age. Spontaneous CSF rhinorrhea arising from the middle cranial fossa is less frequent[15] and will be discussed in Chapter 13. MR Gd-DTPA intrathecal technique has been proposed and, as yet, no in- trathecal MR contrast agents have been approved.[16]

References

1. Dolinskas CA. Intracranial trauma. In Gonzalez CF, Grossman CB, Masdeu JC (Eds): *Head and Spine Imaging.* New York: John Wiley & Co., 1985; 357–395.
2. Chuang SH, Fitz CR. Computed tomography of head trauma. In Gonzalez CF, Grossman CB, Masdeu JC (Eds): *Head and Spine Imaging.* New York: John Wiley & Co., 1985; 523–536.
3. Gentry LR, Godersky JC, Thompson B, Dunn V. Prospective com- parative study of intermediate-field MR and CT in the evaluation of closed head trauma. *AJNR* 1988; 9:91–100.

4. Hesselink JR, Dowd CF, Healy ME, et al. MR imaging of brain contusions: A comparative study with CT. *AJNR* 1988; 9:269–278.
5. Gentry LR, Godersky JC, Thompson B. MR imaging of head trauma: Review of the distribution and radiopathologic features of traumatic lesions. *AJNR* 1988; 9:101–110.
6. Zimmerman RA, Bilaniuk LT. Computed tomographic staging of traumatic epidural bleeding. *Radiology* 1982; 144:809–812.
7. Cohen RA, Kaufman RA, Myers PA, Towbin RB. Cranial computed tomography in the abused child with head injury. *AJNR* 1985; 6:883–888.
8. Kapila A, Trice J, Spies WG, et al. Enlarged cerebrospinal fluid spaces in infants with subdural hematomas. *Radiology* 1982; 142:669–672.
9. Reed D, Robertson WD, Graeb DA, et al. Acute subdural hematomas. Atypical CT findings. *AJNR* 1986; 7:417–421.
10. Franklin J, Belkin R, Howieson J, Gallo A. Posterior fossa chronic subdural hematoma in the neonate. *AJNR* 1986; 7:1099–1100.
11. Smith WP Jr, Batnitsky S, Rengatchary SS. Acute isodense subdural hematomas: A problem in anemic patients. *AJNR* 1981; 136:543–546.
12. Osborn AG, Anderson RE, Wing SD. The false falx sign. *Radiology* 1980; 134:421–425.
13. Adams JH, Mitchell DE, Graham DI, Doyle D. Diffuse brain damage of immediate impact type: Its relationship to primary brain stem damage in head injury. *Brain* 1977; 100:489–502.
14. Manelfe C, Cellerier P, Sobel D, et al. Cerebrospinal fluid rhinorrhea: Evaluation with metrizamide cisternography. *AJNR* 1982; 3:25–30.
15. Yeates AE, Blumenkoph B, Drayer BP, et al. Spontaneous CSF rhinorrhea arising from the middle cranial fossa: CT demonstration. *AJNR* 1984; 5:820–821.
16. DiChiro G, Girton ME, Frank JA, et al. Cerebrospinal fluid rhinorrhea: Depiction with MR cisternography in dogs. *Radiology* 1986; 160:221–222.

CHAPTER 8

Infections and Inflammatory Diseases

Introduction

Intracranial inflammatory conditions are classified in this chapter according to etiology and location. The offending organism and the host response greatly affect the pathological process. Depressed host immunity is frequently the underlying cause of intracranial infection and significantly affects the appearance of the lesion. For example, opportunistic organisms such as *Aspergillus, Nocardia,* and *Cryptococcus* are often responsible for intracranial infections in the immunosuppressed patient. Other organisms such as toxoplasmosis have a fulminant course in acquired immune deficiency syndrome (AIDS) patients as compared to a self-limited benign course in the immunocompetent adult.[1–3]

Very often, the clinician suspects an inflammatory etiology of the patient's presenting complaints before requesting a scan. For example, a febrile illness, presence of a known nidus of infection, or immune compromise is very useful information for scan interpretation. Often, a study is ordered for a known condition such as meningitis in order to evaluate potential complications such as abscess and infarct. The radiologist interpreting these images should focus attention to these potential complications.

As with the imaging of other clinical conditions, the question arises as to the choice of CT or MR as the first order examination. Given that there are no MR contraindications for a particular patient, we feel that MR, most likely, will prove to have the advantage over CT. This preliminary judgment is based on MR sensitivity for tissue water content, hemorrhage detectability, improved brain structural detail, orthogonal plane imaging, and lack of tissue-bone interface image degradation. If detection of calcification is necessary such as in cytomegalovirus en-

cephalitis, CT is the more specific study. Both i.v. contrast CT and Gd-DTPA i.v. contrast MR are very effective for identification of blood-brain barrier (BBB) breakdown. MR contrast technique is superior for investigation of inflammatory disease due to lack of tissue-bone interface obscuration that occurs with CT.

Bacterial Infections

CEREBRITIS AND BRAIN ABSCESS

Cerebritis may resolve with appropriate antibiotics or may develop into a cerebral abscess. The characteristic edema, petechial hemorrhage, and vascular congestion of cerebritis produces nonspecific MR and CT findings. CT and MR evidence of cerebritis is most often found in patients with other recognized cerebral infections such as intracranial abscesses and subdural and epidural empyemas. CT demonstrates a poorly delineated hypodense mass with slightly heterogeneous enhancement (Fig. 8.1). MR not only demonstrates edema but is also likely to demonstrate the petechial hemorrhages.[1,2]

Brain abscess develops when fibroblasts surround the inflamed area and central liquefaction develops. The fibroblast is derived from vascular endothelial cells and helps build the three-layer abscess wall. From within-out, this wall is formed of granulation tissue, collagen, and reactive glial tissue.[1] The weakest portion of the capsule faces the white matter, which likely explains why daughter abscesses tend to develop medially toward the ventricles. For this reason, intraventricular rupture and pyogenic ventriculitis may develop with an often lethal outcome.[1] Marked degree vasogenic edema typically surrounds the abscess. The source of the infection may be hematogenous spread, open trauma, and direct extension from contiguous structures such as paranasal and mastoid sinuses. Those at risk include immunosuppressed, valvular and septal heart defect, and i.v. drug abuse patients. In the absence of the special risk factors described above, brain abscesses most commonly occur in infants, children, and the elderly. Hematogenous origin abscesses are usually solitary and are most frequent in the frontal and temporal lobes at the corticomedullary junctions. Direct parenchymal extension from meningitis and epidural abscess may result in a brain abscess. Adult hematogenous origin

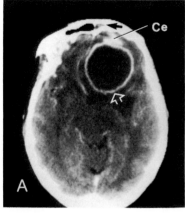
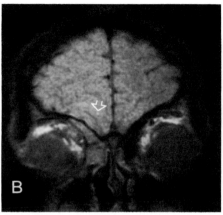
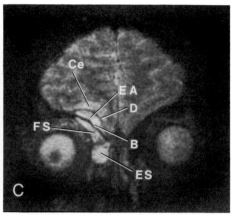

Figure 8.1.   Cerebritis. *A and B, C are two different cases. Axial i.v. contrast supraorbital level CT scan (A), coronal orbital level SE 2000/20 (B) and 2000/80 (C) MR scans. A, Frontal sinusitis, cerebritis, and frontal abscess. Hyperdense left frontal sinus (closed arrow). Thin smooth ring contrast-enhanced left frontal lobe abscess (open arrow). Connecting contrast-enhanced cerebritis (Ce). B and C, Frontal* and ethmoid sinusitis, epidural abscess, and cerebritis. Ethmoid *(ES)* and frontal *(FS)* sinusitis. Anterior fossa floor bone *(B)*. Epidural abscess *(EA)* elevating the dura *(D)*. Adjacent cerebritis *(Ce)*. T1-weighted image hyperintensity *(open arrow)* possibly representing a hemorrhagic focus.

abscesses are usually caused by mixed aerobic and anaerobic organisms. Staphylococci, pneumococci, and streptococci are often responsible for abscesses in children. Staphylococci are usually responsible for traumatic origin brain abscesses.[1,2] In the immunosuppressed patient and particularly in patients with AIDS, organisms such as *Toxoplasma, Cryptococcus, Candida, Nocardia,* and *Aspergillus,* which would not ordinarily be the cause of abscess formation, are often responsible.[3]

CT and MR demonstrate the developmental spectrum of cerebritis through mature abscess (Figs. 8.1–8.3). Poorly defined, heterogeneous hypodense lesions (usually maximum at corticomedullary junctions) in the early phase of cerebritis can be seen by CT. Edema then increases producing a CT hypodense mass effect. Patchy areas of CT heterogeneous contrast enhancement and, occasionally, ring contrast enhancement can be demonstrated. As the process continues, BBB breakdown increases and thick and irregular ring contrast enhancement develops.[2] MR is superior to CT for demonstration of cerebritis due to its greater sensitivity for detection of tissue water content and its orthogonal plane imaging capability. MR characteristically demonstrates T2 abscess capsule hypointensity (Figs. 8.2 and 8.3) and contrast enhancement. The capsular hypointensity has been attributed to blood products[1] but recently investigators have shown that it probably is not[1a]. This smoothly marginated thin T2-hypointense contrast enhancing rim is valuable for distinguishing abscess from tumor[1a]. Intravenous Gd-DTPA is recommended for MR investigation of inflammatory disease at any stage.

A smoothly marginated thin ring of contrast enhancement surrounding a homogeneous central hypodense necrotic core is typical of a mature cerebral abscess (Figs. 8.2 and 8.3). Other lesions such as gliomas, metastases, lymphoma, infarcts, and hema-

tomas may have a similar appearance. Steroid therapy reduces capsular contrast enhancement.[1,4] A differential diagnosis for CT ring contrast-enhancing lesions appears in Chapter 2.

Both the CT and MR methods demonstrate abscess healing with reduction of the cavity size and surrounding edema. Capsular contrast enhancement diminishes but may persist for months and focal atrophy secondary to encephalomalacia may develop.

VENTRICULITIS

Infection of the ventricular ependymal lining may be caused by intraventricular rupture of a parenchymal abscess, meningitis, and ventricular shunt infections. CT usually demonstrates some degree of hydrocephalus and ventricular (ependymal) contrast enhancement. CSF density is increased due to the purulent fluid.[1] Periventricular edema may develop and ventricular septation may occur (Fig. 8.4).[2,5] Transit of i.v. contrast into the ventricles through the inflamed ependyma occasionally can be recognized.[6]

MR of ventriculitis demonstrates ependymal contrast enhancement, T1 CSF hyperintensity due to the purulent fluid, ventricular enlargement, and periventricular edema. The ependyma may appear as an isointense band between the hyperintense purulent ventricular CSF and the periventricular edema on T2-weighted images. Further experience with MR imaging of ventriculitis is necessary in order to determine imaging characteristics of the pathological process. Follow-up examination may demonstrate ventricular septation from scarring and hydrocephalus (Fig. 8.4).

Differential diagnosis of ventriculitis includes subependymal tumor spread (Fig. 5.4). The diagnosis is usually suspected or known before the scan. Evidence of meningitis, the offending abscess, or shunt, is usually present on the scan.

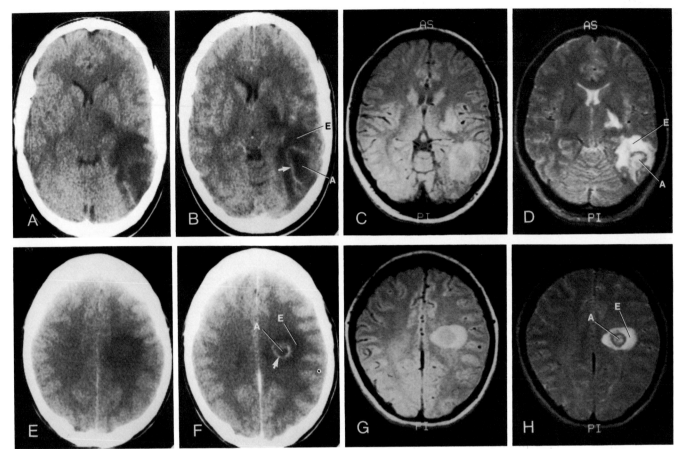

Figure 8.2. Multiple cardiac origin pyogenic abscesses. Incompletely developed and mature abscesses. Same case same day CT and MR scans. *Axial lateral ventricle frontal horn-level noncontrast **(A)** and i.v. contrast **(B)** 37/100 CT scans and SE 2000/20 **(C)** and 2000/80 **(D)** MR scans. Axial centrum semiovale noncontrast **(E)** and contrast **(F)** CT scans and SE 2000/20 **(G)** and 2000/80 **(H)** MR scans.*

The immature abscess **(A-D)** demonstrates an incompletely formed irregularly contoured rim contrast-enhanced abscess capsule *(arrow)* surrounding the central necrotic abscess *(A)* with surrounding edema *(E)*. Note the relatively round sharply T2 hypointense marginated contrast-enhanced mature abscess **(E-H).**

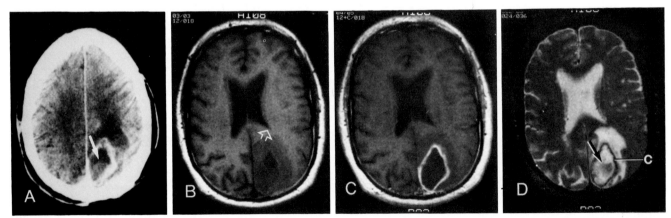

Figure 8.3. Pyogenic abscess posterior left parietal lobe. *Axial i.v. contrast enhanced low centrum-level supraorbitomeatal plane 30/100 CT scan **(A)**. Canthomeatal plane lateral ventricle body-level SE 600/25 noncontrast **(B)**, 600/25 i.v. contrast **(C)** and 2000/100 **(D)** MR scans.* A thin, smooth, even T2 hypointense contrast enhanced capsule **(C)** surrounds centrally necrotic fluid signal. A fluid-fluid

level *(closed arrows)* is seen by CT and long TR MR technique. Note the water-signal of the surrounding edema. Mass-effect causes "pointing" of the left lateral ventricle atrium *(open arrow)*. Of the four MR characteristics (edema, mass, central necrosis, capsule), the capsular characteristics are the most unique for abscess diagnosis.

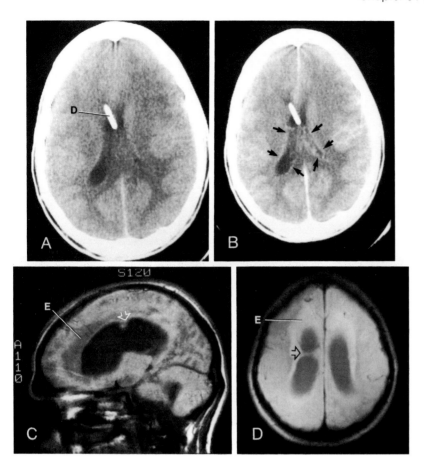

Figure 8.4. **Ventriculitis—shunt infection.** MR scan 1 month after CT scan. *Axial lateral ventricle body-level 37/100 noncontrast* **(A)** *and i.v. contrast* **(B)** *CT scans. Sagittal lateral ventricle body-level SE 600/25* **(C)** *and axial latereal ventricle body-level SE 2000/20* **(D)** *MR scans.* Right lateral ventricle drain *(D).* Periventricular abnormal contrast enhancement *(closed arrows).* Hydrocephalus, periventricular edema, and lateral ventricle septation *(open arrow)* has developed 1 month after ventricle drain withdrawal.

PURULENT MENINGITIS

These infections can be classified as leptomeningitis when only the pia and arachnoid membranes are involved and pachymeningitis when the dura is involved. The collective term "meningitis" will be used, however. Meningitis can be conveniently categorized as purulent (acute bacterial) meningitis, granulomatous (tubercular, fungal, and sarcoid) meningitis and viral meningitis (often diagnosed as "aseptic meningitis.") Purulent meningitis will be discussed in this section. Granulomatous meningitis will be principally discussed etiologically, e.g., under tuberculosis, sarcoidosis, etc.

Purulent meningitis may be of hemotogenous origin, a result from direct extension of paranasal and mastoid sinusitis or may complicate CSF rhinorrhea. In the adult population, meningitis occurs most frequently in the immunosuppressed or debilitated patient. The responsible organism in bacterial meningitis is age-dependent. For example, in neonatal infants, gram-negative rods are usually responsible. *Hemophilus influenza* is seen in infants and young children with upper respiratory infections whereas *Staphylococcus, Pneumococcus,* and *Meningococcus* are most commonly responsible in adults but may occur at all ages.

The infected pia and arachnoid membrane become congested and hyperemic and the exudate may initially distend the subarachnoid space. Blood vessels traversing the exudate may become occluded by the inflammatory process with the development of cortical infarcts. The pia and arachnoid membranes serve as barriers to the spread of infection, however. A combination of factors including ischemia, toxins, and direct infection may cause pial and arachnoid necrosis.

Arachnoid necrosis may be responsible for subdural fluid collections and pia necrosis may lead to cerebritis and abscess. Usually, treatment has been given by the time that the subdural effusions have developed and they are sterile. Pyogenic subdural collections (empyemas) may occur, however. Dural venous sinus thrombosis is also a complication of meningitis. The meningitic inflammatory exudate frequently causes communicating hydrocephalus due to blockage of the CSF pathways. Ventriculitis can also develop. In the neonate, multiple infarcts may produce a multicystic brain imaging appearance.[1,2,5]

Granulomatous meningitis is usually caused by tuberculosis, fungi, and sarcoidosis. Tuberculous meningitis usually results from hematogenous spread. Fungi most likely responsible for meningitis include *Cryptococcus, Coccidiodes* and *Blastomyces.*[4] The sulci may initially distend, however, cerebral edema commonly develops resulting in sulcal compression. Granulomatous meningitis preferentially involves the

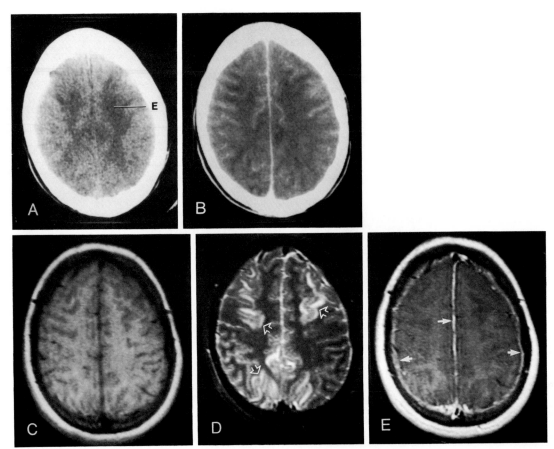

Figure 8.5. Supportive bacterial meningitis with edema and/or cortical infarcts. *Axial centrum semiovale noncontrast (A) and i.v. contrast (B) CT scans. Same level SE 600/25 (C), 2800/80 (D), and Gd-DTPA i.v. contrast 600/25 (E) MR scans 2 days later. Although there is some evidence for white matter edema (E) and gyral pattern* contrast enhancement *(B),* the CT scan only suggests a generalized diffuse pathological process. The MR scan demonstrates multifocal T2 cortical gyral pattern edema *(open arrows)* and meningeal Gd-DTPA contrast enhancement *(closed arrows).*

basal cisterns. A predominantly basal cistern location favors the diagnosis over purulent meningitis. The characteristic thick exudate causes reactive fibrosis with resultant hydrocephalus. Tuberculous meningitis often results in basal arteritis and subsequent infarction.[4]

Intravenous contrast MR is more sensitive than i.v. contrast CT for identification of acute bacterial meningitis. As already stated, the major role of both CT and MR is to diagnose the development of complications such as abscess, ventriculitis, hydrocephalus, infarction, venous thrombosis, and subdural effusion.

The initial CT scan is often normal. There may be cisternal hyperdensity and contrast enhancement. Abnormal marked meningeal contrast enhancement is often seen adjacent to the anterior interhemispheric fissure. The ventricles may appear small due to diffuse cerebral edema (Fig. 8.5). Hydrocephalus, cortical infarcts, subdural fluid collections, cerebral abscess, ventriculitis, and dural sinus thrombosis may be present. Pyogenic subdural infections tend to be of higher density than the sterile collections that appear CSF isodense. Contrast CT can also enhance the subdural empyema membrane, the abscess wall, the

delta sign of sinus thrombosis, and the inflamed ependyma of ventriculitis.[1,2,7]

CT differential diagnosis of meningeal contrast enhancement includes carcinomatous meningitis and, very rarely, rheumatoid pachymeningitis.[8] Both of these latter conditions present in patients in whom the underlying disease process is already known. Granulomatous meningitis, as already mentioned, preferentially involves the basal cisterns. Hydrocephalus frequently develops. Infarcts commonly occur and CT-detectable calcification may develop with tuberculous meningitis.[4]

MR with Gd-DTPA is more accurate for the diagnosis of meningitis than CT due to lack of bone obscuration of meningeal contrast enhancement and due to Gd-DTPA sensitivity for inflamed pia-arachnoid tissue (Fig. 8.5). The greatest value of MR for imaging of meningitis cases, like that of CT, is for investigation of infection involving other intracranial tissues and consequences of such spread of infection as cortical and subcortical infarction and subdural fluid collections. Despite reliance upon i.v. contrast MR techniques for imaging evidence of meningitis, the T2-weighted image is necessary for identification of complications such as infarct and edema.[1]

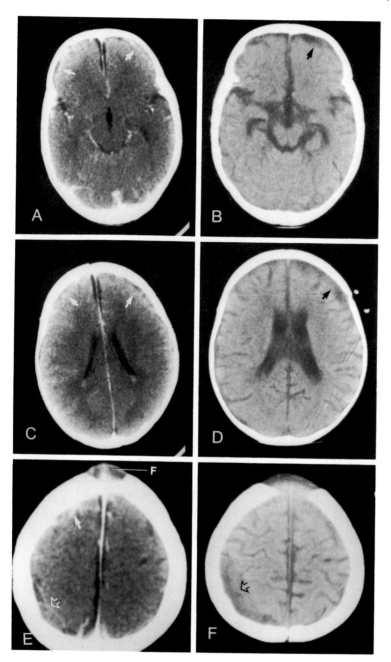

Figure 8.6. *Hemophilus influenza* meningitis. **B, D,** and **F** are 10 days after **A, C,** and **E.** Midbrain level (**A** and **B**), lateral ventricle body level (**C** and **D**), and centrum semiovale level (**E** and **F**) axial CT scans. **A, C,** and **E** are i.v. contrast enhanced. The widened extracerebral spaces with arachnoid, and possibly cortical, contrast enhancement *(closed arrows)* represent small subdural effusions. A larger posterior high convexity effusion is present *(open arrows)*. Note the small anterior interhemispheric effusion. The anterior fontanel *(F)* is bulging **(E).** Diffuse atrophy is already present at 10 days.

EPIDURAL AND SUBDURAL EMPYEMA

Epidural and subdural empyema (abscess) usually develops from an adjacent sinus infection or, less commonly, from adjacent skull osteomyelitis. Subdural empyemas may develop as a complication of meningitis. As already mentioned, the subdural fluid collections often associated with meningitis are usually sterile. The dura is a resistant barrier to the spread of infection, however, spread may occur along venous channels. Subdural empyemas are more likely to cause parenchymal spread of infection than are epidural empyemas.[4] Cerebritis and brain abscess may result. Interhemispheric extension of subdural empyema commonly occurs.[1,2,4] Two features serve to

distinguish the epidural from the subdural empyema that should be looked for on MR or CT images: one is the location of the MR hypointense dura and the other is an interhemispheric component.

CT of epidural empyemas (Fig. 8.7) demonstrates the underlying sinus or skull infection and the subjacent lenticular isodense or hypodense fluid collection. Intravenous contrast CT often demonstrates contrast enhancement of the inflamed displaced dura. A centrally located epidural empyema will displace the superior sagittal sinus.[4] CT of subdural empyemas (Fig. 8.8) may demonstrate similar findings of underlying sinus disease and an isodense or hypodense mass. Subdural empyemas may have a crescentric shape instead of lenticular and often extend

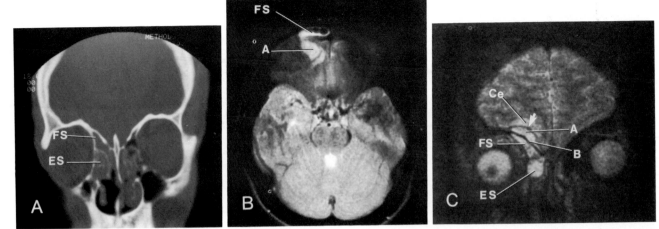

Figure 8.7.   Epidural abscess. Acute frontal and ethmoid sinusitis. *Coronal 3-mm thickness +295/3000 orbital level CT scan **(A)**. Axial supraorbital level **(B)** and coronal orbital level **(C)** SE 2000/80 MR scans.* Note the CT hyperdense and MR hyperintense frontal *(FS)* and ethmoid *(ES)* sinuses. The axial section **(B)** demonstrates con-

tinuity of the frontal sinus infection with the epidural abscess *(A)*. The coronal section **(C)** shows a portion of intact bony floor of the anterior fossa *(B)*. There is a contiguous frontal orbital gyrus focus of cerebritis *(Ce)*. The upward convex curved line *(arrow)* is the displaced dura.

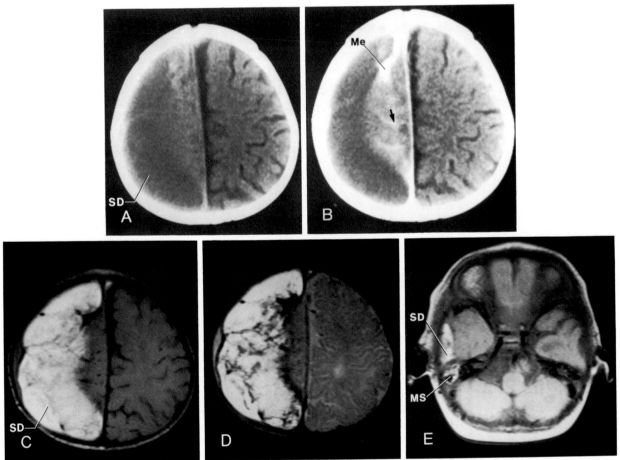

Figure 8.8.   Subdural empyema and mastoid sinusitis. *Axial low centrum semiovale noncontrast **(A)** and i.v. contrast **(B)** CT scans and SE 2000/20 **(C)** and 2000/80 **(D)** MR scans. Axial petrous bone level SE 2000/20 MR scan **(E)**.* Note the CT homogeneous hypodense and the MR heterogeneous T1/T2 enormous hyperintense subdural abscess *(SD)*. There is membrane *(Me)* contrast enhance-

ment and there is also gyral pattern contrast enhancement *(arrow)* possibly indicating underlying cerebritis. The empyema is continuous with the mastoid sinus inflammation *(MS)*. The size of the subdural empyema in this case is unusually large. The purpose of using this case is to demonstrate the contiguity of the mastoid sinusitis to the subdural empyema.

into the interhemispheric fissure. Intravenous contrast CT of active cases that are of at least 1 week's duration will demonstrate a medial enhancing rim of granulation tissue or of inflamed subjacent membranes and cortex.[4]

MR demonstrates the extracerebral T2 hyperintense epidural and subdural masses and the epidural T2 hypointense displaced dural membrane can often be identified. The epidural mass is usually lenticular and the subdural empyema can be either lenticular or crescentric. The inward displaced dura distinguishes the epidural from the subdural empyema. Adjacent sinus inflammation, edema, cerebritis, or parenchymal abscess can also be demonstrated (Figs. 8.7 and 8.8).[1] MR i.v. contrast enhances inflamed leptomeninges, abscess capsules, and subdural "capsules."

Other unusual meningeal bacterial infections such as *Actinomyces*[10] and meningovascular syphilis[11] occur but will not be further mentioned in this text.

Granulomatous Diseases

TUBERCULOSIS

Although intracranial tuberculosis is an uncommon disease in the United States, it is common in Third World countries. It is the most frequent intracranial granulomatous disease. The two forms of intracranial tuberculosis are meningitis and tuberculoma. Tuberculous meningitis is by far the most common manifestation.[12]

Blood-borne granulomatous infiltration of the meninges produces basal fibrogelatinous exudates leading to cisternal block of the CSF pathways, hydrocephalus, and arteritis. The arteritis may lead to cerebral infarction. Cranial nerve palsies may develop. The hydrocephalus may or may not remit after drug therapy.[13] Tuberculomas (tuberculous granulomas) may result from tuberculous meningitis or may be the cause of the latter condition.[12] Intracranial tuberculomas are often located infratentorially in patients less than 20 years of age. They may occupy an extra-axial location. They usually occur in white matter and may be located either peripherally or deep.[2]

The CT findings of tuberculous meningitis include isodense or hyperdense cisterns, marked sulcal and cisternal contrast enhancement, edema, and hydrocephalus (Fig. 8.9). Cerebral infarcts may be seen. Marked cerebral cortical enhancement may occasionally occur without evidence for cerebral infarct.[12] There may be coexisting tuberculomas. Calcification of the basal meninges may occur late in the disease course.[4,14]

MR findings in tuberculous meningitis include hy-

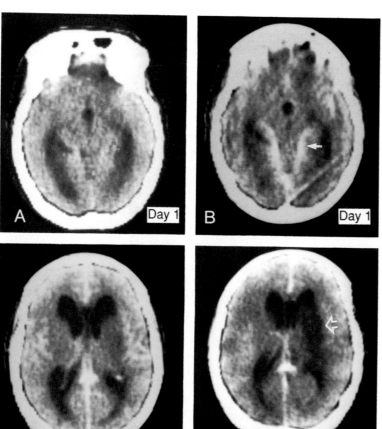

Figure 8.9. Tuberculous meningitis. Basilar meningitis with left middle cerebral artery infarct. *Axial midbrain-level noncontrast (A) and i.v. contrast (B) and internal cerebral vein-level (C and D) i.v. contrast CT scans. A–C* are at day 1 of clinical presentation and **D** is at day 3. There is marked thick contrast enhancement along the tentorial edge *(closed arrow).* Left middle cerebral artery infarct at day 3 *(open arrow).*

Figure 8.10. Tuberculous abscess—tuberculoma in an immunosuppressed lymphoma patient. *Axial superior lateral ventricle body-level (A) and centrum semiovale-level (B) 37/100 i.v. contrast CT scans.* There is a slightly irregular ring contrast-enhanced granuloma *(open arrow)* and a contiguous smaller lesion *(closed arrow)* representing a "microring". There is marked edema *(E)*.

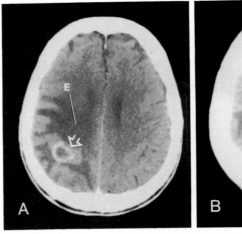 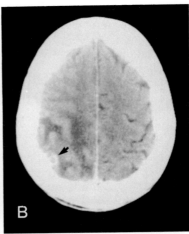

drocephalus and infarcts.[1] Intravenous contrast MR techniques are required paralleling the CT need of a contrast injection supplement to noncontrast CT techniques for investigation of inflammatory conditions. MR is more sensitive than CT for identification of infarction.

CT of tuberculomas demonstrates two types of lesions. One type demonstrates singular or multiple small masses with ring contrast enhancement, i.e., "microrings." The other type is nodular, markedly contrast enhances, and is typically found at corticomedullary junctions. There may be surrounding edema (Fig. 8.10).[14] Older lesions frequently demonstrate calcifications that tend to be larger than those found with toxoplasmosis and cysticercosis. The combined microrings and basilar meningitis represents strong evidence for tuberculosis. Differential diagnosis includes primary tumor, metastasis, pyogenic or fungal abscess and, in cases of extra-axial tuberculoma, meningioma.[2]

MR demonstrates T2 hyperintensity of tuberculomas and may demonstrate focal hemorrhage in the lesions.[1] More experience with MR imaging of intracranial tuberculosis, especially i.v. contrast MR techniques, is necessary in order to establish the MR characteristics of the disease process.

SARCOIDOSIS

Sarcoidosis involving the central nervous system is a rare occurrence. The disease may present as diffuse granulomatous meningitis and/or cerebral granulomas, as does tuberculosis. Cranial nerve palsies, hydrocephalus, and hypothalamic dysfunction may develop.[15]

CT demonstrates hyperdensity and i.v. contrast enhancement of the basal cisterns. Mass-like meningeal involvement may resemble enplaque meningiomas with i.v. contrast. Nodular parenchymal slightly hyperdense masses with varying degrees of edema and with homogeneous contrast enhancement also commonly occur. Occasionally, granulomatous extension of the meningeal process into the perivas-

cular (Virchow-Robin) spaces results in cortical linear and nodular contrast enhancement extending deeply into the white matter.[15,16]

Lack of nodule central necrosis represents evidence against tuberculosis. Diffuse meningeal contrast enhancement may be indistinguishable from carcinomatous or pyogenic meningitis.[15,16]

The majority of neurosarcoid lesions demonstrate T2 hyperintensity. MR i.v. contrast technique should be particularly accurate for demonstration of meningeal and parenchymal lesions. MR imaging of hypothalamic, basal cistern, posterior fossa, and cortical lesions is superior to CT due to lack of bone-induced artifact, absent MR cortical bone signal, and multiplanar imaging. Periventricular white matter T2 hyperintensity may also occur.[15]

Fungal Infections

Cryptococcus and *Coccidiomyces* can be responsible for a clinical syndrome not unlike tuberculosis. Both organisms can cause basilar meningitis and parenchymal granulomas. Ventriculitis, hydrocephalus, focal infarcts, and cortical atrophy may result with calcifications late in the course.[2]

CT may demonstrate contrast enhancement of the basal cisterns, hydrocephalus, contrast-enhancing nodules with possible ring enhancement, infarcts, and atrophy. Late calcifications may be present. The CT pattern is similar, if not identical, to that of tuberculosis.

Chemotherapy, steroid therapy, and AIDS are usually responsible for the virulent infectious processes caused by otherwise relatively harmless ubiquitous organisms. *Nocardia, Aspergillus,* and *Candida* may cause brain abscesses in immunocompromised patients. *Aspergillus* intracranial infection may result from direct spread of a sinus infection or may arise from hematogenous spread—the infectious route for *Nocardia* and *Candida*. In general, these lesions are similar to those caused by pyogenic organisms. Vascular thrombosis within the

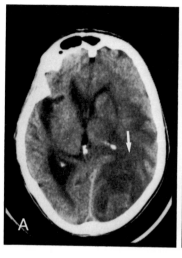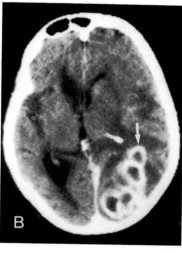

Figure 8.11. *Nocardia* **brain abscess.** Immunosuppressed lymphoma patient. *Axial third ventricle-level non-contrast* **(A)** *and i.v. contrast* **(B)** *37/100 CT scans.* The "multiring" contrast-enhancing mass with marked surrounding edema are indistinguishable from the so-called "microrings" of tuberculous abscess. The ring-like marginated abscesses *(arrows)* are barely perceptible without i.v. contrast.

abscess cavity may develop and may lead to massive subarachnoid hemorrhages. *Aspergillus* may extend to the subarachnoid space producing meningitis and may invade the cavernous sinus producing venous or arterial thrombosis.[2]

CT of parenchymal lesions of *Nocardia* (Fig. 8.11), *Aspergillus,* and *Candida* may initially demonstrate ill-defined hypodensity with or without contrast enhancement. When an abscess develops, ring contrast enhancement is seen. Direct spread from an infected sinus can be demonstrated and favors the diagnosis of aspergillosis in the immunosuppressed patient. Infarction and hemorrhage may be present. Steroid therapy is known to diminish contrast enhancement, presumably by partial restoration of the BBB.[2]

MR imaging of fungal parenchymal infection may have greater sensitivity for early stage detection than CT. Direct sinus extension from the paranasal sinuses can be well demonstrated in orthogonal planes.[1]

Intracranial mucormycosis is an uncommon, often fatal fungal infection usually occurring in diabetic and immunosuppressed patients. Isolated cerebral mucormycosis is rare. The *Mucor* fungi invade blood vessel walls and usually gain entrance to the cranium by destruction of a paranasal sinus or an orbit. There is frequent development of meningitis, arteritis, and cerebrovascular thrombosis. Extensive tissue necrosis with hemorrhage develops. CT and MR demonstrate bone destruction, a possibly hemorrhagic mass, and edema. Contrast enhancement may be present.[17] MR may detect cavernous venous sinus or arterial thrombosis (see Chapter 13).

Parasitic Infections

INTRODUCTION

Parasitic diseases of the central nervous system are uncommon in the United States. Increased foreign travel and recent increased immigration to the United States have caused an increased incidence of cysticercosis. The most common CNS parasitic disease in the United States is likely to be toxoplasmosis, which has three types of clinical presentations: *(a)* congenital, *(b)* acquired (immunocompetent), and *(c)* acquired (AIDS).

TOXOPLASMOSIS

Toxoplasma gondii is a protozoan with a worldwide distribution. The reservoir is an infected cat and also other animals. In the congenital form, the organism is transmitted to the fetus by the mother infected during pregnancy. This form produces meningitis, encephalitis, chorioretinitis encephalomalacia, and atrophy.[2] CT will show periventricular and basal ganglionic calcifications, microcephaly, and large ventricles (Fig. 8.12). Periventricular contrast enhancement due to ependymitis may be present.[7] CT has an advantage over MR for imaging of congenital toxoplasmosis due to the characteristic calcification.

In the acquired (immunocompetent) form of the disease, the CNS is uninvolved and the affliction is minor and self-limited after causing adenopathy and fever. Toxoplasmosis in AIDS patients is a fulminant, devastating CNS disease process that will be described later in this chapter.

CYSTICERCOSIS

CNS cysticercosis is a parasitic disease caused by ingestion of tapeworm *(Taenia solium)* eggs (oncospheres) that penetrate the intestine and encyst in tissues that include the brain. The cysts are found primarily in the cerebral gray matter, within the subarachnoid space adherent to the meninges and within the ventricles. The cyst initially contains a living larva. When the larva dies, it incites an inflammatory response leading eventually (years) to calcification of the larva. Reinfection may result in the presence of both dead and living larvae in the same patient. Cyst rupture can cause diffuse vasculitis, which may result in thrombosis and infarctions. Praziquantel therapy has been effective for treatment of cysticercosis. CT and MR are effective means of monitoring therapy.

Figure 8.12.   Congenital toxoplasmosis. Hyperextended semiaxial lateral ventricle frontal horn **(A)** and body **(B)** 35/100 noncontrast CT scans in a newborn. Note the basal ganglia and periventricular calcifications *(arrows)*, the ventricular enlargement, subdural effusions, and microcephaly.

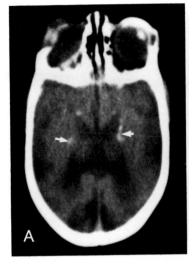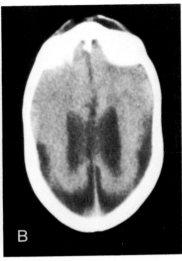

The three types of CNS cysticercosis (intraventricular, parenchymal, and arachnoidal) result in different CT and MR appearances. The parenchymal location appears to be the most common.[18,19] The intraventricular cysts most often occur in the fourth ventricle. They may be attached to the ependyma or they may be free floating. Intraventricular cysticercosis is a potentially lethal form of disease due to acute ventricular obstruction.[20] Solitary cysts are 1 cm or slightly larger and can be mistaken for colloid cysts and intraventricular tumors.[1,18]

Degenerative "racemose" cysts occur with arachnoidal cysticercosis. This cyst is multilobular and nonviable, lacking a larva "scolex." It is often several centimeters in size and is associated with chronic meningitis. The cerebellopontine (CP) angle and the suprasellar cisterns are common locations for racemose cysts. The local inflammatory changes associated with these cysts may involve adjacent cranial nerves. These cysts may erode the internal auditory canal. Hydrocephalus is common due to blockage of the subarachnoid pathways.[18]

Viable cyst fluid is CT water-isodense. The cysts usually do not contrast enhance (Fig. 8.13). CT is often unable to identify an arachnoidal or intraventricular cyst without intrathecal contrast. Occasionally, the larvae may be demonstrated within the ventricle with lack of distinction of the cyst wall.[18] Despite lack of cyst identification, the location of an obstructive lesion can be determined. CT of live parenchymal cysticerci usually demonstrates cysts containing larvae without detectable edema or contrast enhancement. Many of these "parenchymal" cysts are actually deep within sulci but appear to be parenchymal. When the larvae die, cyst wall contrast enhancement and edema develop. The edema may be severe and lead to cerebral damage.[19] Calcification finally develops. The calcified cysts measure 7–11 mm in diameter.[18]

MR is superior to CT for recognition of the cyst wall, the contained larva, and edema (Fig. 8.13). The cyst wall may be inflamed demonstrating a thin rim of increased T2 signal. The fourth ventricle can be expanded by a cyst or because of outlet obstruction by arachnoiditis. In the latter case, no cyst wall or scolex is recognized.[18,20] Due to relative water isodensity (CT) and intensity (MR), the fluid of the racemose cyst can be difficult to differentiate from the cistern. Focal cisternal widening and, occasionally, cyst rim signal hyperintensity may be helpful to identify the cyst.[18] MR analysis of T1, proton density, and T2-weighted images can usually identify the cyst.

OTHER PARASITES

Hydatid disease usually occurs (75%) in children. It is endemic in sheep-raising regions of poorer nations and is rare in the United States. The brain echinococcal cyst most always results from hematogenous spread from the liver or lung. CT demonstrates the mass usually in a cortical location in the distribution of the middle cerebral artery. Extradural location is a very rare event.[21] The water density mass is usually clearly defined without edema or contrast enhancement. Daughter cysts are not unusual. Leakage is rare but, when it does occur, edema and contrast enhancement may develop. Thinning of the calvarium may result with inner table erosion. Calcification in the wall of a degenerative cyst may occur.[2,22]

Toxocariasis canis develops when ingested larva from dog stool produce granulomas in the human. Eye and brain involvement can occur although brain involvement is uncommon. CT demonstrates white matter calcifications surrounded by areas of decreased density. MR demonstrates T2 hyperintensity. These CT and MR findings are nonspecific.[1]

Other parasitic intracranial infections such as coenurosis[24] and schistosomiasis[25] will not be discussed in this text.

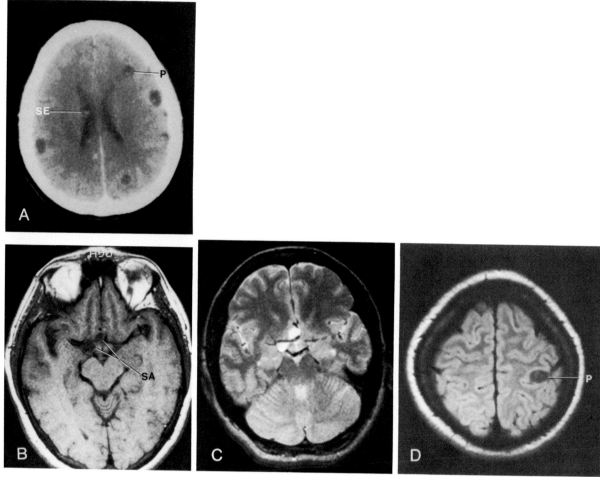

Figure 8.13.   Cysticercosis. A and **B–D** are different cases. *Axial lateral ventricle-body level i.v. contrast CT scan* **(A).** *Axial chiasmatic cistern-level SE 600/25* **(B)** *and SE 2000/80* **(C)** *MR scans. Axial vertex SE 2000/20 MR scan* **(D).** Note the subependymal *(SE),* subarachnoid *(SA),* and parenchymal or deep sulcal *(P)* location cysts.

They contain CT and MR water-signal fluid with CT isodense and MR proton density **(D)** hyperintense larvae (scolices). No evidence of edema or hydrocephalus is seen. The chiasmatic cistern cysts may be classified as racemose ("bunch of grapes").

Viral Encephalitis

Viral encephalitis can produce necrosis, hemorrhage, edema, and vascular congestion. Pathological features vary with the type of virus and host response. Host factors include patient age and immune status.

Prenatal infection with cytomegalovirus [cytomegalic inclusion disease (Fig. 8.14)], herpes simplex, and rubella may result in encephalomalacia and meningeal and ependymal inflammation. [Toxoplasmosis (a protozoan) can produce similar pathological changes.] Multicystic changes, atrophy, and microcrania may result with associated brain parenchymal calcification. Because these diseases present similar CT changes, they are often considered in the gamut: "TORCH" (Toxoplasmosis, Rubella, Cytomegalovirus, Herpes simplex). Extracerebral CSF collections may develop. CSF pathway obstruction may cause hydrocephalus.

Neonatal herpes simplex encephalitis produces different changes than in the adult. This form of the disease is usually a rapidly progressive diffuse bihemispheric process that may affect the cerebellum[26] (Fig. 8.15). In the adult form, the disease principally affects one or both temporal lobes, insula, inferomedial frontal lobes, and cingulate gyrus.

CT of neonatal herpes simplex encephalitis demonstrates widespread rapidly progressive white matter patchy hypodensity with minimal degree meningeal pattern contrast enhancement. The cortex becomes hyperdense and may remain that way for months. At approximately 3 weeks, atrophy becomes apparent. Calcification patterns vary from punctate to gyral.[26]

CT of adult herpes simplex encephalitis usually fails to identify abnormality until approximately the fifth day. Temporal or bitemporal edema is frequently detected at that time, occasionally associated with hemorrhagic foci (Fig. 8.16). There may be variable

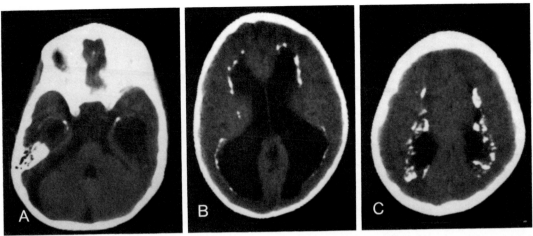

Figure 8.14. Cytomegalovirus encephalitis. Five-year-old child. *Axial fourth ventricle-level **(A)**, lateral ventricle body-level **(B)**, and atrial level **(C)** CT scans.* Note ventriculomegaly and marked periventricular calcification.

degrees of contrast enhancement that usually do not appear before the second week.[1]

MR appears to be more accurate for early diagnosis of herpes simplex encephalitis and, therefore, should be helpful for earlier initiation of medical treatment. T2-weighted images can demonstrate early stage high signal abnormalities in the inferior frontal and temporal lobes. Medial temporal lobe and insular edema are seen in orthogonal planes without the artifact that hinders CT imaging adjacent to bone.[1]

Subacute sclerosing panencephalitis is a rare, usually fatal disease occurring in older children and young adults after a measles infection. CT may be normal in the acute phase. CT usually demonstrates cerebral atrophy but may demonstrate diffuse or focal white matter hypodensity. The lesions do no contrast enhance.[2,27]

Progressive multifocal leukodystrophy is a progressive demyelinating disease caused by a papovavirus that usually occurs in immunosuppressed or immunodeficient patients. The disease is character-ized by multifocal areas of demyelination varying in size within the subcortical hemispheric white matter, cerebellum, and brainstem. Coalescence of these areas may form cysts. CT demonstrates white matter hypodensity and MR demonstrates proton-signal and T2 hyperintensity (Fig. 8.17). This condition is further discussed in Chapter 10 under the category of secondary demyelinating disorders.

AIDS

The HIV (human immunodeficiency virus) virus causes dysfunction of cell-mediated immunity. The population at greatest risk includes homosexual and bisexual men and their sexual partners, intravenous drug abusers, and patients such as hemophiliacs who require multiple blood or blood product transfusions. Up to 60% of AIDS patients have neurological complications. Despite this high frequency of neurological complications in AIDS, identification of a particular opportunistic organism is relatively uncommon. The HIV virus directly causes an encephalitis, "subacute encephalitis," producing moderate to marked atrophy involving the white matter, basal ganglia, cerebellum, and brainstem with relative sparing of the cortical gray matter.[1,3,28] The AIDS virus also causes focal encephalitis and meningitis. As has been already mentioned in this chapter, infectious agents producing CNS involvement in AIDS include *Toxoplasma gondii, Cryptococcus neoformans, Candida albicans,* herpes simplex, and cytomegalovirus.[1,3] A high incidence of intracerebral lymphoma and Kaposi's sarcoma also occurs in these patients.

Both CT and MR are relatively insensitive to early-phase AIDS encephalitis. Cortical atrophy due to subacute encephalitis is eventually seen in virtually all of these cases. In the minority of cases, CT findings include white matter hypodense foci of demyelization without evidence of mass effect or abnormal contrast enhancement. CT findings in AIDS encephalitis are often indistinguishable from progressive

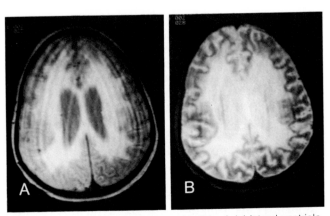

Figure 8.15. Neonatal herpes encephalitis. Axial lateral ventricle body-level proton density-weighted **(A)** and T2-weighted **(B)** MR images. There is extensive bilateral white matter hyperintensity. (Courtesy of Richard D. Smith, M.D., Indiana University Medical Center, Indianapolis, IN).

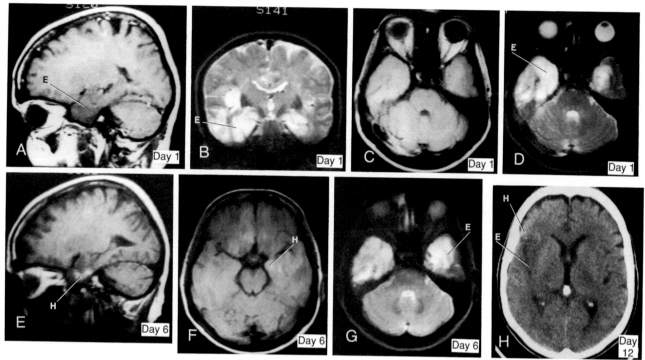

Figure 8.16.   Herpes encephalitis—adult. A–D are at day 1, **E–G** are at day 6, and **H** is at day 12. ***A–D*** *at day 1: Sagittal right temporal insular-level SE 600/25* ***(A)*** *and coronal third ventricle-level SE 2000/80* ***(B)*** *MR scans. Axial sella-level SE 2000/20* ***(C)*** *and 2000/80* ***(D)*** *MR scans.* **E–G** *at day 6: Sagittal left hippocampal-level SE 600/25* ***(E)*** *MR scan. Axial hippocampal-level SE 2000/20* ***(F)*** *and sella-level SE 2000/80* ***(G)*** *MR scans.* **H** *at day 12: Axial third ventricle-* *level 37/100 noncontrast CT scan* **(H).** Note the day 1 T1 hypointense and proton signal/T2 hyperintense bitemporal and right insular edema *(E).* MR evidence for hemorrhage *(H)* and increased left temporal edema is seen on day 6. The day 12 CT scan suggests a right frontal opercular area of hemorrhage and edema. Vague insular and opercular hypodensity *(E)* is noted, associated right Sylvian fissure and convexity sulci compression (compare to left hemisphere of **H**).

multifocal leukoencephalopathy (PML) and cytomegalovirus (CMV) encephalitis, which may also occur in these patients. Although the lack of mass effect and failure to contrast enhance tends to exclude toxoplasmosis and lymphoma, the diagnosis is uncertain without biopsy. CT of AIDS viral meningitis is indistinguishable from suppurative or granulomatous meningitis.[28]

MR of AIDS viral encephalitis also identifies the almost universal atrophy. MR demonstrates with greater frequency than CT the demyelinated areas. These appear as periventricular and centrum semiovale T2 hyperintensity (Fig. 8.18).[28]

Toxoplasmosis is the most frequent opportunistic organism causing intracerebral lesions in AIDS patients. CT shows often multiple hypodense homoge-

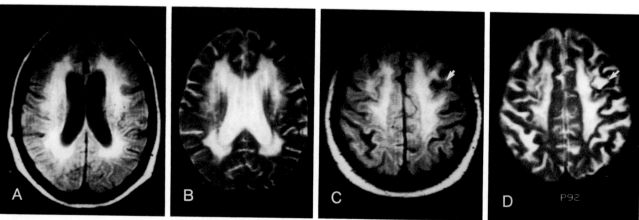

Figure 8.17.   Progressive multifocal leukodystrophy. Immunosuppressed patient. *Axial lateral ventricle body-level SE 2000/20* ***(A)*** *and 2000/80* ***(B)*** *MR scans. Axial centrum semiovale-level* ***(C)*** *SE 2000/ 20 and 2000/80* ***(D)*** *MR scans.* Note the marked proton density and T2 signal periventricular hyperintensity. A deep posterior left frontal area of focal atrophy or cystic encephalomalacia *(arrow)* of approximately water-isointensity is noted. There is atrophy and ventriculomegaly.

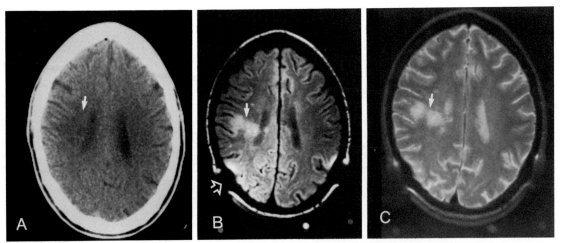

Figure 8.18.   AIDS viral encephalitis. *Axial lateral ventricle body-level noncontrast CT scan* **(A).** *Same level SE 2000/20* **(B)** *and SE 2000/80* **(C)** *MR scans 4 days later.* An abnormal right corona radiata and deep frontoparietal CT hypodense and proton density/T2 neous or mixed density masses at the ganglionic or corticomedullary junctional regions (Fig. 8.19). There is usually contrast enhancement, often of the ring type, and edema is common (Fig. 8.20).[1,3] These lesions may respond to pyrimethamine and sulfadiazine but usually recur with cessation of therapy.[1,3]

MR is more sensitive but not more specific than

MR hyperintense lesion lacks mass effect *(closed arrows).* The patient is scanned within an MR stereotactic biopsy device, which causes screw metal artifact *(open arrow).*

CT for demonstrating the lesions (Fig. 8.19). CT and MR ring contrast-enhanced masses in AIDS patients are not necessarily of infectious etiology. Primary lymphoma and metastatic Kaposi's sarcoma can present with similar findings or may even coexist with infectious intracerebral processes.[1,28]

Figure 8.19.   Toxoplasmosis in an AIDS patient (noncontrast enhancing). *Axial vertex-level i.v. contrast 37/100 CT scan* **(A).** *Left parasagittal SE 600/25* **(B)** *and vertex SE 2000/20* **(C)** *and 2000/80* **(D)** *MR scans.* This case is unusual because of the lack of toxoplasma abscess rim contrast enhancement. Perhaps this lesion has been detected and treated before abscess formation. The CT hypodense and MR T1 hypointense and proton density/T2 hyperintense irregularly contoured mass is identifiable on all images *(arrows).* The mass displaces and deforms the marginal sulcus *(MS).* The T2-weighted MR sequence best defines the lesion and the CT technique is least effective. The presence of mass effect is presumptive evidence against AIDS encephalitis.

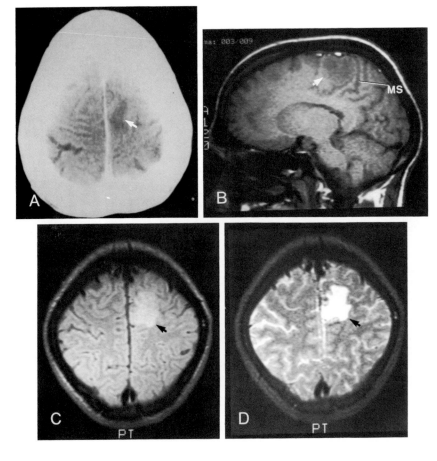

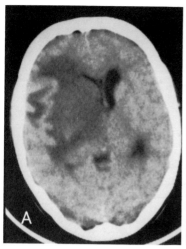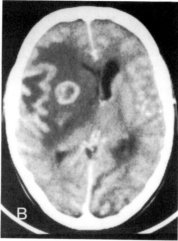

Figure 8.20. Toxoplasmosis in an AIDS patient (contrast enhancing). *Axial foramen of Monro-level noncontrast (A) and i.v. contrast (B) CT scans.* There is a hypodense round mass obscured by the marked right hemispheric edema **(A)** that demonstrates "signet ring" marked contrast enhancement **(B)**. There is marked mass effect with compression, displacement, and distortion of the right lateral ventricle frontal horn. Clinical history is necessary to distinguish this lesion from a pyogenic abscess. Lymphoma would be expected to be iso- or hyperintense. Metastases have an identical appearance. Courtesy of Mary K. Edwards, M.D., Indianapolis, IN.

References

1. Zimmerman RA, Bilaniuk LT, Sze G. Intracranial infection. In Brant-Zawadzki M, Norman D (Eds). *Magnetic Resonance Imaging of the Central Nervous System.* (Chapter 15) New York: Raven Press, 1986; 235–257.
1a. Haimes AB, Zimmerman RD, Morgello S, et al. MR imaging of brain abscesses AJNR 1989; 10:279–291.
2. Gonzalez CF, Palacios E. Infections and inflammatory diseases. In Gonzalez CF, Grossman CB, Masdeu JC (Eds). *Head and Spine Imaging.* New York: John Wiley & Sons, 1985; 397–434.
3. Levy RM, Rosenbloom S, Perrett LV. Neuroradiologic findings in AIDS: A review of 200 cases. *AJNR* 1986; 7:833–839.
4. Williams AL. Infectious diseases. In Williams AL, Haughton VM (Eds). *Cranial Computed Tomography.* St Louis: CV Mosby Co, 1985; 269–315.
5. Edwards MK, Brown DL, Chua GT. Complicated infantile meningitis: Evaluation by real-time sonography. *AJNR* 1982; 3:431–434.
6. Sullivan WT, Dorwart RH. Leakage of iodinated contrast material into the cerebral ventricles in an adult with ependymitis. *AJNR* 1983; 4:1251–1253.
7. Fitz CR. Inflammatory disease. In Gonzalez CF, Grossman CB, Masdeu JC (Eds). *Head and Spine Imaging.* New York: John Wiley & Sons, 1985; 537–554.
8. Allison DJ, Marano GD. Computed tomography of rheumatoid pachy meningitis: In correspondence. *AJNR* 1985; 6:976–977.
9. Zimmerman RD, Leeds NE, Canzinger A. Subdural empyema: CT findings. *Radiology* 1984; 150:417–422.
10. Atri M, Robertson WD, Durity FA, Dolman CL. Actinomycotic granuloma of the trigeminal ganglion. *AJNR* 1987; 8:167–169.
11. Holland BA, Perrett LV, Mills CM. Meningovascular syphyllis: CT and MR findings. *Radiology* 1986; 158:439–442.
12. Suss RA, Resta S, Diehl JT. Persistent cortical enhancement in tuberculous meningitis. *AJNR* 1987; 8:716–720.
13. Rovira M, Romero F, Torrent O, Ibarra B. Study of tuberculous meningitis by CT. *Neuroradiology* 1980; 19:137–141.
14. Whelan MA, Stern J. Intracranial tuberculoma. *Radiology* 1981; 138:75–81.
15. Hayes WS, Sherman JL, Stern BJ, et al. MR and CT evaluation of intracranial sarcoidosis. *AJNR* 1987; 8:841–847.
16. Mirfakhraee M, Crofford MJ, Guinto FC Jr, et al. Virchow-Robin space: A path of spread in neurosarcoidosis. *Radiology* 1986; 158:715–720.
17. Ginsberg F, Peyster RG, Hoover Ed, Finkelstein SD. Isolated cerebral mucormycosis: Case report with CT and pathologic correlation. *AJNR* 1987; 8:558–560.
18. Suss RA, Maravilla KR, Thompson J. MR imaging of intracranial cysticercosis: comparison with CT and anatomopathologic features. *AJNR* 1986; 7:235–242.
19. Rodriguez-Carbajal J, Salgado P, Gutierrez-Alvarado R, et al. The acute encephalitic phase of neurocysticercosis: Computed tomographic manifestations. *AJNR* 1983; 4:51–55.
20. Zee C-S, Segal HD, Apuzzo MLJ, et al. Intraventricular cysticercal cysts: further neuroradiologic observations and neurosurgical implications. *AJNR* 1984; 5:727–730.
21. Ba'assiri A, Haddad FS. Primary extradural intracranial hydatid disease: CT appearance. *AJNR* 1984; 5:474–475.
22. McCorkell SJ, Lewall DB. Computed tomography of intracerebral echinococcal cysts in children. *J Comput Tomogr* 1985; 9:514.
23. Edwards MG, Pordell GR. Ocular toxocariasis studied by CT scanning. *Radiology* 1985; 157:685–686.
24. Schellhas KP, Norris GA. Disseminated human subarachnoid coenurosis: Computed tomographic appearance. *AJNR* 1985; 6:638–640.
25. Schils J, Hermanus N, Flament-Durant J, VanGansbeke D, Baleriaux D. Cerebral schistosomiasis. *AJNR* 1985; 6:840–841.
26. Noorbehesht B, Enzmann DR, Sullender W, et al. Neonatal herpes simplex encephalitis: Correlation of clinical and CT findings. *Radiology* 1987; 162:813–819.
27. Duda EE, Huttenlocher PR, Patronas NJ. CT of subacute sclerosing panencephalitis. *AJNR* 1980; 1:35–38.
28. Post MJD, Tate LG, Quencer RM, et al. CT, MR and pathology in HIV encephalitis and meningitis. *AJNR* 1988; 9:469–476.

CHAPTER

9

Congenital Brain Malformations and Neonatal Disorders

Introduction

This categorization of congenital brain malformations and neonatal disorders is based upon that already used by other authors and our own experience. The etiology of some of these conditions is speculative but it is hoped that the utility of the classification overcomes the inevitable pathological inaccuracies of their grouping.

MR produces superior images of most of these conditions; however, CT usually suffices and the CT scan is easier to obtain. Intravenous contrast injection is generally unnecessary for work-up of congenital anomalies. MR parenchymal detail, particularly of gyri, nuclei, and tracts, is unsurpassed. CT is superior for diagnosing those conditions in which the type of calcification is unique. The role of each method will be discussed under each disease category.

Neural Tube Closure Defects

CHIARI II MALFORMATIONS

The Chiari II malformation is a complex congenital anomaly characterized by an abnormal caudal elongation of the cerebellum and brainstem. The patients almost always have myelomeningoceles. Hydrocephalus requiring shunting is usually present and may be due to aqueduct compression or stenosis.[1–4] Shunted infants usually have normal intelligence but have sensory and motor deficits.[1–3] The Chiari II malformation is frequently associated with dysgenesis of the corpus callosum. Hydromyelia commonly occurs (20–70%)[2] and other associated spinal anomalies include diastematomyelia and diplomyelia.[4]

A "vermial" peg of caudally positioned vermis projects below the foramen magnum behind the partially cervical medulla. A "medullary kink" is formed by the buckled medulla behind the cervical spinal cord. The falx and tentorium are hypoplastic. The tentorium has a low occipital insertion and a wide

incisura. Because the posterior compartment is enclosed by this hypoplastic tentorium, it is small. Not only is there cerebellar downward transforaminal extension (the vermial peg) but there is upward transincisural extension. The cerebellum characteristically bulges upward through the hiatus and anteriorly wraps around the pons. The medial cerebral hemisphere convexities abut one another because the hypoplastic falx is shallow resulting in "gyral interdigitation." Collicular fusion results in "beaking" of the quadrigeminal plate-collicular complex. Prominent fused thalami cause a large massa intermedia and a small diverticulum of the anterior third ventricle may be present.[4]

Small crowded gyri may occur in 50% of Chiari II patients and appear on gross inspection to be identical with polymicrogyria. These small, crowded gyri differ from polymicrogyria, however, because they do not lack cellular layers. They have been distinguished from polymicrogyria for this reason and are called "stenogyria."[4] Gray matter heterotopia and gyral dysplasias may also occur.[2,4]

Osseous abnormalities also occur with a high frequency in the Chiari II malformation. Leukenschädel skull is almost always present at birth. Convex anterior bowing of the posterior petrous and clivus margins ("scalloping") and foramen magnum enlargement is almost always present.[4] The posterior C1 arch may be absent.

CT of Chiari II demonstrates the Leukenschädel skull, which is present at birth and no longer present at several months of age, scalloping of the posterior clivus and petrous bone, and a large foramen magnum (Fig. 9.1). CT also demonstrates the myelomeningocele, the elongated caudal fourth ventricle, and hydrocephalus. The upward cerebellar bulge and gyral interdigitation can usually be demonstrated on axial images. Frontal horn indentation by prominent caudate nuclei is noted on axial images and coronal imaging (difficult in the infant) demonstrates pointing of the inferior frontal horns. The third ventricle has an hourglass shape due to the large connected massa intermedia. Some degree of hydrocephalus is almost always present before shunting and is more marked in the occipital horns and atria. The commonly seen postshunt lateral ventricular

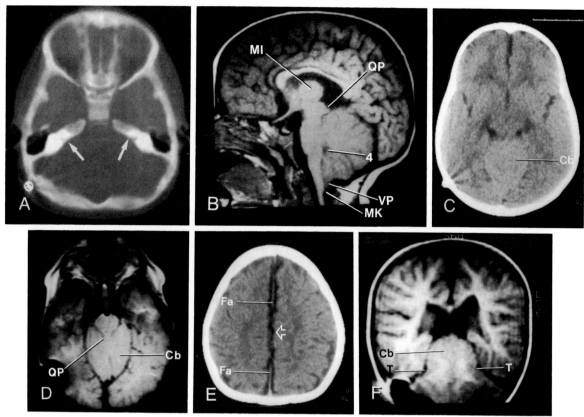

Figure 9.1. Chiari II malformation (ventriculoperitoneal shunt). *Axial petrous pyramid 200/3000* **(A)**, *cerebellar vermis-level 37/100* **(C)**, *and centrum semiovale 37/100* **(E)** *CT scans. Midsagittal SE 600/25* **(B)**, *axial midbrain-level SE 2000/20* **(D)**, *and coronal cerebellar-level SE 600/25* **(F)** *MR scans.* There is an upward cerebellar bulge *(Cb)* through the wide tentorial hiatus with characteristic tentorial *(T)* indentations and scalloping of the posterior petrous pyramids *(closed arrows)*. Note the tectal beaking of the quadrigeminal plate *(QP)*. The fourth ventricle *(4)* has only a slightly low position but may be elongated. A vermial peg *(VP)* extends below the foramen magnum and there is a medullary kink *(MK)*. There is interhemispheric gyral "interdigitation" *(open arrow)* caused by approximation of medial convexity apposing gyri under the abnormally shallow hypoplastic falx *(Fa)*. There is absence of the septum pellucidum. The massa intermedia is enlarged *(MI)*. There is a ventriculoperitoneal shunt and possible aqueductal stenosis (the cerebral aqueduct is not visualized).

"wrinkled" appearance may be caused partly by gray matter heterotopia.[2] There may be absence of the septum pellucidum.[1–3]

MR better demonstrates all but the bone changes due to orthogonal plane imaging and better parenchymal, posterior fossa, and spinal cord detail. Sagittal imaging has particular advantage for demonstrating the craniocaudal elongated low position fourth ventricle and cerebellum (Figs. 9.1 and 9.2).[4] The vermial peg, tectal beaking (collicular fusion), corpus callosal dysgenesis, and medullary kinking are clearly seen on the MR sagittal image.

The CT differential diagnosis may include cerebellar mass due to the high position cerebellar hemispheres. The diagnosis is obvious by MR.

ENCEPHALOCELE

This rare malformation is characterized by a skull defect that is usually midline through which meninges, CSF, and varying amounts of neural tissue protrude. The infants are often microcephalic and evidence markedly varied clinical deficits from minimal[2] to severe.[1,2] Varying degrees of brain dysgenesis may be present in the encephalocele and/or the cranial vault.[1–3] Although occipital and cervical encephaloceles with cerebellar herniation are often classified as "Chiari III malformations," we prefer the simpler classification "encephalocele." Occipital encephaloceles are the most common type in Europe and North America and are more common is female patients. Encephaloceles occur in other locations such as parietal, frontal, nasal, and nasopharyngeal.[1–3]

CT and MR demonstrate the cranial defect. MR better identifies normal and abnormal intracranial and extracranial tissues and associated anomalies (Fig. 9.3).

Cerebral Hemisphere Formation Defects

The five defects within this category that will be discussed are dysgenesis of the corpus callosum, interhemispheric lipoma, holoprosencephaly, septo-optic dysplasia, and hemimegalencephaly.

Figure 9.2 Chiari II malformation with corpus callosum dysgenesis and stenogyria. *Parasagittal SE 600/25 (A) and (B), SE 2000/25 centrum semiovale-level (C), and midbrain-level (D) MR scans.* Parieto-occipital dysgenesis and posterior corpus callosal dysgenesis *(CC)* results in an interhemispheric cyst-like cavity *(IHC).* "Gyral interdigitation" and a "meandering" hemispheric fissure *(IHF)* result from falx hypoplasia. Note the radially oriented, closely spaced stenogyria of the medial posterior frontal and medial parietal convexity *(Sg).* An abnormal temporal gyral lobule projects into the interhemispheric cyst *(TG).* Note the tectal breaking of the quadrigeminal plate *(QP).* The upward herniated cerebellum has a characteristic axial image "heart shape" and the cerebellar hemispheres "cuff" around the pons *(solid arrow).* There is a ventriculoperitoneal shunt *(Sh).* There is no aqueductal visualization. Note the collapsed low position fourth ventricle *(4).*

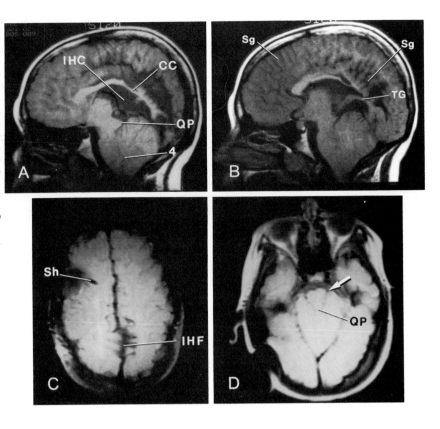

DYSGENESIS OF THE CORPUS CALLOSUM

This category of anomalies includes maldevelopment (dysgenesis) and absence (agenesis) of the corpus callosum. Patients may be relatively asymptomatic but most present before 3 years of age with developmental delay or seizure disorder. Severe cases often have associated interhemispheric cysts.[2] Other associated anomalies include Dandy-Walker malformation, Chiari II malformation, lipoma, encephalocele, trisomy 13–15 and 18, and Aicardi syndrome.[2,5]

Approximately 50% of patients with lipoma of the corpus callosum have corpus callosal dysgenesis.[2]

The largest fiber tract in the human brain is appropriately named the "corpus callosum." It is connected to the fornix by the septum pellucidum. Limbic system development is intimately related to development of the corpus callosum. Limbic maldevelopment such as cingulate gyrus, fornix, or hippocampal dysgenesis frequently accompanies callosal maldevelopment. The severity of maldevelopment of

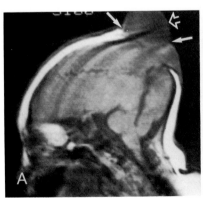
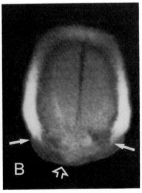
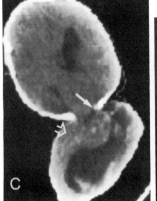
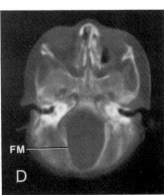

Figure 9.3. Encephaloceles. Parieto-occipital encephalocele **(A and B)** and occipital encephalocele **(C and D).** Different cases. **A** and **B,** *Parasagittal SE 600/25 (A) and axial centrum semiovale-level SE 2000/ 20 (B) MR scans.* Note the skull defect *(closed arrows),* microcephaly, and herniated parietal lobes within the encephalocele sac *(open arrows).* There is lack of normal gyration and presence of bi- zarre fissures. **C** and **D,** occipital encephalocele—Chiari III malformation. *Axial lateral ventricle body-level 35/100 (C) and foramen magnum-level 564/3000 (D) CT scans.* Note the occipital defect *(solid arrow)* and the herniated partially cystic brain *(open arrow).* There is enlargement of the foramen magnum *(FM).*

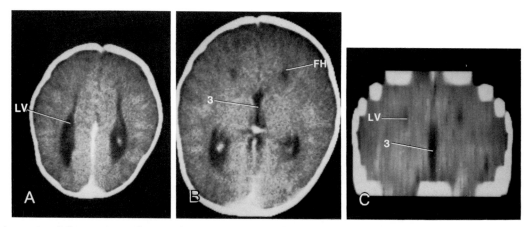

Figure 9.4. Agenesis of the corpus callosum—CT. *Axial lateral ventricle body-level (**A**) and frontal horn-level (**B**) 37/100 i.v. contrast injection CT scans and coronal third ventricle-level reformation (**C**).* Note the widely separated lateral ventricle bodies *(LV)* and frontal horns *(FH)*. The elevated third ventricle or cyst *(3)*.

the corpus callosum ranges from dysgenesis (Fig. 9.2) to agenesis associated with limbic dysgenesis and associated anomalies. The characteristic nondecussated longitudinal callosal bundles associated with agenesis of the corpus callosum are called "Probst bundles."

Although both CT (Fig. 9.4) and MR (Fig. 9.5) are diagnostic, MR is the preferred technique due to the ease of imaging orthogonal planes and superior parenchymal detail. The midsagittal section demonstrates absence of the entire corpus callosum. The lateral ventricles are separated, the foramina of Monro are elongated, the frontal horns are small and the atria, the temporal, and the occipital horns are usu-

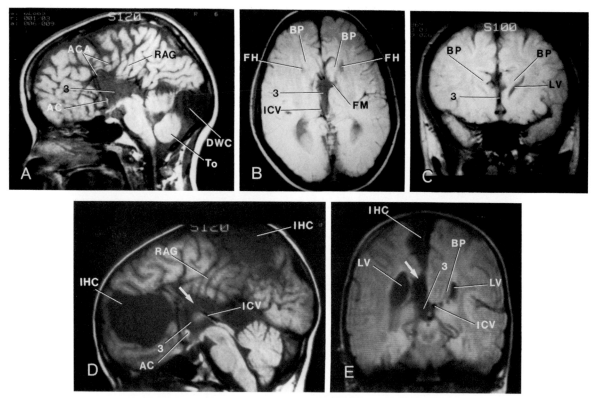

Figure 9.5. Agenesis of the corpus callosum—MR. *A–C and D–E are different cases. Midsagittal SE 600/25 (**A** and **D**), axial SE 2000/20 lateral ventricle frontal horn-level (**B**), and coronal SE 2000/20 third ventricle-level (**C** and **E**) MR scans. Case 1 (**A–C**) has an associated Dandy-Walker cyst (DWC) and case 2 (**D–E**) has associated interhemispheric cysts (IHC). The corpus callosum and cingulate gyrus are absent in both cases. An abnormally high third ventricle (3) displaces the internal cerebral veins (ICV) and separates the lat-* eral ventricle frontal horns *(FH)* and bodies *(LV)*. The third ventricle in case 2 is continuous with a cyst *(arrows)* which, in turn, is continuous with the interhemispheric cyst. There is resultant stretching of the foramina of Monro *(FM)*. Bundles of Probst *(BP)* are easily recognized adjacent to the medial surfaces of the lateral ventricles. The anterior commissures *(AC)* are normal. Cerebellar tonsil *(To)* resembles an inferior vermis in case 1. Note the radially arranged gyri *(RAG)*.

ally enlarged. Usually the third ventricle is dilated, has an abnormally high position, and is often continuous with an interhemispheric cyst or the interhemispheric fissure. MR better demonstrates the abnormal callosal bundles (bundles of Probst) that are adjacent to the medial margins of the lateral ventricular frontal horns and bodies. Cingulate gyrus and fornix dysgenesis is often associated with medial hemisphere, radially arranged gyri "sunburst." There is often lack of recognition or lack of anterior convergence of the parieto-occipital and calcarine gyri. The internal cerebral veins are separated and the anterior cerebral arteries "wander." Associated agyria, pachygyria, polymicrogyria, and heterotopic gray matter that may occur are far more clearly demonstrated by MR.[1,2,5]

INTERHEMISPHERIC LIPOMA

Interhemispheric lipoma is a rare condition characterized by collections of primitive and mature fat within or adjacent to the corpus callosum.[1] Up to 50% of cases are associated with agenesis of the corpus callosum.[1,2] These lesions may be asymptomatic although seizures and mental retardation are common. The nearly symmetrical midline mass is usually at or in the genu of the corpus callosum. The lipoma may extend posteriorly to the splenium and laterally through the choroid fissure to the choroid plexus. Other common intracranial lipoma locations include

pericallosal (Fig. 5.6) quadrigeminal plate and the tuber cinereum (see Fig. 9.17).[1] There may be marginal calcification. Encasement of anterior cerebral artery branches may occur.[1,2]

CT has the advantage of accurately identifying the calcification (Fig. 9.6). Both CT and MR readily identify the fat although CT number measurement quantitatively confirms fat presence. The major MR imaging advantage is orthogonal plane imaging, particularly of associated agenesis of the corpus callosum. MR also best demonstrates vascular encasement.[1]

HOLOPROSENCEPHALY

Holoprosencephaly is a condition characterized by the failure of brain hemispherization (the holoprosencephalon) that occurs in different degrees of severity and is divided into three types: alobar, semilobar, and lobar forms (Table 9.1 and Figs. 9.7–9.10). These types vary according to degree of abnormality. Craniofacial abnormalities frequently occur with this anomaly. The craniofacial anomalies, generally, increase in severity paralleling the severity of the brain defect. Severe brain defects, however, may be unaccompanied by severe facial deformity.[1–3,6]

Several conditions can be confused with holoprosencephaly such as hydranencephaly, Dandy-Walker cyst, and severe hydrocephalus. Absence of or incomplete formation of the falx and interhemispheric fis-

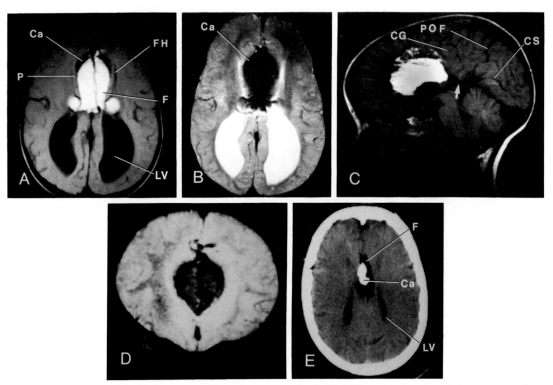

Figure 9.6. Corpus callosum lipoma. A–D and **E** are different cases. *Axial lateral ventricle atria-level SE 2000/20* **(A)**, *2000/80* **(B)** *MR scans. Midsagittal SE 600/25* **(C)** *and coronal frontal horn-level SE 2000/80* **(D)** *MR scans and 36/100 noncontrast CT scan* **(E)**. There are large fat intensity and density *(F)* corpus callosum lipomas with calcified

portions *(Ca).* There is absence of the corpus callosum splenium *(arrow).* Cingulate gyrus *(CG).* There is a normal relationship of the parieto-occipital fissure *(POF)* and calcarine sulcus *(CS).* There is lateral ventricle atrial dilatation *(LV)* resembling colpocephaly. Note how much more anatomic detail is seen by the MR technique.

Table 9.1. Holoprosencephaly

Type	Alobar (Fig. 9.7)	Semilobar (Figs. 9.8 and 9.9)	Lobar (Fig. 9.10)
Clinical	Hypotelorism-cyclopia, microcephaly, most are still-born	Hypotelorism, microcephaly	Nearly normal facies, may be asymptomatic
Interhemispheric fissure	Absent	Posterior interhemispheric fissure may be developed	Nearly complete, deficient anteriorly
Falx	Absent	Partially absent	Near normal, deficient anteriorly
Hemisphere formation	Holoprosencephalon, absent corpus callosum, "pancake-, cup-, or ball-" shaped brain, pachygyria, possible large dorsal cyst	Partial hemisphere formation, pachygyria, developing Sylvian fissures	Nearly complete hemisphere formation posteriorly, anterior frontal lobe fusion
Lateral ventricles	"U"-shaped, monoventricle, no temporal horns	Temporal and occipital horns with anterior fused frontal horns	Near normal slightly dilated with absent septum pellucidum, "squared off" frontal horns
Third ventricle	Absent	May be present but rudimentary	Near normal
Basal ganglia and thalamus	Fused	May be near normal, variable degrees of fusion	Near normal
Vascular anomalies	Absent or hypoplastic midline veins and dural sinuses, possible azygous anterior cerebral artery; possible hypoplastic "wandering," middle cerebral artery	Lesser severity, vascular anomalies	Possible azygous anterior, cerebral artery
Facial anomalies	May have: hypotelorism, absent nasal septum, cleft lip and palate, microphthalmia, anophthalmia, micrognathia, trigonencephaly, or cyclopia	Less severe	Usually none, may have mild form of cleft lip or palate

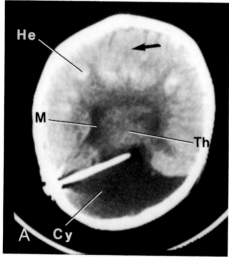 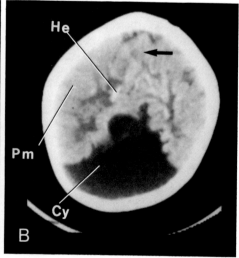

Figure 9.7. Alobar holoprosencephaly. *Axial ventricular level* **(A)** *and higher level* **(B)** *37/100 CT scans.* Note the lack of a falx or interhemispheric fissure *(arrow)* and the fused thalamus and basal ganglia *(Th)*. There is a cup-shaped monoventricle *(M)* and a large dorsal cyst *(Cy)* within which there is a shunt. There is abnormal hyperdense tissue *(He)* adjacent to the central white matter which probably represents heterotopic gray matter. Bizarre large gyri *(Pm)* probably represent polymicrogyria. The holoprosencephalon (brain) is anteriorly displaced by the dorsal cyst.

Figure 9.8. Severe semilobar holoprosencephaly. **A–B,** *Semilobar holoprosencephaly (severe). Axial CT scan at "third ventricle" level* **(A)** *and at petrous level* **(B).** There is a cup-shaped ventricle *(V)* continuous with a primitive third ventricle *(3)* that divides the thalamus *(Th).* There are primitive lateral ventricle temporal horns *(TH)* and there is a shallow anterior falx *(F).* The cerebral aqueduct *(A)* is surrounded by the midbrain tectum around which is the quadrigeminal plate cistern *(QPC).* (Courtesy of Mary K. Edwards, M.D., Indianapolis, IN.

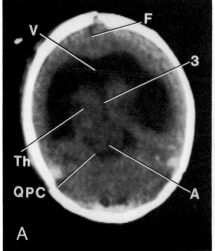
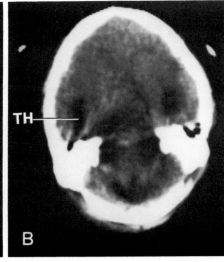

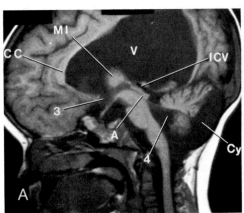
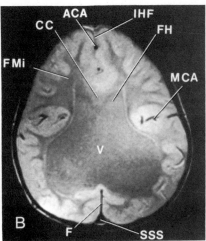
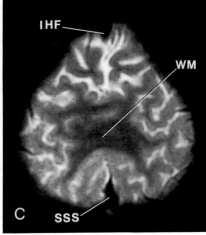

Figure 9.9. Semilobar holoprosencephaly. **A–C,** Semilobar holoprosencephaly and Dandy-Walker variant. *Midsagittal SE 600/25* **(A),** *axial "ventricular" frontal horn-level SE 2000/30* **(B),** *and "supraventricular" level SE 2000/80* **(C)** *MR scans.* There are primitive frontal horns *(FH)* of the undivided "ventricle" *(V).* Between the frontal horns is a thin corpus callosum *(CC)* which is continuous with the forceps minor *(FMi).* The primitive third ventricle *(3)* is joined to the undivided ventricle by a patulous foramen of Monro. The partially divided thalamus presents as a massa intermedia *(MI).* The cerebral aqueduct *(A)* joins the third and fourth *(4)* ventricles. Shallow anterior and posterior interhemispheric fissures *(IHF)* are noted. Azygous anterior cerebral artery branch *(ACA)* within the interhemispheric fissure. Undivided central white matter *(WM)* occupies the high convexity. A shallow falx *(F)* is seen in the posterior interhemispheric fissure. There is development of a superior sagittal sinus *(SSS)* and an internal cerebral vein *(ICV).* Middle cerebral artery branches *(MCA)* are within the primitive Sylvian fissures. There is posterior cerebellar vermis dysplasia and a retrocerebellar cyst *(Cy)* representing a Dandy-Walker variant.

Figure 9.10. Septo-optic dysplasia in a patient with lobar holoprosencephaly. *Intravenous contrast direct coronal frontal horn-level* **(A)** *and axial midorbital* **(B)** *CT scans.* There is absence of the septum pellucidum *(open arrow),* hypoplastic optic nerves *(closed arrows),* squaring of the lateral ventricle frontal horns *(FH),* and dilatation of the third ventricle anterior recesses *(3).* Note also the shallow falx and interhemispheric fissure *(IHF)* just beneath the contrast-filled superior sagittal sinus.

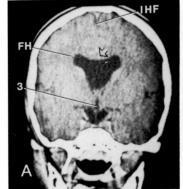
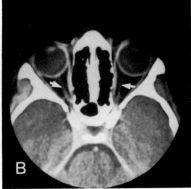

sure is diagnostic of holoprosencephaly. Hydranencephaly has a formed falx as does the uncomplicated Dandy-Walker cyst. Falx hypoplasia of the Chiari II malformation should not be confused with holoprosencephaly due to Chiari lobar differentiation and typical findings already described.[1,2,6]

SEPTO-OPTIC DYSPLASIA

Septo-optic dysplasia (deMorsier's disease) is a condition characterized by absence of the septum pellucidum, hypoplasia of the optic nerve, chiasm, and disk, and enlarged third ventricle anterior recesses. Females are more frequently affected and the patients may suffer from seizure disorder, blindness, and growth retardation.[1-3] Septo-optic dysplasia may be regarded as a mild form of lobar holoprosencephaly.[1,2] The frontal horns of the lateral ventricles appear angular or "squared off" similar to their appearance in lobar holoprosencephaly. Unlike lobar holoprosencephaly, there is usually a well-developed interhemispheric fissure and falx.[1,2] The case shown here is a combined septo-optic dysplasia and lobar holoprosencephaly.

Both CT (Fig. 9.10) and MR accurately identify the hypoplastic optic nerves, the absent septum pellucidum, the "squared off" lateral ventricle frontal horns, and the enlarged third ventricle anterior recesses. MR, because of its greater parenchymal definition and multiplanar capability, is the imaging system of choice for diagnosis of septo-optic dysplasia and distinguishing it from lobar holoprosencephaly.

HEMIMEGALENCEPHALAY

Hemimegalencephaly is a rare condition characterized by cerebral hemihypertrophy and cortical dysplasia. Microscopic examination shows loss of horizontal lammation and disorganized cytoarchitecture. The patients present in infancy with seizure disorder, encephalopathy, and focal neurological signs.

MR is the imaging procedure of choice and demonstrates an ipsilateral enlarged cerebral hemisphere, ipsilateral lateral ventricle dilatation, abnormal gyral pattern, and an ipsilateral thick cortex. The ipsilateral sulci are shallow and the gyri are excessively wide. There is periventricular white matter T2 hyperintensity.[7]

CT demonstrates ipsilateral lateral ventricular dilatation and cerebral hemisphere enlargement.

This condition is not to be confused with Dyke-Davidoff hemiatrophy where the large lateral ventricle is on the *contra*lateral side. The appearance suggests focal areas of agyria and pachygyria.

Aqueductal Obstruction

Although obstructive anomalies of the aqueduct are often classified as stenosis, forking, and atresia, it is not possible to identify the cause with imaging techniques. Aqueductal obstruction is often associated with other congenital anomalies such as the Chiari II malformation. Aqueduct compression in certain circumstances may actually result from ventricular en-

largement due to midbrain compression by the temporal and occipital horns. Aqueductal stenosis (narrowing without occlusion) as an isolated lesion is a rare condition.[3]

Both CT and MR demonstrate marked enlargement of the lateral and third ventricles and a small fourth ventricle. There is often associated periventricular edema. MR better visualizes the cerebral aqueduct and the third ventricle outlet (Fig. 9.11) and MR studies including i.v. contrast injection best exclude obstruction caused by tumor.

Cerebral Cortex Dysplasias

This group of rare conditions includes agyria, pachygyria, polymicrogyria, and cortical heterotopias. They are thought to result from abnormal migration of neuroblasts from the subependymal germinal matrix to the cerebral cortex. By the end of the second gestational month, neurons migrate from the germinal matrix in the wall of the lateral ventricle to the cortical plate. The neuronal migration continues for another 2 months. The degree of clinical severity parallels the degree of cortical dysplasia. Agyria is associated with microcephaly, severe mental retardation, seizure disorder, and less than a 2-year life expectancy. Patients with only focal areas of polymicrogyria may be asymptomatic.

Agyria refers to absence of cortical gyri. Pachygyria refers to abnormal, broad, flat, shallow gyri. Lissencephaly ("smooth brain") is a term sometimes used as a synonym for agyria. Because both agyria and pachygyria are characterized by a smooth brain surface and a four cellular layer (instead of six) cortex, we will consider both agyria and pachygyria within the category of lissencephaly. MR is superior to CT for identification of cortical gyri and sulci and is, therefore, the imaging method of choice for investigation of cerebral cortex dysplasia.[1]

MR of lissencephaly demonstrates smooth brain surfaces lacking gyration, particularly at fissures and sulci associated with hypoplastic structures such as the operculae, insula, corpus callosum, pyramids, and olives (Fig. 9.12).[1] MR may demonstrate the characteristic thick cortical broad band of gray matter surrounding the relatively small white matter region—the so-called "gray to white matter ratio reversal." A T2-weighted peripheral cortical hyperintense band may be seen.[8]

CT of lissencephaly may demonstrate a figure-of-eight appearance on axial section due to the smooth hypoplastic cortical surface with primitive Sylvian and interhemispheric fissures. A smooth interface of the gray and white matter is seen instead of the normal interdigitation that has been described as smooth subsurface lines.[2]

Polymicrogyria is characterized by excessive cerebral convolutions, increased cortical thickness, and an abnormal four cellular layer cortex. A paradoxical smooth cortical surface results because the multiple small gyri typically have fused surfaces with-

Figure 9.11. Aqueductal obstruction. *Midsagittal (rotated head) SE 600/25* **(A)**, *coronal pineal-level SE 600/25* **(B)**, *and axial third ventricle-level SE 2000/20* **(C)** *MR scans. Axial third ventricle-level CT scan* **(D)**. The third ventricle outlet (iter) is dilated and abruptly ends *(open arrow)*. No evidence of a cerebral aqueduct is noted *(closed arrows)*. There is marked dilatation of the lateral and third *(3)* ventricles. Normal detail of the posterior third ventricle including the posterior commissure *(PCo)*, precentral cerebellar veins *(PCV)* and internal cerebral veins *(ICV)*, and lack of abnormal periaqueductal signal is evidence against a tumor. MR is far more specific for the exclusion of periaqueductal tumor than is CT. An additional contrast CT scan, not done in this case, is necessary if CT is the sole method of diagnosis. MR i.v. contrast technique is recommended for exclusion of tumor and would have been used in this case had it been approved by the FDA at the time of this examination.

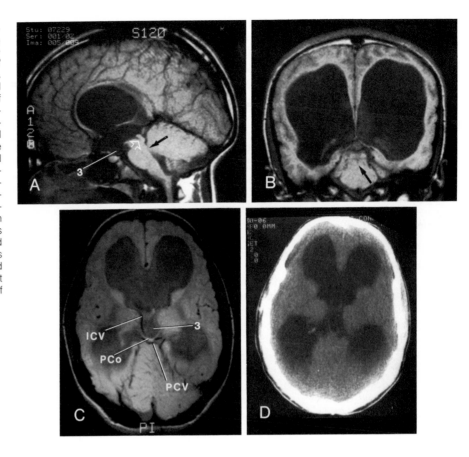

out sulcal clefts. For this reason, the appearance is unlike the stenogyria found in the Chiari malformation but polymicrogyria can be easily confused with pachygyria.[1,8] The condition may be relatively asymptomatic and isolated to a single hemisphere, often involving the opercular region. On the other hand, it may be associated with severe congenital anomalies such as schizencephaly.[1,8]

MR of polymicrogyria demonstrates a paradoxically smooth, thickened cortex lacking the normal white matter digital appearance. There is characteristically opercular involvement.[1,8] The thickened cor-

tical gray matter and diminished white matter digitations may sometimes also be detected by CT (Fig. 9.13).

Cortical heterotopias are islands of gray matter that form along the route of neuroblast migration and can be found anywhere from the germinal matrix subependymal zone to the cortex.[1] Patients with a mild form of cortical heterotopia may be asymptomatic or may present with seizures. Severe cases may be mentally retarded. Cortical heterotopia and polymicrogyria may coexist with other conditions such as Chiari II and Dandy-Walker malformations,[2] agene-

Figure 9.12. Agyria (lissencephaly). Six-week-old full-term infant with a parietal encephalocele and microcephaly. *SE 600/25 sagittal convexity* **(A)** *and axial quadrigeminal plate-level* **(B)** *MR scans.* There is complete absence of gyration. The primitive Sylvian fissure *(SF)* and the temporal-cerebellar cleft *(closed arrow)* represent the only surface landmarks. The parietal encephalocele *(open arrow)*.

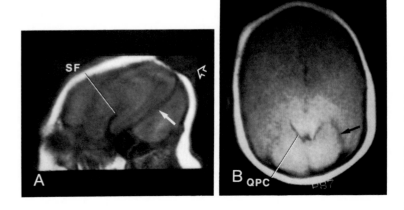

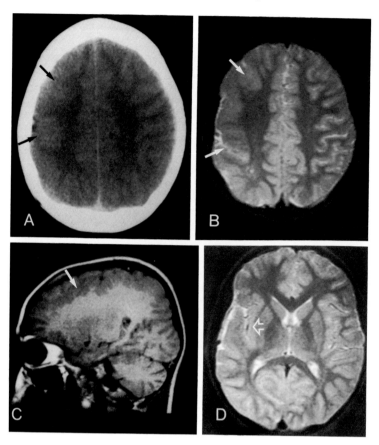

Figure 9.13. Polymicrogyria. *Axial centrum semiovale-level 37/100 CT scan* **(A)** *and SE 2800/30 MR scan* **(B).** *Insular level parasagittal SE 600/25* **(C)** *and axial 2800/80* **(D)** *MR scans.* Note the smooth right hemisphere cortical surface, increased cortical thickness *(arrows),* diminished white matter digitation, and lack of insular gyration *(open arrow).* The lesion conspicuity is far superior by MR. CT does demonstrate the abnormalities in this case, however.

sis of the corpus callosum,[1] and neurofibromatosis.[9] Heterotopias and polymicrogyria may coexist in the same patient.

MR easily detects the islands of gray matter signal within white matter structures such as the centrum semiovale (Fig. 9.14). The size of the abnormal gray matter regions varies from punctate to several centimeters in diameter. CT is far less sensitive than MR for diagnosis of heterotopia.[8]

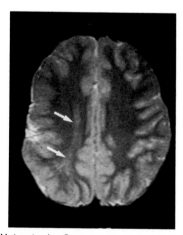

Figure 9.14. Heterotopia. Same case as Figure 9.13. Axial centrum semiovale-level 2800/80 MR scan. Note the "island" of gray matter within the centrum *(arrows).*

Cerebellar Dysplasias
POSTERIOR FOSSA CYSTS

This group of anomalies includes Dandy-Walker cysts, Dandy-Walker variants, retrocerebellar arachnoid cysts, and cystic dilatation of the fourth ventricle.

Dandy-Walker Cysts

Dandy-Walker cysts are characterized by absence of the inferior vermis, massive cystic dilatation of a fourth ventricle, or wide communication of the fourth ventricle and the cyst, and hypoplastic cerebellar hemispheres. The foramina of Luschka and Magendie are absent. The ballooned cystic fourth ventricle is continuous with a large primitive cyst, which anteriorly displaces the hypoplastic cerebellar hemispheres producing petrous pyramid pressure erosion. The tentorium has a supralambdoid abnormally high insertion (torcular lamboid inversion).[1,2] There is absence of paramedian retrocerebellar septae. These patients present with macrocephaly, hydrocephalus, and raised intracranial pressure. Mental retardation is common even after shunting, probably secondary to the high incidence of associated anomalies. These anomalies include dysgenesis of the corpus callosum (15–20%), holoprosencephaly (10–25%), and and cerebrocerebellar cortical dysplasias (20–25%).[1,2]

Although both CT and MR can easily establish the

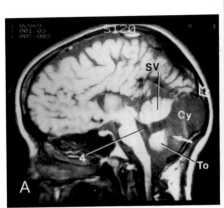
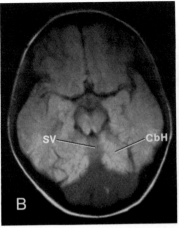
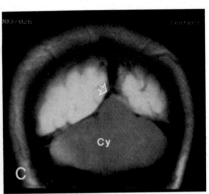

Figure 9.15.   Dandy-Walker cyst. Associated agenesis of the corpus callosum. Same case as Figure 9.5. *Midsagittal SE 600/25 (A), axial midbrain-level SE 2000/20 (B), and coronal SE 2000/20 occipital-level (C), MR scans.* The enlarged fourth ventricle (4) freely communicates with the large posterior fossa cyst (Cy) that anteriorly displaces the dysplastic cerebellar hemispheres (CbH); superior vermis (SV). There is absence of the posterior inferior vermis (closed arrow) and torcular labdoid inversion (open arrow). Note that the cerebellar tonsil (To) has a shape similar to an inferior vermis and can be easily mistaken for it. Analysis of the axial inferior cerebellar sections and coronal sections confirmed the absence of the inferior vermis.

diagnosis, MR is the imaging method of choice due to better parenchymal anatomical detail and orthogonal plane imaging (Fig. 9.15). Postventricular shunt or cyst shunt imaging can lead to confusing appearances and comparison to preshunt images is necessary.

The principal MR finding in Dandy-Walker cyst is dysgenesis of the vermis. The sagittal section demonstrates the vermis abnormality, the posterior fossa cyst, the high tentorial insertion, and possible associated abnormalities of the corpus callosum. The hypoplastic cerebellar hemispheres are well-demonstrated by orthogonal views.

CT lacks a satisfactory direct sagittal technique but can still accurately diagnose Dandy-Walker malformation. Vermis dysgenesis, enlarged fourth ventricle (alone or widely patent with a posterior fossa cyst), hypoplastic cerebellar hemispheres, and possible associated corpus callosum agenesis can be accurately demonstrated. Sagittal reformations are quite helpful for analysis of the vermis.[2]

Dandy-Walker Variant

The Dandy-Walker variant is more common than the Dandy-Walker cyst. There may[1] or may not[2] be torcular lambdoid inversion, the inferior vermis is often dysplastic, and the cystic fourth ventricle is often smaller. The foramen of Magendie is present with the variant anomaly (Fig. 9.16). There is presence of paramedian retrocerebellar septae.[1,2]

Retrocerebellar Arachnoid Cyst or Pouch

The retrocerebellar arachnoid cyst or "pouch" is formed by evagination of the fourth ventricle telchloroidea above and behind the intact vermis. The pouch communicates with the fourth ventricle and the subarachnoid space. Frequently, there is a falx cerebelli that may be bifid producing vertical parallel divi-

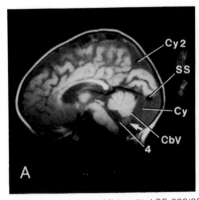
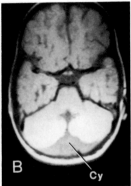
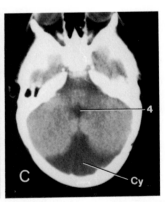

Figure 9.16.   Dandy-Walker variant. *Midsagittal SE 600/25 (A) and axial fourth ventricle-level SE 2000/20 (B) MR scans. Same axial level 36/100 CT scan (C).* Note the slight inferior cerebellar vermis hypoplasia (CbV) and the large posterior fossa cyst (Cy). The moderately enlarged fourth ventricle (4) communicates with the cyst at the widely patent foramen of Magendie. The straight sinus (SS) curves upward to the high torcula. An additional supratentorial communicating cyst (Cy2) is also present. All lobules of the cerebellar vermis are represented. The cerebellar tonsil (arrow).

sions of the cyst (Fig. 4.31C). This condition is probably responsible for many cases of "mega cisterna magna."[1] There are usually no adverse clinical sequellae. MR orthogonal plane imaging (particularly sagittal) is superior to CT for diagnosis of retrobulbar arachnoid pouch although the latter method is usually sufficient.[1,2]

Cystic Dilatation of the Fourth Ventricle

Cystic dilatation of the fourth ventricle is secondary to a variety of unrelated congenital and acquired conditions including atresia of the outlet foramina, ependymal cyst, and it may present as an acquired condition secondary to intraventricular hemorrhage.[10] The "isolated" fourth ventricle secondary to shunting will be described in Chapter 10.

Fourth ventricle cyst dilatation causes upward transtentorial herniation. The tentorial edge produces a notch ("keyhole") on axial sections at the base of the herniated portion. Since the keyhole is seen only with an expansile noncommunicating cystic structure, the notch indicates lack of free communication with the ventricular system.[10]

The differential diagnosis of cystic posterior fossa lesions includes a large cisterna magna, a retrocerebellar cyst, a Dandy-Walker cyst and variant, and a cystic tumor. The imaging distinction between a large cisterna magna and a retrocerebellar cyst is unclear and depends upon size. The diagnosis of a Dandy-Walker cyst depends upon recognition of vermis dysplasia, enlarged fourth ventricle, absent foramen of Magendie, absent paramedian septae, and associated anomalies such as agenesis of the corpus callosum and holoprosencephaly. Cystic tumor lacks the smooth, thin, even cystic wall and usually has areas of contrast enhancement. Sagittal MR imaging has proven to be very valuable for vermis and corpus callosal detail. An intact vermis excludes Dandy-Walker malformations. These findings are more difficult to recognize by CT imaging and, therefore, MR is the imaging method of choice for evaluation of cyst-like posterior fossa lesions. Shunt ventriculography may be helpful to demonstrate lack of cisternal communication of a cystic fourth ventricle but is seldom performed.

CEREBELLAR VERMIS DYSPLASIA

Recently, the association between isolated cerebellar vermis dysplasia and autism has been described. How frequently this association occurs has yet to be reported (Fig. 9.17).

CHIARI I MALFORMATIONS

This anomaly presents with caudal elongation of the cerebellar tonsils into the spinal canal and a small "tight" cisterna magna. It is often associated with craniocervical osseous anomalies and hydromyelia. Hydrocephalus may be present. The cerebellar caudal extent below the foramen magnum is greater than 2 mm.[11] The craniovertebral anomalies include oc-

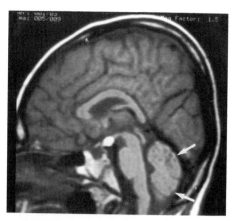

Figure 9.17. Vermis dysplasia in an autistic patient. *Midsagittal SE 600/25 MR scan.* Note the small smooth-surfaced cerebellar vermis lacking the characteristic folia *(arrows).* An incidental tuber cinereum lipoma is present.

cipitalization of the atlas, small foramen magnum, and block C2-3 vertebral body. Chiari I malformation is not associated with meningomyelocele and is unrelated to Chiari II or Chiari III malformations.[1,2] It has a confusing clinical presentation with onset usually in early adulthood.

MR is clearly superior to CT for demonstrating the full spectrum of these findings (Fig. 9.18) with the exception of occipitalization the atlas (Chapter 16). Assimilation of C1 to the occiput (occipitalization) and block vertebral body can be detected accurately by both the MR and CT techniques. The CT technique requires use of intrathecal contrast material and direct coronal and sagittal reformation for diagnosis of tonsillar herniation and delayed CT myelography for demonstration of hydromyelia (see Fig. 15.21). Both of these latter CT techniques are far less accurate than MR imaging.

Neurocutaneous Syndromes

These uncommon hereditary diseases of dyshistiogenesis are also called "phakomatoses." They include both nervous system and skin disorders. The most common disorders in this group are tuberous sclerosis, neurofibromatosis, and Sturge-Weber syndrome.

TUBEROUS SCLEROSIS (BOURNEVILLE'S DISEASE)

The overgrowth of astrocytes characterizes tuberous sclerosis. Multifocal tubers (hamartomas) consisting of bizarre astrocytes and neurons occur in the subependymal, cortical, subcortical, and white matter locations. Heterotopias and myelination defects may also occur. Hamartomas at the foramen of Monro are quite common and can cause obstructive hydrocephalus. Ventricular enlargement may also result from cerebral dysgenesis. Up to 15% of tubers (hamartomas) undergo malignant degeneration into giant cell astrocytomas—a slow-growing glioma. The foramen of Monro location is a common site of malignant

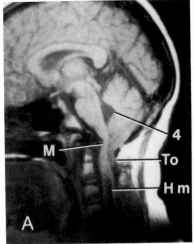
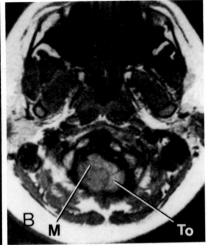

Figure 9.18.   Chiari I malformation. *Midsagittal* **(A)** *and foramen magnum-level axial* **(B)** *SE 600/25 MR scans.* The cerebellar tonsils *(To)* are caudally elongated to the C2 level and are seen tightly compressing the medulla *(M)* in the foramen magnum. There is a hydro- myelia *(Hm).* The fourth ventricle *(4)* is normal in size and position. Note the lack of a tectal break or a medullary kink that are seen in Chiari II malformations. The massa intermedia is unusually prominent, however.

transformation. Follow-up examinations have been recommended to detect malignant tuber degeneration.[1–3]

Renal angiomyolipomas are very commonly associated and hamartomas of heart, spleen, lungs, GI tract, skeleton, and eye also occur.[3] A cerebrovascular occlusive condition similar to Moya Moya may develop.[1] Although some cases are transmitted as an autosomal dominant trait of variable expression, the majority appear to occur spontaneously.[1] The clinical childhood triad of adenoma sebaceum, mental retardation, and seizures is well known.

Noncontrast and contrast CT is an excellent method for imaging these patients. The noncontrast scan identifies the characteristic calcifications (Fig. 9.19). The nodules are usually located along the lateral margins of the lateral ventricles and anterior third ventricle. The benign tubers do not CT contrast enhance. The giant cell astrocytoma is usually CT isodense or slightly hyperdense, is partially calcified, and uniformly contrast enhances.[2]

The CT differential diagnosis principally involves toxoplasmosis and cytomegalic inclusion disease. Of course, the clinical triad is usually known and a genetic inheritance is often suspected. The characteristic subependymal nodular appearance differentiates this condition from the others. It is important to recognize the lateral location of the subependymal tumors as to differentiate them from a lateral ventricle calcified choroid plexus that is almost always adjacent to the medial ventricular wall.[2,12]

MR not only can demonstrate the subependymal hamartomas and giant cell tumors (Fig. 9.19), but it can detect the hamartomas of more centrifugal locations as well as heterotopias and areas of demyelination. The subependymal nodules are best seen on T1-weighted images.[1,12,13] Calcified hamartomas are T1/T2 markedly hypointense.

MR is the preferred method for investigation of tu- berous sclerosis due to its detectability of noncalcified and peripheral hamartomas, heterotopias, demyelination, and arterial occlusions. MR can directly identify arterial occlusions and both CT and MR are sensitive to cerebral infarct.[1,12,13]

NEUROFIBROMATOSIS

Neurofibromatosis is a dyshistiogenesis of neuroectodermal and mesodermal tissue. There are two principal types: neurofibromatosis 1 (NF-1 or von-Recklinghausen's disease) and neurofibromatosis 2 (NF-2). Both are autosomal dominant diseases with different chromosome locations. NF-1 is associated with optic glioma and intracranial astrocytoma. NF-2 is associated with intracranial tumors of Schwann cells and meninges. Cranial nerve tumors other than cranial nerve II in NF-1 patients and occurrence of optic glioma in NF-2 patients is, at most, a rare occurrence. The dianositic feature of NF-2 is almost always bilateral acoustic neuromas. Approximately 90% of neurofibromatosis patients are NF-1 which is approximately 10x as common as NF-2. Intracranial "hamartomas" and skeletal dysplasias are exclusive to NF-1. Plexiform craniofacial neurofibromas and vascular dysplasias occasionally occur in NF-1. Both NF-1 and NF-2 are associated with spinal tumors. Other subdivisions of neurofibromatosis have been described; some of which overlap[9].

The intracranial disease will be discussed in this section. The reader is referred to Chapters 11 and 14 for discussion of optic gliomas, Chapter 12 for discussion of cranial nerve schwannomas, Chapter 13 for discussion of sphenoid dysplasia and to Chapter 15 for discussion of spinal and paraspinal neurofibromatosis.

Optic glioma is the most common intracranial tumor arising in neurofibromatosis patients occurring in up to 35% of afflicted NF-1 children[9]. Neurofibro-

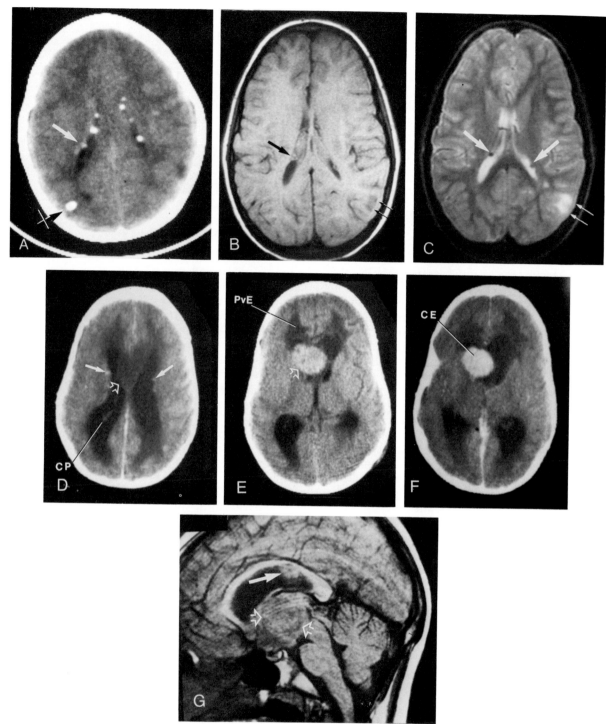

Figure 9.19. Tuberous sclerosis. A–C, D–F and G are different cases. Case 1: Axial ventricular body-level non-contrast 35/85 CT scan (9.19A) and SE 800/25 (9.19B) and 2500/80 (9.19C) MR scans. There are calcified subependymal (closed arrows) and a deep right parietal (crossed arrow) hamartomas. The subependymal lesions are more conspicuous by CT than by MR and have a characteristic lateral location. The noncalcified left parietal hamartoma (double arrows) is MR T1 gray matter-isointense and T2 water-isointense. Two of the calcified subependymal hamartomas are clearly seen on the T2-weighted image but they can be confused with the signal void of the subependymal veins. Case 2: **D–F** giant cell astrocytoma. *Axial i.v. contrast lateral ventricle body-level* **(D),** *noncontrast third ventri-* *cle-level* **(E)** *and same level i.v. contrast* **(F)** *CT scans.* The giant cell astrocytoma (open arrows) has a superior relatively hypodense portion **(D)** and fairly homogeneously hyperdense calcified foramen of Monro level portion **(E)** which homogeneously contrast enhances *(CE,* **(F)**)*. Subependymal calcified hamartomas *(closed arrows)* provide evidence to support the diagnosis of tuberous sclerosis. Note the hydrocephalus with periventricular edema *(PvE).* **(G)** Case 3. Hamartoma and giant cell astrocytoma in a case of tuberous sclerosis. *Midsagittal SE 600/25 MR scan.* The subependymal hamartoma *(closed arrow)* and foramen of Monro location giant cell astrocytoma *(open arrows)* are well seen on this T1-weighted image.

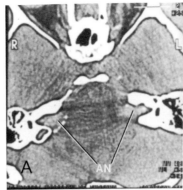

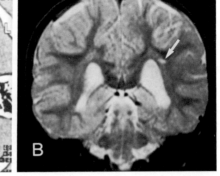

Figure 9.20. Neurofibromatosis. **A** and **B** are different cases. *Axial internal auditory canal-level i.v. contrast 59/400 edge enhancement filter CT scan (A).* Contrast enhanced bilateral acoustic neuromas *(AN)* erode the internal auditory canals. *Coronal lateral ventricle atrial level SE 2800/80 MR scan (B).* A T2 hyperintense left parietal white matter lesion is noted *(arrow)* in this 2-year-old male.[9]

matosis may account for as much as 50% of all optic gliomas. Most of the rare childhood occurrences of meningiomas, schwannomas and "acoustic neuromas" are associated with neurofibromatosis (NF-2). Sphenoid dysplasia (NF-1) commonly causes partial absence of the sphenoid greater wing. This results in hypoplasia and elevation of the lesser sphenoid wing and enlargement of the superior orbital fissure. Pulsatile exophthalmos occurs in a minority of these patients. Foci of proton density and T2-weighted hyperintensity "hamartomas" are common in NF-1 patients (Fig. 9.20B). The lack of mass effect and of CT contrast enhancement help distinguish the "hamartoma" from an astrocytoma. Occasionally, an arterial vascular occlusive process develops in NF-1 patients resembling moyamoya disease (Fig. 6.21)[1,3,9]

Both CT and MR (Fig. 9.20) demonstrate the multiple manifestations of this disease. Acoustic neuromas are more easily detected by MR than by CT due to the CT need of intrathecal contrast for demonstrating intracanalicular lesions. Intravenous contrast MR is the most sensitive method for detecting small meningiomas, however, i.v. contrast CT is also effective. Optic chiasmal tumors are better detected by MR than CT although both methods are effective. MR sagittal sections are particularly helpful. The

sphenoid wing defects are best seen by CT. MR is superior to CT for detecting the vascular occlusive changes that may resemble moyamoya.[2,3] The lack of mass effect and of contrast enhancement help distinguish the "hamartoma" from an astrocytoma.

STURGE-WEBER SYNDROME (ENCEPHALOTRIGEMINAL ANGIOMATOSIS)

This phakomatosis has no known hereditary pattern. It is characterized by usually unilateral angiomatosis of the face and leptomeninges with an underlying superficial layer of gyral cortical calcification and ipsilateral atrophy.[3,14] Abnormal local venous drainage occurs with nonfunctional or absent cortical veins and patent deep veins. The facial portwine stain is usually in a distribution approximating the innervation of the trigeminal nerve superior division. More than two-thirds of cases have seizure disorder. Mental retardation, ipsilateral glaucoma, hemilegia, and homonymous hemianopsia are common[1]

Plain skull x-ray, CT localizer view, and CT establish the diagnosis. CT and MR can establish the degree of atrophy (Fig. 9.21). CT has an advantage over MR of detecting the characteristic parieto-occipital calcification that follows the pattern of cerebral con-

Figure 9.21. Sturge-Weber syndrome. *Lateral skull x-ray (A) and axial corona radiata level 36/200 i.v. contrast CT scan (B).* Note the characteristic unilateral posterior convexity serpentine calcification following the convolution contours.

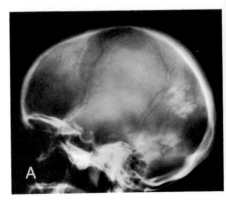

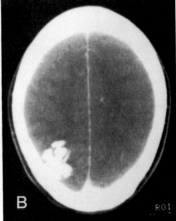

volutions of a single hemisphere. Wide window technique best demonstrates the cortical calcification pattern.[2,3,14] The calcifications can appear as early as 3 months of age. Enlargement and increased contrast enhancement of the ipsilateral choroid plexus is a very common finding.[14] Nonvisualization of the superior sagittal sinus with contrast CT may occur. MR demonstrates superficial leptomeningeal angiomas and also absence (or paucity) of cortical veins with patent deep veins.[1] The calcifications may easily be confused with flow-void phenomenon by MR technique, particularly with spin-echo sequences.

CT differential diagnosis of cortical pattern calcification includes calcification secondary to intrathecal methotrexate therapy and meningitis—neither of which would fit the unilateral specific geographic localization. Since a port-wine nevus is necessary for diagnosis, the other conditions are excluded.

Destructive Lesions

Hydranencephaly and schizencephaly are included in this category although they may have different etiological mechanisms. Cerebral hemiatrophy (Dyke-Davidoff-Masson syndrome) has already been discussed (Fig. 6.25).

HYDRANENCEPHALY

This condition is characterized by incomplete or total absence of the cerebral hemispheres (carotid artery distribution) with preservation of structures supplied by the basilar artery distribution. The meninges and cranial vault are usually intact.[2,3] The falx is preserved. CT demonstrates virtually total cerebral hemisphere absence with a normal diencephalon, midbrain, cerebellum, and brainstem. CSF fills the void normally occupied by the cerebral hemispheres (Fig. 9.22).[2,3] We have no MR experience with hydranencephaly. Our most recent case was studied by our cine CT scanner to obtain a stop-motion scan and to avoid anesthesia in a critical neonate.

CT and MR can exclude consideration of hydrocephalus and holoprosencephaly because of the almost total lack of hemispheric tissue associated with falx, diencephalon, and brainstem and cerebellar preservation.

SCHIZENCEPHALY

This anomaly may be a form of porencephaly[2] or may be a disorder of sulcation and migration.[3] It resembles porencephaly and appears as a cone-shaped defect pointing inward with its base at the cortex. It is usually bilateral, often asymmetrical, and usually involves the frontal and parietal lobes. Associated abnormalities such as agenesis of the corpus callosum and absent septum pellucidum may occur. Polymicrogyria[2] and pachygyria within the cleft may be present.[15,16]

CT and MR demonstrate the CSF-filled cavities that may communicate with the ventricles (Fig. 9.23). MR may detect polymicrogyria within the cleft. Porencephaly and arachnoid cysts are two major differential diagnostic possibilities. Porencephaly is unusual

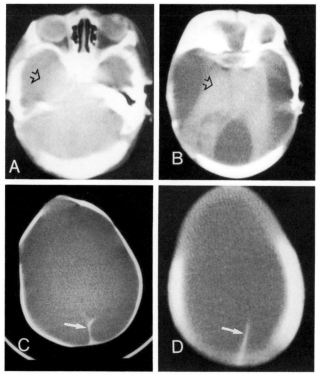

Figure 9.22. Hydranencephaly. *Axial 30/136 0.8-sec scanning electron beam posterior fossa* **(A)**, *supraorbital level* **(B)**, *low convexity* **(C)**, *and vertex* **(D)** *CT scans. The falx (closed arrow) is present. Cerebellum, thalamus, diencephalon, and portions of the inferior* temporal, occipital, and parietal lobes are preserved *(open arrows)*. The cerebellum is relatively intact. There is no cortical mantle and CSF fills the rest of the calvarial space.

Figure 9.23. Schizencephaly. A and B are different cases. *Noncontrast axial lateral ventricle level* **(A)** *CT scan and T2-weighted MR scan* **(B).** Note the brain structural coronal cleft from rostral to caudal including the lateral ventricles at level "B." (**A** is courtesy of Mary K. Edwards, M.D., Indianapolis, IN.)

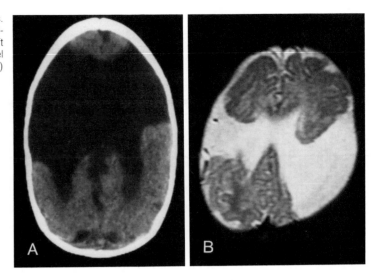

in the neonate and most often occurs after infection producing the characteristic pattern of multiple cysts associated with encephalomalacia. Arachnoid cysts have a characteristic middle fossa location with a flat, posterior margin (Fig. 5.7).

Miscellaneous Anomalies

Arachnoid cysts, porencephalic cysts, and ependymal cysts belong in this category. Arachnoid cysts have been discussed in Chapter 5 and porencephalic cysts will be discussed in Chapter 10.

Ependymal cysts are rare and extremely difficult to diagnose by CT without positive contrast ventriculography. MR may be successful in differentiating the cyst fluid from the surrounding CSF (Fig. 5.38).

References

1. Naidich TP, Zimmerman RA. Common congenital malformations of the brain. In Brandt-Zawadzki M, Norman D (Eds). *Magnetic Resonance Imaging of the Central Nervous System.* New York: Raven Press, 1987: 131–150.
2. Fitz CR. Congenital and neonatal disorders. In Gonzalez CF, Grossman CB, Masdeu JC (Eds). *Head and Spine Imaging.* New York: John Wiley & Sons, 1985; 555–573.
3. Ludwin SK, Norman MG. Congenital malformations of the nervous system. In Davis RL, Robertson DM (Eds). *Textbook off Neuropathology.* Baltimore: Williams & Wilkins, 1985; 176–242.
4. Wolpert SM, Anderson M, Scott RM. Chiari II malformation: MR imaging evaluation. *AJNR* 1987; 8:783–792.
5. Atlas SW, Zimmerman RA, Bilaniuk LT, et al. Corpus callosum and limbic system: Neuroanatomic MR evaluation of developmental anomalies. *Radiology* 1986; 160:355–362.
6. Altman NR, Altman DH, Sheldon JJ, Leborgne J. Holoprosencephaly classified by computed tomography. *AJNR* 1984; 5:433–437.
7. Kalifa GL, Chiron C, Sellier N, et al. Hemimegalencephaly: MR imaging in five children. *Radiology* 1987; 165:29–33.
8. Barkovich AJ, Chuang SH, Norman D. MR of neuronal migration anomalies. *AJNR* 1987; 8:1009–1017.
9. Aoki S, Barkovich AJ, Nishimura K, et al. Neurofibromatosis types 1 and 2: cranial MR findings. Radiology 1989; 172; 527–534.
10. Wolfson BJ, Faerber EN, Truex RC Jr. The "keyhole": A sign of herniation of a trapped fourth ventricle and other posterior fossa cysts. *AJNR* 1987; 8:473–477.
11. Barkovich AJ, Wippold FJ, Sherman JL, Citrin CM. Significance of cerebellar tonsillar position on MR. *AJNR* 1986; 7:795–799.
12. Altman NR, Purser RK, Post MJD. Tuberous sclerosis: Characteristics at CT and MR imaging. *Radiology* 1988; 167:527–532.
13. McMurdo SK, Moore SG, Brant-Zawadzki M, et al. MR imaging of intracranial tuberous sclerosis. *AJNR* 1988; 8:77–82.
14. Stimac GK, Solomon MA, Newton TH. CT and MR of angiomatous malformations of the choroid plexus in patients with Sturge-Weber disease. *AJNR* 1986; 7:623–627.
15. Bird CR, Gilles FH. Type 1 schizencephaly: CT and neuropathologic findings. *AJNR* 1987; 8:451–454.
16. Barkovich AJ, Norman D. MR imaging of schizencephaly. *AJNR* 1988; 9:297–302.

10

Hydrocephalus and Atrophic and Degenerative Disorders

Introduction

Hydrocephalus and atrophic and degenerative disorders are often associated with dementia and movement disorders, particularly in the elderly. The classification, as outlined here, of this group of diseases might offend the neuropathologist due to the diverse etiologies of these conditions. Despite the dissimilar (and in some cases, unknown) etiologies, they are considered together here because of their clinical similarities and for imaging differential diagnostic purposes.[1,2]

MR, in general, provides more diagnostic information in this group of diseases than does CT due to greater gray-white matter discrimination and lack of bone-related artifacts.

Hydrocephalus

The simplest definition of hydrocephalus is enlargement of the cerebral ventricles; however, this chapter excludes ventricular dilatation associated with atrophy from the hydrocephalus classification. Much controversy exists regarding classification of types of hydrocephalus. Some authors believe that the term "hydrocephalus" should be used only in the presence of raised intracranial pressure. We disagree with that usage because, frequently, there is lack of proof of raised pressure in these cases. Raised intracranial pressure (possibly intermittent) may play a dominant role in nonatrophic ventricular enlargement.

Obstructive hydrocephalus includes communicating and noncommunicating types. Noncommunicating hydrocephalus is caused by intraventricular or fourth ventricle outlet obstruction. Obstruction anywhere along the extraventricular CSF pathways between the fourth ventricle outlet foramina and the arachnoid granulations may occur in communicating hydrocephalus.[1,3,4]

NONCOMMUNICATING HYDROCEPHALUS

Noncommunicating hydrocephalus is caused by blockage or compression of ventricles, foramina, and the cerebral aqueduct. Since the ventricles dilate proximal to the obstruction, the level of obstruction is quite clear with CT or MR. The most common levels of obstruction are the foramen of Monro (Fig. 5.18), the cerebral aqueduct (Fig. 9.11), and the fourth ventricle (Fig. 10.1).

The most common cause of obstructive hydrocephalus is a mass compressing, displacing, or invading the fourth ventricle, the aqueduct, the third ventricle, or the foramina of Monro. Foramen of Monro obstruction causes lateral ventricular enlargement with small third and fourth ventricles. With aqueductal obstruction, the lateral and third ventricles dilate and the fourth ventricle usually becomes quite small. Foramen of Monro and third ventricle region masses include colloid cysts, subependymal giant cell astrocytomas, ependymomas, and lymphomas. Suprasellar tumors such as adenomas and craniopharyngiomas can also produce foramen of Monro obstruction. Posterior third ventricle-pineal region masses include pineal tumors, cerebellar vermis tumors, and corpus callosum (splenium) tumors. Aqueductal stenosis may be of congenital, postmeningitic, postintraventricular hemorrhagic, or neoplastic origin. Fourth ventricle outlet obstruction may be of congenital (Dandy-Walker cyst), neoplastic, or postinfectious origin. Ventricular shunting may result in an "isolated fourth ventricle"—a relatively rare condition in which the fourth ventricle behaves as an expansile cyst.

All cases of noncommunicating hydrocephalus demonstrate ventricular enlargement terminating at the level of obstruction and sulcal compression. There is usually prominent and often disproportionate lateral ventricle temporal and frontal horn dilatation and periventricular (interstitial) edema.[1,3]

Both MR and CT of noncommunicating hydrocephalus (intraventricular blockage) (Fig. 10.1) demonstrate markedly dilated temporal and frontal horns, compressed cisterns and sulci, and transependymal CSF resorption "periventricular" interstitial edema.[4,5] The periventricular edema may render the lateral ventricle margins difficult to detect by CT and T2-weighted MR. The T1/proton density-weighted image (e.g., SE 2000/20) best contrasts the hypointense intraventricular CSF against the moderately hyperintense interstitial fluid. Although the interstitial

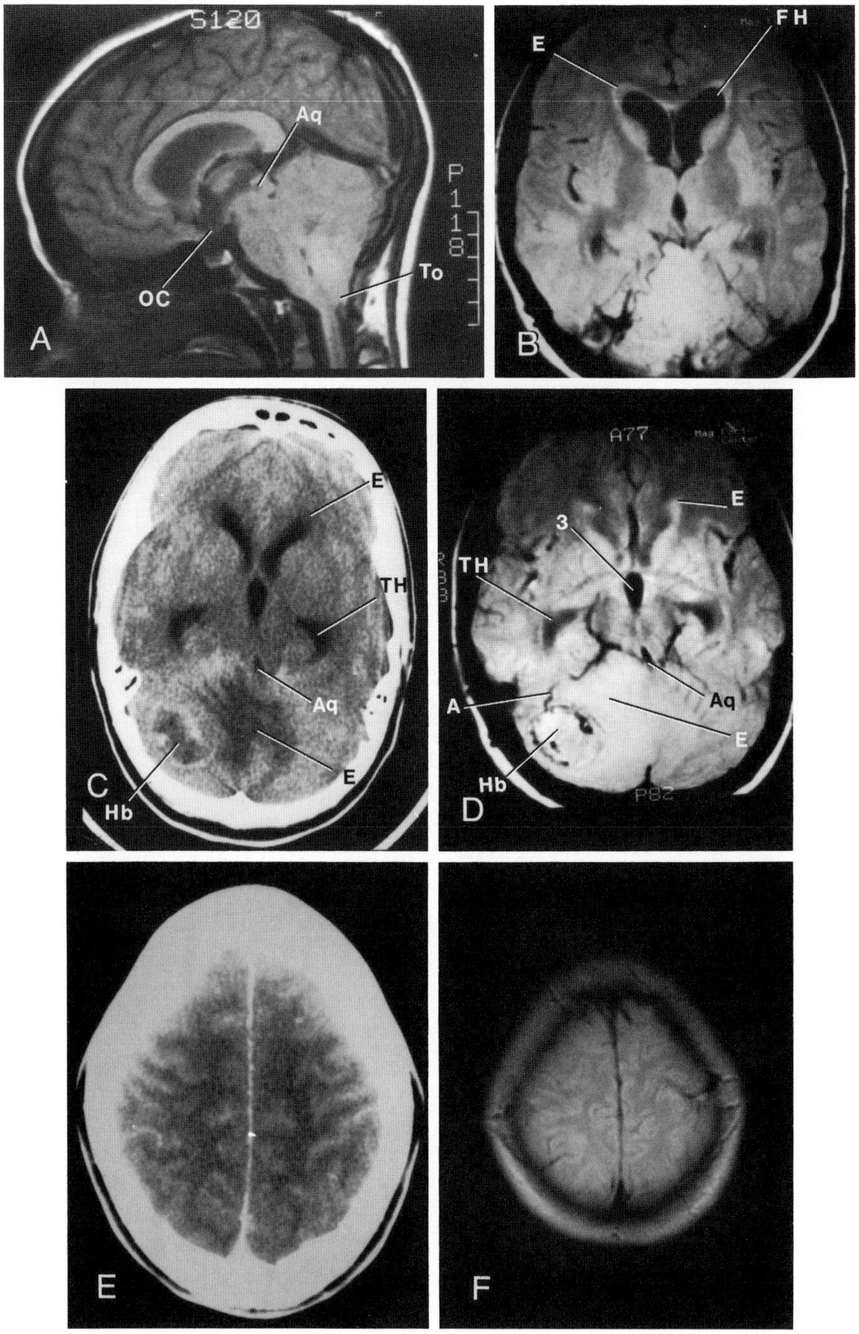

Figure 10.1. Noncommunicating hydrocephalus cerebellar hemangioblastoma. *Midsagittal SE 600/25 (A) and axial lateral ventricle frontal horn-level SE 2000/20 (B) MR scans. Axial temporal horn-level 36/100 i.v. contrast CT scan (C) and same level SE 2000/20 MR scan (D). Axial 36/100 centrum semiovale-level i.v. contrast CT scan (E) and SE 2000/20 MR scan (F).* A cerebellar hemangioblastoma *(Hb)* and associated edema *(E)* has displaced and compressed the fourth ventricle and aqueduct *(Aq)* and has caused tonsillar herniation *(To).* There is a moderate to marked degree of lateral ventricle frontal horn *(FH),* temporal horn *(TH),* and third ventricle *(3)* dilatation. Interstitial edema *(E)* surrounds the frontal horns. There is dilatation of the proximal aqueduct. There is lack of prominence of convexity sulci and perimesencephalic cisterns. Optic chiasm (OC).

edema fluid origin is CSF, much of the water approximates myelin protein that causes the T1/proton density-weighted imaging hyperintensity.[4] The characteristic relatively smooth layer of interstitial edema that almost always surrounds the ventricles in acutely elevated intracranial pressure may linger indefinitely after relief following shunting.[4] MR can identify an obstructing fourth ventricle cystic tumor or epidermoid tumor that may be inconspicuous because of water density and noncontrast enhancement by CT.[1–4]

COMMUNICATING HYDROCEPHALUS

Communicating hydrocephalus results from extraventricular CSF pathway obstruction at the basal cistern, lateral convexity, or at the pacchionian granulation levels. This condition may follow subarachnoid hemorrhage, trauma, meningeal infections, carcinomatosis, or intracranial surgery. Hurler's syndrome and achondroplasia also may be associated with communicating hydrocephalus.[3] Communicating hydrocephalus may also develop as a result of markedly raised CSF protein that presumably blocks the CSF pathways—Froin's syndrome.

Normal pressure hydrocephalus may be considered as a form of communicating hydrocephalus in which evidence of raised intracranial pressure is lacking. Raised intracranial pressure, however, may have been present during the developmental stage of the condition. Patients with normal pressure hydrocephalus may present with the classic triad of dementia, gait apraxia, and urinary incontinence.

MR, again, is the preferred method of investigation due to its superior tissue discrimination and imaging detail in orthogonal planes.[5] Both CT and MR (Fig. 10.2) demonstrate enlargement of the entire ventricular system. We agree with authors who require the presence of small sulci for diagnosis (distinction from cerebral atrophy).[3] Interstitial periventricular edema is often detected by both CT and MR but is best identified by the MR proton density technique.

The "aqueductal flow-void sign" results from the pulsatile motion and flow of CSF through the aqueduct resulting in dephasing and signal loss.[4] The flow-void sign is particularly prominent with ventricular and aqueductal dilatation. Directional flows and "to and fro" flow both produce the flow-void sign and cannot be differentiated. Signal void from pulsatile flow can also be seen in the third ventricle [particularly in the regions of the foramina of Monro (Fig. 10.3)].[4] The aqueductal flow-void sign does not appear to be very useful for clinical diagnosis.

Noncommunicating hydrocephalus proximal to the fourth ventricle outlets can usually be differentiated from communicating hydrocephalus by identifying the proximal ventricular enlargement due to obstruction of the foramen of Monro or the cerebral aqueduct (Fig. 10.1). Fourth ventricle outlet obstruction is difficult to distinguish from communciating hydrocephalus due to the presence in both conditions of a dilated fourth ventricle.

Degenerative, Toxic, and Metabolic Diseases Affecting Primarily the Gray Matter

GENERALIZED CEREBRAL ATROPHY AND SENILE DEMENTIA OF THE ALZHEIMER TYPE (SDAT)

Generalized cerebral atrophy frequently occurs in elderly patients (>65 years) with or without dementia. Many elderly patients exhibit no MR or CT evidence for atrophy, however. Atrophy is also seen in many other conditions, such as Alzheimer's disease, Pick's disease, Creutzfeldt-Jakob disease, Binswanger's disease, diffuse small vessel disease, amyloid angiopathy, alcoholism, and in the late stages of Parkinson's disease and Huntington's chorea. It may occur as a sequella of trauma, meningitis, malnutrition, and whole brain therapeutic radiation.[1,6,7] MR or CT evidence for or against atrophy may not correlate at all with the clinical findings. For example, a normal elderly patient may have imaging findings of atrophy and a severely demented patient may have normal imaging findings. Patients with CT or MR evidence of severe atrophy, however, are usually demented. Associated prominent dilatation of the third ventricle appears to correlate with dementia.[2]

MR and CT of diffuse cerebral atrophy demonstrate enlargement of ventricles, sulci, fissures, and cisterns (Fig. 10.4). There may be associated evidence for perivascular demyelination (diffuse small vessel disease) with its characteristic CT periventricular hypodensity and MR proton density/T2-weighted irregular periventricular conglomerate and punctate hyperintensity.[8–10]

Interstitial edema should not be confused with perivascular demyelination. The former is relatively continuous and smoothly marginated, associated with disproportionate frontal and temporal horn dilatation and lack of atrophic changes. The latter is discontinuous, irregular, patchy or punctate, and associated with atrophy.[11]

The incidence of severe dementia increases rapidly with age from approximately 1% at 65 years to 15% by 85 years of age.[2,12] Senile dementia of the Alzheimer type, a primary degenerative disorder, is the most common cause of progressive memory loss in the elderly patient.[2,12] It presents clinically with progressive failure of memory (particularly recent), confusion, disorientation, and apathy. The disease may progress slowly over many years and is remarkable for sparing of the corticospinal and cerebellar functions.

The term "presenile dementia" for Alzheimer's disease has been discarded because the disease has the same clinical and pathological characteristics regardless of the age of onset. It has a shorter course in younger patients, however. The disease is now called "senile dementia of the Alzheimer type"

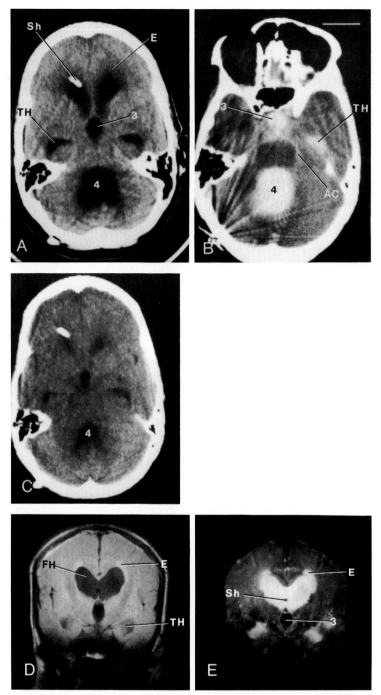

Figure 10.2. Communicating hydrocephalus. *A* and *B* shunt malfunction: axial fourth ventricle-level 37/100 CT scans without contrast
(A) and after shunt ventriculogram ***(B). C,*** shunt revision: same level
and technique axial CT scan. ***D*** and ***E,*** shunt malfunction—second
episode: SE 2000/20 ***(D)*** and 2000/80 ***(E)*** coronal frontal horn-level
MR scans. Marked dilatation of the ventricular system including the
fourth ventricle *(4)*, third ventricle *(3)*, lateral ventricle frontal horns
(FH), and temporal horns *(TH)* occurs during episodes of shunt malfunction and remits ***(C)*** after shunt *(Sh)* revision. Interstitial edema

(E) also occurs during episodes of shunt malfunction. The ventriculogram demonstrated ventricular and cisternal (ambient cistern =
AC) contrast confirming patency of the fourth ventricle outlets and
confirming the diagnosis of *communicating* hydrocephalus. Ventriculography is seldom used to confirm the diagnosis of communicating hydrocephalus. Note the convexity sulcal compression (or lack
of prominence) on the coronal sections. The MR appearance of interstitial edema may remain for a prolonged period after successful
shunting.

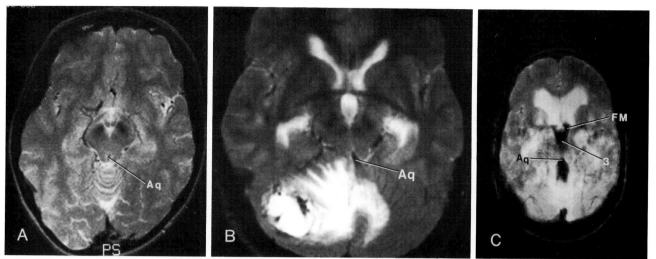

Figure 10.3.   The aqueductal flow-void sign. *Three different cases. All with axial SE 2000/80 axial scans without flow-compensation techniques demonstrating aqueductal signal void.* **A** *is a normal patient.* **B** *is a patient with hemangioblastoma and midaqueduct level* obstruction; **C** is a patient with communicating hydrocephalus. There is profound third ventricle *(3)* and foramen of Monro *(FM)* signal void in the latter case.

(SDAT). Grossly, Alzheimer's disease is characterized by gyral atrophy, which is particularly prominent in the frontal and temporal lobes. Microscopic examination demonstrates widespread neuronal loss, neuritic (senile) plaques, neurofibrillary tangles, and granulovacuolar degeneration, which is most prominent in the hippocampal pyramidal cell layer.[1]

CT of Alzheimer's disease may demonstrate generalized cerebral atrophy but it is not specific. Normal CT and MR studies do not exclude Alzheimer's disease.

In addition to generalized and particularly frontal and temporal cerebral atrophy, Alzheimer's patients often demonstrate a "halo" or smooth, thick T2-weighted image periventricular hyperintensity. Hippocampal and insular cortex T2 hyperintensity may also be present.[11] Faint peripheral gyral bands of T_2 hypointensity may be found in Alzheimer's patients, particularly in the parietal lobes (Fig. 10.5).[2] Whether these recently described MR changes found in Alzheimer's patients can reliably establish the diagnosis requires additional investigation.

Pick's disease, another primary degenerative disorder causing dementia, is far less common than senile dementia of the Alzheimer type. Severe frontal and temporal atrophic changes in a demented patient should include Pick's disease among the differential diagnostic considerations. Inasmuch as the imaging characteristics of Pick's disease are similar to, and not reliably distinguishable from, nonspecific generalized cerebral atrophy, it will not be further discussed.[2]

Wernicke-Korsakoff syndrome is usually a clinically obvious cause of dementia. It almost always presents in an alcoholic patient with characteristic associated ophthalmoparesis and gait ataxia. It is due to thiamine deficiency and may also occur in severely malnourished nonalcoholic patients. Microscopic capillary hyperplasia and proliferation, petechial hemorrhages, and astrocytic and microglial proliferation with relative neuronal sparing are characteristic. The mamillary bodies are the most frequently affected structures, however, the periventricular thalamic and hypothalamic tissues and the periaqueductal gray matter are also frequently involved. T2 signal hyperintensity in the periaqueductal gray matter and medial thalamus may be present. Atrophy of the mamillary bodies, superior cerebellar vermis, and generalized cerebral atrophy can be identified by MR.[2]

Reversible "atrophy-like" changes in alcoholics can be seen by both CT and MR. These changes are presumably caused by dehydration but brain regeneration or healing in abstinent patients may also play a role in decreasing the sulcal enlargement.[13]

The diagnosis of multi-infarct dementia is given to demented patients who clinically present with an episodic and progressively more severe confusional state in whom there is evidence for multiple, small ganglionic infarcts (lacunae) and often perivascular demyelination [diffuse small vessel disease (Fig. 10.6)].[11] These findings are not specific, however.[2] MR and CT evidence for diffuse small vessel disease does not accurately predict the severity of the patient's mental deterioration (Figs. 10.7 and 6.19).[8] Surprisingly, patients with SDAT uncommonly have marked degree perivascular demyelination.[2]

Less commonly, the more severe changes of Binswanger's subcortical arteriosclerotic encephalopathy may be present (Fig. 10.8).[2,14] Binswanger's disease is characterized by central white matter demyelination sparing the subcortical arcuate fibers

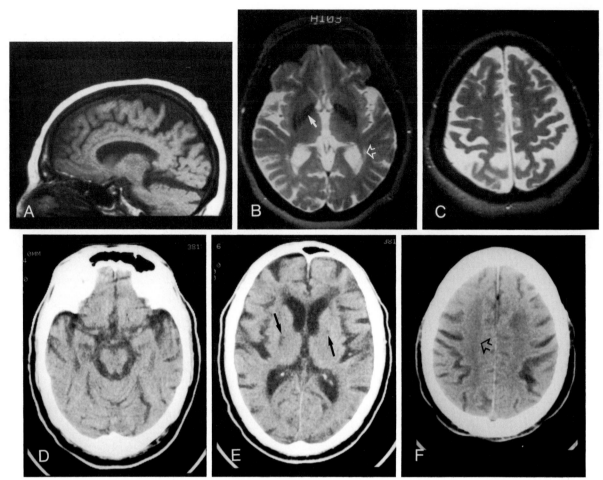

Figure 10.4. Generalized cerebral atrophy. A–C and **D–F** are different cases. **A–C:** *a 62-year-old demented man. Parasagittal SE 600/25* **(A),** *axial foramen of Monro-level* **(B),** *and convexity-level* **(C)** *SE 2000/80 MR scans.* There is marked gyral atrophy and compensatory marked sulcal enlargement with only a moderate degree of third and lateral ventricle dilatation. There is no disproportionate frontal horn or temporal horn enlargement or interstitial edema. There is a small amount of small vessel disease *(open arrow)* without evidence for a periventricular "halo" or for abnormal bands of cortical signal hypointensity, which may be seen in SDAT. The globus pallidus signal hypointensity *(closed arrow)* is more marked than that of the putamen (normal relationship). **D–F:** Generalized cerebral atrophy; a 68-year-old man with slight memory loss. *Axial midbrain-level* **(D),** *third ventricle-level* **(E),** *and centrum semiovale-level* **(F)** *36/100 CT scans.* There is generalized enlargement of fissures, cisterns, and sulci. The lateral and third ventricles are normal. Two lacunar infarcts are noted *(closed arrows).* Frontal periventricular and centrum semiovale hypodensity *(open arrow)* indicates a degree of perivascular demyelination ("small vessel disease"). This degree of atrophy can be present in the normally functioning elderly patient, however, it is moderately exaggerated for a patient of this age.

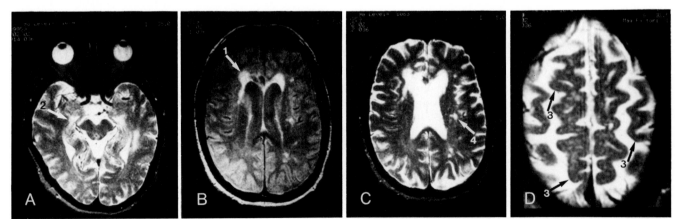

Figure 10.5. Alzheimer's disease. *Axial midbrain-level SE 2800/80* **(A),** *lateral ventricle body-level SE 2800/30* **(B)** *and 2800/80* **(C),** *and axial convexity-level 2800/80* **(D)** *MR scans.* There is a pronounced periventricular halo *(arrow 1),* medial temporal T2 hyperintensity *(arrow 2),* parietal and frontal gyral hypointense bands *(arrow 3),* and subcortical white matter hyperintensity *(arrow 4).*

Figure 10.6. Multi-infarct dementia. *Axial SE 2000/80 foramen of Monro (A) and lateral ventricle frontal horn (B) MR scans.* There are multiple basal ganglia foci of T2 signal hyperintensity that vary in size and that include the lenticular and caudate nuclei. The thalamus is also involved. There is generalized cerebral atrophy without evidence of severe perivascular demyelination. Note that the ganglionic signal and detail at the higher level *(B)* is obscured by the multiple hyperintense foci.

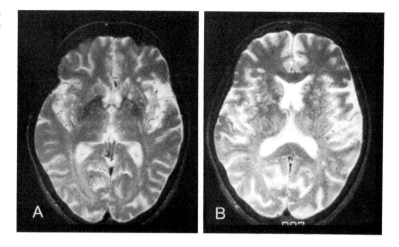

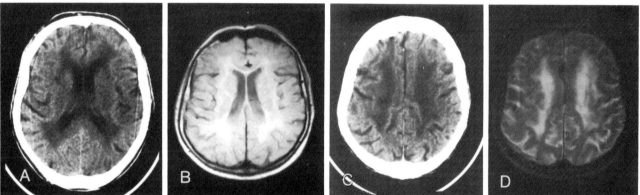

Figure 10.7. Perivascular demyelination "small vessel disease." *Axial lateral ventricle body-level 35/100 noncontrast CT scan (A) and SE 2000/20 MR scan (B). Axial low centrum semiovale-level 35/100 CT scan (C) and SE 2000/80 MR scan (D).* Prefrontal horn and atrial periventricular and deep white matter CT hypodensity and proton density/T2-weighted image MR hyperintensity is present. There is a minimal to moderate degree of cerebral atrophy.

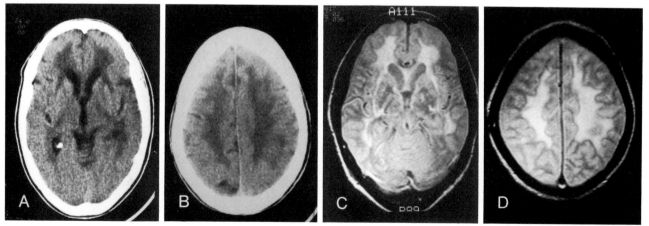

Figure 10.8. Binswanger's disease (subcortical arteriosclerotic encephalopathy); same case as Figure 6.20. *Axial basal ganglionic-level (A) and centrum semiovale-level (B) noncontrast CT 36/100 scans and same levels (C–D) SE 2000/30 MR scans.* Note the extreme basal ganglia and subcortical proton density signal hyperintensities and the CT subcortical white matter hypodensity.

Table 10.1. MR Characteristics of Diseases and Conditions Causing Dementia (Adapted from Drayer[2])[a]

Disease	Atrophy	Morphological Characteristics	T1 Intensity Characteristics	T2 Intensity Characteristics
Senile dementia of the Alzheimer type	+	Disproportionate frontal and temporal lobe atrophy		Periventricular hyperintense halo, parietal gyral hypointense bands, medial temporal hyperintensity
Wernicke-Korsakoff	+	Gyral, superior vermis and mamillary body atrophy		Periaqueductal gray matter and medial thalamus hyperintensity
Binswanger's disease[b]	+	Basal ganglia lacunae	Hypointense basal ganglia lacunae	Subcortical white matter, basal ganglia, thalamus and pons hyperintensity
Multi-infarct dementia[b]	+	Basal ganglia lacunae	Hypointense basal ganglia lacunae	Periventricular (irregular) basal ganglia lacunae
Normal pressure hydrocephalus	−	Hydrocephalus, compressed cisterns and sulci		Periventricular interstitial edema

[a]Pick's disease: Not reliably distinguishable from nonspecific atrophy. Atrophy may be severe ("knife-like gyri") in frontal and temporal lobes.
[b]"Vascular dementias": Binswanger's disease may be the more severe form of a continuum including multi-infarct dementia.

and by multiple basal ganglia, thalamus, and pons lacunar infarcts.[2] This condition is also discussed in Chapter 6. It is likely that multi-infarct dementia and Binswanger's disease is a continuum of the same process that can be included under the term "vascular dementia."[2,11]

Creutzfeldt-Jakob disease is caused by a viral-like particle known as a "prion" or a "slow virus" that causes rapidly progressive generalized cerebral atrophy. Micropathological changes include nerve cell loss, glial proliferation, and spongiform degeneration. The basal ganglia are often affected. The victims develop rapidly progressive dementia over a 6-month period associated with motor signs such as myoclonus and rigidity leading to coma and death. CT and MR will demonstrate changes typical of generalized cerebral atrophy. The late stages of other degenerative conditions such as Parkinson's disease, Huntington's chorea, and the late stages of leukodystrophies also demonstrate generalized cerebral atrophy.[1]

MR is clearly superior to CT for the investigation of dementia due to improved sensitivity for detection of gray and white matter, water and iron, due to the lack of bone-induced artifact that degrades CT images in regions adjacent to bone and due to orthogonal plane imaging. Table 10.1 summarizes the MR imaging characteristics of diseases causing dementia.

FOCAL CEREBRAL ATROPHY

Focal atrophy is the result of local brain injury. It may be secondary to cerebral infarction, hemorrhage, cerebritis or abscess, contusion, or surgery.

Wallerian degeneration (progressive demyelination and disintegration of distal axonal segments after axon transection or destruction) commonly occurs after infarcts (Fig. 6.6) and trauma and can also be seen in demyelinating diseases.[15] Postsurgical encephalomalacia and leukotomy ("frontal lobectomy") are iatrogenic causes of focal cerebral atrophy. Bilateral burr holes associated with bifrontal white matter encephalomalacia is characteristic of leukotomy.[1] Focal cerebral atrophy is discussed in Chapter 6.

PORENCEPHALY

The term "porencephaly" describes a cavity within the brain that may or may not communicate with a ventricle or cistern. It usually develops later in life most often after cerebral infarction or hemorrhage. It occasionally develops as a singular lesion in a neonate after an intracerebral hemorrhage. Multifocal porencephalic cysts may occur in the infant most commonly after intrauterine and postnatal infections.

Both CT and MR demonstrate these lesions (Fig. 10.9). Differential diagnosis includes arachnoid cyst, schizencephaly, cystic tumor, and cerebral hemiatrophy.

CEREBRAL HEMIATROPHY

Cerebral hemiatrophy is a condition in which one cerebral hemisphere is smaller than the other. This condition is usually the result of infarct in utero or in the perinatal period (Fig. 6.25). It may occur in the adult after a large infarct. A full discussion of this condition is found in Chapter 6.

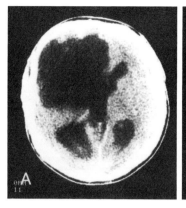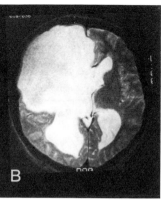

Figure 10.9. Porencephaly. Remote right internal carotid artery infarct. *Axial lateral ventricle-level 36/100 CT scan **(A)** and SE 2000/80 MR scan **(B)**.* There is a middle and anterior cerebral artery distribution large water isodense and isointense cyst openly communicating with the enlarged right lateral ventricle.

MOVEMENT DISORDERS

Diseases characterized as movement disorders include Parkinsonisms, Huntington's chorea, Wilson's disease, Hallervorden-Spatz disease, Leigh's disease and Fahr's disease. Parkinsonisms include Parkinson's disease and the Parkinson-plus group of diseases.[2,16–21] The most common diseases of the Parkinson-plus group are the multiple system atrophies that include striatonigral degeneration, Shy-Drager orthostatic hypotension, and olivopontocerebellar atrophy. Progressive supranuclear palsy is an uncommon condition also belonging to this group.[2,22]

Table 10.2 summarizes the MR basal ganglia iron-induced signal hypointensity observed in movement disorders according to Drayer.[2] One may conclude from his findings that putamen T2 signal is more markedly hypointense in the Parkinson-plus multi-system atrophy group and that globus pallidus T2 signal hypointensity is most marked in Hallervoerden-Spatz disease. More experience is necessary in order to confirm the early data. Atrophy and severe T2 basal ganglia signal hypointensity also occur with

hypothyroidism.[2] CT findings in movement disorder patients will be discussed under the specific disease process.[22,23]

Parkinson's Disease

Parkinson's disease presents clinically as cogwheel rigidity, bradykinesia, postural instability, and resting tremor. Dementia similar to that in Alzheimer's disease is commonly seen in chronic cases. Chronic cases demonstrate generalized cerebral atrophy in addition to iron-induced T2-weighted basal ganglia signal depletion.[2,16] Secondary Parkinson's disease develops from multiple causes such as demyelination, infarct, trauma, and exposure to toxic substances such as manganese, carbon monoxide, and phenothiazines.

Parkinson-Plus Syndrome

Parkinson-plus syndrome patients as a group experience poor response to anti-Parkinsonian therapy. They frequently exhibit decreased putamen T2 signal equal to that of a normal 80-year-old (Fig. 10.10). Putaminal marked T2 hypointensity is not characteristic of primary Parkinson's disease.[2,16,19] The pu-

Table 10.2. T2 Signal Abnormality in Movement Disorders (Adapted from Drayer[2])

Disease	Location or Structure	Signal Intensity T2[b]
Parkinson	Putamen, substantia nigra	+/−
Parkinson-plus		
Striatonigral degeneration[a]	Putamen, substantia nigra (pars compacta)	↓
Shy-Drager[a] (idiopathic orthostatic hypotension)	Putamen and substantia nigra (pars compacta)	↓
Olivopontocerebellar atrophy[a]	Putamen	↓
Progressive supranuclear palsy	Dentate nucleus	↓
Halvervorden-Spatz	Globus pallidus, red nucleus, substantia nigra	↓ ↓

[a]Striatonigral degeneration, Shy-Drager, and olivopontocerebellar atrophy can be classified as "multiple system atrophy."[2]
[b] ↓ =decreased; ↓ ↓ =markedly decreased; +/− =sometimes decreased.

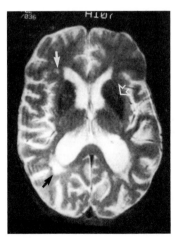

Figure 10.10. Putamen hypointense signal in an 81-year-old man with slight memory loss. *Axial SE 2000/80 MR scan.* The marked signal hypointensity of the putamen *(open arrow)* equals that of the globus pallidus. There is evidence of diffuse small vessel disease *(closed arrows)*. Compare to Figure 10.4**B**.

tamen hypointensity is due to iron-laden macromolecule deposition and may serve as a predictor of poor response to anti-Parkinsonian therapy.[2,16–20]

Huntington's Chorea

Huntington's chorea is an autosomal dominant disease that is characterized by choriform movements and severe dementia in the late stages of disease. Caudate nucleus atrophy is caused by nerve cell loss. MR and CT demonstrate caudate nucleus atrophy and resultant lateral ventricle frontal horn dilatation (Fig. 10.11). Caudate nucleus and, to a lesser extent, putamen, T2 signal hypointensity, can be detected by MR.[16] It should be noted, however, that putamen iron in normal patients increases with age and approaches the fairly constant globus pallidus iron concentration in the eighth decade.[2,17] Chorea acanthocytosis and Sydenham's chorea patients may also have abnormal T2 ganglionic signal. Hemiballismus may result from subthalamic nucleus of Luys infarction.[16]

Wilson's Disease

Wilson's disease (hepatolenticular degeneration) has a hepatic and a cerebral form. Only the cerebral form will be discussed here. This autosomal recessive dystonic disease is responsible for abnormally low levels of serum ceruloplasm. It is characterized by basal ganglionic copper deposition that primarily affects the putamen.[23] CT will often demonstrate lenticular nucleus hypodensity and may also demonstrate dentate nucleus, frontal lobe, and cerebellar hemisphere hypodensity.[1,3,24] MR demonstrates lenticular nucleus, thalamic, caudate nucleus, dentate nucleus, and brainstem T2 hyperintensity.[16,21]

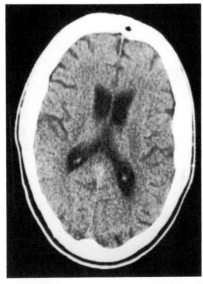

Figure 10.11. Huntington's chorea in a 30-year-old man. *Axial frontal horn-level 36/100 CT scan.* There is lack of the normal caudate nucleus impression upon the lateral ventricle frontal horns. The frontal horn rectangular appearance has been called "boxcar ventricles." There is a moderate degree of atrophy evidenced by ventricular and sulcal enlargement.

Hallervorden-Spatz Disease

Hallervorden-Spatz disease is a rare dystonic childhood-onset hereditary disease with abnormal globus pallidus iron deposition, dementia, and extrapyramidal signs. MR may detect marked globus pallidus T2 signal hypointensity and both CT and MR may demonstrate caudate nucleus atrophy.[1,3,16]

Leigh's Disease (Subacute Necrotizing Encephalomyelopathy)

Leigh's disease is a rare fatal hereditary dystonic progressive condition affecting infants and young children producing brain and spinal cord degeneration. A variety of clinical manifestations includes decreased levels of consciousness and respiration, blindness, and nystagmus. CT shows bilateral small putamen and centrum semiovale hypodensities.[3,25] MR demonstrates irregular bilateral basal ganglia T2 hyperintensities as well as other multifocal lesions that can occur in the brainstem, periventricular white matter, and cerebral cortex.[26]

Fahr's Disease

Fahr's disease (ferrocalcinosis) is a dystonic disease characterized by calcium, iron, and other metallic deposition in cerebral and cerebellar blood vessel walls, particularly those of the basal ganglia. It is thought to be a hereditary disorder. Marked basal ganglia and dentate calcifications are detected by CT (Fig. 10.12).[1]

In summary, Fahr's disease is the only movement disorder that appears to have imaging findings specific enough to arrive at a diagnosis by CT. The role of MR imaging in arriving at the correct diagnosis in movement disorders has yet to be firmly established. It should also be remembered that the diagnosis of most of these conditions is known before scanning. The scans are often ordered to exclude complications such as infarcts and hematomas and to evaluate the degree of atrophy. MR and CT are certainly helpful for establishing the cause of secondary Parkinson's disease. Whether marked putamen T2 signal hypointensity can reliably establish the diagnosis of Parkinson-plus disease has yet to be determined. Although choreic disorders may demonstrate caudate nucleus T2 signal hypointensity, there are not sufficient data to establish the reliability of the finding.[2,16]

CT findings are generally not characteristic of these diseases except for Fahr's disease (familial basal ganglia calcification or ferrocalcinosis). Wilson's and Leigh's disease may demonstrate basal ganglia CT hypodensities similar to that of anoxic and carbon monoxide changes.[21] The caudate nucleus atrophy of Huntington's chorea disease is not a reliable finding for this disease and is not specific.

CEREBELLAR ATROPHY AND SPINOCEREBELLAR ATROPHY

Cerebellar atrophy may be associated with diffuse cerebral atrophy, particularly of the Alzheimer type.

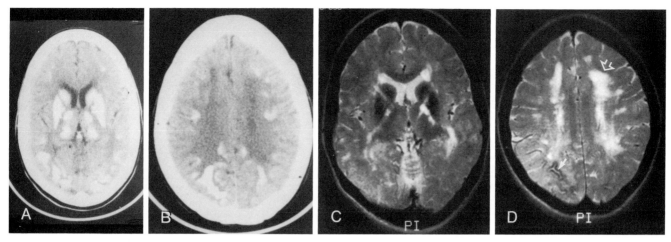

Figure 10.12. Fahr's disease (ferrocalcinosis) in a 29-year-old woman. *Axial lateral ventricle frontal horn-level (A) and low centrum semiovale-level (B) noncontrast 36/100 CT scans and same levels SE 2000/80 MR scans (C and D).* There is CT evidence of marked basal ganglia and gyral calcification without evidence for atrophy.

Marked ganglionic, but not gyral, T2 hypointensity is present possibly indicating increased ganglionic iron deposition. The internal capsules are markedly signal-hyperintense. In addition, there may be perivascular demyelination *(open arrow)* and gyral iron deposition *(closed arrow).*

Cerebellar atrophy in younger patients occurs with alcohol abuse and as a result of phenytoin toxicity. It also occurs in patients with ovarian and bronchogenic carcinoma and Hodgkin's disease and may even be the first manifestation of the malignant process (carcinomatous cerebellar degeneration). Alcoholic cerebellar atrophy is principally confined to the cerebellar vermis.[1,27]

The term "spinocerebellar degeneration" includes Friedrich's ataxia, olivopontocerebellar atrophy, and other conditions. *Friedrich's ataxia* is a hereditary condition usually presenting in late childhood with limb and trunk ataxia, absent tendon reflexes, and propioreception loss.[28,29] *Olivopontocerebellar atrophy* is probably sporadic and usually presents in middle age. Both conditions result in spinal cord atrophy.

The brainstem and cerebellum are often grossly preserved in Friedrich's ataxia although the dentate nuclei are often involved. Friedrich's spinal cord degenerative changes are localized to the dorsal half.[28] CT of Friedrich's ataxia often is normal although cerebellar hemisphere and vermis atrophy may be present.[27] MR demonstrates spinal cord atrophy and occasional associated cerebellar and pons atrophy.

Olivopontocerebellar atrophy results in marked atrophy of the cerebellum, pons, inferior olives, and spinal cord (Fig. 10.13). The marked involvement of the pons and olives should establish the diagnosis. CT without intrathecal contrast shows nonspecific brainstem and cerebellar atrophy.[27] MR changes include atrophy of the cerebellar vermis and hemisphere (particularly inferior), pons (anterior flattening), inferior olives, medulla, and spinal cord. Cerebral atrophy may also be present. Abnormally decreased putamenal signal on T2-weighted images is common.[2,19]

Diseases Affecting Primarily the White Matter

The various white matter diseases are classified here within two categories: dysmyelinating and demyelinating disorders. Dysmyelinating disorders involve abnormal myelination and demyelinating disorders involve myelin destruction. MR, due to its very sensitive gray-white matter resolution, is the method of choice for investigation of these conditions. CT is relatively insensitive to small foci of abnormal my-

Figure 10.13. Olivopontocerebellar atrophy. Midsagittal *(A)* and coronal fourth ventricle-level *(B)* SE 600/25 MR scans. There is marked atrophy of the pons with anterior flattening *(solid arrow).* Cerebellar vermis and hemisphere atrophy is evidenced by enlarged sulci, small folia, and enlarged fourth ventricle. The medullary olives could not be identified.

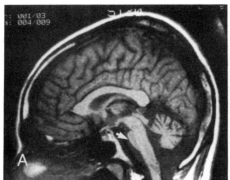

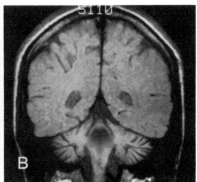

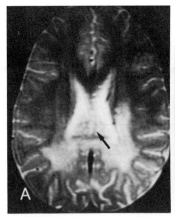
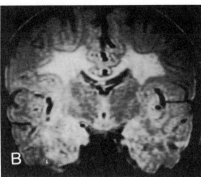
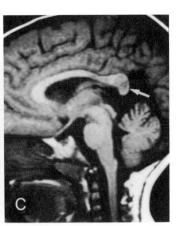

Figure 10.14. Metachromatic leukodystrophy. Axial T2-weighted **(A)**, coronal proton density-weighted **(B)**, and midsagittal T1-weighted **(C)**, images. The forceps major, parietal centrum semiovale, splenium of the corpus callosum *(arrows)* and the periventricular white matter are markedly involved. The dysmyelinated structures are T1-hypointense/T2- and proton density-hyperintense. (Courtesy of Richard D. Smith, M.D., Indianapolis, IN).

elin and cannot effectively image the spinal cord directly.[6]

DYSMYELINATING DISEASES

The dysmyelinating diseases include metachromatic leukodystrophy (Fig. 10.14), adrenoleukodystrophy, globoid leukodystrophy (Krabbe disease), Canavan's disease, and Alexander's disease. Of these diseases, metachromatic leukodystrophy is the most common. These clinically devastating diseases have in common abnormal myelin that has been either malformed or has been formed and not maintained. The majority are genetic in origin, have infantile clinical onset, lead to severe mental and neurological deterioration with death occurring in childhood. Adrenoleukodystrophy is an exception with symptoms usually appearing in childhood rather than infancy. Abnormal lipid accumulation in metachromatic leukodystrophy and galactocerebroside accumulation in globoid leukodystrophy occurs.[1,3,30]

CT is less sensitive than MR to dystrophic white matter abnormalities.[31] The reported CT findings of these conditions demonstrate few distinguishing characteristics to help differentiate one from the other. All demonstrate white matter hypodensity. The low density foci may vary and may be characteristic of certain diseases. Generally, bilateral periventricular distribution is the most common, however, bilateral parieto-occipital involvement is characteristic of adrenoleukodystrophy.[1,3,6,31] Early hyperdensity involving the basal ganglia and other sites has been described in globoid leukodystrophy. Contrast enhancement occurs in adrenoleukodystrophy and Alexander's disease and may demonstrate an active phase or region of the disease process.[31]

MR is more sensitive to white matter changes of leukodystrophy as it is in other abnormal myelination processes. White matter T2 hyperintensity occurs in regions of dysmyelination.

DEMYELINATING DISORDERS

The demyelinating (myelinoclastic) disorders include primary diseases of unknown etiology such as multiple sclerosis (MS) and secondary disorders that follow infectious, toxic, or vascular insults. MR is the superior imaging method for detection of these disease processes; particularly for small lesions such as are commonly seen in multiple sclerosis.[6,32]

Primary Demyelinating Disorders

Multiple sclerosis is, by far, the most common disorder within this group. This condition produces remission and exacerbation of clinical signs and symptoms that commonly include paresis, paresthesias, impaired vision, and diploplia. Women are twice as likely to be afflicted and the peak incidence is the third and fourth decade. Multiple focal lesions varying in size from 1 mm to several centimeters occur predominantly in the periventricular white matter but are also found in the cortex, cerebellum, brainstem, and spinal cord.[1,6] Each plaque develops as a small focus of inflammation associated with edema, blood-brain barrier breakdown, and perivascular lymphocytic infiltration. It becomes a chronic plaque of glial cell infiltration with myelin sheath resorption. These chronic plaques lack edema.[33]

CT demonstrates lesions in less than half of the patients with known multiple sclerosis as compared to MR, which demonstrates lesions in greater than 75% of the patients with known disease. T2- and proton density-weighted sequences are most effective (Fig. 10.15).[1,6]

The MR abnormal foci probably represent MS demyelination and plaque and appear as proton density/T2-weighted image hyperintense well-circumscribed homogeneous lesions varying from 3 mm to 3 cm in size. More than two lesions are identified in the majority of cases. Relative putamen and thalamus-decreased T2 signal intensity occurs in the ma-

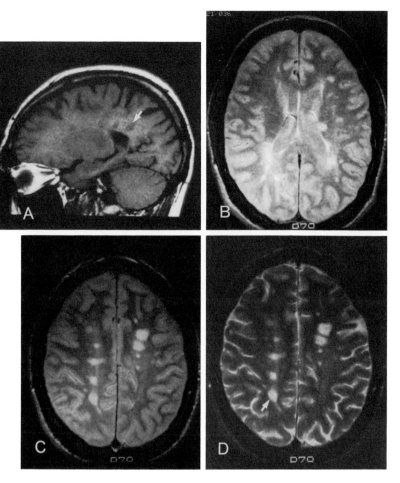

Figure 10.15.   Multiple sclerosis. *Sagittal right lateral ventricle atrial-level SE 600/25* **(A),** *axial atrial-level* **(B)** *and centrum semiovale-level* **(C)** *SE 2800/30, and centrum-level 2800/80* **(D)** *MR scans.* Note how the proton-density image **(B)** identifies the periventricular hyperintense lesions while demonstrating the relatively hypointense lateral ventricles and best identifying gray and white matter detail. The lesions, plaques, are T1 hypointense and proton density/T2 hyperintense *(arrows).*

jority of multiple sclerosis patients, which correlates with the degree of white matter abnormality.[32] Care must be exercised not to misdiagnose such normal findings as the periatrial normal T2 hyperintensity (Fig. 4.28). In addition to the periventricular foci, additional plaques may be identified in the subcortical white matter; the internal capsule and temporal lobe white matter (Fig. 10.15). Corpus callosal and subcallosal-periventricular lesions are common (Fig. 10.16). Pontine, midbrain, or cerebellar white matter lesions are seen in almost half of the cases (Fig. 10.17). Generalized cerebral atrophy is usually present in advanced cases (Fig. 10.16).[6]

Positive MR findings in the cerebral convexities and posterior fossa correlate more closely with clinical findings than do periventricular lesions. MR i.v. contrast scans may serve as effective indicators of MS activity,[33] however, a contrast-enhanced MS lesion can be mistaken for a neoplasm. MR of spinal cord MS will be discussed in Chapter 15.

Those lesions detectable by CT are usually multifocal, nonconfluent, hypodense, moderately well-defined, and juxtaventricular. There may be associated atrophy. Contrast enhancement is probably related to acute-onset plaques and may be homogeneous or "ring-like" (Fig. 10.18).[3]

Even though MR is the more sensitive technique for multiple sclerosis imaging, CT effectively excludes other conditions such as tumors or vascular malformations that may mimic the clinical findings. CT is indicated only if MR cannot be done. Contrast-enhancing lesions may resemble metastasis although there is a characteristic lack of surrounding edema and mass effect.[1,3,33]

Secondary Demyelinating Disorders

This group includes disorders caused by toxic, anoxic, and infectious agents. The toxic and anoxic group includes methotrexate encephalopathies, central pontine myelinolysis, anoxia, and Binswanger's disease.[1] The infectious group includes progressive multifocal leukoencephalopathy (PML), subacute sclerosing panencephalitis, and acute disseminated encephalomyelitis.

Anoxia and Binswanger's disease (subcortical arteriosclerotic encephalopathy) have already been discussed in Chapter 6 and Binswanger's disease has been discussed in this chapter and is shown in Figure 10.8.

Radiation brain treatment may cause radiation necrosis and combined radiation-intrathecal methotrexate brain treatment may cause a more severe

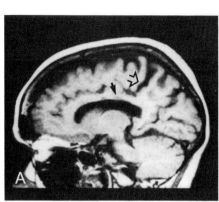
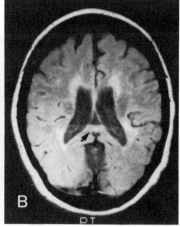
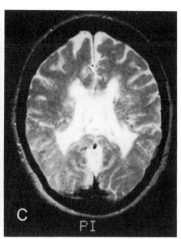

Figure 10.16. Chronic MS with cerebral atrophy in a 63-year-old woman. *Parasagittal SE 600/25 **(A)**, axial lateral ventricle atrial-level SE 2000/20 **(B)**, and SE 2000/80 **(C)** MR scans.* T1-weighted image hypointense and proton density/T2-weighted image hyperintense corpus callosum lesions are seen *(closed arrows).* Enlargement of the marginal sulcus *(open arrow)* is prominent. Note the proton density/T2 periventricular hyperintensity. This case is indistinguishable from diffuse small vessel disease with the possible exception of the T1-weighted corpus callosal hypointensities.

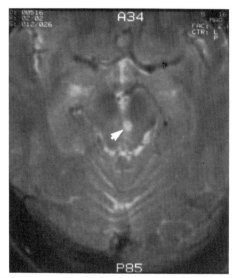

Figure 10.17. Midbrain (central tegmental tract) MS plaque. *Axial midbrain-level SE 2000/80 MR scan.* Note the round hyperintense lesion *(arrow).*

condition (subacute disseminated necrotizing leukoencephalopathy).

Radiation brain injury can be divided into three chronological phases—acute reactions, transient intermediate reactions, and severe delayed reactions. Transient acute reactions may occur during the course of irradiation. These usually mild reactions are probably caused by cerebral edema. Reactions occurring from a few weeks to a few months postirradiation probably result from demyelination and result in a moderate degree of cerebral atrophy. Despite these changes, symptoms are usually transient and minor.

Delayed severe and often fatal dose-related reactions resulting from ischemia and necrosis (coagulation necrosis) develop from several months to years after irradiation. A wide range of symptomatology from slight reduction of intellectual function to coma and from ataxia to decerebration occurs. The risk of severe reactions increases with high dose (more than 6000 rads), improper dose fractionation, and patient age.[7,34,35] Pathologically, there is endothelial hyper-

Figure 10.18. Multiple sclerosis contrast-enhancing plaques. *Different patients. Axial lateral ventricle body-level i.v. contrast CT scan **(A)** and SE 800/22 motion compensation MR scan **(B)**.* There is CT ring contrast enhancement and MR homogeneous enhancement *(arrows).*

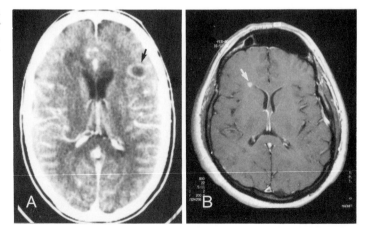

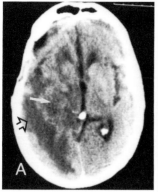
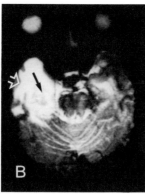
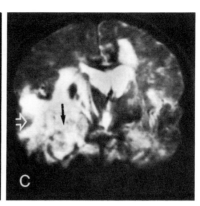

Figure 10.19. Radiation necrosis (proven central coagulation necrosis) in a 76-year-old, 3 years postirradiation for a craniopharyngioma. *Axial noncontrast third ventricle-level 36/100 CT scan (A), midbrain-level SE 2000/80 MR scan (B), and coronal third ventricle-level SE 2000/80 MR scan (C).* A heterogeneous CT hypodense and MR T2 mixed intensity temporal mass *(closed arrows)* is surrounded by marked edema *(open arrows).* There is a large mass effect with displacement of the septum pellucidum, third ventricle, and pineal gland to the left. In addition, there are left hemispheric abnormal T2 signal hyperintensities that include a large homogeneous forceps minor lesion **(C)** and generalized frontal and temporal lobe punctate and conglomerate T2 hyperintensities. MR is clearly superior to CT in this case for distinguishing mass and edema and for recognition of left hemispheric abnormalities.

trophy, medial hyalinization, adventitial thickening, and fibrosis of small and medium-sized cerebral arteries. Perivascular collagen deposition causes cerebral ischemia and necrosis, which is usually more severe in the white matter than in the cortex.[7]

CT of radiation necrosis demonstrates coagulation necrosis as a hypodense mass within the irradiated region (Fig. 10.19). There may be an irregular ring of contrast enhancement. CT is not sensitive to the less severe forms of brain radiation effect but may demonstrate findings similar to those seen in small vessel disease. Delayed (several months to years) postradiation proton density- and T2-weighted images frequently demonstrate bilateral symmetrical periventricular hyperintensity similar to that of small vessel disease.[35] This could represent acceleration of involutional white matter changes associated with aging.[35] MR of less common radiation necrosis demonstrates focal cerebral edema, mild cerebral atrophy, and necrosis (Fig. 10.19) corresponding to the field of radiation. The necrotic mass appears T2 hyperintense and may cause structural displacement and midline shift. Despite the superior sensitivity of MR for radiation changes, the method still cannot differentiate radiation necrosis from tumor regrowth.

Mineralizing microangiopathy occurs more frequently than does necrotizing leukoencephalopathy in response to combined methotrexate and whole brain irradiation therapy. It is less debilitating than necrotizing leukoencephalopathy. Symptoms include headache ataxia and seizure disorder. Calcification within and around small cerebral blood vessels is responsible for the characteristic CT appearance. CT demonstrates bilateral symmetrical corticomedullary junction and basal ganglia calcifications. Minimal degree atrophy may coexist.[7]

Central pontine myelinolysis occurs predominantly in alcoholics and is usually associated with hyponatremia, which has been rapidly corrected. Initial neurological improvement is followed by clinical deterioration including quadraparesis, pseudobulbar signs, and the locked-in syndrome. Death usually occurs within the first few weeks, however, some patients survive.[36] CT demonstrates central pontine, (4–10 mm diameter) hypodense lesions without brainstem enlargement.[37] These lesions are MR T1 hypointense and T2 hyperintense (Fig. 10.20). Differential diagnosis includes brainstem infarct and multiple sclerosis. Glioma, encephalitis, and abscess are less likely due to the lack off mass effect.[6]

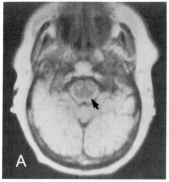
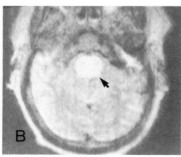

Figure 10.20. Central pontine myelinolysis. *Axial pontine level 550/32 (A) and 2000/120 (B) MR scans in a 0.15 T resistive scanner.* There is a large T1 hypointense/T2 hyperintense central pontine lesion with only minor mass effect *(arrows).* (Courtesy of Mary K. Edwards, M.D., Indianapolis, IN.)

Marchiafava-Bignami disease is a rare condition of uncertain etiology that results in medial zone corpus callosal demyelination and necrosis. It most commonly occurs in alcoholics. There are striking MR changes of corpus callosal T2 hyperintensity. CT may show corpus callosal hypodensity.[6]

Subacute sclerosing panencephalitis may present up to 6 years after exposure to measles virus. Acute disseminated encephalomyelitis may present 1 week after exposure to varicella or influenza virus. The demyelination caused by these diseases produces nonspecific CT and MR findings that include the cortical and subcortical white matter and deep gray matter.[6]

Progressive multifocal leukoencephalopathy is a progressive demyelinating disease caused by the DNA-containing papovavirus. It occurs principally in patients with AIDS, patients receiving immunosuppressive therapy, and patients with leukemia and lymphoma. There are focal areas of demyelination varying markedly in size that have origin in the subcortical hemispheric white matter, the cerebellum, and the brainstem. These areas may coalesce to form large atrophic regions. The parietal and occipital lobes are most commonly affected. There is visual disturbance and paresis with progressive deterioration of mental functions leading to coma and death that usually occurs within 3–6 months after onset of symptoms.[1,6]

CT demonstrates subcortical white matter hypodensity with scalloped edges. The lesions are often asymmetric and in a parietal-occipital location. Cortical enhancement similar to that seen in infarction may occur and there may be mass effect (Fig. 10.21). CT differential diagnosis includes dysmyelinating diseases, primary and other secondary demyelinating disorders, cerebritis, and metastasis.[1,3,6]

MR of progressive multifocal leukoencephalopathy demonstrates T2 hyperintensity of the lesions also detected by CT. MR is more sensitive to these pathological changes than CT but may not be more specific. In AIDS patients, these changes cannot be distinguished from cytomegalovirus or AIDS virus encephalitis.[6]

Ventricular Shunting

Ventricular shunts are almost always placed in a lateral ventricle, usually for the relief of obstructive hydrocephalus (noncommunicating or communicating). On occasion, a catheter is placed in a lateral ventricle so that chemotherapeutic agents can be directly injected into the ventricle via a subcutaneous reservoir. If there is bilateral foramen of Monro obstruction, a shunt tube must be placed in each lateral ventricle in order to avoid subfalx and tentorial herniation. The foramina of the fourth ventricle and the aqueduct may occlude. The resulting "isolated fourth ventricle" may then behave as a posterior fossa cyst.[38] Ventricular complications include a malfunctioning shunt with hydrocephalus, ventriculitis, chronic subdural hematomas, and an isolated fourth ventricle.[38,39]

Shunts can also be placed in cysts such as those in the posterior fossa and they can drain to the spinal subarachnoid space rather than to the peritoneum depending upon the surgeon's choice. Subdural drains are quite common if the subdural hematoma continues to reaccumulate.

Both CT and MR effectively monitor shunt patients and detect complications. Ventricular asymmetry ocurs in 30% of shunted patients, is usually minor, asymptomatic, and usually requires no shunt revision. Shunt malfunction, subdural hematomas, ventriculitis (Fig. 10.22), and an isolated fourth ventricle are well demonstrated by both the CT and MR methods.

References

1. Gonzalez CFF, Reyes PF. Hydrocephalus, atrophic and degenerative disorders. In Gonzalez CF, Grossman CB, Masdeu JC (Eds). *Head and Spine Imaging.* New York: John Wiley & Sons, 1985; 435–450.
2. Drayer BP. Imaging of the aging brain. Part II: pathologic conditions. *Radiology* 1988; 166:797–806.
3. Haughton VM. White matter and basal ganglia diseases. In Williams AL, Haughton VM (Eds). *Cranial Computed Tomography.* St. Louis: CV Mosby Co, 1985; 257–268.

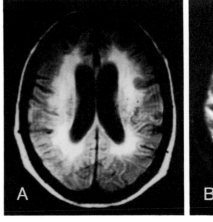
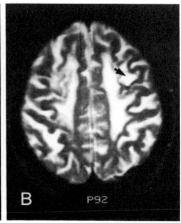

Figure 10.21. Progressive multifocal leukodystrophy. *Axial lateral ventricle body-level SE 2000/20* **(A)** *and centrum-semiovale-level SE 2000/80* **(B)** *MR scans.* Same case as shown in Figure 8.17. There is marked periventricular and subcortical white matter hyperintensity, atrophy, and a small irregular necrotic lesion *(arrow).*

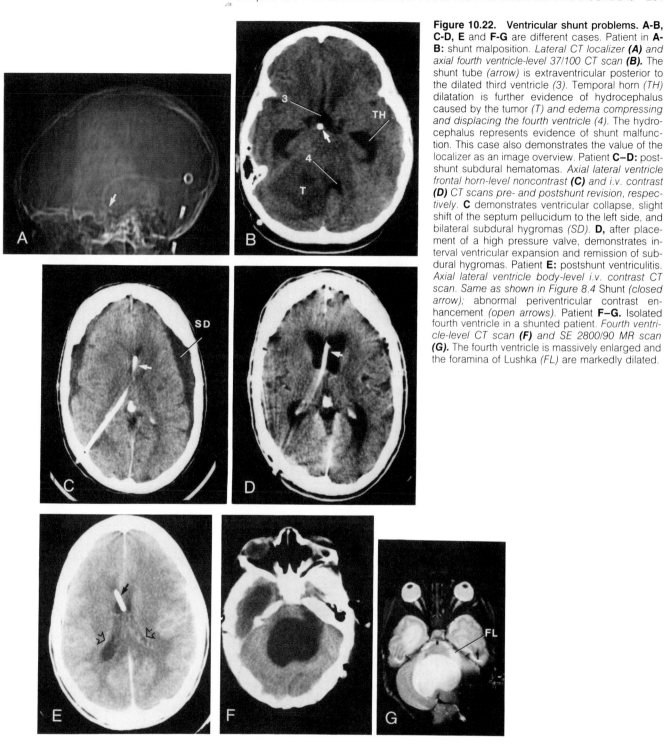

Figure 10.22. Ventricular shunt problems. A-B, C-D, E and **F-G** are different cases. Patient in **A-B:** shunt malposition. *Lateral CT localizer **(A)** and axial fourth ventricle-level 37/100 CT scan **(B)**.* The shunt tube *(arrow)* is extraventricular posterior to the dilated third ventricle *(3)*. Temporal horn *(TH)* dilatation is further evidence of hydrocephalus caused by the tumor *(T)* and edema compressing and displacing the fourth ventricle *(4)*. The hydrocephalus represents evidence of shunt malfunction. This case also demonstrates the value of the localizer as an image overview. Patient **C–D:** postshunt subdural hematomas. *Axial lateral ventricle frontal horn-level noncontrast **(C)** and i.v. contrast **(D)** CT scans pre- and postshunt revision, respectively.* **C** demonstrates ventricular collapse, slight shift of the septum pellucidum to the left side, and bilateral subdural hygromas *(SD)*. **D,** after placement of a high pressure valve, demonstrates interval ventricular expansion and remission of subdural hygromas. Patient **E:** postshunt ventriculitis. *Axial lateral ventricle body-level i.v. contrast CT scan. Same as shown in Figure 8.4* Shunt *(closed arrow)*; abnormal periventricular contrast enhancement *(open arrows)*. Patient **F–G.** Isolated fourth ventricle in a shunted patient. *Fourth ventricle-level CT scan **(F)** and SE 2800/90 MR scan **(G)**.* The fourth ventricle is massively enlarged and the foramina of Lushka *(FL)* are markedly dilated.

4. Bradley WG Jr. Pathophysiologic correlates of signal alterations. In Brant-Zawadzki M, Norman D (Eds). *Magnetic Resonance Imaging of the Central Nervous System.* New York: Raven Press, 1987; 23–42.

5. El Gammal T, Allen MB Jr, Brooks BS, Mark EK. MR evaluation of hydrocephalus. *AJNR* 1987; 8:591–597.

6. Holland B. Diseases of white matter. In Brant-Zawadzki M, Norman D (Eds). *Magnetic Imaging of the Central Nervous System.* New York: Raven Press, 1987; 259–277.

7. Williams AL. Tumors. In Williams AL, Haughton VM (Eds). *Cranial Computed Tomography.* St Louis: CV Mosby Co, 1985, 1148–239.

8. Kirkpatrick JB, Hyman LA. White matter lesions in MR imaging of clinically healthy brains of elderly subjects: Possible pathologic basis. *Radiology* 1987; 162:509–511.

9. George AE, deLeon MJ, Gentes CI, et al. Leukoencephalopathy in normal and pathologic aging: I. CT of brain lucencies. *AJNR* 1986; 7:561–566.

10. George AE, deLeon MJ, Kalnin A, et al. Leukoencephalopathy in normal and pathologic aging: II. MRI of brain lucencies. *AJNR* 1986; 7:567–570.

11. Fazekas F, Chawluk JB, Alavi A, et al. MR signal abnormalities at 1.5TG in Alzheimer's dementia and normal aging. *AJNR* 1987; 8:421–426.

12. Drayer BP. Degenerative brain disorders and brain iron. In Brant-Zawadzki M, Norman D (Eds). *Magnetic Resonance Imaging of the Central Nervous System.* New York: Raven Press, 1987; 123–130.

13. Artmann H, Gall MV, Hacker H, Herrlich J. Reversible enlargement of cerebrospinal fluid spaces in chronic alcoholics. *AJNR* 1981; 2:23–27.

14. Lotz PR, Ballinger WE Jr, Quisling RG, Subcortical atherosclerotic encephalopathy: CT spectrum and pathological correlation. *AJNR* 1986; 7:817–822.

15. Cobb SR, Mehringer CM. Wallerian degeneration in a patient with Schilder disease: MR imaging demonstration. *Radiology* 1987; 162:521–522.

16. Rutledge JN, Hilal SK, Silver AJ, et al. Study of movement disorders and brain iron by MR. *AJNR* 1987; 8:397–411.

17. Drayer B, Burger P, Darwin R. Magnetic resonance imaging of brain iron. *AJNR* 1986; 7:373–380.

18. Pastakia B, Polinsky R, DiChiro G, et al. Multiple system atrophy (Shy-Drager syndrome): MR imaging. *Radiology* 1986; 159:499–502.

19. Drayer BP, Olanow W, Burger P. Parkinson plus syndrome: Diagnosis using high field MR imaging of brain iron. *Radiology* 1986; 159:493–498.

20. Ambrosetto P. CT in progressive supranuclear palsy. *AJNR* 1987; 8:849–851.

21. Aisen AM, Martel W, Gabrielson TO. Wilson disease of the brain: MR imaging. *Radiology* 1985; 157:137–141.

22. Masucci EF, Borts FT, Smirniotopoulos JG, et al. Thin-section CT of midbrain abnormalities in progressive supranuclear palsy. *AJNR* 1985; 6:767–772.

23. Starosta-Rubinstein S, Young AB, Kluin K, et al. Clinical assessment of 31 patients with Wilson's disease. Correlations with structural changes on magnetic resonance imaging. *Arch Neurol* 1987; 44.

24. Kvicala V, Vymazal J, Nevsimalova S. Computed tomography of Wilson disease. *AJNR* 1983; 4:429–430.

25. Paltiel JH, O'Gorman AM, Meagher-Villemure K, et al. Subacute necrotizing encephalomyelopathy (Leigh's disease): Ct study. *Radiology* 1987; 162:115–118.

26. Davis PC, Hoffman JC Jr, Braun IF, et al. MR of Leigh's disease (subacute necrotizing encephalomyelopathy). *AJNR* 1987; 8:71–75.

27. Ramos A, Quintana F, Diez C, et al. CT findings in spinocerebellar degeneration. *AJNR* 1987; 8:635–640.

28. Rosenberg RN. Hereditary ataxias. In Rowland LP (Ed). *Merritt's Textbook of Neurology.* Philadelphia: Lea & Febiger, 1984; 499–508.

29 Fitz CR. Congenital and neonatal disorders. In Gonzalez CF, Grossman CB, Masdeu J (Eds). *Head and Spine Imaging.* New York: John Wiley & Sons, 1985; 555–573.

30. Becker LE, Yates A. Inherited metabolic disease. In Davis RL, Robertson DM (Eds). *Textbook of Neuropathology.* Baltimore: Williams & Wilkins, 1985; 284–371.

31. Kumar AJ, Rosebaum AE, Naidu S, et all. Adrenoleukodystrophy: Correlating MR imaging with CT. *Radiology* 1987; 165:497–504.

32. Drayer B, Burger P, Hurwitz B, et al. Reduced signal intensity on MR images of thalamus and putamen in multiple sclerosis: Increased iron content? *AJNR* 1987; 8:413–419.

33. Grossman RI, Braffman BH, Brorson JR, et al. Multiple sclerosis: Serial study of Gadolinium-enhanced MR imaging. *Radiology* 1988; 169:117–122.

34. Brant-Zawadzki M, Kelly W. Brain tumors. In Brant-Zawadzki M, Norman D (Eds). *Magnetic Resonance Imaging of the Central Nervous System.* New York: Raven Press, 1987; 151–185.

35. Tsuruda JS, Kortman KE, Bradley WG, et al. Radiation effects on cerebral white matter: MR evaluation. *AJNR* 1987; 8:431–437.

36. Poser CM, Alter M, Sibley WA, Scheinberg LC. Demyelinating diseases. In Rowland LP (Ed). *Merritt's Textbook of Neurology.* Philadelphia: Lea & Febiger, 1984; 7:593–615.

37. Rosenbloom S, Buchholz D, Kumar AJ, et al. Evolution of central pontine myelinolysis on CT. *AJNR* 1984; 5:110–112.

38. Scotti G, Musgrave MA, Fitz CR, Harwood-Nash DC. The isolated fourth ventricle in children: CT and clinical review of 16 cases. *AJR* 1980; 135:1233–1238.

39. Schellinger D, McCullough DC, Pederson RT. Computed tomography in the hydrocephalic patient after shunting. *Radiology* 1980; 137:693–704.

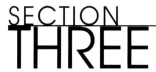

SECTION
THREE

The Skull Base, the Skull, and Face

CHAPTER

11

The Sella Region

Introduction

MR has become our imaging method of choice for the sella region. Although CT still does a credible job, there are certain advantages of MR. These advantages include exquisite tissue detail, excellent blood vessel definition, direct orthogonal plane imaging, absence of petrous and dental hardware sella artifact, lack of necessity of i.v. x-ray contrast, and lack of radiation exposure. Currently, 3-mm thickness sections and less than 1-mm pixel sizes enable high spatial MR resolution. The MR and CT differential diagnostic features of sella region abnormalities are summarized in Table 11.1 on pages 255–257. The use of this table avoids unnecessary repetition and duplication.

MR Technique

Contrary to methods of image analysis elsewhere, the T1-weighted image is usually all that is necessary for MR sella imaging. This is due to the readily recognizable intraglandular anatomy and pathology seen by the T1-weighted technique. Our current sella method includes sagittal and coronal T1-weighted images using a circumferential head coil and variable axial sections parallel to the canthomeatal plane (10° "Towne" to Reid's baseline). Two NEX, 18-cm FOV and 3-mm thickness sections are obtained on a 256×256 matrix at 1.5 T. Interleaving technique obtains contiguous sections without intervening unscanned "gaps" or image degrading "cross-talk." Intravenous contrast injection may be used for MR pituitary investigation.

CT Technique

A generally accepted technique is 5-mm noncontrast and contrast axial canthomeatal plane sella-suprasellar sections followed by 3-mm direct coronal sections. Prone positioning may be most helpful to avoid dental artifacts that obscure detail with the routine supine technique.[1] Both bone and soft tissue windows are obtained with a soft tissue algorithm. Intrathecal sellar CT cisternography can document communication of a cyst with the subarachnoid space but it is rarely used.

Normal MR and CT Anatomy

PITUITARY

The anterior lobe (adenohypophysis) and posterior lobe (neurohypophysis) of the pituitary gland have separate embryological origins. The anterior lobe arises from Rathke's pouch in the roof of the primitive oral cavity. The posterior lobe arises from the floor of the third ventricle. The pars intermedia is between the anterior and posterior lobes.

Since the pituitary gland lacks a blood-brain barrier, it normally contrast enhances. The normal pituitary gland has a subtle CT noncontrast and contrast heterogeneity due to several factors including the hypodense pars intermedia and the anterior and posterior lobe stromal inhomogeneities. The pars intermedia hypodensity is partly the result of contained small "colloid" cysts. This causes varying noncontrast and contrast heterogeneous patterns. These heterogeneities can be central, bilateral, and asymmetrical.[1-3] Noise artifacts from thin section, soft tissue CT technique also contributes to pituitary gland density heterogeneity. Further contributing to the normal CT heterogeneity is a 3–4 mm ovoid, normal posterior pituitary lobe hypodensity seen on axial contrast scans.[4] These normal heterogeneities and hypodensities should not be confused with microadenomas. Also, care must be taken not to misinterpret a thin or asymmetrical sella floor as evidence of an intrasellar mass. The sella floor may be slanted due to an eccentric sphenoid sinus septum.

The normal glandular heterogeneity demonstrated by CT is not obvious by the MR technique (Fig. 11.1).[5] The anterior lobe of the pituitary gland is of intermediate homogeneous intensity on T1- and T2-weighted MR images. A strong fat MR signal is almost always present in the normal posterior pituitary lobe due to fat-laden pituicytes.[5] This fat signal

Table 11.1. The Differential Diagnosis of Sella Region Abnormalities

Lesion	Lesion Characteristics	Lesion Characteristics for Group (Column 4) Exclusion	Differential Diagnostic Disease Group	Exclusionary Characteristics of Column 1 Lesion in Addition to Column 3
Microadenoma (<10 mm)	Intrasellar <10 mm hypodense/T1 hypointense mass Pituitary gland height >9 mm Eccentric upper surface convex gland bulge		Incidental cyst	Stalk tilt; eccentric glandular height increase >9 mm; contrast enhancement of ACTH variety
Macroadenoma (>10 mm)	Intrasellar origin mass ± suprasellar extension; ballooned sella; T1 hypointensity		Intrasellar craniopharyngioma	Rare in childhood; ballooned sella; lacks calcification; cysts unusual
			Intrasellar meningioma	No hyperostosis; usually lacks calcification; lacks T1/T2 isointensity
			Intrasellar aneurysm	No signal void; no peripheral calcification
			Rathke's cleft cyst	Usually not cystic; hemorrhage uncommon but may not be distinguished from mucoid type
			Lymphocytic adenohypophysitis	Not distinguishable
Craniopharyngioma Difficult to distinguish from hypothalamic glioma, dermoid cyst, and mucoid type Rathke's cleft cyst	Calcified cystic usually suprasellar mass; contrast enhances		Hypothalamic glioma	Calcification; no history of neurofibromatosis
			Mucoid type Rathke's cleft cyst	Calcification primarily suprasellar
			Macroadenoma	Common in children; calcification and cystic
			Meningioma	Lacks T1/T2 isointensity; cystic; lacks hyperostosis
			Germinoma	Calcification; cystic
			Dermoid tumor	Lacks fat
Rathke's cleft cyst Difficult to distinguish mucoid type from craniopharyngioma and hemorrhagic pituitary adenoma	Predominantly intrasellar cyst Two types: CSF and mucoid May ring contrast enhance		Macroadenoma	Cystic; mucoid type resembles hemorrhagic pituitary adenoma
			Craniopharyngioma	Lacks calcium; lacks shallow sella
			Arachnoid cyst	Primarily an intrasellar cyst
			Abscess	Possible ballooned sella; lacks symptoms
			Empty sella	Displaced infundibulum
Arachnoid cyst Difficult to distinguish from epidermoid tumor	Suprasellar smoothly marginated water density/intensity mass		Rathke's cleft cyst	Primarily suprasellar; CSF density/intensity
			Empty sella	Displaced infundibulum
			Epidermoid tumor	Lacks interstices; lacks diploic space involvement; difficult to differentiate No fat or calcification
			Dermoid tumor Cysticercosis	No cranial calcifications or lesions, lacks travel history to endemic area
Empty sella Easy to distinguish from other sellar cystic lesions	Intrasellar cistern Posterior position infundibulum stalk and pituitary gland	Intact infundibulum	Arachnoid cyst Rathke's cleft cyst	An intrasellar process CSF density/intensity

Table 11.1.   The Differential Diagnosis of Sella Region Abnormalities (continued)

Lesion	Lesion Characteristics	Lesion Characteristics for Group (Column 4) Exclusion	Differential Diagnostic Disease Group	Exclusionary Characteristics of Column 1 Lesion in Addition to Column 3
Abscess (intrasellar) Difficult to distinguish from other pituitary cystic masses	Intrasellar centrally necrotic mass CT central hypodensity with ring contrast enhancement	History of meningitis	Pituitary adenoma	Lacks ballooned sella; ring contrast enhancement central necrosis
			Craniopharyngioma	Lacks calcification and ballooned sella
			Metastasis	Lacks bone destruction
			Rathke's cleft cyst	Lacks hyperintensity of mucoid type; may not be distinguishable from CSF type; symptomatic
Lymphocytic Adenohypophysitis Not distinguishable from pituitary macrodenoma	CT shows contrast-enhancing intrasellar mass	Regression of lesion on hormonal therapy	Pituitary adenoma	Not distinguishable
			Intrasellar meningioma	No hyperostosis or calcification
			Intrasellar craniopharyngioma	No cystic change or calcification intrasellar
			Abscess	No cystic change
Meningioma	CT hyperdense contrast enhancing MR T1/T2 isointense Cleft separating tumor from displaced tissue Hyperostosis	Hyperostosis T1/T2 isointensity	Pituitary adenoma	Relative T1 and T2 isointensity; may be calcified
			Craniopharyngioma	Adult occurrence; uncommonly cystic; lacks a shallow sella
			Epidermoid tumor	Contrast enhancement; noncontrast hyperdensity
Epidermoid tumor	CT hypodense non-contrast-enhancing mass MR water-intensity mass with interstices		Arachnoid cyst	Interstices possible diploic space origin; difficult to differentiate
			Dermoid tumor	Lacks fat and usually lacks calcium
			Craniopharyngioma	Lacks calcium; no contrast enhancement; homogeneous hypodensity and CSF-like intensity; lacks shallow sella
			Meningioma	Hypodensity, CSF-like intensity; no hyperostosis
			Cysticercosis	Usually no hydrocephalus; no intracranial calcifications; no endemic travel history
Hypothalamic glioma	Invasive solid suprasellar tumor; usually occurs in children. Neurofibromatosis often present.	Neurofibromatosis (exclusion not applicable to meningioma)	Craniopharyngioma	Lacks calcification
			Meningioma	Lacks isointense T1 and T2; lacks hyperostosis; lacks calcification; invasive
			Metastasis	Lacks bone destruction; most common in children
			Germinoma	Lacks associated pineal region tumor
			Hamartoma	Larger lesion not confined to tuber cinereum; not associated with precocious puberty
Hamartoma	Small solid tuber cinereum mass projects into chiasmatic cistern	Childhood precocious puberty; small masses (≤2 cm)	Hypothalamic glioma	Small (≤2 cm) tuber cinereum mass; no history of neurofibromatosis
			Germinoma	No associated pineal mass; small mass at tuber cinereum

Lesion	Lesion Characteristics	Lesion Characteristics for Group (Column 4) Exclusion	Differential Diagnostic Disease Group	Exclusionary Characteristics of Column 1 Lesion in Addition to Column 3
Hamartoma (continued)			Granuloma	No bone lysis; no history of sarcoid; small mass at tuber cinereum; no diabetes insipidus
Granuloma	A suprasellar solid mass	History of sarcoid or diabetes insipidus Sarcoid regression on steroids Hand-Christian-Schüller osteolysis in children	Germinoma Hamartoma	No associated pineal mass Possibly greater than 2 cm; no precocious puberty
			Hypothalamic glioma	No history of neurofibromatosis
			Craniopharyngioma	No calcification; no shallow sella
			Meningioma	No hyperostosis; no isointensity; Hand-Christian-Schüller disease occurs in children
			Metastasis	No adult osteolysis; no history of metastatic disease. If Hand-Christian-Schüller disease, occurs in children
Aneurysm	CT suprasellar hyperdense contrast-enhancing mass MR virtually diagnostic	MR flow effects Peripheral curvilinear calcification CT homogeneous lumen	Pituitary adenoma Meningioma	Often eccentric location Lacks hyperostosis; lacks T1/T2 isointensity
			Craniopharyngioma	Lacks globular calcification and cystic changes; lacks mixed intensities
			Germinoma	Lacks associated pineal region mass; usually occurs in older adults; sharply marginated
Vascular malformation Easy in most circumstances to distinguish from other lesions because of tortuous vessels	CT contrast-enhancing suprasellar mass with serpentine vessels MR flow effects with serpentine vessels Little mass effect unless hemorrhage Associated subarachnoid hemorrhage	Serpentine vessel MR flow phenomenon and CT enhancement	Meningioma	No hyperostosis; no MR isointensity
			Metastasis	No bone destruction; calcifications
			Germinoma	No pineal involvement
			Aneurysm	Multiple flow voids; more irregular shape
			Craniopharyngioma	No cysts (calcifications can be mistaken for signal-void)
Cysticercosis Difficult to distinguish from epidermoid and arachnoid cyst	Cyst-like suprasellar cistern lesions Near-water-density/intensity Possible associated intracranial lesions	Frequent associated hydrocephalus Travel to endemic regions Scolex	Arachnoid cyst	Density/intensity may reflect protein content
			Epidermoid cyst	Lacks cyst margin interstices
Chordoma Difficult to distinguish from metastasis	Bone destruction Sella region mass	Calcification	Metastasis	Osteolysis origin at clivus
Metastasis	Bone destruction	Lacks calcification	Chordoma	No calcification; osteolysis not centered at clivus

correlates to the CT posterior pituitary lobe hypodensity. Disruption of hypothalamic secretory or axonal transport mechanisms to the neurohypophysis may cause lack of the posterior lobe hyperintensity.[5] The disruption can be caused by a hypothalamic tumor, large intrasellar tumor, an empty sella that compresses posterior lobe tissue, and by surgical section of the infundibulum.[6] Absence of the T1 hyperintensity is seen in patients with diabetes insipidus. It should be noted, however, that some normal patients lack this hyperintense signal.[5,6] The neonatal anterior hypophysis has a higher T1 signal than that of the adult and there is a lack of intensity difference between anterior and posterior lobes in these in-

Figure 11.1.   The normal pituitary gland. *Intravenous contrast axial* **(A)** *and coronal* **(B)** *CT scans. Midsagittal noncontrast* **(C)** *and i.v. contrast* **(D)** *MR scans of different patients. Coronal noncontrast* **(E)** *and i.v. contrast* **(F)** *MR scans of the same patient. Axial noncontrast MR scan* **(G).** *All MR scans are SE 600/25 3 mm in thickness.* The sagittal MR scans demonstrate the optic chiasm *(OC)* between the optic *(3-OR)* and infundibular *(3-1R)* recesses of the third ventricle *(3)*. The pituitary gland *(P)* is also identified in some sections as pars anterior *(PA)* and pars posterior *(PP)*. The pituitary gland demonstrates noncontrast MR homogeneity and subtle CT and MR i.v. contrast heterogeneity *(arrows)*. The infundibular stalk *(I)* contrast enhances by both the i.v. CT and MR methods. It is seen at the diaphragma sellae hiatus in **A.** The pars posterior demonstrates characteristic T1 hyperintensity on sagittal MR sections. Contrast of the infundibular stalk *(I)* is apparent on the coronal section **(F).** The internal carotid artery *(ICA)* signal void is seen within the contrast-enhanced cavernous sinus *(CS)* by the MR method but is obscured on the coronal CT. The MR dorsum sella *(DS)* marrow signal can blend with the pars posterior T1 signal hyperintensity.

NOTE: (1) CT identifies the sella floor, which MR (in absence of sphenoid sinus fluid or mucosal hypertrophy) does not. (2) The dorsum sella, easily identified by CT, can also be identified by MR due to fat within the marrow space. (3) The diaphragma sellae is not identifiable by CT or T1-weighted MR in the normal patients.

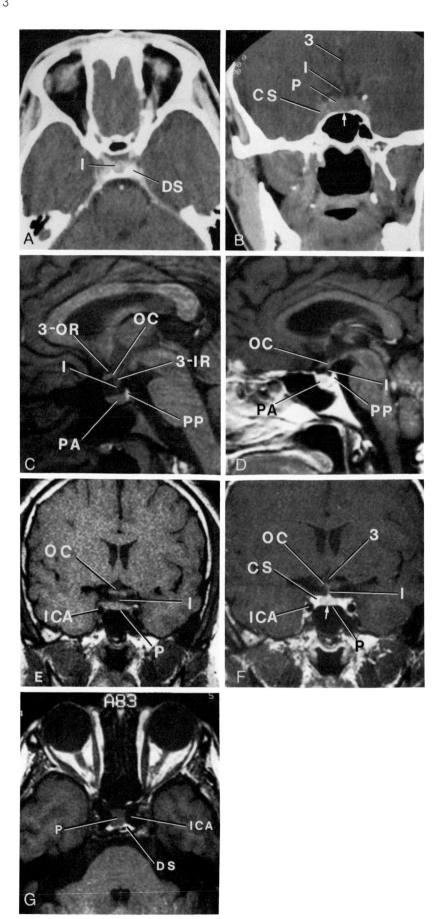

fants.[7] The gland height should be at least 3 mm and may exceed 8 mm in young women (particularly during pregnancy)[8] and the height may vary with the menstrual cycle. A height of 9 mm is the upper limit of normal and is common in pubescent children.[8,9] The normal gland may have a cephalic convexity.[5,6,9]

The pituitary stalk (hypophyseal stalk, infundibulum) is easily identified by MR and CT (particularly with contrast injection). It arises from the hypothalamic tuber cinereum and slopes anteriorly to the posterior pituitary gland. The stalk passes behind the optic chiasm maintaining a central position. It has a more posterior position in patients with the empty sella syndrome. It should be identified by MR in sagittal, axial, and coronal planes in all patients. The normal stalk measures 2–4.5 mm in thickness.[10–12] It and the tuber cinereum contrast enhance with Gd-DTPA.

CHIASMATIC CISTERN

The chiasmatic cistern lies directly above the diaphragma sellae. The diaphragma is not distinctly visualized by CT but may be seen by MR in the normal state as a thin band of negligible signal.[13] The chiasmatic cistern has a five-pointed star shape (pontine level) or six-pointed star (midbrain level) shape on axial sections and is clearly seen by both the CT and MR techniques (Fig. 11.2). Within the cistern, the optic chiasm lies anterior to the pituitary stalk. MR in all orthogonal planes more sharply visualizes the

chiasm and adjacent optic nerves and tracts than does CT.

The chiasmatic cistern may herniate through a deficient diaphragma sellae resulting in an intrasellar cistern, "the empty sella." There is a "primary" and "secondary" type of empty sella. The primary type occurs spontaneously and the secondary type occurs after surgery or irradiation for an intrasellar mass. The primary type is usually asymptomatic; however, CSF rhinorrhea may rarely develop. Primary empty sellas are usually incidentally detected as an expanded sella on skull or sinus x-rays, or CT or MR scans that have been obtained for various clinical indications. The demonstration of the infundibulum inserting into the posterior positioned gland within the often expanded balloon-contoured sella confirms the diagnosis of empty sella and excludes an intrasellar cyst (Fig. 11.3).[14] Presence of a small portion of the chiasmatic cistern within the superior portion of the sella turcica is a normal finding (Fig. 11.4). The secondary form may very rarely cause visual disturbance due to intrasellar herniation of the optic chiasm.[15]

CAVERNOUS SINUS

The cavernous sinus is a dura-enclosed septated venous channel containing an approximately 2-cm segment of the internal carotid artery, the oculomotor nerve (n.III), trochlear nerve (n.IV), the ophthalmic (n.V[1]) and maxillary (n.V[2]) divisions of the trigeminal nerve, and the abducens nerve (n.VI).[16] The cra-

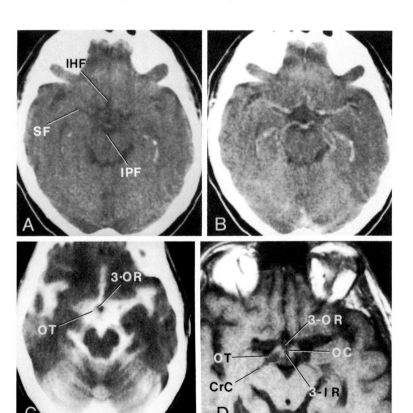

Figure 11.2 Chiasmatic cistern. *Axial noncontrast chiasmatic cistern-level 36/150* **(A)** *and i.v. contrast 36/100* **(B)** *CT scans. Same level iopamidol CT cisternogram* **(C)** *and SE 600/25 MR scan* **(D).** *The chiasmatic cistern has the shape of a "six-pointed star" due to the interhemispheric fissure (IHF) anteriorly, the interpeduncular fossa (IPF) posteriorly, and the paired Sylvian fissures (SF) and the crural cisterns (CrC) laterally. The optic tracts (OT) join at the optic chiasm (OC). The third ventricle optic recess (3-OR) is anterior to the infundibular recess (3-IR). MR has replaced positive contrast cisternography for investigation of the chiasmatic cistern.*

Figure 11.3. Empty sella turcica. *Midsagittal SE 600/25 MR **(A)** scan. Axial sellar-level SE 2000/ 20 MR **(B)** and i.v. contrast 36/100 CT **(C)** scans. Coronal midsellar-level SE 600/25 MR **(D)** and i.v. contrast 36/100 CT **(E)** scans. The sella is enlarged ("ballooned") by an intrasellar cyst. The infundibular stalk (I) lies posteriorly within the sella and is sharply outlined by the intrasellar CSF. The "remodeled" pituitary gland (P) lies posteriorly against the dorsum sella (DS).*

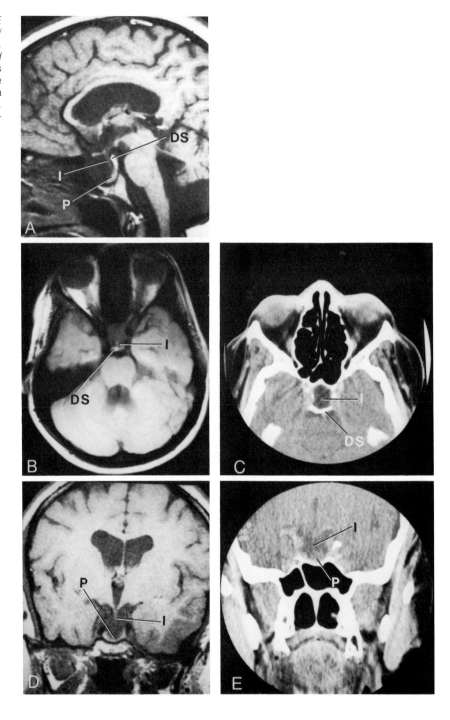

nial nerves are identifiable in their characteristic locations. It also contains the carotid sympathetic plexus. The cavernous sinus connects with the ophthalmic, central retinal, middle and inferior cerebral, middle meningeal and pterygoid veins, and the petrosal sinuses.[17]

Both MR and contrast CT (Fig. 11.5) demonstrate excellent cranial nerve detail on coronal sections. The trochlear nerve (n.IV), because of its small size and proximity to the occulomotor nerve (n.III), is not routinely seen. The Meckel's cave is seen abutting the

most posterior portion of the sinus on orthogonal plane sections. The major advantages of the MR technique are distinction of the internal carotid artery with the sinus, carotid artery and cavernous venous flow estimation and dependable orthogonal plane views.[16,17]

Our current MR technique requires small (18-mm) FOV, thin section (3 mm), coronal heavily T1-weighted spin-echo image sequences. Intravenous MR contrast is used to investigate tumor involvement, i.e., meningioma. Gradient echo MR technique can be useful to identify intracavernous tumor and to help

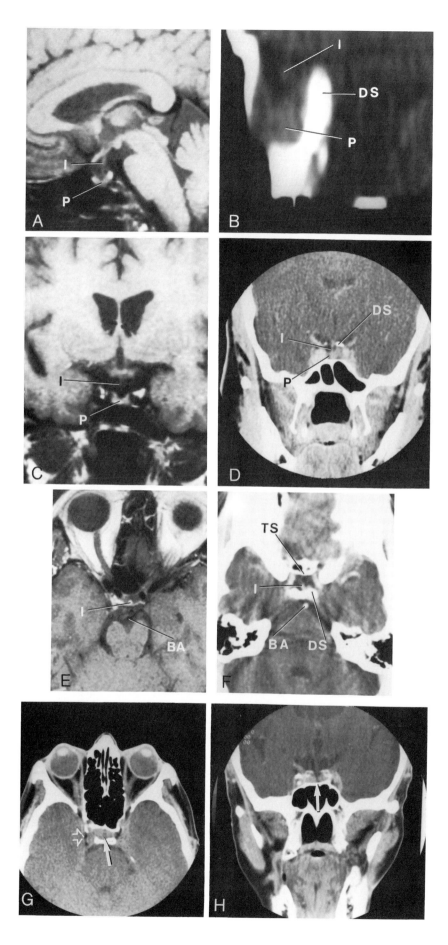

Figure 11.4. Normal variants. A–F demonstrate the presence of a small portion fo the chiasmatic cistern in the superior aspect of the sella turcica ("partial empty sella"). **G** and **H** demonstrate pars intermedia cysts producing pituitary tissue CT inhomogeneities. **A–F:** "Partial empty sella." The MRs and CTs are of different patients. *Midsagittal (A), coronal mid-pituitary-level (C) and Gd-DTPA contrast axial sella-level (E) SE 600/25 MR scans. CT midsagittal reformation (B). Same level direct coronal (D) and axial (F) i.v. contrast CT scans.* Note the presence of a small portion of the chiasmatic cistern outlining the infundibulum *(I)* in the superior sella. The pituitary gland *(P)* has a concave upward shape. The infundibulum is particularly sharply outlined when contrast enhanced. The dorsum sella *(DS)* and tuberculum sella *(TS);* basilar artery *(BA).* G–H: Pars intermedia cysts. *Axial (G) and direct coronal (H) i.v. contrast sella-level CT scans.* Note the central pars intermedia cysts *(closed arrows).* Incidental juxtadural fatty tissue is present *(open arrow).* The scan was done for visual disturbance.

Figure 11.5. The normal cavernous sinus. *Intravenous contrast SE 600/25 MR scans and 36/200 CT scans. Coronal midpituitary level. MR **(A)** and direct coronal CT **(B)** scans. Posterior cavernous sinus MR **(C)** and direct coronal CT **(D)** scans. Axial inferior cavernous sinus-level MR **(E)** and CT **(F)** scans. Coronal GRE 125/12 30° flip-angle MR image **(G).*** Both the MR and CT methods clearly identify the cavernous sinus *(CS).* The oculomotor nerve *(n3),* the opthalmic nerve *(n5.1),* and the maxillary nerve *(n5.2)* are well defined surrounded by contrast-enhanced venous blood. The coronal CT pituitary gland *(P)* heterogeneous signal is due to noise as well as glandular inhomogeneity. The Meckel's cave *(MC)* is located at the posterior aspect of the cavernous sinus lateral to the internal carotid artery **(F).** Note the contrast-enhanced tuber cinereum *(TC)* and the proximal infundibular stalk; dorsum sella *(DS);* basilar artery *(BA);* sphenoid sinus *(SS).* The signal-void left internal carotid artery and (probably) the right third nerve are seen surrounded by hyperintense cavernous sinus venous blood on the gradient echo image **(G).**

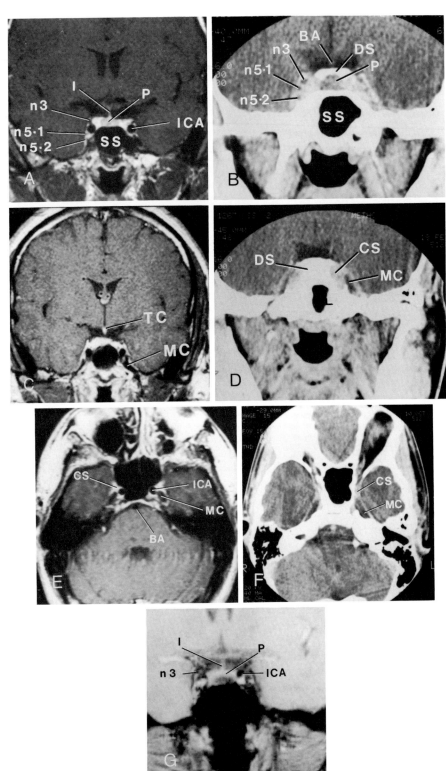

estimate blood flow.[16] In addition, we obtain axial infraorbitalmeatal plane 5-mm variable echo sections. This series of imaging parameter enables us to analyze different signals from the same structures in orthogonal planes. Internal carotid artery aneurysm and occlusion and venous sinus displacement by tumor are conditions easily analyzed by these techniques.

CT cavernous sinus imaging requires direct coronal i.v. contrast, small FOV (16 mm) zoom, soft tissue filter technique.[17,18]

Lesions Originating in the Sella

PITUITARY ADENOMA

These histologically benign tumors that arise from the adenohypophysis represent from 10–15% of all intracranial neoplasms. They are, by far, the most common intrasellar tumor. Tumor size determines whether an adenoma is classified as a microadenoma (less than 10 mm in diameter) or a macroadenoma (greater than 10 mm in diameter).[19]

Microadenomas clinically present due to hormonal production—usually prolactin—but, not uncommonly, adrenocorticotrophic hormone (ACTH) or growth hormone.[5] Because nonfunctioning occult microadenomas may be very common (up to 25% of the general population at autopsy), a lesion defined by CT or MR may not be clinically significant.[19,20] A hormonal function classification defines whether the adenoma is a nonsecreting or secreting "functioning" type. This latter type of pituitary adenoma may secrete prolactin (amenorrhea, galactorrhea), growth hormone (gigantism or acromegaly), ACTH (Cushing's syndrome), or, far less commonly, a variety of other hormones. In general, macroadenomas are clinically nonfunctional although 50–60% of cases may have laboratory evidence of prolactin secretion. This explains the "clinical silence" of macroadenomas before reaching a large enough size to compress critical structures.

The clinical presentation of a pituitary adenoma depends on its functional status (hormonal production), its size, and its extrasellar extent. Pituitary insufficiency often results from compression by a large intrasellar mass component and bitemporal hemianopsia often results from suprasellar extension compressing the optic chiasm. Rarely, compression of the foramen of Monro by even larger tumors may cause hydrocephalus. The cavernous sinus is often laterally displaced. Cavernous sinus invasion is less common and is difficult to document by CT or MR. MR gradient recalled echo (GRE) technique helps identify cavernous sinus invasion by analysis of venous sinus and carotid artery flow phenomena.[16] Occasionally, the patient presents with pituitary apoplexy due to pituitary tumor infarction, necrosis, and hemorrhage. These patients present with headache, obtundation, nausea, vomiting, visual field loss, and ophthalmoplegia. The apoplectic presentation may mimic the signs of spontaneous subarachnoid hemorrhage. Aggressive large tumors can cause skull base destruction as well as structural displacements.[21] The pituitary stalk (infundibulum) may be enlarged or displaced. The normal infundibulum measures less than 4.5 mm. In young patients, if the stalk is larger than the basilar artery at the dorsum sellar level, it is pathologically enlarged.[22] Lateral extension is also important to document because of its implication for surgical approach and its adverse prognostic implication of potential endocrinological cure.[22] A large off-midline suprasellar component, a large tumor with a small sella, or a "dumb-bell shaped" tumor with a narrow waist at the diaphragma sellae are potential indicators against transsphenoidal surgery.[23] The position of sphenoid sinus septae should be noted for transsphenoidal surgery reference. An incompletely pneumatized sphenoid sinus, nasal infection, sinusitis, or a previous craniotomy for a sellar lesion are potential contraindications for transsphenoidal surgery.[23] The diagnostic scan may be used as a baseline for bromocriptine (a dopamine analog) therapy.[24] Documentation of microadenoma or, on occasion, macroadenoma, with volume reduction several months after treatment confirms that the imaged lesion is responsible for the clinical presentation.[5,22]

MR of macroadenoma often demonstrates sella ballooning on sagittal sections. Suprasellar, sphenoid, and parasellar macroadenoma expansion is easily documented by identification of effects on adjacent structures such as the optic chiasm, the sphenoid sinus, the cavernous sinus, and the foramina of Monro (Fig. 11.6).[25] MR i.v. contrast usually can distinguish the normal pituitary gland, the cavernous sinus, and the pituitary adenoma. Cavernous sinus invasion by tumor often can be detected by coronal plane T1-weighted i.v. contrast MR.[26] MR of pituitary adenomas usually demonstrates T1 hypointensity with less predictable T2 intensity results.[26] MR intravenous contrast injection T1-weighted coronal sequences have become standard for MR pituitary investigation. The coronal scan should immediately follow the contrast injection to avoid possible delayed contrast enhancement of a microadenoma.[26]

Hemorrhage into a pituitary adenoma is occasionally seen and most often is unassociated with pituitary apoplexy (Fig. 11.7). Intratumoral cystic changes are evidenced by T1 hypointense and T2 hyperintense signals.[5] A fluid-fluid level is less common. MR, with its excellent tissue detail, gives better definition of tumor margins and adjacent nonosseous structures than does CT.[16,27] CT is superior for detection of bone detail such as sella floor destruction, however.

The CT scout view of macroadenomas often demonstrates a ballooned sella. CT of macroadenomas demonstrates homogeneous isodensity and diffuse contrast enhancement. Macroadenomas may, rarely,

Figure 11.6. Pituitary macroadenoma (nonfunctioning). *Axial chiasmatic cistern-level noncontrast (A) and i.v. contrast (B) 36/100 CT scans. Same level SE 2000/20 (C) and 2000/80 (D) MR scans. Midsagittal (E) and coronal pituitary-level (F) SE 600/25 MR scans.* A round smoothly marginated CT homogeneously hyperdense and contrast-enhancing mass *(closed arrows)* compresses the foramina of Monro *(open arrows)* causing hydrocephalus with dilatation of the temporal horns *(TH)* and interstitial edema *(IE).* The mass is T1 gray matter-homogeneously isointense and T2 hyperintense. A notch in the tumor is caused by the diaphragma sellae *(DiS).* The intracavernous carotid arteries are laterally displaced. Note that the optic chiasm cannot be identified on the midsagittal scan *(E).*

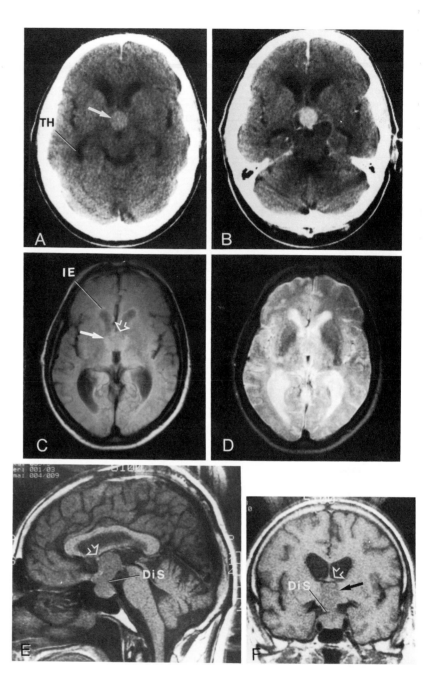

have a curvolinear rim of calcification or globular central calcification.[28] Cystic components occasionally occur and can be detected by CT[29] but MR is far more effective than CT for detection of intratumoral hemorrhage (Fig. 11.7). CT is superior to MR for distinguishing between sella floor remodeling and destruction with inferior extension of a pituitary adenoma (Fig. 11.8).[5]

Microadenomas are usually in a lateral glandular position and appear on MR as a focal area of T1-weighted hypointensity often associated with asymmetrical upward glandular bulge and stalk displacement.[30] The pituitary stalk may not be displaced and, rarely, it may actually be tilted toward the microad-

enoma (paradoxical displacement. Asymmetry of the sella floor is a less valuable sign[30] that can also be related to position of the sphenoid sinus septum. Most microadenomas larger than 3 mm can be accurately localized.[30] The microadenoma, itself, rarely expands above the diaphragm. The most common hormone-secreting microadenoma, the prolactin-secreting adenoma, does not contrast enhance by either the CT or MR methods (Fig. 11.9).[26,31,32] ACTH-producing microadenomas characteristically demonstrate delayed enhancement with i.v. Gd-DTPA. Coronal MR sections obtained immediately (within 5 min) after i.v. injection demonstrate a noncontrast-enhancing cyst-like lesion within the homogeneously enhancing

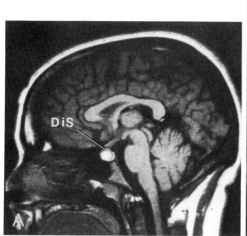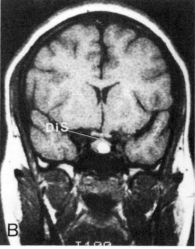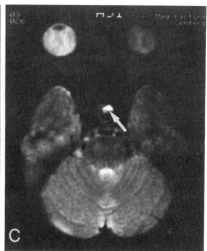

Figure 11.7. Hemorrhagic microadenoma (prolactin-secreting). *Midsagittal (A) and pituitary-level coronal (B) SE 600/25 MR scans. Axial pituitary-level SE 2000/80 MR scan (C).* The T1 homogeneously

hyperintense eccentric 9-mm diameter mass bulges the diaphragma sellae upward and has a T2-weighted image fluid-fluid level *(arrow)* probably due to settling of intracellular methemoglobin.

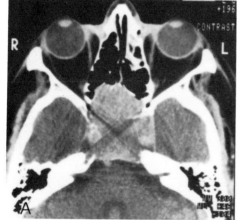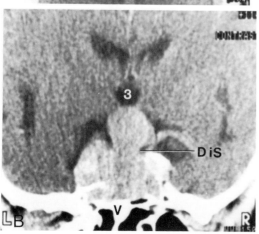

Figure 11.8. Nonfunctioning invasive pituitary adenoma with skull base destruction. *Intravenous contrast sella-level 46/300 (A) and direct coronal 38/150 (B) CT scans.* A fairly homogeneously contrast-enhanced mass has destroyed the sella and sphenoid sinus margins, has filled the sphenoid sinus, has extended above the diaphragma sellae *(DiS),* and elevates the third ventricle *(3);* vomer *(V).*

surrounding normal tissue. Delayed images (1 hour) may demonstrate lesion contrast enhancement and, therefore, decreased lesion/pituitary gland conspicuity. Early scanning after injection is therefore recommended.[31]

CT findings of pituitary adenomas are not only dependent, like MR, upon tumor size but also upon type. Many patients with proven microadenomas have normal high quality CT scans. For instance, an ACTH-secreting microadenoma characteristically contrast enhances as compared to the more usual lack of enhancement of other microadenomas (Fig. 11.9). Since the CT characteristic of most microadenomas is a small, hypodense lesion silhouetted by diffusely contrast-enhanced surrounding pituitary gland, ACTH-producing microadenomas are more difficult to detect by CT and greater reliance is placed on focal hypophyseal stalk displacement, diaphragma sella bulge, and focal sella floor downward convex bulge.[31] Hypodensity and glandular enlargement are the two most important CT criteria of microadenoma detection.

INTRASELLAR CYSTS

Autopsy, CT, and MR evidence of very small (up to several millimeters) pituitary cysts is very common. Larger expansile cysts are uncommon. The two types of the expansile cysts are those that originate from arachnoid membrane rests and those originating from epithelial rests.

Those cysts of arachnoid origin (arachnoid cysts) are usually suprasellar with occasional intrasellar components and, rarely, entirely intrasellar. These are identified by both CT and MR as a water-containing, thin-walled sac expanding the sella and displacing or obliterating the infundibular stalk. They

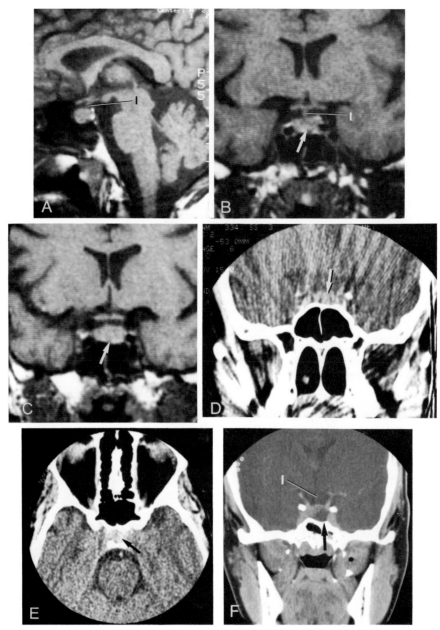

Figure 11.9. **Microadenomas.** **A–E** and **F** are different patients with functioning microadenomas. The first case **(A–E)** is an ACTH-secreting microadenoma. **F** (second case) is a prolactin-secreting microadenoma. *SE 600/25 midsagittal (A) and pituitary-level coronal (B and C) MR scans. B is 4 mm posterior to C. Same level i.v. contrast direct coronal 38/200 (D) and axial pituitary-level 38/130 (E) CT scans. Second case: Direct coronal pituitary-level 3-mm thickness 94/550 i.v. contrast CT scan (F).* First case: ACTH-secreting microadenoma. The diaphgrama sellae is bulged upward, the infundibular stalk *(I)* is displaced to the right side and the sella floor is convexly downward depressed by a left-sided 8-mm maximum diameter pituitary tumor *(arrows).* Dental CT streak artifact markedly obscures detail **(D)** *but tumor contrast enhancement is demonstrated on the axial scan **(E)**. The microadenoma has mixed peripheral hypointense signals with central isointensity.* Second case: Prolactin-secreting microadenoma. There is lack of CT contrast enhancement of the isodense 9 mm height microadenoma **(F).**

are easily differentiated from the empty sella turcica by stalk displacement and the usual typical suprasellar arachnoid cyst appearance (to be described later in this chapter).

The Rathke's cleft cyst is also known as benign intrasellar epithelial cyst, pars intermedia cyst, intrasellar colloid cyst, and Rathke's pouch cysts. The Rathke's pouch has embryological origin in the oropharynx, migrates cephalad, and is responsible for the formation of the anterior and intermediate pituitary lobes. Small remnants of the cleft (epithelial rests) persist. The Rathke's cleft cyst is thought to result from such an epithelial rest. The cyst may be entirely within the sella or have a suprasellar component. It occasionally becomes symptomatic when it attains a very large size.[5,33]

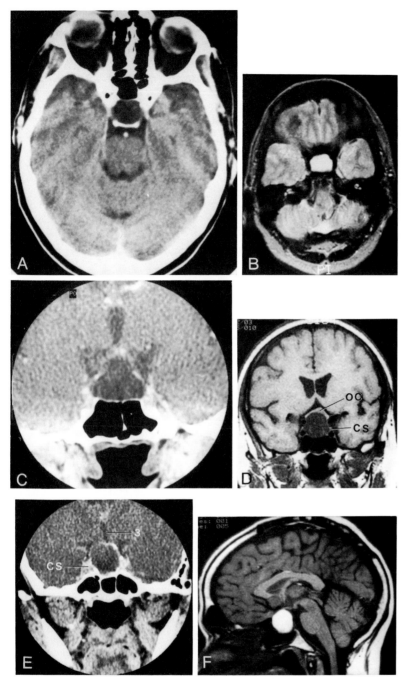

Figure 11.10   Rathke's cleft cyst. A–D and **E–F** are different cases. *Axial pituitary-level 35/90 i.v. contrast CT scan **(A)** and SE 2000/80 MR scan **(B)**. Coronal pituitary-level 40/250 i.v. contrast CT scan **(C)** and SE 600/25 MR scan **(D)**. Coronal pituitary-level i.v. contrast 36/200 CT scan **(E)** and midsagittal SE 600/25 MR scan **(F)**. First case **(A–D):** A water-CT homogeneous isodense mass expands the sella, and elevates the optic chiasm (OC). The lesion is slightly T1 water-hyperintense **(D)** and T2 water-isointense **(B)**. The infundibular stalk cannot be identified. Second case **(E–F):** A tissue CT isointense and MR T1 hyperintense mass expands the sella and elevates the third ventricle (3) anterior recesses. Both cysts laterally displace the cavernous sinus (CS).*

CT demonstrates a hypodense cystic mass within or partially above the sella. Ring-contrast enhancement may occur and may be secondary to aseptic inflammatory changes. The ring contrast-enhanced lesion is difficult to differentiate from a craniopharyngioma, cystic pituitary adenoma, or abscess.[5,33] MR demonstrates two distinct types or Rathke's cleft cysts; one having homogeneous CSF intensity and the other of homogeneous T1 and T2 hyperintensity [mucoid type (Fig. 11.10)].[34] The cyst location of both types appears to be predominantly within the gland rather than predominantly above it as in the case of arachnoid cyst.

INFLAMMATORY LESIONS

Lymphocytic adenohypophysitis is a rare intrasellar possibly autoimmune inflammatory process usually presenting with hypopituitarism. These lesions characteristically lack cavitation and undergo spontaneous regression after hormonal replacement therapy. CT demonstrates an enlarged homogeneously enhancing pituitary gland with possible suprasellar extension not distinguishable from a pituitary adenoma.[28,35] MR changes reported in a single case demonstrated a diffusely enlarged gland with signal isointensity.[5]

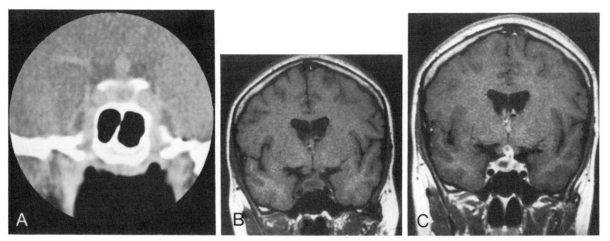

Figure 11.11. Pituitary inflammatory disease. *Direct coronal pituitary-level i.v. contrast 50/550 CT scan* **(A)** *and coronal pituitary-level noncontrast* **(B)** *and contrast* **(C)** *SE 600/25 MR scans.* The partially necrotic irregular rim contrast-enhanced pituitary mass extends up-ward into the infundibular stalk. The surgical biopsy material revealed pus that histologically demonstrated nonspecific chronic inflammatory changes.

Pituitary abscess is a rarely occurring lesion usually associated with a history of meningitis. CT demonstrates a hypodense intrasellar mass with a surrounding thin rim of contrast enhancement. These lesions cannot be differentiated from other cystic-appearing intrasellar masses. One of two cases that we have seen at our hospital with similar appearances of inflammatory disease of the pituitary gland without an organism recovered is presented here (Fig. 11.11).

OTHER INTRASELLAR LESIONS

Although craniopharyngiomas, meningiomas, and metastases may be confined solely within the sella,

Figure 11.12. Craniopharyngioma. Predominantly cystic. *Axial noncontrast pituitary-level 36/150* **(A)** *and chiasmatic cistern-level 36/100* **(B)** *CT scans. Midsagittal SE 600/25 MR scan* **(C).** *Same axial level as* **B**—*SE 2800/80 MR scan* **(D).** The sella is markedly eroded. The third ventricle *(3)* is markedly elevated and deformed. The sharply, irregularly contoured mass is homogeneously CT tissue-hypodense with a surrounding irregularly contoured calcified rim *(Ca).* It is T1 and T2 hyperintense with the exception of the calcified portions.

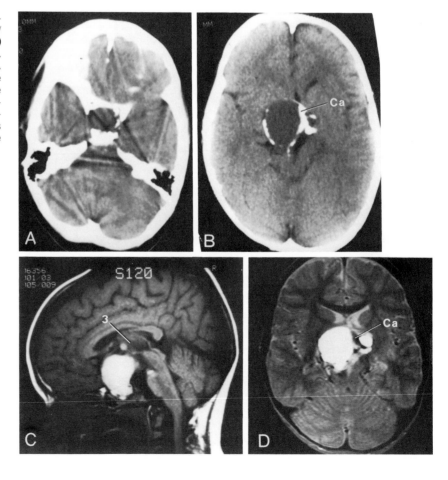

in order to avoid repetition, they will be fully discussed in the next section but reference will be made to these intrasellar lesions in the differential diagnostic table (Table 11.1).

Extrasellar Origin Lesions

CRANIOPHARYNGIOMAS

Craniopharyngioma is the most common tumor arising in the suprasellar cistern. It accounts for 2–3% of all intracranial tumors. The majority of these tumors are discovered during childhood and adolescence; however, there is a smaller second incidence peak in the fifth decade.[19,36] Most cases present with pituitary hypofunction. Visual disturbance may occur due to involvement of the optic chiasm, tracts, or nerves. Diabetes insipidus may occur. Severe hydrocephalus may develop due to obstruction of the foramen of Monro.[37]

Craniopharyngiomas are slow-growing benign tumors that are usually primarily cystic but may be partially cystic or solid. Seventy-five percent of cran-

iopharyngiomas contain calcium and they often have a high cholesterol content.[36] They are thought to have origin as a Rathke's pouch remnant. They are associated with a gliotic reaction with resulting tight adherence to adjacent structures that often precludes total surgical excision.[19]

The vast majority of craniopharyngiomas are suprasellar but occasionally an entirely intrasellar tumor is found. Rarely, an entirely intraventricular (third ventricle) craniopharyngioma may occur. Since pituitary adenomas are uncommon in children, the most common intrasellar tumor of childhood is the craniopharyngioma.[38] The suprasellar tumors tend toward a spherical shape but may be lobulated and irregular.[28,39]

CT findings of calcification, cysts, and contrast enhancement of a suprasellar mass is virtually pathognomonic of craniopharyngioma (Figs. 11.12 and 11.13). CT has an advantage over MR for this diagnosis due to greater CT accuracy for calcification.[5,36] With the exception of identification of calcification,

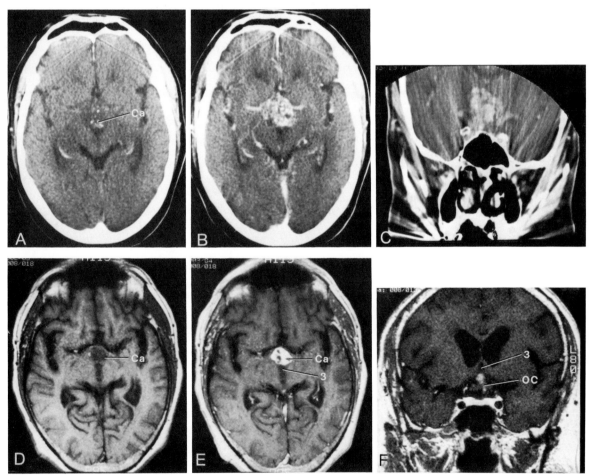

Figure 11.13. Craniopharyngioma. Predominantly solid. *Axial chiasmatic cistern-level 36/100 noncontrast (A) and i.v. contrast (B) and direct coronal pituitary-level i.v. contrast 29/300 (C) CT scans. One year postirradiation, same level axial SE 600/25 noncontrast (D) and Gd-DTPA i.v. contrast (E) and coronal SE 600/25 i.v. contrast (F) MR scans. Marked tumor regression has occurred over the 1-year interval. The irregularly calcified (Ca) suprasellar tumor mark-* edly contrast enhances. Note how the calcifications appear as signal voids within the MR contrast-enhanced tumor. **F** shows contrast-enhanced tumor interposed between the optic chiasm *(OC)* and the third ventricle *(3)*. This tumor was T2 hyperintense with scattered calcific punctate areas of hypointensity. The ease of recognition of the tumor-optic chiasm relationship is a good example of superior MR tissue resolution.

MR is the procedure of choice for craniopharyngioma imaging due to superior tissue discrimination, orthogonal plane imaging, and lack of ionizing radiation. Most craniopharyngiomas have cystic components and contrast enhance by both the CT and MR methods. The contrast enhancement is confined to solid portions including cyst walls. Rarely, the tumor may be entirely solid without CT contrast enhancement.[19,31,39] Erosion of the upper portion of the dorsum sella and a shallow sella turcica that can be seen on a good quality (third generation) CT localizer view or on sagittal MR scans is characteristic of craniopharyngioma. Sagittal and coronal sections most accurately document the suprasellar tumor location and juxtasellar structural displacement. The rare intraventricular craniopharyngioma is usually solid, usually contrast enhances, and is associated with a thickened septum pellucidum.[39]

MR of craniopharyngioma demonstrates T1 hyperintensity of cholesterol-containing cystic tumors or those containing methemoglobin[36] and slight T1 hypointensity in cysts not laden with cholesterol.[5] T2 signal hyperintensity is characteristic of cystic tumors of both T1 intensity types.[34,36] Solid noncalcified portions tend to be T1 tissue-isointense and T2 hyperintense. A heavily calcified lesion may demonstrate T1 and T2 hypointensity.[27,36]

MENINGIOMA

The reader is referred to Chapter 5 for a full discussion of meningiomas.

Meningiomas, on rare occasions, can present entirely within the sella. The common location of sella region meningiomas is suprasellar and parasellar usually arising from the planum sphenoidale or the tuberculum sella. Hyperostosis of the involved planum is common and, occasionally, the tumor is very heavily calcified.[19]

It had been originally thought that MR imaging of small en plaque planum and tuberculum meningiomas, compared to CT imaging, had less detectability and equal specificity for diagnosis. With MR imaging improvements and available i.v. contrast material, we feel that MR offers greater detectability and equal or greater specificity compared to CT. MR specificity for meningiomas is due to the lower T2 signal intensities of the tumor compared to other tumors, the peritumoral cleft and characteristic tumor vessel signal void. Tumor effect upon the diaphragma sellae and optic chiasm,[13] the cavernous sinus,[16] the third ventricle and hypothalamus,[27] and the internal carotid arteries[13] is well demonstrated on variable echo orthogonal planar views (Fig. 11.14). MR imaging of structural compression and displacement is superior to that of contrast CT.[40] CT and MR of the parasellar region requires noncontrast and contrast small FOV, thin section technique (Fig. 11.15).

HYPOTHALAMIC GLIOMA

These tumors are usually low grade astrocytomas that occur predominantly in children but may occur at any age. They usually have a relatively benign course. More malignant gliomas may also occur in this location. They may arise from the hypothalamus or walls of the anterior third ventricle and frequently involve the optic chiasm. Those tumors involving the optic nerves will be discussed in Chapter 14. Patients may develop diabetes insipidus, hypothalamic dysfunction, or optic chiasmal symptoms. There is a high incidence of associated von Recklinghausen's disease.[38]

MR demonstrates an intra-axial, chiasmatic, hypothalamic, or both hypothalamic and optic chiasm mass sometimes involving the thalamus. The T1 signal tends to be isointense or hypointense and the T2 signal tends to be hyperintense. Cystic areas with close-to-CSF signal can be present (Fig. 11.16).[27]

CT demonstrates hypothalamic and/or optic chiasm tumor involvement but not with the same degree of detail as MR. The tumors are of variable size and contour. They usually lack cystic change and are not calcified. They tend to be uniformly isodense and they usually contrast enhance.[38] Lack of calcification and frank invasiveness is evidence against craniopharyngioma.

EPIDERMOID AND DERMOID TUMOR

These relatively rare tumors have been thoroughly discussed in Chapter 5. The parasellar area is a favored location. They are irregularly contoured, sharply marginated chiasmatic cistern irregularly masses that extend within the subarachnoid spaces displacing and encasing structures such as the optic chiasm and the internal carotid arteries.[19]

The MR signal of the epidermoid contents approximates CSF intensity. Lipid contents (more likely of the dermoid tumor) would be expected to give an MR fat signal (Fig. 5.41). CT demonstrates a homogeneous water-density, sharply marginated, noncontrast-enhancing cisternal mass. An area (collar) of enlarged subarachnoid space may surround the tumor (Fig 11.17). Direct coronal images supplement the axial sections.[19] MR is superior to CT for evaluation of structural relationships and displacements although CT does a credible and fully acceptable job for sella region epidermoid and dermoid tumor diagnosis.[41]

GERM CELL TUMORS

These tumors may arise primarily in the suprasellar region or may be the result of spread from the pineal region (Chapter 5). The coexistence of pineal and suprasellar masses is highly suggestive of germinoma. Suprasellar germinomas are more common in women and their peak incidence is in the second and third decades. They are usually fairly smoothly marginated, often involving the optic chiasm and third ventricle.

MR demonstrates T1 isointensity and T2 hyperintensity[27] or isointensity[5] of germinomas. CT usually demonstrates homogeneous isodensity with marked contrast enhancement (Fig. 11.18).[19]

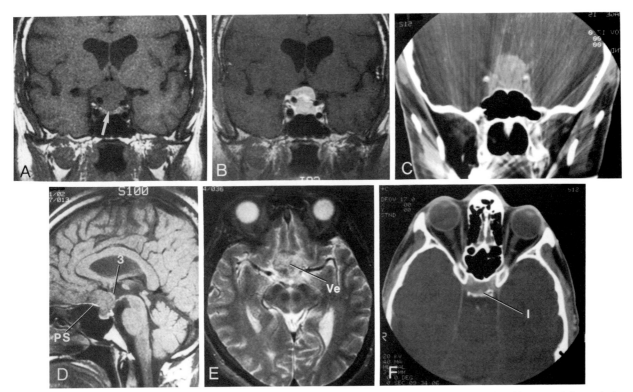

Figure 11.14. Diaphragma sellae and planum sphenoidale meningioma. *Coronal pituitary-level SE 600/25 3-mm thickness 18-mm FOV noncontrast **(A)** and i.v. contrast **(B)** MR scans and direct coronal 100/650 5-mm thickness 17-FOV i.v. contrast CT scan **(C)**. Midsagittal SE 600/25 3-mm thickness 16-mm FOV **(D)** and axial chiasmatic cistern-level SE 2800/80 20-mm FOV 5-mm **(E)** MR scans. Axial pituitary-level 100/500 3-mm thickness 17-mm FOV i.v. contrast CT scan **(F)**. A 21-mm height T1 and T2 gray matter-isointense, contrast-enhancing, smoothly marginated suprasellar and intrasellar mass*

elevates and compresses the optic chiasm and the anterior recesses of the third ventricle (3). It is clearly separated from the compressed slightly hyperintense pituitary gland by a thin hypointense cleft (closed arrow). The mass grows anteriorly over the planum sphenoidale (PS). Hypointense tumor vessels are seen within the tumor on the T2-weighted image (Ve). The infundibular stalk (I) is identified beneath the tumor by CT confirming an extrapituitary origin of the mass.

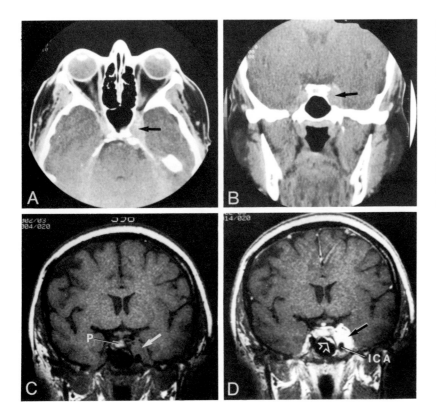

Figure 11.15. Cavernous sinus meningioma. *Axial 50/340 **(A)** and direct coronal 50/550 **(B)** cavernous sinus-level i.v. contrast CT scans. Coronal noncontrast **(C)** and i.v. contrast **(D)** cavernous sinus-level SE 600/25 MR scans. The left cavernous sinus (closed arrows) is expanded by a mass that homogeneously contrast enhances. The hyperintense pituitary gland (P) is displaced to the right side. Carotid artery (ICA) encasement and downward displacement is suggested by the noncontrast study **(C)**. The internal carotid artery is not identified by CT. Because of contrast enhancement of both the lesion and the cavernous sinus, i.v. contrast enhancement does not help determine carotid encasement. There is sphenoid sinus tumor involvement (open arrow).*

Figure 11.16. Hypothalamic glioma. *Axial chiasmatic-level noncontrast 36/100 CT scan* **(A).** *Same level SE 2800/30* **(B)** *and midsagittal SE 600/25* **(C)** *MR scans.* CT demonstrates a round water-density mass in the interpeduncular fossa spreading the cerebral peduncles *(closed arrow).* The mass is T1 water-isointense and is water-hyperintense on the proton density-weighted image. Midbrain and ganglionic tumor infiltration and/or edema is also seen on the proton density MR image. The midsagittal MR scan demonstrates the diaphragma sellae *(open arrow)* separating the tumor from the compressed pituitary gland. The dorsum sella and the tuberculum sella are markedly eroded. Surgical specimens showed solid tumor without gross cystic components.

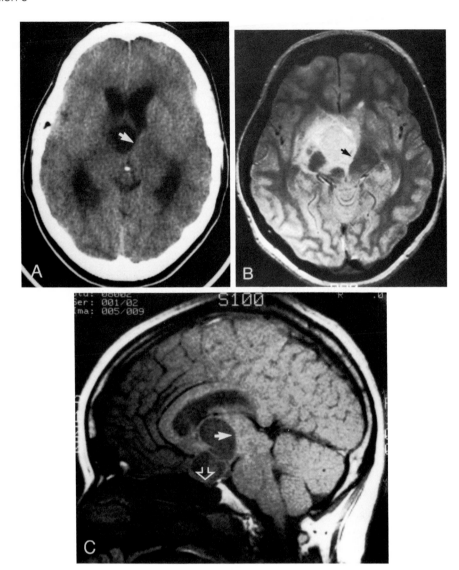

Figure 11.17. Epidermoid tumor in the chiasmatic cistern. *Axial chiasmatic cistern-level i.v. contrast 36/100 CT scan* **(A)** *and SE 2000/80 MR scan* **(B).** Same case as Figure 5.39. A chiasmatic cistern noncontrast-enhancing water-CT density and T2 intensity irregularly and sharply marginated mass markedly compresses and deforms the midbrain *(arrows).*

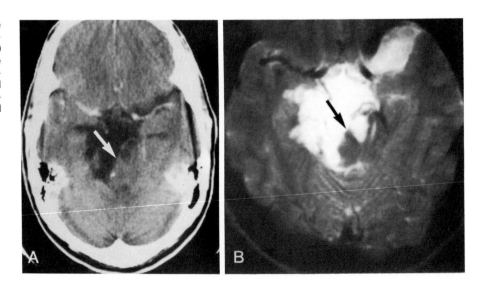

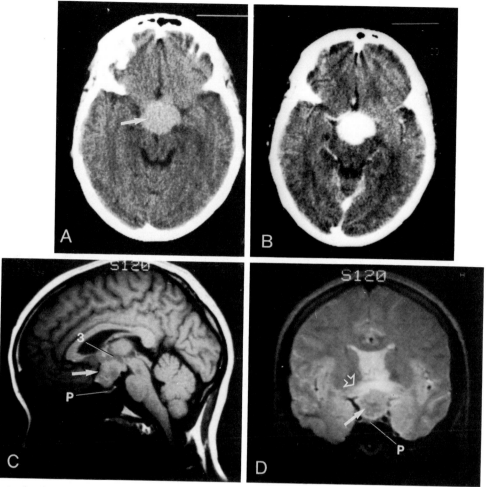

Figure 11.18.   *Suprasellar germinoma "ectopic pinealoma." Axial chiasmatic cistern-level noncontrast* **(A)** *and i.v. contrast* **(B)** *CT scans. Midsagittal SE 600/25* **(C)** *and coronal pituitary-level SE 2000/80 MR* **(D)** *scans. A homogeneously hyperdense and contrast-enhancing slightly irregularly contoured mass (arrows) compresses and distorts* the third ventricle *(3)* and the pituitary gland *(P)* and causes edema in the region of the anterior commissure, anterior perforated substance *(open arrow),* and the optic chiasm. Note the intact hypointense band that includes the diaphragama sellae separating the compressed pituitary gland from the tumor.

HAMARTOMA (TUBER CINEREUM)

Hamartoma of the tuber cinereum is a rare tumor usually found in young boys. It produces isosexual precocious puberty. Those cases documented by CT demonstrate hypothalamic tumors smaller than 2 cm in diameter bulging into the posterior chiasmatic cistern. They are homogeneous, isodense, and do not contrast enhance.[19] A single case studied by MR shows a T1 and T2 isointense mass at the tuber cinereum distorting the anterior third ventricle and optic chiasm and displacing the midbrain on sagittal section. The orthogonal planar technique of MR has decided advantage in the investigation of the region.[5]

GRANULOMA

Histiocytosis and sarcoid can cause a suprasellar granuloma. Histiocytosis occurs in children and sarcoid granulomas occur in adults. Eosinophilic granuloma may produce an isolated suprasellar lesion whereas Hand-Schüller-Christian disease has associated bone destruction. Both histiocytosis and sar-coid lesions cause diabetes insipidus. Sarcoid granulomas are often associated with cranial nerve palsies. Steroid therapy produces marked regression and symptomatic improvement.[19]

On CT, both types of granulomas demonstrate an isodense or minimally hyperdense suprasellar mass with homogeneous contrast enhancement. A small amount of edema may surround the sarcoid granuloma.[19]

ANEURYSMS

The subject of cerebral aneurysms has been discussed in Chapter 6. Specific points with reference to the sellar region are covered here.

Sella region aneurysms occur most frequently in the fourth through sixth decades. Although they are usually of the berry (or congenital) type, atherosclerosis probably plays a role in their development. Cavernous sinus carotid aneurysms may also arise as a result of trauma (Fig. 6.37). Intrasellar and suprasellar carotid aneurysms are accurately identified by MR techniques. In the absence of calcium, there will still remain some doubt as to the diagnosis by CT.

MR demonstrates vascular flow effects of the patent lumen and possible laminated thrombus and is, therefore, diagnostically more accurate than CT. MR of intrasellar masses, by effectively excluding the presence of an intrasellar aneurysm, may obviate the need for arteriography. Coronal sections may demonstrate sella floor asymmetry and origin from the internal carotid artery. CT demonstrates precontrast homogeneous hyperdensity, homogeneous contrast enhancement, and, possibly, curvolinear calcification. Asymmetrical sella floor and/or anterior clinoid erosion is best seen by direct coronal technique (Fig. 11.19).[16,18]

ARTERIOVENOUS MALFORMATIONS

Because these lesions are so rarely present as suprasellar masses, they will not be further discussed in this chapter. The reader is referred to Chapter 6

for a thorough discussion of arteriovenous malformations.

ARACHNOID CYSTS

Suprasellar arachnoid cysts are likely to expand the chiasmatic cistern. Both CT and MR demonstrate these lesions with great accuracy. MR demonstrates a smoothly marginated homogeneous water-isointense mass in orthogonal planes. CT demonstrates a sharply marginated, homogeneous, water-density noncontrast-enhancing mass (Fig. 11.20). CT cisternography can document lack of subarachnoid space communication and smooth margins. A thorough discussion of these lesions is found in Chapter 5.[34]

RATHKE'S CLEFT CYST

Intrasellar Rathke's cleft cysts have already been discussed in this chapter (Fig. 11.10). Those that extend into the suprasellar cistern demonstrate two types of MR findings. One type has serous contents and CSF-like intensities and the other has mucoid

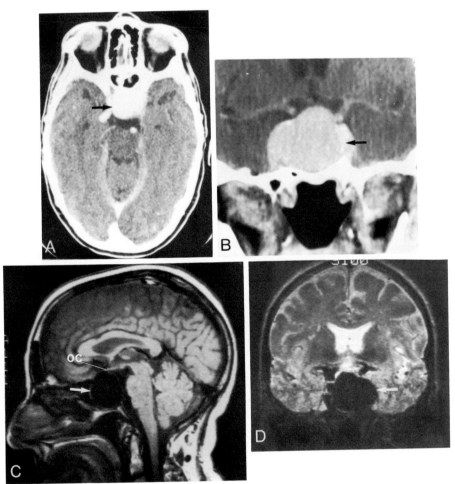

Figure 11.19. Intrasellar cavernous carotid aneurysm. *Pituitary-level axial i.v. contrast 36/100 (A) and direct coronal (B) CT scans. Midsagittal SE 600/25 (C) and coronal pituitary-level SE 2000/80 (D) MR scans.* Same case as Figure 6.32. There is a large CT contrast-enhancing and MR signal-void intrasellar and suprasellar mass *(ar-* rows) laterally displacing the cavernous sinuses, elevating and compressing the optic chiasm *(OC),* markedly expanding the sella, compressing the pituitary gland beyond recognition, and obliterating most of the sphenoid sinus. The MR signal void and bitemporal ghost artifact confirm the lesion as an aneurysm.

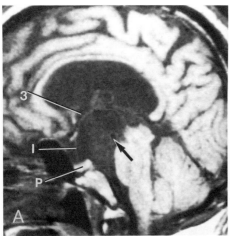
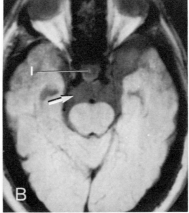
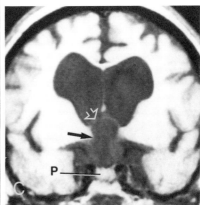

Figure 11.20.   Suprasellar arachnoid cyst. *Midsagittal SE 600/25 (A), axial pituitary-level SE 2000/20 (B) and coronal pituitary-level SE 600/25 (C) MR scans. A large suprasellar cyst (arrows) markedly anteriorly displaces and stretches the infundibular stalk (I). It com-* presses and obstructs the foramina of Monro causing hydrocephalus *(open arrow).* The third ventricle *(3)* is markedly elevated, compressed, and distorted. The pituitary gland *(P)* is intact. The brainstem is posteriorly displaced.

content with T1 and T2 hyperintensities. Both types show a combined intra-extrasellar cyst. CT shows a combined intrasellar-extrasellar homogeneously hypodense mass which may have ring-contrast enhancement.[33]

CYSTICERCOSIS

This topic has been thoroughly discussed in Chapter 8. Cysticercosis cysts may infest the chiasmatic cistern. They are often associated with communicating or obstructive hydrocephalus. An individual cyst measures approximately 1 cm in diameter, contains CSF-isointense fluid, and a 2- to 4-mm mural nodule within which is the scolex.[42] Arachnoidal cysticercosis often causes multilobular degenerative (racemose) cysts. These cysts lack scolexes. They have a predilection for the suprasellar and CP angle cisterns. They often measure several centimeters in size and are associated with chronic meningitis.[19]

CT and MR demonstrates focal cisternal widening with water or near-water-density and intensity, respectively. Occasionally, the cyst rim can be identified by increased density or difference in intensity (Figs. 8.13 and 11.21).[5,19,42]

CHORDOMA

These relentlessly slow-growing tumors are more thoroughly discussed in Chapters 13 and 15. Clivus chordomas may destroy the sella and project into the suprasellar cistern. These tumors can grow quite large and produce extensive skull base destruction with intracranial and nasopharyngeal masses.[19]

CT demonstrates the clival destruction and mass effect. With the exception of frequent calcification, CT densities and MR intensities and are not dependable for diagnosis.[28] MR demonstrates T1 and T2 mixed intensities partially caused by bone and marrow fragments within the tumor. The tumor clival

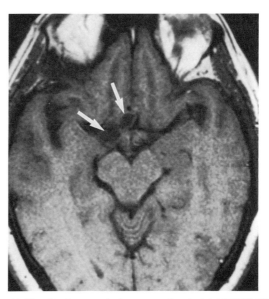

Figure 11.21.   Cysticerocosis (racemose type). *Axial 36/100 SE 600/25 chiasmatic cistern-level MR scan.* Two round smoothly margined centrally hypointense cysts *(arrows)* are present in the chiasmatic cistern.

location is best demonstrated by the MR sagittal section (Fig. 11.22).[5]

METASTASES

Sellar, intrasellar, suprasellar, and parasellar masses may result from metastases via hematogenous and CSF pathways. Sellar region metastatic carcinoma and plasmacytoma are usually associated with bone destruction. The CT and MR appearance of sellar region metastasis varies. Contrast enhancement is probable (Fig. 11.23). Bone destruction, hemorrhage, and necrosis are likely to influence CT densities and MR intensities. Meningeal tumor infiltration may occasionally occur and has been discussed in Chapter 5 (Figs. 5.5 and 11.24).

Figure 11.22. Clivus chordoma. *Axial clivus-level +257/3000* **(A)** *and midbrain-level 36/100 i.v. contrast* **(B)** *CT scans. Midsagittal* **(C)** *and foramen of Monro-level* **(D)** *MR scans.* There is a large partially contrast enhancing *(CE)*, cystic, and hemorrhagic *(H)* destructive mass. The clivus *(Cl)* is the epicenter of the skull base destruction with mass extending through it into the sphenoid sinus anteriorly **(C)**. Bone fragments within the mass present as CT calcifications *(Ca)*. The mass posteriorly displaces and distorts the midbrain *(MB)* and brainstem with marked posterior displacement of the fourth ventricle *(4)*. The right middle cerebral artery *(MCA)* and the internal cerebral vein *(ICV)* are markedly elevated. The pituitary gland *(P)* is intact. There is hydrocephalus probably caused by third ventricle *(3)* compression.

The major differential diagnostic consideration in this case is chordoma vs. metastatic carcinoma to the clivus and skull base. The very large bulk of this lesion favors chordoma.

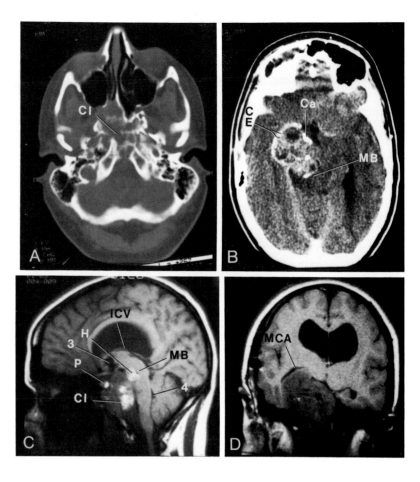

Figure 11.23. Optic chiasm metastasis. A 63-year-old woman with breast cancer and markedly decreased visual acuity. *Axial chiasmatic cistern-level noncontrast* **(A)** *and i.v. contrast* **(B)** *CT scans. The patient was unable to maintain a hyperextended position for direct coronal CT. Midsagittal* **(C)** *and optic chiasm level-coronal SE 600/25* **(D)** *MR scans.* The tumor *(arrow)* deforms the anterior recesses of the third ventricle *(3)*. The optic chiasm is not identified. Between peripheral portions of tumor and tumor-isointense pituitary gland is the diaphragma sellae *(DiS)*. There is lack of pituitary pars posterior hyperintensity. The CT isodense slightly irregular and slightly heterogeneous contrast-enhancing mass has homogeneous T1 gray matter-isodense and T2 hyperintense (not shown) MR signals. Although chiasmal and pituitary gland involvement is suggested by this study, surgery was necessary to confirm chiasmal metastasis and lack of pituitary gland invasion. Note the absence of a recognizable dorsum sella.

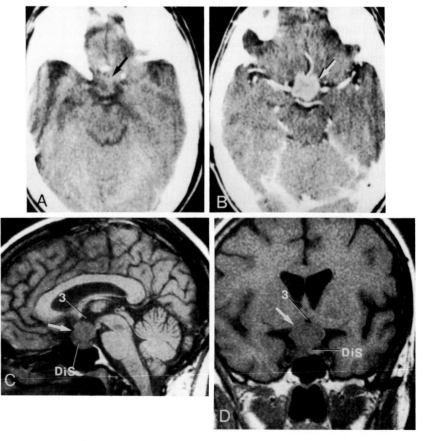

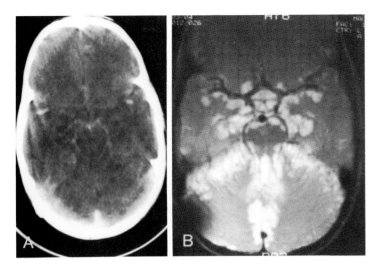

Figure 11.24. Meningeal tumor infiltration. Gliomatous arachnoid tumor deposits. Same case as Figure 5.5. *Axial chiasmatic cistern-level i.v. contrast 35/100 CT scan (A) and SE 2000/80 MR scan (B).* There is marked leptomeningeal MR T2 hyperintensity with only subtle CT contrast enhancement rimming slightly hypodense tumor deposits.

Differential Diagnosis of Sella Region Masses

In order to avoid repetition, a gamut system of differential diagnosis has been devised (Table 11.1, pages 255–257).

Cavernous Sinus Lesions

Pathological conditions involving the cavernous sinus include aneurysm, carotid cavernous fistula, thrombosis, and tumor invasion.

ANEURYSM

The subject of cavernous and suprasellar internal carotid artery aneurysms has already been discussed and illustrated (Fig. 11.19). Traumatic cavernous sinus false aneurysms may occasionally develop (Fig. 11.25). These false aneurysms have been briefly discussed in Chapter 6 (Fig. 6.37).

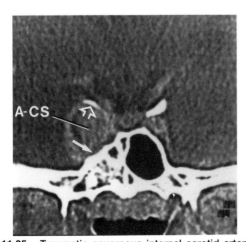

Figure 11.25. Traumatic cavernous internal carotid artery aneurysm (same case as Fig. 6.37). Direct coronal pituitary-level i.v. contrast CT scan of a patient who sustained a skull base fracture 6 months before this scan. There is right cavernous sinus expansion by a contrast-enhancing central aneurysm *(A-CS)* surrounded laterally by clot. Note the right lateral sphenoid sinus wall *(closed arrow)* and anterior clinoid process *(open arrow)* erosion.

CAROTID CAVERNOUS FISTULA

These lesions are spontaneous or acquired connections between the internal carotid artery and the cavernous sinus. They usually occur due to severe facial and skull trauma or a ruptured intracavernous carotid artery aneurysm. They may also be secondary to collagen deficiency syndromes, arterial dissection, fibromuscular dysplasia, and direct trauma.[43]

CT demonstrates enlargement of one or both cavernous sinuses and superior ophthalmic veins (most prominent on the fistula side), and edematous extraocular muscles (Fig. 11.26). The lateral wall of the involved cavernous sinus bulges and maintains a smooth margin.[17] Because the fistula develops slowly (days) after trauma, the immediate post-trauma study is usually normal. The fistula may enlarge to aneurysmal (pseudoaneurysm) size.[28] MR can demonstrate the fistula, flow effects, and identify abnormal, large, draining ophthalmic veins. Catheter balloon embolization is currently the therapeutic procedure of choice.[43]

CAVERNOUS SINUS THROMBOSIS

Cavernous venous sinus thrombosis is almost always caused by septic thrombophlebitis but occlusion can be caused by tumors or aneurysms. Contrast CT demonstrates irregular cavernous sinus filling defects, enlargement of the superior ophthalmic vein, and orbital soft tissue inflammatory change.[44] Sinus expansion and lateral wall bowing can be seen in cases of septic cavernous sinus thrombosis. In unusual cases, air may be seen within the cavernous sinus.[45] Not to be confused with air, fat deposition in the cavernous sinus in patients with Cushing's disease[46] and fat deposits in normal patients at juxtacavernous sinus dural margins can be identified by CT (Figs. 11.4G and 11.4H).

Despite the accuracy of CT and MR for demonstration of cavernous sinus detail, cavernous sinus occlusion is still difficult to document. Internal carotid ar-

Figure 11.26. Carotid cavernous fistula. *Axial cavernous sinus-level (A) and globe-level (B) i.v. contrast −5/400 CT scan.* There is an enlarged left cavernous sinus *(F-CS)* and an abnormal dilated tortuous ophthalmic vein *(open arrow)* and a markedly enlarged superior ophthalmic vein *(closed arrow).*

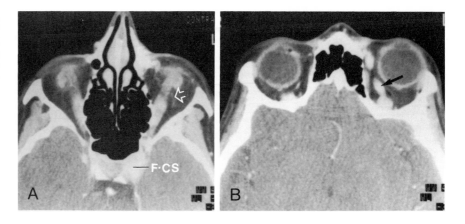

tery flow and tumor contrast enhancement within an occluded cavernous sinus can give the impression of partial patency by the CT technique. MR i.v. contrast enhancement of intracavernous tumor can simulate flow. The use of both gradient reversal and i.v. contrast MR techniques is our current preferred method for investigation of cavernous sinus flow. The gradient reversal MR technique can identify vascular flow as hyperintense regions. Comparison of the noncontrast T1-weighted image, the i.v. contrast T1-weighted image, and the gradient reversal image can then identify normal vessels and vascular spaces, nerves, and masses.[16]

TUMOR COMPRESSION AND INVASION

Tumor compression of the medial cavernous sinus wall is usually caused by pituitary adenoma. Lateral compression can be caused by meningiomas, neuromas, and epidermoid tumors. Internal carotid artery aneurysm, carotid cavernous fistulas, and neuromas may be responsible for intracavernous mass effects that laterally bow the normally straight lateral cav-

Figure 11.27. Sella changes after transsphenoidal hypophysectomy. **A–C** is a different case than **D**. First case: Growth hormone-secreting tumor in an acromegalic patient. *Sagittal 600/25 MR scans.* The preoperative scan **(A)** demonstrates a T1 white matter-isointense intrasellar and suprasellar mass that elevates and deforms the anterior third ventricle and obliterates optic chiasm *(OC)* and infundibulum detail. Three months after transphenoidal hypophysectomy **(B)**, the mass is no longer present, the optic chiasm *(OC)* is now clearly visualized, and the infundibulum *(I)* is surrounded by the CSF within the secondary empty sella. The pituitary gland is small, crescentic, and posterior. Beneath the pituitary gland, fatty tissue *(F)* used to pack the floor has a hyperintense T1 signal. At 1 year after surgery **(C)**, the fat signal has markedly diminished. Second case: *Direct coronal pituitary-level 36/150 i.v. contrast CT scan (D).* Post-transsphenoidal hypophysectomy. A cursor within the surgically introduced sella floor fat measures −74 H. Only a small amount of air *(A)* is seen in the recently postoperative sphenoid sinus. The pituitary gland *(P)* is borderline enlarged on the right side.

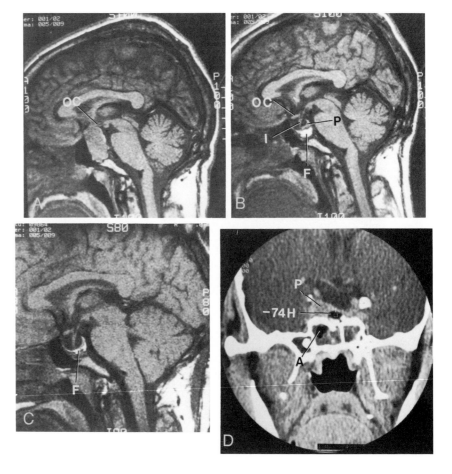

ernous sinus margin.[17] Despite the cavernous sinus distortion and compression, benign processes are associated with preservation of a smooth lateral wall. Metastasis to the cavernous sinus and perineural tumor extension from facial carcinoma produces irregular and lobular margins.[16,17,47]

MR is more effective than CT for demonstrating the internal carotid artery and tumor-related arterial abnormalities such as encasement and displacement.[16]

Postoperative Transsphenoidal Hypophysectomy Changes

Transsphenoidal surgical sella changes may be classified as complications, transient changes, and permanent changes.

Complications include hemorrhage, structural compression by packing material, CSF leak, tension pneumocephalus, and sinusitis. Hematoma and/or surgical packing can produce optic chiasm or cranial nerve compression with visual loss. The sella hematoma is often asymptomatic and its presence in the immediate postoperative period should not necessarily be a cause for alarm. Subarachnoid and paren-

chymal hemorrhage is uncommon. The cartilage used to reconstruct the sella floor may become dislodged. A "plug" of fatty tissue is usually placed in the sella cavity to prevent CSF leak. Tumor surgical resection and/or post-treatment regression in a patient with an enlarged sella may result in a secondary empty sella. The optic chiasm and nerves may herniate downward into the sella cavity, which only rarely leads to visual loss. CSF leak is an occasionally transsphenoidal hypophysectomy complication. Pneumocephalus may occur concurrently, particularly when a shunting procedure has been done for hydrocephalus.

Sella floor reconstruction and packing material produce CT and MR findings that include fat, soft tissue, and bone intrasellar densities and intensities. The fat density/intensity may diminish or disappear with time [months to years (Fig. 11.27)]. Associated permanent sinus changes include disrupted anterior and superior sphenoid sinus walls and sphenoid-ethmoid sinus opacities.[5,23] Sagittal and coronal MR can document optic chiasm and optic nerve herniation into a secondary empty sella (Fig. 11.28). CT may, occasionally, demonstrate this complication but with less detail and with a degree of uncertainty.

Following the surgical removal of a microadenoma, the pituitary gland may not return to normal height for several months.[48] One year after successful surgery of a growth hormone-secreting adenoma, CT (and probably MR) can demonstrate decreased thickness of the skull soft tissues and return to normal size of the extraocular muscles.[22]

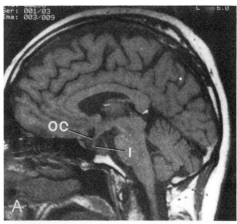

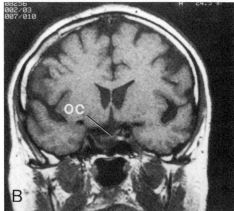

Figure 11.28. Tethered optic chiasm in secondary empty sella. *SE 600/25 midsagittal (A) and sella-level coronal (B) MR scans.* The enlarged sella is filled with CSF. There is an intrasellar optic chiasm *(OC).* The infundibulum *(I)* appears detached. Only a thin rim of possible pituitary tissue appears to line the sella floor.

References

1. Roppolo HMN, Latchaw RE, Meyer JD, Curtin HD. Normal pituitary gland: 1. Macroscopic anatomy—CT correlation. *AJNR* 1983; 4:927–935.
2. Roppolo HMN, Latchaw RE. Normal pituitary gland: 2. Microscope anatomy—CT correlation. *AJNR* 1983; 4:937–944.
3. Chambers EF, Turski PA, LaMasters D, Newton TH. Regions of low density in the contrast enhanced pituitary gland: Normal and pathologic processes. *Radiology* 1982; 144:109–113.
4. Bonneville JF, Cattin F, Portha C, et al. Computed tomographic demonstration of the posterior pituitary. *AJNR* 1985; 6:889–892.
5. Kucharczyk W. The pituitary gland and sella turcica. In Brant-Zawadzki M, Norman D (Eds.). *Magnetic Resonance Imaging of the Central Nervous System.* New York: Raven Press, 1987; 187–208.
6. Colombo N, Berry I, Kucharczyk J, et al. Posterior pituitary gland: Appearance on MR images in normal and pathologic states. *Radiology* 1987; 165:481–485.
7. Wolpert SM, Osborn M, Anderson M, Runge VM. The bright pituitary gland. A normal MR appearance in infancy. *AJNR* 1988; 9:1–3.
8. Peyster RG, Hoover ED, Viscarello RR, et al. CT appearance of the adolescent and preadolescent pituitary gland. *AJNR* 1983; 4:411–414.
9. Wolpert SM, Molitch ME, Goldman JA, Wood JB. Size, shape and appearance of the normal female pituitary gland. *AJNR* 1984; 5:263–267.
10. Peyster RG, Hoover ED, Adler PL. CT of the normal pituitary stalk. *AJNR* 1984; 5:45–47.
11. Peyster RG, Hoover ED. CT of the abnormal pituitary stalk. *AJNR* 1984; 5:49–52.
12. Seidle FG, Towbin R, Kaufman RA. Normal pituitary stalk size in children: CT study. *AJNR* 1985; 6:733–738.

13. Daniels DL, Pojunas KW, Kilgore DP, et al. MR of the diaphragma sellae. *AJNR* 1986; 7:765–769.
14. Haughton VM, Rosenbaum AE, Williams AL, Drayer B. Recognizing the empty sella by CT: The infundibulum sign. *AJNR* 1980; 1:527–529.
15. Kaufman B, Tomsak RL, Kaufman BA, et al. Herniation of the suprasellar visual system and third ventricle into empty sella: Morphologic and clinical considerations. *ANJR* 1989; 10:65–76.
16. Daniels DL, Czervionke LF, Bonneville JF, et al. Magnetic resonance imaging of the cavernous sinus. Value of spin echo and gradient recalled echo images. *AJNR* 1988; 9:947–952.
17. Kline LB, Acker JD, Post MJD, Vitek JJ. The cavernous sinus: A computed tomographic study. *AJNR* 1981; 2:299–305.
18. Hasso AN, Pop PM, Thompson JR, et al. High resolution thin section computed tomography of the cavernous sinus. *Radiographics* 1982; 2:83–100.
19. Maravilla KR. The sella and suprasellar region. In Gonzalez CF, Grossman CB, Masdeu JC (Eds.). *Head and Spine Imaging.* New York: John Wiley & Sons, 1985; 639–673.
20. Turski PA, Newton TH, Horten BH. Sellar contour: Anatomic polytomographic correlation. *AJR* 1981; 137:213–216.
21. Virapongse C, Bhimani S, Sarwar M, et al. Prolactin-secreting pituitary adenomas: CT appearance in diffuse invasion. *Radiology* 1984; 152:447–471.
22. Kaplan HC, Baker HL, Houser OW, et al. CT of the sella turcica after transsphenoidal resection of pituitary adenomas. *AJNR* 1985; 6:723–732.
23. Dolinskas CA, Simeone FA. Transsphenoidal hypophysectomy: Postsurgical CT findings. *AJR* 1985; 144:487–492.
24. Chernow B, Buck DR, Early CB. Rapid shrinkage of a prolactin-secreting pituitary tumor with bromocriptine: CT documentation. *AJNR* 1982; 3:442–443.
25. Scotti G, Yu C-Y, Dillon W, et al. MR imaging of the cavernous sinus involvement by pituitary adenomas. *AJNR* 1988; 9:657–664.
26. Davis PC, Hoffman JC, Malko JA. Gadolinium-DTPA and MR imaging of pituitary adenoma: a preliminary report. *AJNR* 1987; 8:817–823.
27. Karnaze MG, Sartor K, Winthrop JD, et al. Suprasellar lesions: Evaluation with MR imaging. *Radiology* 1986; 161:77–82.
28. Daniels DL. The sella and juxtasellar region. In Williams AL, Haughton VM (Eds). *Cranial Computed Tomography.* St. Louis: CV Mosby Co, 1985; 444–511.
29. Daniels DL, Williams AL, Thornton RS, et al. Differential diagnosis of intrasellar tumors by computed tomography. *Radiology* 1981; 141:697–701.
30. Kucharczyk W, Davis DO, Kelly WM. Pituitary adenomas: High resolution MR imaging at 1.5T. *Radiology* 1986; 161:761–765.
31. Dwyer AJ, Frank JA, Doppman JL, et al. Pituitary adenomas in patients with Cushing's disease: Initial experience with Gd-DTPA-enhanced MR imaging. *Radiology* 1987; 163:421–426.
32. Peck WW, Dillon WP, Norman D, et al. High resolution MR imaging of microadenomas at 1.5T: Experience with Cushing's disease. *AJNR* 1988; 9:1085–1091.
33. Okamoto S, Handa H, Yamashita J, et al. Computed tomography in intra- and suprasellar epithelial cysts (symptomatic Rathke cleft cysts). *AJNR* 1985; 6:515–519.
34. Kjos BO, Brant-Zawadzki M, Kucharczyk W, et al. Cystic intracranial lesions: Magnetic resonance imaging. *Radiology* 1985; 155:363–369.
35. Quencer RM. Lymphocytic adenohypophysitis: Autoimmune disorder of the pituitary gland. *AJNR* 1980; 1:343–345.
36. Pusey E, Kortman KE, Flannigan BD, et al. MR of craniopharyngiomas, tumor delineation and characterization. *AJNR* 1987; 8:439–444.
37. Zimmerman EA. Congenital tumors. In Rowland LP (Ed). *Merritt's Textbook of Neurology.* Philadelphia: Lea & Febiger, 7th ed. 1984; 250–251.
38. Fitz CR. Neoplastic diseases. In Gonzalez CF, Grossman CB, Masdeu JC (Eds). *Head and Spine Imaging.* New York: John Wiley & Sons, 1985; p. 483–521.
39. Lanzieri CF, Sacher M, Sam PM. CT changes in the septum pellucidum associated with intraventricular craniopharyngiomas. *J Computer Assist Tomogr* 1985; 9:507–510.
40. Spagnoli MV, Goldberg HI, Grossman RI, et al. Intracranial meningiomas: High field MR imaging. *Radiology* 1986; 161:369–375.
41. Brant-Zawadzki M, Kelly W. Brain tumors. In Brant-Zawadzki M, Norman D (Eds). *Magnetic Resonance Imaging of the Central Nervous System.* New York: Raven Press, 1987; 151–185.
42. Suss RA, Maravilla KR, Thompson J. MR imaging of intracranial cysticercosis: comparison with CT and anatopathologic features. *AJNR* 1986; 7:235–242.
43. Halbach VV, Hieshima GB, Higashida RT, Reicher M. Carotid cavernous fistulae: indications for urgent treatment. *AJNR* 1987; 8:627–633.
44. Ahmadi J, Deane JR, Seagall HD, Zee CS. CT observations pertinent to septic cavernous sinus thrombus. *AJNR* 1985; 6:755–758.
45. Cunes JT, Creasy JL, Whaley RL, Scatliff JH. Air in the cavernous sinus: A new sign of septic cavernous sinus thrombosis. *AJNR* 1987; 8:176–177 (correspondence).
46. Bachow TB, Hesselin KJR, Aaron JO, et al. Fat deposition in the cavernous sinus in Cushing disease. *Radiology* 1984; 153:135–136.
47. Woodruff WW Jr, Yeates AE, McLendon RE. Perineural tumor extension to the cavernous sinus from superficial facial carcinoma: CT manifestations. *Radiology* 1986; 161:395–399.
48. Teng MMH, Huang C-I, Chang T. The pituitary mass after transsphenoidal hypophysectomy. *AJNR* 1988; 9:23–26.

CHAPTER
12

The Temporal Region

Introduction
Temporal Bone Anatomy
Congenital Anomalies
Trauma
Inflammatory Disease

The Postoperative Ear (for inflammatory conditions)
Neoplasms, Cysts, and Other Masses
Osteodystrophies

Introduction

The dense otic capsule surrounding the hypodense inner ear structures, the contrasting ossicles and air of the tympanum, and the air-bone contrast of the mastoid sinus are reasons that CT still has a primary role for investigation of the petrous pyramid. Furthermore, MR fails to demonstrate contrast between the osseous and air-containing ear structures. MR is the method of choice for investigation of soft tissue abnormalities and CT is the procedure of choice for investigation of osseous abnormalities of the temporal region. The most common indication for imaging the petrous region is for diagnosis of acoustic neuroma, cholesteatoma, or trauma. CT scanning for otosclerosis has recently been a subject of renewed interest in the radiology literature. The preference for MR of acoustic neuroma is quite obvious. Such soft tissue masses, even small ones, can be distinguished from adjacent structures by various MR techniques. Lack of bone-related CT artifact adds to the MR advantage. Intravenous contrast injection MR imaging is the standard method for investigation of acoustic neuroma. On the other hand, the CT-targeted small FOV technique is the standard method for evaluation of cholesteatoma, otosclerosis, and temporal bone fractures because of bone detail of such structures as the otic capsule, ossicles, and the facial nerve canal. The ease and accuracy of the CT method for investigation of acute trauma is an additional advantage over MR. For many circumstances, CT and MR play complementary roles and, for others, they may provide identical information. An example of the complementary role of the two methods is the analysis of acquired cholesteatoma for the condition of the ossicles and petrous pyramids (CT) and for possible intracranial erosion and extension (MR).

This chapter will discuss anatomy and pathology of the temporal region and applications of both the MR and CT methods for structural definition and demonstration of abnormalities.

Before considering normal imaging anatomy, basic anatomy of the petrous bone will be described. The anatomical course of the facial nerve and the eighth cranial nerves will be discussed in some detail due to their great clinical importance and as a way of integrating anatomical relationships of petrous structures (Fig. 12.1). We will look at temporal bone axial sections from caudal to cranial, coronal sections from posterior to anterior, and sagittal sections from medial to lateral. Figures 12.2–12.5 demonstrate CT and MR normal petrous anatomy.

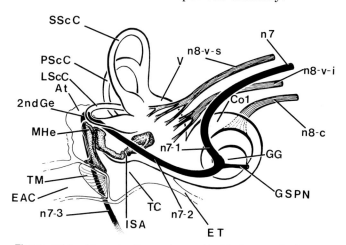

Figure 12.1. Normal otic anatomy. Modified coronal diagram demonstrating the first division of the facial nerve and nervus intermedius *(n7)* superior to the cochlear nerve *(n8-c)* within the anterior internal auditory canal. They are in front of the superior *(n8-v-s)* and inferior *(n8-v-i)* divisions of the vestibular nerve. The cochlear nerve enters the modiolus nucleus of the cochlea and the vestibular nerve enters the vestibule *(V)*. The cochlea is anterior-inferior to the vestibule. The posterior semicircular canal *(PScC)* shares a common crus with the superior semicircular canal *(SScC)*. The tympanic membrane *(TM)* separates the external auditory canal *(EAC)* from the tympanic cavity *(TC)*. The malleus head *(MHe)* in the attic *(At)* and incudostapedial articulation *(ISA)* are labeled. The facial nerve exits the internal auditory canal close to its junction with the vestibule and enters the facial nerve canal as the labyrinthine segment *(n7-1)*. The first segment of the facial nerve canal curves around the cochlear base turn *(Co1)*. The first genu of the facial nerve is at the geniculate ganglion *(GG)*. The greater superficial petrosal nerve *(GSPN)* arises at this point. The horizontal portion of the facial nerve canal *(n7-2)* in the medial tympanic wall is cranial to the oval window and caudal to the lateral semicircular canal *(LScC)*. At this point, it courses downward at the second genu *(2nd Ge)* and becomes the "vertical" or third segment of the facial nerve *(n7-3)*. It exits from the vertical facial canal of the mastoid bone at the stylomastoid foramen. The eustachean tube *(ET)* is shown communicating with the tympanum.

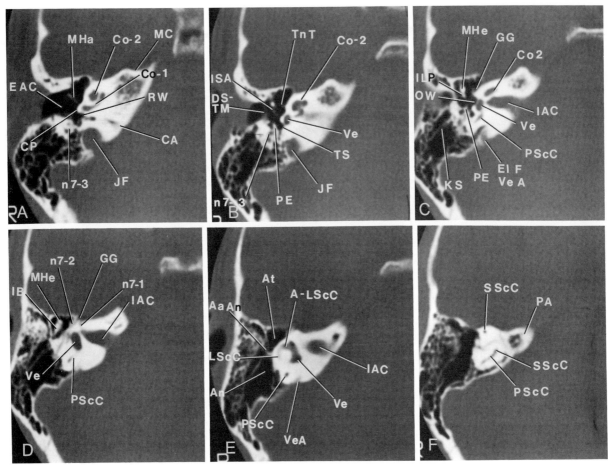

Figure 12.2. *Normal axial 365/4000* **(A–F)** *and direct coronal 1200/ 4000 and 700/3000* **(H–L)** *1.5-mm thickness, 12.8-cm FOV, bone filter, target technique CT scans.* **A–F, G,** *and* **H–L** *are different cases.* The axial sections are presented caudal to cranial and the coronal sections from posterior to anterior. Different WL/WW techniques are required to optimize detail of different structures due principally to bone density and structural size, shape, and thickness. A list of label abbreviations used throughout this chapter appears below. Note how the malleus handle *(MHa)* parallels the tympanic membrane *(dotted lines)*. The round window is seen on coronal sections posterior to the oval window. *AaAn = aditus ad antrum; A-LScC = anterior limb lateral semicircular canal; An = antrum; At = attic or epitympanic recess; CA = cochlear aqueduct; CC = carotid canal; Co = coch-lea; Co1 = cochlea first turn; Co2 = cochlea second turn; CfP = cochleariform process; CP = cochlear prominence; DS = drum spur; EAC = external auditory canal; ElF = endolymphatic fossa; FC = falciform crest; GG = geniculate ganglion; HT = hypotympanum;*

IAC = internal auditory canal; IB = incus body; ILP = incus long process; ISA = incudostapedial articulation; ISP = incus short process; JF = jugular fossa; KS = Koëmer septum or spur; LScC = lateral semicircular canal; Li = limbus; MHa = malleus handle; MHe = malleus head: MC = Meckel's cave; n7-1 = seventh cranial nerve—labyrinthine segment; n7-2 = seventh cranial nerve—horizontal segment; n7-3 = seventh cranial nerve—vertical segment; n8-c = cochlear division—eighth cranial nerve; n8-v = vestibular division—eighth cranial nerve; n8-vi = inferior division vestibular nerve; n8-vs = superior division vestibular nerve; OW = oval window; PA = petrous apex; PE = pyramidal eminence; POS = petro-occipital suture; PS = Prussak's space; PScC = posterior semicircular canal; RW = round window; SScC = superior semicircular canal; TM = tympanic membrane; TS = tympanic sinus; TgT = tegmen tympani; TnT = tensor tympani; Ve = vestibule; VeA = vestibular aqueduct.

The symptoms most responsible for temporal bone imaging are disorders of hearing, vertigo, draining ear, and facial nerve dysfunction. These symptoms draw clinical attention to the petrous pyramid. Studies for the jugular foramen are less common.

Temporal Bone Anatomy

The four major portions of the temporal bone are petrous, tympanic, mastoid, and squamous. The wedge-shaped petrous portion contains the inner ear and the tympanic portion surrounds the tympanic membrane and forms the external auditory canal anterior and inferior wall. The mastoid portion contributes to the posterior external canal, the posterior middle ear, and includes the mastoid antrum and sinus. The squamous portion forms part of the lateral skull. The jugular foramen is bounded anteriorly by the temporal bone and posteriorly by the occipital bone.[1]

Figure 12.1 is a schematic representation of the seventh and eighth cranial nerve course and internal and middle ear structural relationships.

EAR

Inner Ear

The beginning of the internal auditory canal (porus acousticus interna) is defined by closure of the

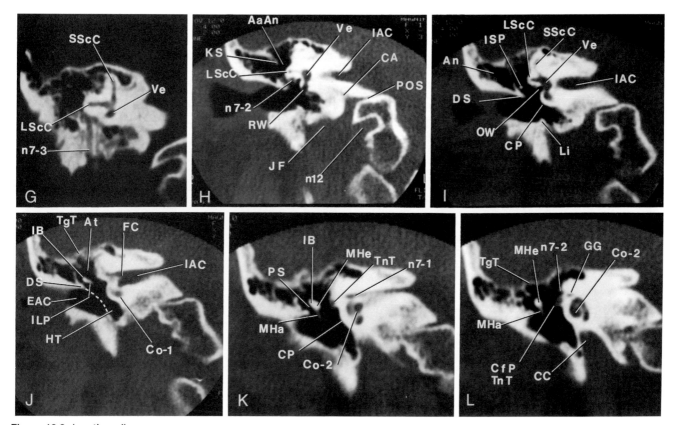

Figure 12.2. (continued)

petrous groove at the canal posterior wall. The internal auditory canal is oriented in approximately the coronal plane as compared to the 45° off-coronal plane of the petrous pyramid. The canal ends at the vestibule. The vestibule is attached to the semicircular canals and the cochlea and, together, this three-part unit is called the labyrinth. The vestibular aqueduct is the bone canal for the endolymphatic duct. The duct begins at the common crus of the posterior and superior semicircular canals and ends at the endolymphatic fossa in the epidural space on the posterior margin of the petrous pyramid (Figs. 12.2C and E).

The cochlea is anteroinferior to the posterosuperior semicircular canals. It has 2½ to 2¾ turns. The cochlear basal turn forms the middle ear cochlear promontory (Figs. 12.2A and K). The round window is a membrane-covered opening in the cochlear basal turn that transmits perilymph vibrations to cochlear endolymph. It is seen on coronal CT sections just posterior to the plane of the oval window (Fig. 12.2H). The cochlear aqueduct (Figs. 12.2A and H) is found below and parallel to the internal auditory canal. It connects the cochlear perilymph with the subarachnoid space at the posterior medial surface of the petrous pyramid. Its functional significance has not been established.[1] The complex cavity within the petrous temporal bone housing these structures is called the osseous labyrinth and the membranous sacs, ducts, and organs within the osseous portion are collec-

tively called the membranous labyrinth. The membranous labyrinth contains endolymph and is surrounded by perilymph.[1]

Sound vibrations are mechanically transferred by the ossicular chain to the stapes footplate at the vestibular oval window. The foot plate conducts the vibrations to the cochlear perilymph which, in turn, transmits them to the cochlear endolymph. The cochlear endolymphatic space contains the organ of Corti where small hair cells convert the vibrations to nerve impulses.[1]

The posterior semicircular canal is parallel to the posterior petrous pyramid [Fig. 12.2D and E (45° "off-coronal")] and the three semicircular canals are perpendicularly arranged. They are sensitive to head position and send sensory equilibrium input to the brain.

Middle Ear

The middle ear (tympanum) is the pneumatized space that lies between the tympanic membrane and the labyrinth and contains the ossicles, the stapedius, and tensor tympani muscles and a portion of the chorda tympani nerve. Vertically, the middle ear is divided into the epitympanum (attic), the mesotympanum, and the hypotympanum. The epitympanum and mesotympanum communicate at the tympanic isthmus, which is at the level of the tensor tympani tendon and stapes (coronal sections, Fig. 12.2).[2] The isthmus is a relatively narrow passage-

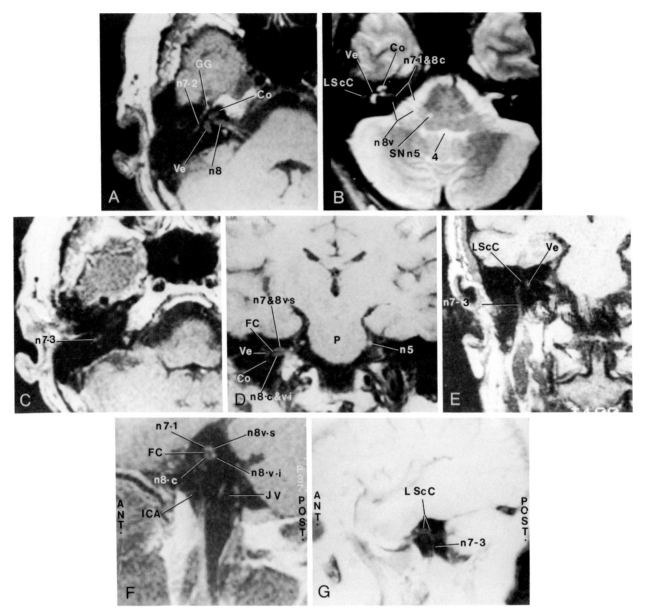

Figure 12.3. Normal petrous temporal MR anatomy. *All but **B** are SE 600/25 images. **B** is a 5-mm SE 2800/80 axial image at the same level as **A**. Axial fourth ventricle-level 3-mm thickness **(A)** and more inferior level **(C)**. Coronal slightly rotated pons-level **(D)** and more posterior level **(E)**. Sagittal 3-mm internal auditory canal-level **(F)** and more lateral **(G)**. The facial nerve (n7) and vestibular (n8-v) and cochlear nerve (n8-c) are seen within the internal auditory canal. The cochlea (Co) is anterior to the vestibule (Ve). The vestibular nerve is divided by the falciform crest (FC). Above the falciform crest is the first segment of the facial nerve (n7-1) anterior and vestibular nerve* superior division (n8-v-s) posterior. Below the falciform crest is the cochlear nerve (n8-c) anterior and the vestibular nerve inferior division (n8-v-i) posterior. The internal carotid artery (ICA) is anterior to the jugular vein (JV). The geniculate ganglion (GG) is seen anterior to the facial canal second segment (n7-2) **(A)**. The lateral semicircular canal (LScC) is seen above the third segment (n7-3) of facial nerve. In **B**, the seventh and eighth nerves approach the region of the spinal nucleus of the fifth nerve (SNn5) in the medulla. The trigeminal nerve root (n5) is seen emerging from the pons in **D**.

way that is particularly susceptible to obstruction in the inflamed tympanum. The narrow communication between the middle ear epitympanum and the mastoid sinus antrum is called the aditus ad antrum (Fig. 12.2E and H). Blockage of the aditus by inflammatory processes frequently occurs in chronic otomastoiditis. The "handle" of the malleus is the arm attached to the tympanic membrane [Fig. 12.2L (eardrum)]. The malleolar neck is between the head

and the handle of the malleus. The tensor tympani inserts on the malleolar neck and is seen on most coronal sections extending from the insertion to the cochleariform process where it often creates a "semicanal" (Fig. 12.2B, K, and L). Medially, parallel to the handle is the long process of the incus that articulates with the stapes (Fig. 12.2B, C, and J). The stapes has two crura that join at the footplate. The stapedius tendon arises in the pyramidal eminence

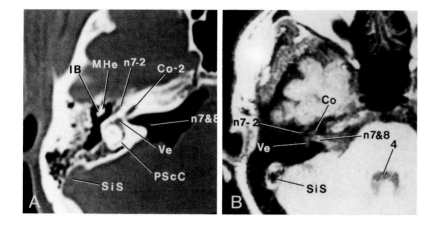

Figure 12.4. CPA air cisternogram compared to the same level MR scan. Same patient. *Axial 600/3200 1.5-mm thickness bone filter CT air cisternogram (A). Same level SE 600/25 3-mm thickness MR scan (B).* The head of the malleus *(MHe)* and body of the incus *(IB)* have an "ice cream cone" relationship. The vestibule *(Ve)* lies between the cochlea *(Co-2)* and the semicircular canals *(PScC).* The horizontal portion of the seventh cranial nerve *(n7-2)* is within tympanic cavity medial wall. The neurovascular bundle *(n7 & 8)* is surrounded by air **(A).** Middle ear detail is absent on the MR scan. There is sigmoid sinus MR flow effect *(SiS);* fourth ventricle *(4).*

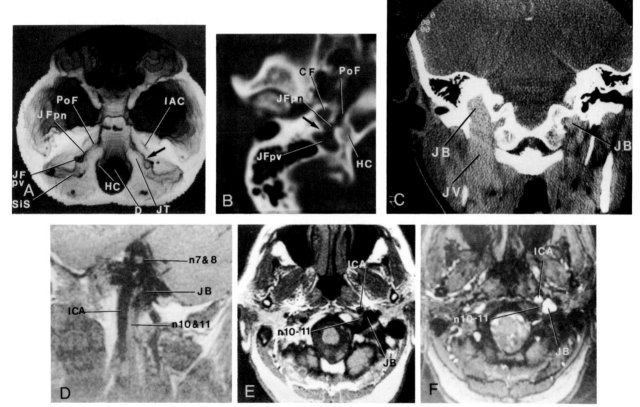

Figure 12.5. The jugular foramen. **A–C** are different cases. **D–F** are the same case. *Axial 3-mm section CT reformation (A) Axial 825/3000 5-mm thickness, 20-cm FOV soft tissue filter (B) and i.v. contrast direct coronal 50/300 3-mm thickness, 16-cm FOV bone filter (C) CT scans. Sagittal (D) and axial (E) SE 600/25 3-mm thickness, 18-cm FOV MR scans. Axial same level as E, 3-mm thickness gradient echo 50/17 30° flip angle 4-NEX, 18-cm FOV MR scan (F).* The 3-D reformation shows the dens of C2 *(D)* at the tip of the foramen magnum just under the clivus inferior lip (basion). The hypoglossal canal *(HC)* is directly under the jugular tubercle *(JT).* The parieto-occipital fissure *(PoF)* contains the inferior petrosal sinus. The jugular foramen is divided by the petrous jugular spine *(arrow)* into the pars venosa *(JFpv)* posteriorly and the pars nervosa *(JFpn)* anteriorly. The sigmoid sinus groove *(SiS)* leads to the pars venosa.

The porus acousticus of the internal auditory canal *(IAC)* is seen in the posterior surface of the petrous pyramid. The carotid foramen *(CF)* is anteromedial to the jugular foramen. **C** demonstrates a very large, high-position right jugular bulb *(JB)* and a more common size and position left jugular bulb. Contrast is demonstrated in both jugular veins *(JV)* including the bulb portions. The jugular bulb is posterolateral to the internal carotid artery *(ICA)* and is separated from the artery at the inferior skull base by a bony ridge which is best demonstrated by gradient echo axial and sagittal technique. The vagus *(n10)* and accessory *(n11)* nerves are immediately anteromedial to the jugular bulb. The glossopharyngeal nerve, not clearly identifiable in this case, is in the pars nervosa posteromedial to the internal carotid artery and is anterior to cranial nerves X and XI *(n10 & 11).*

and inserts on the posterior crus (Fig. 12.2.**B**). The stapes is normally visualized by axial and coronal CT. The head of the malleus articulates with the body of the incus and the combined "ossicular mass" is equidistant from the medial and lateral walls of the epitympanum (Fig. 12.2**D** and **K**). The ossicular mass has the shape of an ice cream cone on axial sections (Fig. 12.2**D**). Prussak's space is a space medial to the scutum (drum spur) and lateral to the malleolar neck (Fig. 12.2**K**). Acquired cholesteatomas most frequently arise in this space.[2]

External Ear

The medial two-thirds of the external auditory canal is osseous and the lateral one-third is cartilagenous. The tympanic membrane is at the medial end of the external auditory canal. It angles medially from top to bottom and laterally from front to back.[1] It inserts superiorly on the drum spur and inferiorly on the limbus (Fig. 12.2**I** and **J**).

SEVENTH AND EIGHTH CRANIAL NERVES

The facial nerve exits the brainstem at the cerebellopontine angle (CPA) accompanied by the intermediate nerve (nervus intermedius or nerve of Wrisberg). It has the longest intraosseous course of any nerve and it is the most frequently paralyzed in the human body.[3] It courses the CPA to enter the internal auditory canal and then, in turn, it enters the facial nerve canal (Figs. 12.1 and 12.2**K**).[3,4]

The facial nerve within the internal auditory canal lies above the falciform crest anterior to the superior vestibular division of the eighth cranial nerve. This segment is called the "canalicular or meatal" portion (not to be confused with that portion in the facial nerve canal).[4] The falciform crest separates the facial nerve above from the cochlear division of the eighth nerve below. The inferior vestibular division is posterior to the cochlear nerve (Figs. 12.1, 12.2**J**, 12.3**B**, and **F**).[3,4]

The facial nerve has three arbitrarily named divisions (segments) within the facial nerve canal: (a) labyrinthine, (b) tympanic or horizontal, and (c) mastoid or vertical. The canal begins close to the internal auditory canal-vestibular junction. The labyrinthine portion of the canal curves around the cochlear base, turns in the intervestibulocochlear groove, and increases in caliber to accommodate the geniculate ganglion (Figs. 12.2**D**, **L**, and 12.3**A**). Transverse temporal fractures commonly compromise the labyrinthine facial nerve segment. The greater superficial petrosal nerve derives from the intermediate nerve at the ganglion to supply the lacrimal and parotid glands, respectively (Fig. 12.1).[3,4]

The tympanic (horizontal) segment of the facial nerve canal begins at the first (or anterior) genu of the facial nerve. The tympanic segment courses along the inner wall of the tympanic cavity (Figs. 12.2**D**, **H**, 12.3**A** and 12.4) posteriorly above the oval window and below the prominence of the lateral semi-

circular canal (Figs. 12.1 and 12.3**A**). The vertical portion of the facial nerve canal begins at the second genu under the lateral semicircular canal (Fig. 12.3**E**). Congenital bone dehiscence of the tympanic segment is common resulting in nerve protrusion into the anterior epitympanic space inferior to the horizontal semicircular canal near the oval window. The tympanic segment is particularly susceptible to erosion by tubotympanic diseases. Due to the roughly horizontal plane of the labyrinthine and tympanic segments of the facial nerve canal, these first two segments are best imaged in the axial projections.[3,4] For petrous axial CT, a $+15°$ image plane is recommended in order to avoid unnecessary lens dose without compromising imaging quality.[5] Gd-DTPA contrast enhancement of facial nerves in some patients with temporal bone, internal auditory canal, or cerebellopontine angle masses has been demonstrated in a small series[6] but we have not found enhancement of normal facial nerves.

The facial canal medial to the ossicles then curves downward (posterior or second genu) in its mastoid or "vertical" portion. The nerve exits the mastoid bone at the stylomastoid foramen. The mastoid segment of the facial nerve gives origin to the nerve of the stapedius muscle and the chorda tympani. The jugular bulb is medial to the stylomastoid foramen.[3,4]

Sagittal and coronal MR imaging of the mastoid segment of the facial nerve and coronal CT imaging is optimal. Although the mastoid "vertical" segment of the nerve (MR) and canal (CT) can be imaged sectionally in the axial plane, sagittal and coronal planar technique best demonstrates its course (Figs. 12.2**G**, 12.3**E**, and **G**).[3] The mastoid segment of the facial nerve canal is more easily demonstrated by CT in poorly pneumatized mastoid sinuses (Fig. 12.2**G**). Because the mastoid segment of the canal is more densely corticated than mastoid air cells, it can often be identified by axial and coronal CT even in patients with normal mastoid sinus pneumatization.[3,4] CPA air or CO_2 cisternography is rarely used in this MR era (Fig. 12.4).

JUGULAR FORAMEN

The jugular foramen lies between the posterior petrous temporal bone and the occipital bone just lateral to the foramen magnum. It is divided into the pars venosa posteriorly and the pars nervosa anteriorly by a fibrous or osseous band between the petrous jugular spine and the jugular process of the occipital bone (Fig. 12.5). The pars nervosa contains cranial nerve IX (glossopharyngeal) and the inferior petrosal sinus. The pars venosa (pars vascularis) contains the jugular bulb, and nerves X (vagus) and XI (spinal accessory). The pars venosa is usually larger on the right side.

Axial and direct coronal CT accurately identifies the jugular foramen (Fig. 12.5). After CT i.v. contrast injection, nerves IX, X, and XI can produce characteristic filling defects in the anteromedial jugular foramen, particularly if scanned 35 sec after i.v. bolus technique.[7]

MR demonstrates the jugular foramen vascular and neural anatomy in orthogonal planes with great accuracy. Thin-section T1-weighted axial MR technique is recommended in order to demonstrate the nerves IX, X, and XI in a horizontal course from the medulla (Fig. 4.10). T1-weighted images, however, do not accurately or dependably distinguish the jugular vein from the osseous jugular foramen margins. Gradient echo axial techniques can produce vascular enhancement, which distinguishes jugular venous flowing blood (markedly hyperintense) from osseous jugular foramen margins (markedly hypointense) and nerves IX, X, and XI (brainstem isointense) (Fig. 12.5). Gradient echo sections demonstrate nerve IX lateral to the inferior petrosal sinus and nerves X and XI medial to the jugular bulb. The carotid artery anteriorly is separated on sagittal sections from the jugular vein at the skull base by a bony ridge.[8] The carotid canal on coronal sections should appear directly below the cochlea (Fig. 12.2L).

Congenital Anomalies

Inner ear development from the primitive otocyst occurs during the second and third fetal month which is earlier than the independent development of the middle and external ear. For this reason, combined inner and middle-external anomalies are unusual with the exception of oval window absence or atresia associated with middle-external anomalies. There is, therefore, earlier fetal development of neurosensory than conductive hearing anomalies. Congenital osseous anomalies of the middle and external ear usually coexist[1] such as ossicular dysplasia and atretic external auditory canal, however, middle ear deformities may occur separately.[9,11]

Inner ear deformities vary in degree from total aplasia (Michel deformity) to different degrees of dysplasia (Fig. 12.6). Sensorineural hearing deficits vary from total deafness to barely detectable compromise. Total labyrinthine aplasia is a rare event. Varying degrees of cochlear, vestibular, and semicircular canal anomalies have been included under the category of "Mondini malformations." Cochlear deformities vary from severe dysplasias such as an unstructured cochlear cavity to a decrease of cochlear turns. Vestibular-semicircular canal anomalies also markedly vary in degree from gross deformity of the osseous labyrinth to only membranous labyrinthine changes that are not detectable by CT. A short broad lateral semicircular canal is fairly common and is often asymptomatic.[10] Inner ear anomalies may occasionally be associated with CSF otorrhea and may be complicated by meningitis.[1] Inner ear dysplasia is rarely associated with external ear anomalies due to their separate embryological origins.

Other congenital inner ear and petrous temporal bone abnormalities may occur without associated labyrinthine anomaly. These include lateral malposition of the internal carotid artery ("ectopic" internal carotid artery) (Fig. 12.7) and jugular bulb malposition and dilatation. The ectopic internal carotid artery bulges into the hypotympanic recess lateral to the cochlear sagittal plane. Jugular bulb dilatation and malposition may cause sensoroneural hearing loss by impinging upon the internal auditory canal or it may cause conductive hearing loss by impinging upon the middle ear compartment (Fig. 12.8).[1] Both the ectopic internal carotid artery and the malpositioned jugular bulb may present clinically as a middle ear mass. Correct diagnosis can obviate potentially very dangerous surgical sequellae.

CT is the imaging study of choice for investigation of inner ear anomalies. These abnormalities include hypoplastic internal auditory canal, saccular cochlea, and dilated deformed semicircular canals.[1]

MR complements the CT osseous labyrinthine findings by demonstrating membranous abnormalities such as atresia or stenosis of the endolymphatic spaces, eighth nerve hypoplasia and abnormal size, shape and position of the cochlea, vestibule, and semicircular canals.

Middle ear deformities cause conductive hearing deficits and can be categorized as ossicular, fenestral, and cholesteatomatous. Ossicular deformities include incudostapedial disconnections (most common), malleoincudal fixations and fusions, stapes fixations, absent stapes, and middle ear dysplasia.[1,9,10]

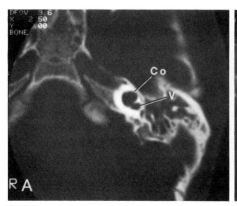
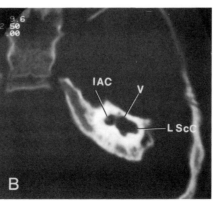

Figure 12.6.   Congenital inner ear dysplasia. *Axial 1.5-mm 850/4000 CT scans.* ***B** is 4 mm cranial to **A.*** There is marked dysplasia of the cochlea *(Co)* and lateral semicircular canal *(LScC)* characterized by lack of cochlear turns and semicircular canal dilatation. The internal auditory canal *(IAC)* has a particularly steep and almost vertical course in this patient resulting in the IAC fundus position directly above the cochlea. (Courtesy of Heun Y. Yune, M.D., Indianapolis, IN.)

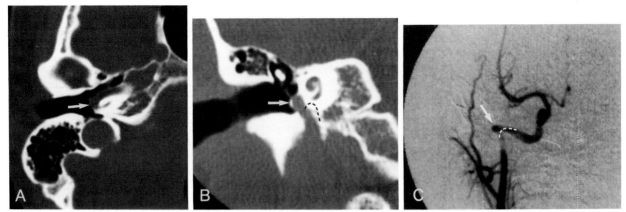

Figure 12.7. Aberrant internal carotid artery. A.*1.2-mm cochlear promontory-level axial 500/4000 and coronal 900/4000 **(B)** CT scans. Digital subtraction AP view right common carotid arteriogram **(C).** The petrous segment of the internal carotid artery courses abnormally laterally and craniad (arrow). It protrudes into the hypotym-* panum. A thin bone septum between the hypotympanum and the petrous carotid artery is seen (arrow, **B**). The theoretical normal course of an internal carotid artery is drawn as a dashed line. (Courtesy of Heun Y. Yune, M.D., Indianapolis, IN.)

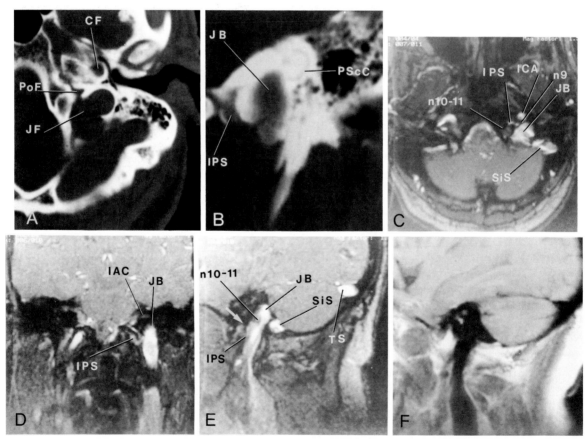

Figure 12.8. Markedly large jugular vein. *Axial **(A)** and direct coronal **(B)** 650/3000 3-mm section 16-cm FOV bone filter CT scans. Axial **(C),** coronal **(D),** and sagittal **(E)** gradient echo 50/17 30° tip-angle, 3-mm thickness 18-cm FOV, 4-NEX MR scans. Sagittal SE 600/25 10-mm thickness, 20-cm FOV MR scan **(F).*** The left jugular foramen (JF) is very large and high in position. It reaches its apex posteriorly where it abuts the ampulla of the posterior semicircular canal (PScC). More anteriorly, the jugular bulb (JB) is just beneath the internal auditory canal (IAC). The inferior petrosal sinus (IPS) within the petro-occipital fissure (PoF) has an unusual downward "kink."

The axial gradient echo MR section demonstrates the large jugular bulb and the relationships of cranial nerves (n9, n10, and n11) to it, to the internal carotid artery (ICA) and to the inferior petrosal sinus. The bony ridge that separates the internal carotid artery and the internal jugular vein at the inferior petrosal margin (arrow) and the distinction between vascular and osseous structures is clear with gradient echo and not with spin-echo technique. More laterally, the internal carotid artery will be seen anterior to the ridge on sagittal images. The sigmoid sinus (SiS) and transverse sinus (TS) are easily identified with gradient echo technique.

Stapes fixations are more common than malleoincudal, however, the stapes fixation may be beyond the limits of CT detection. Malleoincudal fixation usually appears as an attic band attaching the malleus and/or incus to the epitympanic wall (Fig. 12.9).[9] Isolated middle ear fenestral anomalies are rare. Oval window absence or atresia is usually associated with facial nerve canal, ossicular chain, and inner ear anomalies. Middle ear congenital cholesteatomas represent 2% of all middle ear cholesteatomas and are considered to be congenital only if there is an intact tympanic membrane and absence of otitis media. Otherwise, it is similar pathologically and in imaging appearance to acquired cholesteatoma.[9]

CT is the imaging procedure of choice for the osseous ossicular and fenestral and osseous and soft tissue cholesteatomatous abnormalities. MR can provide complementary information, especially for cholesteatoma investigation.

External auditory canal atresia can be osseous or membraneous. These patients usually present clinically with auricular deformity and no visible external auditory canal. The condition may be bilateral in 30% of patients.[11] Malleolar handle (manubrium) hypoplasia is virtually always associated with an atretic plate. Other associated ossicular deformities, particularly malleoincudal fusion in the attic and fusion of the malleus neck to the atretic plate, are common. The thickness of the atretic plate, the severity of ossicular deformity, and the size diminution of the tympanic cavity are important surgical considerations.

CT is the imaging method of choice for external ear congenital malformations (Fig. 12.9). It can determine the degree of severity or correctability of the atretic process and associated (if any) middle ear anomalies. The size of the tympanic cavity (middle ear compartment) and degree of pneumatization is important information for surgical planning.[11] MR plays a minor role in the imaging of external ear congenital anomalies.

Trauma

Temporal bone fractures are classified as longitudinal, transverse, and mixed according to the fracture plane. Approximately three-quarters of temporal fractures are longitudinal. The longitudinal fracture plane traverses the squamous temporal bone through the middle ear external auditory canal ending at the foramen lacerum. Clinical findings include

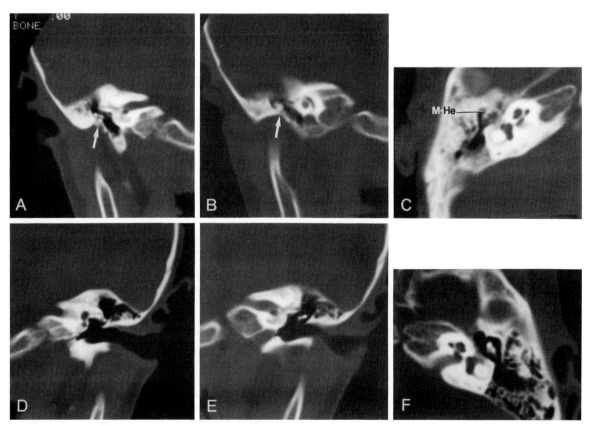

Figure 12.9.   Congenital middle and external ear anomaly. **A–C** are of the affected right ear and **D–F** are of the normal left ear at corresonding levels. Direct coronal **(A, B,** and **D, E)** 700/4000 and axial **(C** and **F)** 1000/4000 1.5-mm thickness, 16-cm FOV bone filter CT scans. There is absence of the right external auditory canal with an ossified moderately thick atretic plate to which the deformed malleus neck is fused *(arrow)*. The head of the malleus *(M-He)* is also fused to the anterior attic wall. The right tympanic cavity is less than half the volume of the left. There is very poor right mastoid pneumatization.

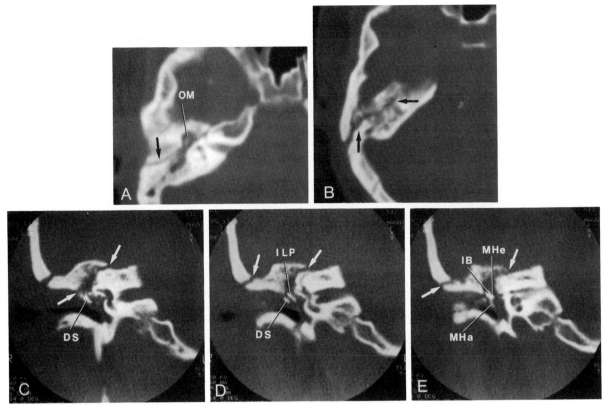

Figure 12.10. Longitudinal fracture. *Axial 3-mm thickness, 22-cm FOV, soft tissue filter, 650/4000 cone-down magnified CT scans (A and B). B is 6 mm cranial to A. Coronal contiguous 1.5-mm, 13-cm FOV bone filter, 650/4000 target technique CT scans (C–E). E is most anterior.* There is fluid in the normally air-filled external auditory canal and tympanum. A petrous longitudinal fracture *(arrows)* isolates the drum spur *(DS)* and traverses the attic and mastoid antrum. The malleus head *(MHe)* and incus body *(IB)* which form the "ossicular mass" *(OM)* are normally related, however, they are abnormally caudal in location. Compare to Fig. 12.2**K.** The incus long process *(ILP)* and malleus handle *(MHa)* appear properly aligned but are probably low in position. There may be an incudostapedial fracture or dislocation. Blood in the middle ear obscures detail.

hemorrhage in the external auditory canal, otorrhea, hearing loss, and torn tympanic membrane. Facial nerve injury is common, may not occur immediately, and usually recovers spontaneously.[1,12]

CT is the method of choice for imaging petrous temporal bone trauma (Fig. 12.10). Axial and coronal 1.5-mm targeted, small FOV sections using bone filtration are recommended.[11] Coronal sections are necessary to identify fractures of the tegmen tympani, drum spur, facial nerve canal, and to identify the ossicles in an orthogonal plane. Petrous fractures are often missed on wide window standard head technique 10-mm thickness, 22-cm FOV soft tissue filter technique. A valuable clue is the presence of mastoid sinus opacity, however.

Ossicular dislocation, usually the incus, occasionally occurs. Malleus and stapes fracture or dislocation is usually associated with injury to the more loosely fixed incus. Axial sections demonstrate dislocation of the malleolar head and incus body such that the ice cream cone appearance is no longer present. Separation of the malleolar handle and long process of the incus also occurs. On axial projection, the "ossicular mass" is no longer equidistant from the medial and lateral attic wall. The stapes CT image is obscured when surrounded by tympanic hemorrhage. Facial nerve canal involvement with longitudinal petrous fractures is usually near the geniculate ganglion. CT cisternography is not used for the investigation of otorrhea. A large tegmen tympani fracture may result in external and middle ear temporal lobe herniation. Petrous temporal gunshot wounds are also accurately imaged by the CT technique.[1,12]

Transverse fractures are more likely associated with trauma to the occiput as compared with longitudinal fractures that are more likely associated with direct petrous trauma. Transverse fractures of the temporal bone are clinically more severe (and fortunately less common) than the longitudinal variety. Deafness and/or facial paralysis may occur in approximately half of patients. This fracture most commonly traverses the internal auditory canal and osseous labyrinth (Fig. 12.11).[1,12]

Labyrinthitis ossificans may develop after trauma, infection, severe otosclerosis, surgery, or tumors. In this condition, the labyrinthine structures become ossified with decreased or obliterated structural definition.[1] Isolated external auditory canal anterior wall fractures may occur associated with posterior thrust

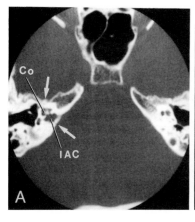 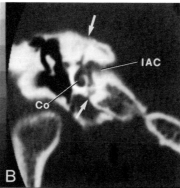

Figure 12.11.   Transverse petrous fracture. Total sensorineural hearing loss. *Axial internal auditory canal 22-FOV 1.5-mm bone filter 400/3000 **(A)** and direct coronal target technique 400/3000 **(B)** CT scans.* A fracture *(arrows)* traverses the petrous apex, the cochlea *(Co)*, and the internal auditory canal *(IAC)*.

of the mandibular condyle in cases of mandibular trauma.[1]

MR will probably not be particularly helpful in acute and subacute petrous temporal bone trauma with respect to adding additional information concerning the condition of the petrous temporal structures. MR is useful, however, for evaluation of adjacent brain structures such as epidural hematoma, contusion, etc.

Inflammatory Disease

CT is the imaging method of choice for petrous temporal inflammatory disease. Conditions such as otitis, cholesterol granuloma, and cholesteatoma are accurately diagnosed by CT axial and coronal images. MR is the imaging method of choice for identification of intracranial spread of inflammatory disease and it plays a secondary role such as confirmation of the diagnosis of petrous apex cholesterol cyst.

Inflammatory conditions will be discussed regionally with respect to the external, middle, and inner ear. However, it should be noted that infections in any of these three regions can spread intracranially resulting in meningitis, lateral or sigmoid sinus thrombosis, and epidural, subdural, or brain abscess.[1] Intravenous contrast MR technique as described in Chapter 8 is used for investigation of intracranial spread of petrous temporal inflammatory disease.

EXTERNAL EAR

Radiological examination of simple (uncomplicated) external otitis is seldom performed. Malignant external otitis is a serious life-threatening necrotizing disease, which occurs mostly in elderly diabetics and is almost always caused by *Pseudomonas aeruginosa*. The early stage of the disease is mostly confined to soft tissue changes. These patients present with ear pain, drainage, decreased hearing, and external auditory canal granulation tissue. Bone destruction occurs in the late stage of the disease with extension of the infection outside of the external auditory canal. Spread of infection may involve the temporomandibular joints, mastoid sinus, middle ear,

petrous apex, skull base, parapharyngeal space, and intracranial space (epidural abscess). Meningitis and/or venous sinus thrombosis may occur. In addition to the symptoms described above, patients may have facial paralysis, other cranial nerve palsies, or temporomandibular pain and swelling. Facial nerve paralysis is a poor prognostic sign indicating a lethal outcome in as many as half of the cases. Nuclear scanning with Gallium-67 citrate may be helpful to determine continuing activity under treatment.[1,13] Intravenous contrast MR is recommended.

Malignant external otitis CT findings include soft tissue within the external auditory canal, canal wall osteolysis, abnormal soft tissue in the mastoid sinus and middle ear, skull base destruction (osteomyelitis), nasopharyngeal inflammatory mass and subtemporal space mass (Fig. 12.12). The obliteration of the masticator and parapharyngeal space fat planes is a CT finding indicating inflammatory disease extending beyond the mastoid bone.[13] Noncontrast and i.v. contrast MR accurately identifies bone and vascular involvement at the skull base, the temporomandibular joint, and intracranial involvement (epidural abscess, venous sinus thrombosis). MR may detect osteomyelitis before CT demonstration of osteolysis (Fig. 12.13 C–E)[1,13]

MIDDLE EAR

The site of middle ear inflammatory involvement distinguishes two types of disease process-tubotympanic and atticoantral. Tubotympanic disease is a chronic eustachean tube, nasopharyngeal, and mesotympanum mucositis. Attico-antral disease is confined to the attic and mastoid air cells and is mainly caused by chronic inflammatory changes that occlude the tympanic isthmus. These two processes often coexist, however.[14,15]

A spectrum of varying severity of inflammatory pathological changes of the middle ear and surrounding tissues may result ranging from acute otitis to chronic otitis and acquired cholesteatoma. Erosion through the tegmen tympani can result in intracranial infection.

Middle ear effusion probably occurs by decreasing

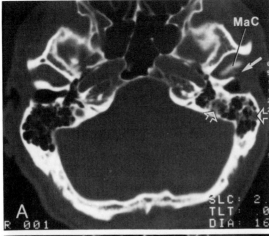

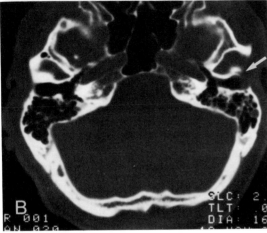

Figure 12.12. Malignant otitis externa. Elderly diabetic male with *Pseudomonas* otitis externa. *Axial 2-mm thickness 400/4000 CT scans.* ***B*** *is 2 mm cranial to* ***A.*** Soft tissue fills the lateral external auditory canal with destruction of its anterior margin *(closed arrow).* A small bone fragment of the anterior canal wall is seen just posterior to the mandibular condyle *(MaC).* Fluid in mastoid air cells *(open arrows)* represents evidence of acute mastoiditis. Comparison to the normal side of contiguous levels is often necessary so that patient positional tilt in the scanner does not lead to an erroneous positive diagnosis. (Courtesy of Heun Y. Yune, M.D., Indianapolis, IN.)

intratympanic pressure with resultant serous or mucoid transudation and may be present as an isolated abnormality. Acute mastoiditis may result. CT of acute otomastoiditis demonstrates a tympanic air-fluid level or an opaque tympanic cavity. A bulging tympanic membrane may be present without evidence for middle ear bone abnormality or other middle ear changes seen in chronic mastoiditis that will be described below (Fig. 12.13).[14–18]

Chronic otitic middle ear changes include effusion, mucosal thickening, tympanosclerosis, granulation tissue accumulation, tympanic retractions, and acquired cholesteatoma.[14–16]

Tympanosclerosis is a postinflammatory ossicular fixation that can be caused by fibrosis, hyalin degeneration and calcification, and new bone formation. Although most cases involve only the tympanic membrane,[16] a generalized tympanic process may occur characterized by multifocal punctate or web-like calcifications. New bone formation is uncommon. Ossicular fibrous fixation may result in an eccentric position and irregular contour of the malleus head and incus body (ossicular mass) wall. There may also be ossicular fibrosis. Scarring of the malleus long arm and the tympanic pars tensa can produce the appearance of a combined calcific mass (Fig. 12.14). Thick calcific webs or generalized calcific debris may be identified by CT. Tympanosclerotic involvement of the oval window may be indistinguishable from fenestral otosclerosis.[15,16]

Granulation tissue accumulating in the middle ear is friable and has a tendency to bleed. This tissue can be soft, fibrous, or granulomatous (cholesterol granuloma) and it can cause hemotympanum. A cholesteatoma may coexist. CT usually demonstrates nonspecific tympanic soft tissue density, but may demonstrate clot and fluid in the presence of a hemorrhage.[15]

Tympanic membrane retractions may result from decreased tympanic pressure pulling the membrane medially. Retraction pockets of the posterior superior tympanic membrane (pars flaccida) are difficult to distinguish clinically from a cholesteatoma, thus requiring CT. Ossicular erosion may develop most often of the long process of the incus. Severe retractions can cause ossicular discontinuity resulting in tympanic membrane adherence to the stapes "nature's myringostapediopexy").[15]

Acquired cholesteatomas usually occur in the middle ear. They may result from middle ear ingrowth of external ear keratinizing squamous epithelium through a tympanic membrane defect. They usually occur in conjunction with infection and eustachian tube dysfunction. Bone demineralization and resorption characteristically occurs probably due to collagenase elaboration by the lesion rather than pressure erosion. Pars flaccida cholesteatomas (most common) spread from the Prussak space of the attic through the aditus to the antrum and the medial wall of the middle ear. Pars tensa cholesteatomas more frequently involve the hypotympanum and erode the incus. Both the "pars flaccida" and the "pars tensa" types can create a lateral semicircular canal fistula.[15,17] They also may become infected with resultant suppurative mastoiditis.[18]

CT findings in cholesteatoma vary according to the disease location extent and bone erosion and destruction. Thin-section 1.5-mm axial and coronal section noncontrast target bone filter technique is used. Additional smooth filter coronal images to evaluate intracranial involvement are recommended. Bone erosion usually affects the drum spur and the incus long process. Lateral semicircular canal erosion can be diagnosed if no thin contiguous section demonstrates lateral cortication of the canal. Fluid and/or granulation tissue is usually present in the tympanum. Tympanosclerosis and tympanic membrane retrac-

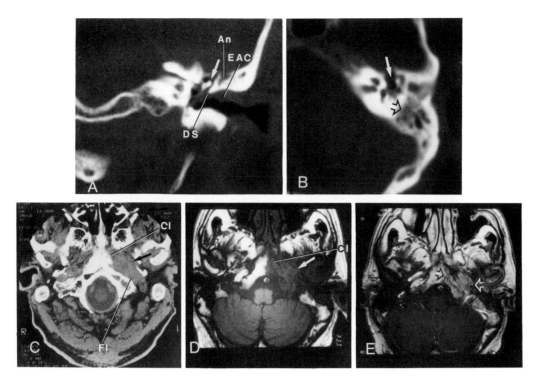

Figure 12.13.   Otitis and apical petrositis. Figures A-B and C-E are different cases. A-B:. Adult otitis media and externa and mastoiditis. *Direct coronal 12.8-cm FOV 1.5-mm target technique 511/ 3000 and axial 22-cm FOV 1.5-mm thickness soft tissue filter 973/ 4000 CT scans. Fluid and/or soft tissue fills the tympanum (closed arrows).* There is mucosal thickening with irregular contour of the external auditory canal roof *(EAC).* There is lack of sharpness of the drum spur *(DS)* raising the possibility of erosion by a cholesteatoma. Fluid and/or mucosal thickening in the mastoid antrum *(An)* and in

mastoid sinus air spaces *(open arrow)* is present. **C–E:** Apical petrositis. A 60 year old diabetic patient with pseudomonas otitis externa and media. *Axial petrous level 84/500 CT scan **(C)** and SE 480/15 **(D)** and i.v. contrast MAST 480/22 **(E)** MR scans.* A mass erodes the clivus lateral margin (Cl), the margins of the foramen lacerum (Fl) and destroys muscular fat planes *(closed arrows).* The left clivus marrow signal is replaced by the T1 contrast enhancing muscle-isointense inflammatory mass *(open arrows).*

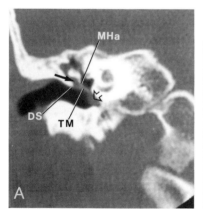
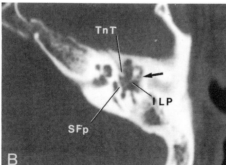
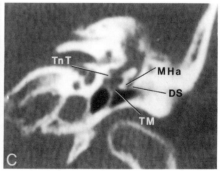

Figure 12.14.   Tympanic membrane retraction. A and **B** and **C** are different cases. **A:** Tympanic membrane retraction. *Direct coronal 1.5-mm 650/4000 CT scan.* An attic *(closed arrow)* and a hypotympanic *(open arrow)* retraction pocket retract the abnormally thickened tympanic membrane medially and upward *(TM).* The malleus handle *(MHa)* is eroded and medially fixated and the drum spur *(DS)* is eroded. The drum spur erosion raises the possibility of early or "incipient" cholesteatoma.[14] (Courtesy of Heun Y. Yune, M.D., Indianapolis, IN.) **B** and **C:** Tympanic membrane retraction and tympanosclerosis, *1.5-mm 800/4000 14-cm FOV target technique axial **(B)** and direct coronal **(C)** noncontrast CT scans.* There is thickening

and medial calcification of the tensor tympani *(TnT),* web-like calcifications of tissue folds *(arrow)* between the lateral attic wall and the laterally fixed malleus head and neck, and incus body. Other calcification is present in the anterior attic **(B).** The calcifications contrast against the tissue-density epitympanum. Stapes footplate thickening is indistinguishable from fenestral otosclerosis *(SFp).* The incus long process *(ILP)* is slightly demineralized and the drum spur *(DS)* is slightly eroded, raising the possibility of an early cholesteatoma. The thickened tympanic membrane *(TM)* is slightly retracted toward the attic, thus displacing the attached malleus handle *(MHa).* Note the lack of normal mastoid sinus pneumatization.

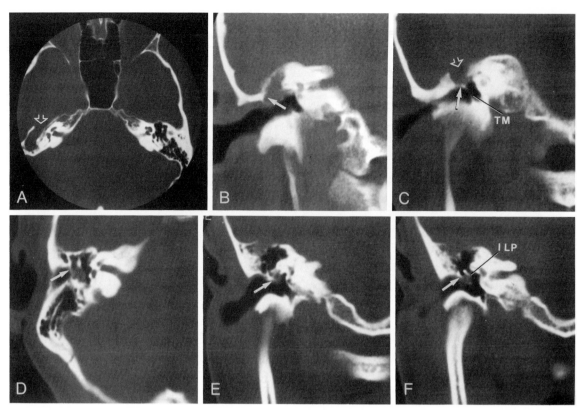

Figure 12.15. Acquired cholesteatoma. A–C and **D–F** are different cases. Target technique has not been used. **A–C:** Pars flacida type acquired cholesteatoma. *Axial 16-cm FOV 1.5-mm thickness (A) and direct coronal 17-cm FOV contiguous 5 mm thick (B and C) 850/4000 CT scans.* The drum spur *(closed arrow)* and ossicles are absent and there is destruction of the roof of the external auditory canal and tegmen tympani *(open arrows)* by a smoothly marginated Prussak's space and mastoid antrum soft tissue mass. The tympanic membrane *(TM)* is thickened. **D–E:** *Pars tensa-type acquired cholesteatoma. Axial (D) and direct coronal (E and F) 17-cm FOV 3-mm thickness 830/4000 CT scans.* A mesotympanic soft tissue mass erodes the drum spur *(closed arrow)* and the incus long process *(ILP)* and extends toward the hypotympanum. The attic and antrum are normal. Lack of involvement of the hypotympanum is evidence against a glomus tympanicum tumor—the principal differential diagnostic consideration.

tion are also frequently seen.[1] There is usually associated paucity of mastoid sinus pneumatization (Fig. 12.15).

MR of acquired cholesteatoma may be very helpful to determine intracranial involvement as well as distinguishing a vascular lesion such as a glomus tumor or ectopic carotid artery from a cholesteatoma.

The CT differential diagnosis of the opacified middle ear (principally) depends on presence or absence of, and location of, bone destruction. The glomus tympanicum tumor is characteristically located in the hypotympanic recess, contrast enhances by CT, and demonstrates a vascular stroma by MR. Differential diagnostic considerations of middle ear masses will be considered after the discussion of glomus tympanicum tumors at the end of this chapter.

INNER EAR

"Acute labyrinthitis" is a frequent empirical clinical diagnosis for patients with vertigo of unknown etiology. It is not known how many of the cases are actually inflammatory in origin. Toxins, viruses, or bacteria may be responsible. Acute viral labyrinthitis from known viral infections (mumps, measles) is unlikely to cause CT abnormalities. Bacterial laby-

rinthitis (suppurative labyrinthitis) may spread from the middle ear, bloodstream, or meninges to the labyrinth. It may progress to labyrinthitis ossificans.[1]

Middle ear and mastoid infection can spread to the petrous apex only in those 30% of patients who have petrous apex pneumatization. Gradenigo's syndrome (otitis media, fifth cranial nerve pain, and sixth cranial nerve palsy) may result. CT demonstrates petrous air cell opacification, evidence of otitis, and evidence of bone destruction (Fig. 12.13).[1,18]

Cholesteatomas can involve the labyrinth by lateral semicircular canal and more uncommonly, oval window fistulization. Cholesteatomas can also extend medially along the facial nerve canal producing facial nerve palsy and medial petrous erosion. CT demonstrates petrous erosion with associated tympanic changes suggesting cholesteatoma. MR or CT contrast injection technique is recommended to exclude a contrast-enhancing neoplasm.[17] MR can be particularly helpful for the evaluation of possible intracranial extension.

MASTOID SINUS

Acute otomastoiditis usually develops de novo and responds well to antibiotics. It may occur as a complication of acute or chronic otitis media or cholesteatoma. Chronic cases progress from mucoperiosteal disease to coalescent mastoiditis. Coalescent mastoiditis is a destructive inflammatory process involving demineralization, trabecular resorption, and resultant air cell coalescence into a single cavity. The cavity often represents an empyema and this, in turn, commonly progresses to subperiosteal abscess. Abscess spread may develop in any direction but it is an unusual condition in the antibiotic era. Lateral and sigmoid sinus thrombosis, leptomeningitis, brain abscess, suppurative labyrinthitis, and petrous apicitis may develop.[18] Brain abscess secondary to mastoiditis usually occurs in the temporal lobe or cerebellar hemisphere.[18]

Both CT (Fig. 12.13C) and MR are useful for investigation of acute otomastoiditis. CT is the usual method of investigation because study of the tympanum is an integral part of the mastoid examination. If intracranial involvement is suspected, MR becomes the procedure of choice for investigation of parenchymal or epidural abscess and for venous sinus thrombosis. Contrast CT should be performed if MR is not available.

Postoperative Ear

CT images of the postinflammatory disease postoperative ear require the analysis of three factors for interpretation:

1. the preoperative state,
2. the surgical changes, and
3. the postsurgical changes.

Previous CT scans are necessary for comparison. The degree of external canal resection during mastoidectomy, placement of middle ear-external canal tympanostomy tubes, and history of ossicular reconstructions is necessary clinical information.[1,19]

Tympanoplasty is usually performed to repair tympanic perforations. Patients with a normal ossicular chain undergo a simple repair. The malleus, the incus, and the stapes can be bypassed with different procedures that are designed to transfer mechanical sound conduction from the tympanic membrane eventually to the oval window. For the first postoperative month, the tympanic membrane will appear thick by CT.[19]

Mastoidectomy is usually performed for colesteatoma. It produces a defect called the mastoid bowl (Fig. 12.16). Closed cavity and open cavity are the two major types of mastoidectomy. Recurrent cholesteatoma occurs more frequently with the closed cavity type. The extent of the surgical procedure depends upon the extent of the pathological process. The closed cavity procedure has a maintained external auditory canal wall often with a tympanoplasty. Open cavity procedures are subdivided into modified radical and radical mastoidectomy. The modified radical procedure preserves or reconstructs middle ear structures and is usually performed if the disease is limited to the attic and antrum. The radical mastoidectomy procedure removes the tympanic membrane remnants, the malleus and the incus, and is used for extensive disease with involvement of the mesotympanum.[19]

The postoperative changes for fenestral otosclerosis will be discussed later in this chapter.

Neoplasms, Cysts, and Other Masses

Since the most common indication at our institution for temporal bone MR is acoustic neurinoma, the regional approach used here for the discussion of petrous region tumors will begin with the inner ear.

INNER EAR AND CEREBELLOPONTINE ANGLE (CPA)

Acoustic (neuromas), other CPA tumors and tumors and cholesterol granulomas of the petrous apex

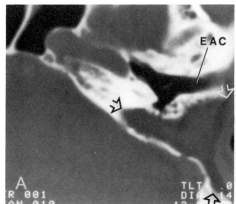 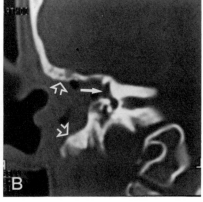

Figure 12.16. Postmastoidectomy changes. A and **B** are different cases. **A:** Closed cavity type. Intact external auditory canal posterior wall mastoidectomy for translabyrinthine approach to an acoustic neuroma. *Axial cochlear base turn-level 2-mm thickness 400/4000 CT scan.* The mastoid sinus has been removed *(open arrows).* The posterior wall of the external auditory canal *(EAC)* is intact. (Courtesy of Heun Y. Yune, M.D., Indianapolis, IN.) **B:** Open cavity type. The mastoid sinus and the posterior wall of the external auditory canal have been removed for treatment of a cholesteatoma and mastoiditis leaving a large mastoid bowl *(open arrows).* The cavity communicates with the tympanum and forms a fistula with the lateral and the superior semicircular canals *(closed arrow).*

will be described in some detail in this section. Brief mention will be made of rarer lesions. The MR and CT techniques described for acoustic neuroma are generally used for workup of any suspected CPA mass.

Acoustic Neuroma ("Schwannoma or Neurilemoma")[a]

Acoustic neuroma is the most common tumor of the CPA and the most common tumor in the temporal bone.[1] Presenting signs usually include hearing loss, tinnitus, and dysequilibrium. When the lesion extends into the CPA, decreased corneal sensation facial paresis and posterior fossa signs also occur. This common benign tumor usually arises from vestibular nerve Schwann cells frequently within the internal auditory canal. It is more prevalent in older age groups (fifth to sixth decades) and is commonly seen earlier in von Recklinghausen's disease.[1] Its occurrence is rare in children, even those with neurofibromatosis.[20] It is usually unilateral and almost all bilateral cases arise in adults with neurofibromatosis (Fig. 12.17). Almost all acoustic neuromas have a significant portion within the internal auditory canal and purely intracanalicular lesions commonly occur. The tumor usually grows medially into the CPA with expansion of the internal auditory canal.[1,21,22]

MR is the diagnostic procedure of choice for investigation of acoustic neuroma because of lack of dependence on intrathecal contrast injection for diagnosis, relatively artifact-free orthogonal plane imaging, and superior detectability. Following a routine variable echo (SE 2800/30 and 2800/80) MR scan, T1-weighted SE 600/25 thin (3-mm) axial 18-cm FOV noncontrast and i.v. contrast MR scans are our present routine. If a lesion is identified, a coronal T1-weighted thin section series is then obtained.

MR accurately demonstrates both the intracanalicular and extracanalicular portions. Generally, tumor signals are homogeneous and slightly T1 hypointense compared to brainstem (Fig. 12.18). Cystic portions may occur; particularly in larger tumors. The CPA tumors are smoothly marginated with ipsilateral cisternal enlargement. They are more likely to exhibit T2 hyperintensity than meningioma. An unexplained central thin horizontal band of low signal intensity may be seen in the intracanalicular portion. This likely represents truncation artifact. Although, noncontrast MR documents the extra- and intracanalicular portion of the tumor in most cases, Gd-DTPA will better document the extent of intracanalicular involvement and increase the conspicuity of the extracanalicular portion of the mass.[22–24] The marked i.v. contrast-enhancement of acoustic neuroma is particularly important for detection of small intracanalicular lesions.

CT usually demonstrates homogeneous isodense, smoothly marginated, homogeneous contrast-enhancing CPA masses with ipsilateral cisternal enlargement. Lack of enhancement occurs occasionally, in cystic portions, however. Bone windows demon-

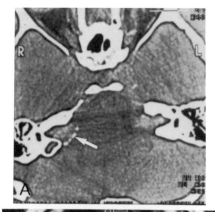

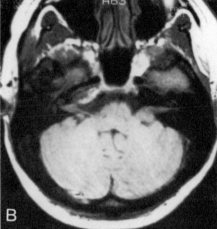

Figure 12.17. Bilateral acoustic neuromas in patients with neurofibromatosis. *Axial i.v. contrast 59/400 bone filter CT scan (A). Another patient with axial SE 600/25 MR scan (B).* Bilateral intracanalicular acoustic neuromas are seen eroding the internal auditory canals and extending into the CPAs in **A**. There is calcification (unusual) of the right acoustic neuroma medial margin *(arrow)*. The tumors contrast enhance. **B** demonstrates a right-sided intracanalicular and a left-sided principally extracanalicular tumor. **A** is the same case as Figure 9.20**A**.

strate internal auditory canal erosion.[1] Gas CPA cisternography is necessary for CT demonstration of intracanalicular tumors (Fig. 12.19).[25] Axial noncontrast and i.v. contrast 3-mm soft tissue filter scans are our present routine. Bone and soft tissue window images are then copied to film.

Fifth Nerve Neuromas

Fifth nerve neuromas are rare schwannomas of the fifth cranial nerve that usually originate at the trigeminal (gasserian) ganglion. CT demonstrates a smoothly marginated tissue isodense or partially cystic contrast-enhancing mass causing bone erosion at Meckel's cave and, often, of the foramen ovale.[1] MR demonstrates a brainstem-T1 hypointense or isointense and T2 hyperintense mass that contrast enhances. Cystic changes may be present (Fig. 12.20), Meckel's cave erosion or identification of fifth nerve branches emanating from the tumor are strong diagnostic clues.[26]

CPA Meningiomas

CPA meningiomas (Fig. 12.21) have similar CT and MR features to those described in Chapter 5. They

---

[a]The terms neuroma, schwannoma, neurilemoma and neurimoma are often used interchangably.

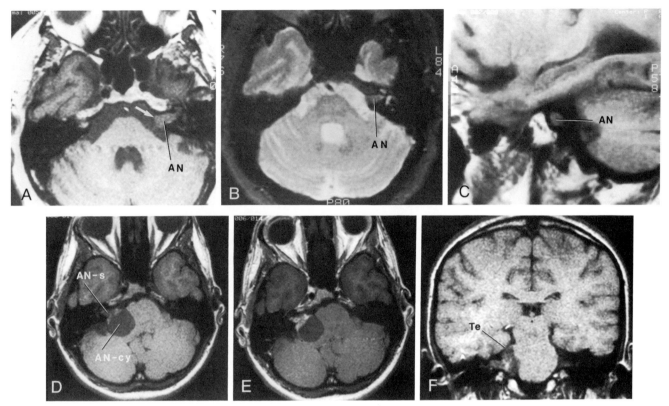

Figure 12.18. Acoustic neuroma—MR. **A–C** and **D–F** are different cases. *Axial SE 600/25 3-mm thickness* **(A)** *and SE 2000/80 5 mm thickness* **(B)** *and sagittal SE 600/25 internal auditory canal-level* **(C)** *MR scans. Axial SE 600/25 non-contrast* **(D)** *and i. v. contrast* **(E)** *and coronal noncontrast* **(F)** *3 mm thick internal auditory canal-level MR scans.* **A–C:** Mostly intracanalicular acoustic neuroma *(AN)* projecting into the CPA *(arrow)*. Note that on the T2-weighted image, the cisternal tumor portion is isointense with CSF and is not recog-

nized. The sagittal section demonstrates the T1 gray matter-isointense intracanalicular tumor that expands the internal auditory canal. **D–F:** Partially cystic acoustic neuroma. The tumor solid portion *(AN-s)* is T1 gray matter-isointense with the exception of a small hyperintense portion seen on the coronal section. The solid portion homogeneously contrast enhances. The cystic portion *(AN-cy)* is homogeneously CSF-isointense and does not contrast enhance. The coronal section shows the tumor relationship to the tentorium *(Te)*.

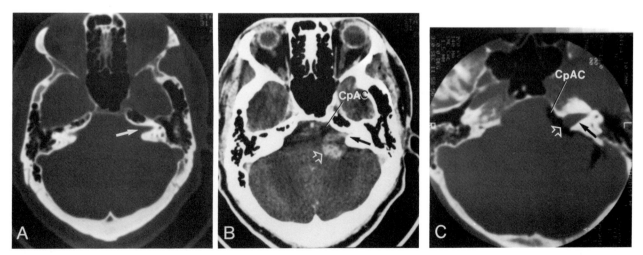

Figure 12.19. Acoustic neuroma—CT. **A–B** and **C** are different cases. *A and B: Axial i.v. contrast 5 mm 843/3000 and 62/200.* There is erosion causing enlargement of the left internal auditory canal *(closed arrow)* by a contrast-enhancing tumor *(open arrow)*. The acoustic neuroma is present within the canal and extends into and enlarges the left cerebellopontine angle cistern *(CpAC)*. The non-

contrast scan at this level failed to identify this isodense tumor partly due to interpetrous artifact. *C: Axial 1.5-mm 125/3600 air cisternogram.* Cerebellopontine angle air *(CpAC)* outlines a protruding extracanalicular portion *(open arrow)* of a mass that erodes and expands the left internal auditory canal *(closed arrow)*.

Figure 12.20.   Fifth nerve neuroma. A–B and **C–D** are different cases. *Axial Meckel's cave-level 39/450 i.v. contrast bone filter CT scan **(A)** and SE 1000/30 MR scan **(B)**. Pontine-level coronal SE 600/25 **(C)** and axial SE 2000/80 **(D)** MR scans.* **A–B** demonstrate ring contrast enhancement *(open arrow)* of a partially cystic mass with a fluid level *(closed arrow)* eroding Meckel's cave *(MC)*. The lower specific gravity fluid is T2-hyperintense due to methemoglobin and/or proteinaceous content. A solid portion is seen laterally and, on other sections, the lesion is predominantly solid with homogeneous contrast enhancement. **C–D** shows a homogeneous T1 pons-isointense T2 heterogeneous hyperintense mass displacing and deforming the medial temporal lobe and pons. On the T2 image, CSF in the cerebellopontine cistern-tumor margin cannot be accurately identified due to T2 tumor hyperintensity.

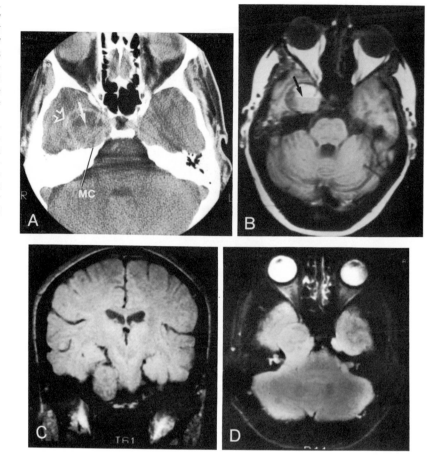

rarely, if ever, expand the internal auditory canal. They may have an epicenter at the internal auditory canal or at Meckel's cave and they may have an "en-plaque" component.[26]

CPA differential diagnostic considerations are shown in Table 12.1.

Petrous Bone Cholesterol Cysts

Petrous bone cholesterol cysts (cholesterol granulomas) are much less common than acoustic neuromas, however, they are the most common benign lesions of the petrous apex.[27] They are different from the cholesteatomas with which they are often confused. The cholesterol cyst contains fibrous tissue enclosing cholesterol clefts, inflammatory infiltrate, and chronic hemorrhagic products, which include hemosiderin-laden macrophages. Cholesteatoma, on the other hand, is composed of squamous epithelium and desquamated keratin. The petrous cholesterol cyst in some patients is thought to be caused by chronic obstruction to ventilation and drainage of pneumatized spaces. They are less likely caused by congenital rests of epidermal cells ("primary cholesteatomas"). Inflammatory reaction to cholesterol crystals and mul-

Figure 12.21.   Cerebellopontine angle meningioma. A and **B** are different cases. *Axial sella turcica-level i.v. contrast CT scan **(A)** and internal auditory canal-level SE 600/25 MR scan **(B)**.* **A:** A round homogeneously contrast-enhanced mass *(arrow)* with a broad-based attachment to the posterior petrous apex. **B:** A gray matter-isointense prepontine meningioma *(arrow)* extends into the left cerebellopontine angle abutting the facial nerve before its entrance into the internal auditory canal.

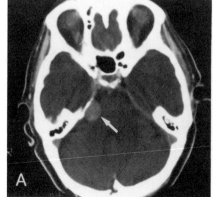
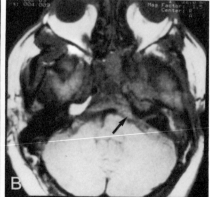

tiple hemorrhages appear to be a common denominator for the continued evolution of these lesions independent of initiating causes. The lesion epicenter is usually the petrous apex. They are usually expansile and can be quite extensive with frequent erosion beyond the petrous apex including the lateral aspect of the clivus, the jugular tubercle, the anterior carotid canal, and the internal auditory canal. They may also involve the labyrinth.

CT demonstrates a sharply and smoothly marginated expansile petrous apex isodense noncontrast-enhancing lesion with a petrous apex epicenter (Fig. 12.22). The mass is principally identified by bone erosion. It usually erodes the internal auditory canal to some degree and may extend into the posterior fossa as an extradural mass resembling a CPA mass. These lesions should not be confused with fatty marrow of a nonpneumatized petrous apex or giant air cells of the petrous pyramid.[27] CT cannot effectively exclude a petrous apex cholesteatoma.

MR usually demonstrates a smoothly and sharply marginated T1- and T2-weighted hyperintense petrous apex mass with T1 and T2 signals suggesting extracellular methemoglobin. In addition, evidence of

peripheral magnetic susceptibility effects on T2-weighted images is seen probably due to hemosiderin-laden macrophages in the fibrous wall. Analysis of T1- and T2-weighted signals excludes petrous apex marrow fat and the usual T1-hypointense petrous apex cholesteatoma. Not only is MR more specific than CT for diagnosis of petrous apex cholesterol cyst before surgery but can document postsurgical lack of reaccumulation of cholesterol cyst content. Reaccumulation documented by a return to T1 and T2 signal hyperintensity indicates lesion recurrence.[27]

Primary Petrous Apex Cholesteatomas

Primary petrous apex cholesteatomas (epidermoid cysts) are rare lesions over which there is much controversy. These lesions, centered in the petrous apex, have a squamous epithelial wall and contain friable kerototic material. There may even be an associated small cholesterol granuloma. The major reason for controversy in considering this disease type in a separate category is that some investigators believe that the primary petrous apex cholesteatoma is simply an extension of a secondary cholesteatoma or an inflam-

Table 12.1. Cerebellopontine Angle and Petrous Temporal Masses: Summary of Comparative CT and MR Findings

	Margination	CT Density	CT Contrast	Calcification	MR T1/T2 Intensity	Gd-DTPA Contrast	Features
Acoustic neuroma[a]	Smooth sharp	Homogeneous isodense	Usually homogeneous	No	T1 brainstem-hypointense; T2 hyperintense	Very marked	Involves internal auditory canal
Meningioma	Smooth sharp	Homogeneous hyperdense	Usually homogeneous	Diffuse or flecks	T1/T2 gray matter-isointense with heterogeneous texture	Marked	MR interface and feeding vessels, CT hyperostosis
Epidermoid tumor	Irregular	Homogeneous hypodense	No	No	T1 water-isointense or slightly hyperintense T2 water-isointense	No	Possible diploic erosion; May arise in petrous apex as a "primary cholesteatoma"
Arachnoid cyst	Smooth sharp	Homogeneous hypodense	No	No	T1/T2 CSF isointense	No	Local skull base expansion
Fifth nerve neuroma	Smooth sharp	Usually homogeneous isodense	Usually homogeneous	No	T1 brainstem-hypointense or isointense; T2 hyperintense	+	Does not involve internal auditory canal; centered at Meckel's cave; possible eroded foramen ovale
Uncommon: petrous bone cholesterol cyst	Smooth sharp	Isodense	No	No (possible bone fragments)	T1/T2 hyperintensity		Petrous apex epicenter expansile process; may also involve internal auditory canal
Uncommon: intratemporal vascular tumor	Smooth or irregular	Isodense	Yes	Flecks	May show flow effect		May involve internal auditory canal; CT may show bone expansion irregular margins; honeycombing and spicules

[a] Large tumors may contain smooth walled cystic portions.

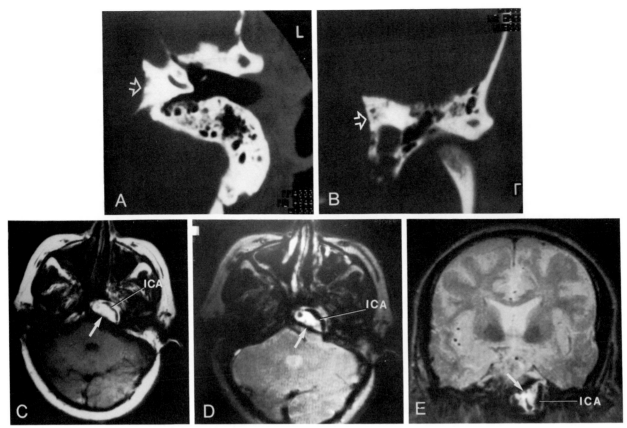

Figure 12. 22. Petrous bone cholesterol cyst. *Axial (A) and direct coronal (B) 1.5-mm thicknes 7.5-cm FOV target technique 600/4000 CT scans. Petrous-level axial SE 800/25 (C), 2000/80 (D), and coronal SE 2000/80 (E) MR scans. There is marked erosion of the petrous apex (open arrow) by a T1 and T2 hyperintense lesion (closed arrows) within which are T1 and T2 hypointense signals. The displaced and stretched encased internal carotid artery (ICA) appears as a signal-void within the hyperintense mass. (Courtesy of Heun Y. Yune, M.D., Indianapolis, IN.)*

matory cholesteatoma in an unusual location. Most believe, however, that some of these lesions are of the primary type that arise from cellular rests.[28]

The lesions have identical pathological, CT, and MR characteristics to other intracranial cholesteatomas (Fig. 5.39). CT is important for identification of petrous apex involvement and to document the lack of inflammatory changes in the middle ear and mastoid sinus that could give origin to the apex lesion (Fig. 12.23). CT demonstrates petrous apex erosion and a water-isodense or slightly hyperdense CPA mass. MR demonstrates a sharply marginated, irregularly, contoured, T1 hypointense and T2 hyperintense (water-intensity) mass. It is conceivable that one of these lesions could be of the dermoid type and, therefore, lipid-containing.[26,28] MR would, in that case, demonstrate typical fat-T1 and T2 signals that could easily be differentiated from the T1 and T2 hyperintense cholesterol granuloma signals.

Arachnoid cysts, similar to those in other locations, may present as smoothly marginated CSF density and intensity masses abutting and eroding the petrous pyramid and displacing structures of the CPA (Fig. 12.24).

Other Uncommon Inner Ear Tumors

Other uncommon tumors or masses also involve the petrous temporal bone. "Intratemporal vascular tumors" is a category that includes intratemporal hemangiomas, vascular hamartomas, and blood vessel malformations.[29,30] These uncommon lesions have a tendency to involve the facial nerve in the geniculate region, the second genu, or in the internal auditory canal location. They have a tendency to produce irregular margins, to have a "honeycombed" matrix, to expand bone to contain flecks of bone, and to contrast enhance.[29,30] These lesions have been termed "ossifying" hemangiomas due to the high frequency of contained calcific flecks.[29]

Masses in the internal auditory canal may project into the CPA. The differential diagnosis of CPA tumors is discussed in the next section.

Facial nerve neuromas can be found anywhere along the course of the facial nerve including the internal auditory canal[24] and the first and second genu locations.[1] The facial nerve neuroma within the facial nerve canal tends to produce smooth erosion that should help to distinguish it from vascular tumors in

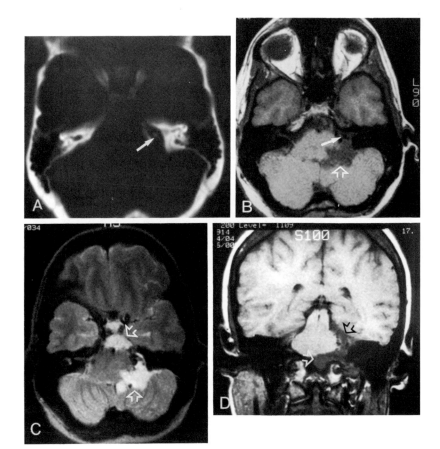

Figure 12.23. Petrous apex primary cholesteatoma. *Axial petrous-level 1760/4000 CT san (A). Same level SE 600/25 3-mm section (B) and SE 2000/80 5-mm section (C) MR scans. Coronal SE 600/25 pons-level MR scan (D).* There is an irregularly "frond-like" contoured T1 water-(slightly) hyperintense and T2 water-isointense CPA and prepontine mass *(open arrows).* There is erosion of the left petrous pyramid with a central bone spicule *(closed arrow).*

most cases. The intratemporal vascular tumor is probably more common than the facial nerve neuroma.[29,30] Cholesterol cysts, primary cholesteatomas, intratemporal vascular tumors, and facial nerve neuromas are the most common benign intratemporal "masses" involving the facial nerve.[30] Meningiomas of the facial nerve are very rare. Acquired cholesteatoma can also cause erosions at the facial nerve genus but should be excluded by characteristic middle ear CT changes.[17]

Other benign lesions such as osteochondroma may involve the inner ear. Direct spread to the inner ear of malignant tumor, particularly nasopharyngeal carcinoma, and metastases may also occur.[1]

Differential Diagnosis of Cerebellopontine Angle Tumors

Differential diagnosis of CPA tumors includes acoustic neuroma, meningioma, fifth nerve neuoma, epidermoid tumors, and petrous bone choles-

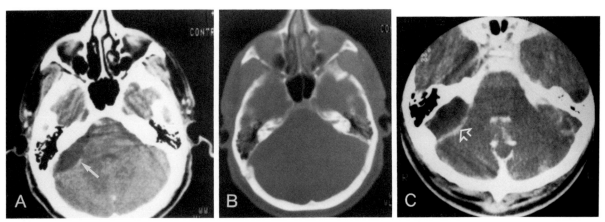

Figure 12.24. CPA arachnoid cyst. *Axial fourth ventricle level i.v. contrast 34/200 (A) and 136/3200 (B) 6-mm thickness CT scans. Same level iopamidol 49/2000 cisternogram (C).* A water density smoothly marginated biconvex mass erodes the posterior petrous pyramid. There is a displaced CPA vein *(closed arrow)* and subarachnoid iopamidol outlines a smooth cyst margin *(open arrow).* The cyst does not communicate with the subarachnoid space. Compare to the petrous apex primary cholesteatoma (Fig. 12.23).

terol cysts.[31,32] Table 12.1 summarizes comparative CT and MR findings. In this group of CPA masses, an often difficult diagnostic problem is the distinction between arachnoid cyst and epidermoid tumor. Associated middle fossa involvement and middle fossa skull expansion are findings favoring arachnoid cyst. Identifying irregular epidermoid margination is difficult due to relative T1 and T2 lesion CSF-isointensity; however, there is a likelihood that analysis of T1-, proton density, and T2-weighted images will identify water-contrasting, slightly heterogeneous signals and that the frond-like margin will be identified. Intrathecal CT contrast can document the fronds and lack of communication with the subarachnoid space, however, we have found no use for the intrathecal contrast CT method since we have successfully used MR noncontrast imaging instead.[28] CT demonstration of bone expansile erosion is seen with both epidermoid tumor and petrous bone cholesterol cyst. The erosion epicenter for cholesterol cyst is usually the petrous apex whereas that for epidermoid tumor is more often the lateral margin of the middle fossa. MR T1 and T2 signal hyperintensity best identifies the cholesterol cyst.

Acoustic neuroma and petrous bone cholesterol cyst are so different by both MR and CT that there should ordinarily be no confusion in differentiating tumor involvement of the internal auditory canal. Another rare lesion that can involve the internal auditory canal and CPA is the intratemporal vascular tumor (hemangiomas and vascular malformations). They may protrude into the CPA and be indistinguishable by CT from acoustic neuroma unless they have characteristic irregular margins and contained bone spicules. MR findings have not been adequately described for these lesions.

MIDDLE EAR TUMORS

Glomus Tumors

Glomus tumors are the most common middle ear and the second most common temporal bone tumors. These benign neoplasms arise from extra-adrenal paraganglia (chemoreceptor cells) and are also known as chemodectomas or nonchromaffin paragangliomas. They occur mainly in middle-aged adults. Temporal bone glomus tumors are divided into those with origin at the middle ear cochlear promontary (glomus tympanicum) and those at the jugular bulb (glomus jugulare). Both of these tumors arise from glomus bodies along Jacobsen's nerve (tympanic division of cranial nerve IX) or Arnolds' nerve (auricular branch of cranial nerve X), respectively.[33] Since these two sites are in close proximity, the glomus jugulare tumor can erode into the middle ear and since glomus tumors may arise between these two sites, it is not always clear to which of the two categories the tumor belongs. The glomus jugulare is more common than the glomus tympanicum.[34]

The glomus tympanicum chemodectomas are more common in women and characteristically present with pulsatile tinnitus and diminished hearing. Rarely, they occur together with other chemodectomas and are usually unassociated with elevation of serum neuroendocrine compounds, possibly because of their small size. The glomus tympanicum characteristically begins as a small vascular mass in the hypotympanic recess. Growth of the tumor may completely fill the middle ear cavity, occlude the eustachian tube, extend into the mastoid sinus, grow through the tympanic membrane, and may extend into the external auditory canal. Osseous destruction is not typical of glomus tympanicum tumors as it is of glomus jugulare. For example, despite encasement, the ossicles remain intact.[34]

Glomus jugulare chemodectomas produce expansion, permeation, and destruction of the jugular fossa with frequent invasion of the tympanic cavity. Tympanic cavity involvement typically involves the eustachian tube, tympanic sinus (hypotympanic recess), and may include the ossicular chain. Parapharyngeal spread of tumor is common. Intracranial extension through osteolytic skull base defects usually remains extradural. Caudal extension causes destruction of the hypoglossal canal and occipital condyles. Occasionally, bilateral glomus jugulare tumors are found.[34]

The CT and MR investigative method for each of these conditions is similar due to the clinical fact that glomus jugulare lesions may extend to the middle ear and that the diagnosis of glomus tympanicum tumor is made by exclusion, of jugular origin. The CT technique includes soft tissue filter, i.v. contrast, axial and coronal thin sections, with a small FOV, soft tissue, and bone windows.

MR technique includes thin-section orthogonal plane, small FOV (17-cm) noncontrast and i.v. contrast T1- and T2-weighted orthogonal plane images. CT technique includes axial and coronal bone filter target technique and soft tissue filter small FOV noncontrast and i.v. contrast technique.

The glomus tympanicum tumor's degree of CT contrast enhancement is equal to that of the temporalis muscle. CT detects hypotympanic recess tumors as small as 3 mm (Fig. 12.25). Tumor growth may surround the ossicular chain, bulge or protrude through the tympanic membrane, fill the middle ear compartment, and block the eustachian tube orifice or aditus ad antrum.[33] CT may be more specific than MR for these small lesions.[34]

CT of glomus jugulare tumors demonstrates destruction of the walls of the jugular foramen, the jugular tubercle, and the hypoglossal canal. Extension into the middle ear cavity is common. Enhancement of subtemporal tumor components is frequently seen (Fig. 12.26).[34]

MR demonstrates signal void of high flow serpentine tumor vessels producing a characteristic "salt and pepper" pattern. The salt and pepper appearance is characterized by multiple punctate and serpiginous areas of signal void within a matrix to T1 muscle-

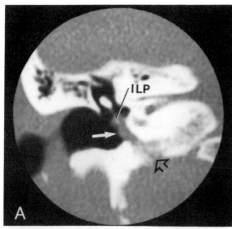

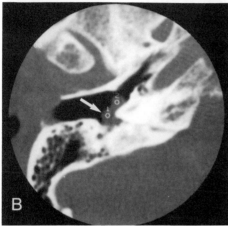

Figure 12.25.   Glomus tympanicum tumor. *Both scans are 1.5-mm thickness 15-cm FOV target technique. Direct coronal −100/4000* **(A)** *and axial 350/4000* **(B)**. *Circular cursors in Figure 12.25B measure tissue isodensity. The lobular hypotympanic and mesotympanic mass (closed arrow) is associated with a slight degree of osteolysis of the jugular fossa (open arrow). The incus long process (ILP), surrounded by tumor, is still recognizable. There was lack of a mass in the jugular fossa on other studies (not shown) representing evidence against glomus jugulare tympanic extension. The presence of mass filling the hypotympanic recess is evidence against cholesteatoma—the other main differential diagnostic consideration.*

isointensity and T2 muscle-hyperintensity[34] on both T1- and T2-weighted images. Heterogeneous contrast enhancement can be seen. MR can best identify the tumor relationship to the internal carotid artery and internal jugular vein and intracranial extension (Fig. 12.26). Ipsilateral tongue atrophy is commonly seen. Invasion of the jugular vein can be demonstrated.[33,34]

Conditions for Differential Diagnosis Consideration

Conditions for differential diagnosis consideration for glomus tympanicum include glomus jugulare extension, aberrant internal carotid artery, and cholesteatoma. Jugular foramen regional osteolysis and tumor excludes glomus tympanicum. Internal carotid artery position under, and not lateral to, the cochlea by CT or MR coronal technique with an intact lateral carotid canal margin excludes the aberrant in-

ternal carotid artery (Fig. 12.7). Acquired cholesteatoma is usually destructive of bone located in Prussak's space and usually spares the hypotympanic recess.[33]

Major differential diagnostic considerations for glomus jugulare tumors include a giant jugular fossa (Fig. 12.8), neuromas of cranial nerves IX, X, XI, and XII, nasopharyngeal malignancies, and metastasis. A giant jugular canal has smooth margins without osteolysis by CT and CT contrast enhancement is homogeneous and contiguous with the sigmoid sinus. MR flow effects of spin-echo and gradient echo images distinguish jugular patency from tumor. Neuromas lack the salt and pepper MR appearance, produce smooth erosion rather than osteolysis, and cause extraluminal rather than intraluminal venous compression. They may be of "dumb-bell" type both above and below the jugular foramen and do not invade the tympanum. Neuromas may have a cystic component (Figs. 12.17 and 12.18). Nasopharyngeal malignancies usually demonstrate characteristic nasopharyngeal involvement. Metastases are very aggressive with respect to osteolysis and to the rapid clinical production of cranial nerve palsies. They do not follow typical patterns for glomus jugulare growth. Most often, the primary site is known. [34]

EXTERNAL AUDITORY CANAL BENIGN TUMORS

This category includes exostoses, osteomas, and gland cell tumors. Exostoses are often multiple and may significantly narrow the canal. Osteomas are usually solitary and may, unlike exostoses, invade adjacent bone. They are readily diagnosed by CT axial and coronal imaging. They appear as dense ovoid masses contiguous with the external canal walls.[1] Gland cell tumors, including ceruminomas, are rare. Simple squamous debris "ear wax" may mimic a soft tissue external auditory canal mass by CT.

MALIGNANT TUMORS OF THE EXTERNAL AND MIDDLE EAR

The most frequent primary malignant tumor of the external canal is squamous carcinoma. Other primary malignancies also include cystic carcinoma and adenocarcinoma. They tend to occur in the late middle-aged adult, often those with a history of chronic suppurative otitis media. The facial nerve is commonly involved. Metastatic carcinoma from direct extension and distal sites also occurs. The most common middle ear malignant tumor is extension of external ear squamous carcinoma.[1]

These external ear primary and metastatic carcinomas share similar CT characteristics that include marked osteolysis and contrast-enhancing soft tissue masses (Fig. 12.27). The tumors tend to spread early to superficial areas such as the parotid gland, temporomandibular joint, and mastoid air cells before extension through the external auditory canal to the middle ear. Middle ear involvement by primary carcinomas is a bad prognostic sign. Intracranial extension is an ominous development.[1,35]

Figure 12.26. Glomus jugulare tumor. *Direct coronal 600/ 3000 bone filter CT scan* **(A)***. Coronal i.v. contrast SE 600/25 MR scan* **(B)***. Axial same technique CT scan* **(C)***. Axial same level SE 600/25 noncontrast MR scan* **(D)***. Left jugular vein-level sagittal 600/25 MR scan* **(E)***. Axial 2800/80 MR scan* **(F)***.

There is marked erosion *(arrows)* of the jugular fossa bulging the tympanic membrane *(TM)*. The MR heterogeneous intensity mass contains signal-void vessels resulting in a "salt and pepper" appearance. The mass markedly contrast enhances and invades the petrous bone not reaching the internal auditory canal *(n7–8)*. It fills the jugular vein. Compare to the normal right jugular vein *(JV)*.

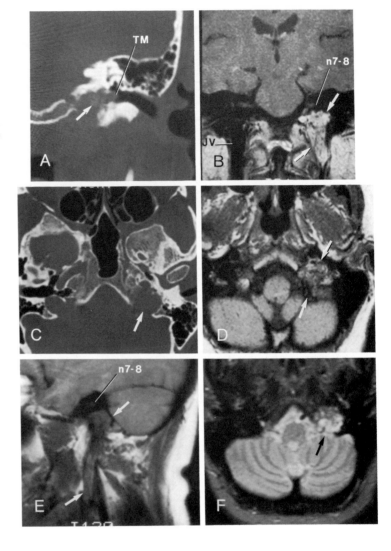

Figure 12.27. Squamous carcinoma of the external ear. *Axial 1.5-mm 650/4000 internal auditory canal-level CT scan* **(A)** *and coronal external auditory canal-level SE 600/25 i.v. contrast 3-mm thickness MR scan* **(B)***. Mastoid osteolysis involves the superoposterior wall of the external auditory canal *(closed arrow)*. There is meningeal contrast enhancement with sulcal effacement *(open arrow)* indicating invasion of the pia-arachnoid membranes. Subcutaneous air bubbles have been introduced by a biopsy at another level.

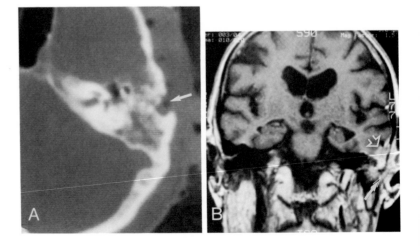

MR identification of intracranial extension and of involvement or lack of involvement of the internal carotid artery and internal jugular vein justifies MR scanning as a valuable adjunct to the CT method.

Differential diagnosis includes malignant external otitis, which usually occurs in elderly diabetics, and cholesteatomas, which are characteristically more confined with a mesotympanic epicenter.

Osteodystrophies

Osteodystrophic ear conditions include otosclerosis (otospongiosis), Paget's disease (osteitis deformans), and other rare conditions such as fibrous dysplasia, osteogenesis imperfecta, and osteopetrosis. Most attention in this section will be directed to otosclerosis.

OTOSCLEROSIS

Otosclerosis is a disease of unknown etiology resulting in tinnitus and hearing loss. It favors young adults and is twice as frequent in women as men. It is frequently bilateral and may be hereditary. This disease occurs when abnormal development of highly vascular haversian bone tissue develops within the normally ivory-hard otic (labyrinthine) capsule. The focus ("site of predilection") where this spongifying process develops is usually just anterior to the oval window and the next most common are the round window borders. Oval and round window otosclerosis are considered the "fenestral" form of the disease. The initial lytic phase (otospongiosis) is followed by a reparative sclerotic phase (otosclerosis) that may be so extensive that it obliterates the oval window niche. The process is virtually confined to the otic capsule. As the process progresses, the stapes footplate may be fixated resulting in a progressive conductive hearing loss (stapedial otosclerosis). Cochlear degeneration with typical subchondral spongiform degeneration at the cochlear base turn may develop producing sensorineural hearing loss (cochlear otosclerosis). Later, obliterative labyrinthine ossification may produce irregular caliber osseous stenosis of the cochlear membranous labyrinth. Cochlear otoscle-

rosis is almost always associated with some degree of stapedial otosclerosis producing mixed conductive and sensorineural hearing loss (mixed hearing loss).[1,36,37]

Contiguous 1.5-mm noncontrast axial and coronal, small FOV, edge-enhancement "bone" filter CT technique is used. A 15° head rotation toward the site of interest has been recommended for coronal investigation of stapedial otosclerosis. The anterior and posterior oval window margins are well seen on axial sections and the superior and inferior margins are well seen on coronal sections.

CT changes of oval window otosclerosis depends upon the type and extent of the disease. Active stapedial otosclerosis results in indistinct oval window margins and a "wide window" appearance. Mature (inactive) otosclerosis appears as marginal or diffuse thickening of the stapes footplate (Fig. 12.28). The characteristic CT appearance of cochlear otosclerosis is a lucent halo "double ring sign" around the cochlea (Fig. 12.29). This results from an enchondral band of spongioform demineralization in the medial aspect of the cochlear capsule.[35,36] The value of MR for studying otosclerosis has yet to be established.

Stapedectomy with prosthesis insertion is performed to relieve oval window closure due to otosclerosis or postinflammatory sclerosis. CT is effective for evaluating the poststapedectomy ear. Prosthesis ankylosis in the oval window, prolapse through the oval window (Fig. 12.30), incudoprosthetic dislocation, reparative granuloma formation, regrowth of obliterative otosclerosis, and incus long process necrosis can be identified.[38] Overlapping 1.5-mm axial sections may be necessary for CT identification of thin Teflon and thin wire devices.[38]

CT is useful for evaluation of cochlear implant candidates by accurately detecting normal cochlear formation and fenestral and membranous labyrinthine patency (Fig. 12.31). The presence of a cobalt magnet in the cochlear implant is a contraindication for MR scanning. CT can also identify the least compromised ear and can establish a preoperative baseline. Contraindications for implants include ob-

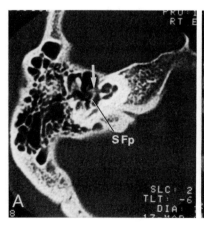
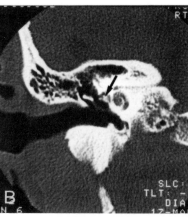

Figure 12.28. Stapedial otosclerosis. *Axial* **(A)** *and coronal* **(B)** *2-mm thickness 600/495 CT scans. The stapes foot plate (SFp) is thickened. There is demineralization of the otic capsule at the cochleariform process (arrow on **B**) and anterior oval window margin* **(A).** (Courtesy of Heun Y. Yune, M.D., Indianapolis, IN.)

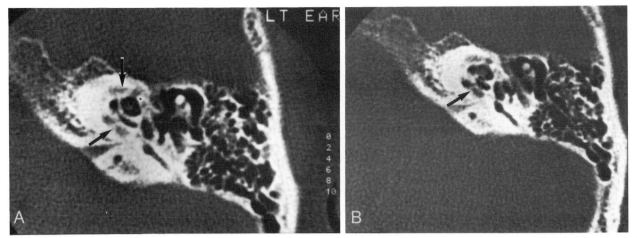

Figure 12.29. **Cochlear otosclerosis.** *Axial 2-mm thickness 600/ 4000 CT scans.* ***B*** *is 2 mm cranial to* ***A****.* There is a band of demineralization in the otic capsule parallel to the cochlear base turn *(arrows).* (Courtesy of Heun Y. Yune, M.D., Indianapolis, IN.)

Figure 12.30. **Stapes prosthesis.** *Direct coronal* ***(A)*** *and axial* ***(B)*** *1.5-mm targeted 886/4000 CT scans.* The stainless steel device *(arrow)* is prolapsed into the vestibule. No evidence for otosclerosis regrowth around the oval window is seen nor is there endosteal sclerosis of the cochlear basal turn. Ideally, the prosthesis should not be prolapsed.

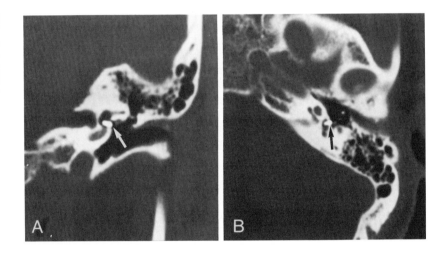

Figure 12.31. **Cochlear prosthesis.** *Axial* ***(A)*** *and coronal* ***(B)*** *target technique 1.5-mm thickness 400/ 3000 CT scans.* The cochlear implant wire enters the round window and is well-positioned in the cochlear base turn *(closed arrows).* A portion of the device at the aditus ad antrum *(open arrows)* is seen.

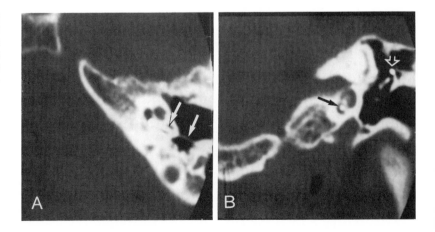

literative labyrinthine ossification, congenital malformation, and severe fenestral otosclerosis—all of which are accurately detected by CT. Postoperative scans show implant location but can be compromised by metallic artifact with certain devices. Although experience with MR is limited, the size of the cochlear nerve and assessment of fluid signal within the membranous labyrinth may prove to be a useful adjunct to CT for evaluation of cochlear implant candidates.[39]

OTHER DISEASES

Paget's disease, osteogenesis imperfecta, fibrous dysplasia, and osteopetrosis may affect the petrous temporal bone and compromise hearing and equilibrium. Paget's disease of the temporal bone is usually accompanied by severe skull changes. Stapes fixation and cochlear involvement may mimic severe otosclerosis (otospongiosis) but the diagnosis is obvious due to the easily identified skull changes. Patients with osteogenesis imperfecta also have changes similar to otospongiosis in a setting of diffuse skull changes. Fibrous dysplasia may rarely affect the temporal bone, producing characteristic homogeneous dense hyperostosis with canalicular stenosis. Patients with osteopetrosis may have severe canalicular stenosis (see Chapter 13).

Bell's palsy is an idiopathic, usually unilateral, facial palsy that has a rapid onset and a spontaneous recovery. Gadolinium contrast enhancement of the involved facial nerve prior to the recovery phase is common. The labryrinthine segment most frequently contrast enhances, however, the entire intratemporal portion of the facial nerve may be enhanced. Gadolinium contrast enhancement of the facial nerve in cases of facial nerve paralysis following temporal bone surgery also occurs. Contrast enhancement of a paralyzed facial nerve is, therefore, a nonspecific finding and adds to the difficulty of detecting a facial nerve neuroma[6,40].

References

1. Shaffer KA. The temporal bone. In Williams AL, Haughton VM (Eds). *Cranial Computed Tomography.* St. Louis: CV Mosby Co, 1985; 512–554.
2. Swartz JD. High resolution computed tomography of the middle ear and mastoid. *Radiology* 1983; 148:449–454.
3. Daniels DL, Haughton VM. The temporal bone. In Daniels DL, Haughton VM, Naidich TP (Eds). *Cranial and Spinal Magnetic Resonance Imaging—an atlas and guide.* New York: Raven Press, 1987; 197–234.
4. Swartz JD. The facial nerve canal: CT analysis of the protruding tympanic segment. *Radiology* 1984; 153:443–447.
5. Chakeres DW, Spiegel PK. A systematic technique for comprehensive evaluation of temporal bone by computed tomography. *Radiology* 1983; 146:97–106.
6. Daniels DL, Czervionke LF, Pojunas KW, et al. Facial nerve enhancement in MR imaging. *AJNR* 1987; 8:605–607.
7. Daniels DL, Williams AL, Haughton VM. Jugular foramen: Anatomic and computed tomographic study. *AJR* 1984; 142:153–158.
8. Daniels DL, Czervionke LF, Pech P, et al. Gradient recalled echo MR imaging. *AJNR* 1988; 9:675–678.
9. Swartz JD, Glazer AO, Faerber EN. Congenital middle-ear deafness: CT study. *Radiology* 1983; 159:187–190.
10. Mafee MF, Selis JE, Yannias DA, et al. Congenital sensorineural hearing loss. *Radiology* 1984; 150:427–343.
11. Swartz JD, Faeber EN. Congenital malformations of the external and middle ear: High resolution CT findings of surgical import. *AJR* 1985; 144:501–506.
12. Holland B, Brant-Zawadzki M. High resolution CT of temporal bone trauma. *AJNR* 1984; 5:291–295.
13. Rubin J, Curtin HD, Yu VL, Kamerer DB. Malignant external otitis: utility of CT in diagnosis and follow up. *Radiology* 1990; 174:391–394.
14. Mafee MF, Aimi K, Kahen HL, et al. Chronic otomastoiditis: A conceptual understanding of CT findings. *Radiology* 1986; 160:193–200.
15. Swartz JD, Goodman RS, Russell KB, et al. High resolution computed tomography of the middle ear and mastoid. Part II: Tubotympanic disease. *Radiology* 1983; 148:455–459.
16. Swartz JD, Wolfson RJ, Martowe FI, Popky GL. Post-inflammatory ossicular fixation: CT analysis with surgical correlation. *Radiology* 1985; 154:697–700.
17. Silver AJ, Janecka I, Wazen J, et al. Complicated cholesteatomas: CT findings in inner ear complications of middle ear cholesteatomas. *Radiology* 1985; 155:391–397.
18. Mafee MF, Singleton EL, Valvassori GE, et al. Acute otomastoiditis and its complications: Role of CT. *Radiology* 1985; 155:391–397.
19. Swartz JD, Goodman RS, Russell KB, et al. High resolution computed tomography of the middle ear and mastoid. Part III: Surgically altered anatomy and pathology. *Radiology* 1983; 148:461–464.
20. Hernanz-Schulman M, Welsh K, Strand R, Ordia JI. Acoustic neuromas in children. *AJNR* 1986; 7:519–521.
21. Gentry LR, Jacoby CB, Turski PA, et al. Cerebellopontine angle-petromastoid mass lesions: Comparative study of diagnosis with MR imaging and CT. *Radiology* 1987; 162:513–520.
22. Valvassori GE, Morales FG, Palacios E, Dobben GE. MR of the normal and abnormal internal auditory canal. *AJR* 1988; 9:115–119.
23. Daniels DL, Miller SJ, Meyer GA. MR detection of tumor in the internal auditory canal. *AJNR* 1987; 8:249–252.
24. Breger RK, Papkej RA, Pojunas KW. Benign extra-axial tumors: Contrast enhancement with Gd-DTPA. *Radiology* 1987; 163:427–429.
25. Pinto RS, Kricheff II, Bergeron RT, Cohen N. Small acoustic neuromas: Detection by high resolution gas CT cisternography. *AJR* 1982; 139:129–132.
26. Yuh WTC, Wright DC, Barloon TJ, et al. MR imaging of primary tumors of trigeminal nerve and Meckel's cave. *AJNR* 1988; 9:665–670.
27. Greenberg J, Oot RF, Wismer GL, et al. Cholesterol granuloma of the petrous apex. MR and CT evaluation. *AJNR* 1988; 9:1205–1215.
28. Latock JT, Kartash JM, Kemink JL, et al. Epidermoidomas of the CP angle and the temporal bone: CT and MR aspects. *Radiology* 1985; 157:361–366.
29. Curtin HD, Jensen JE, Barnes L Jr, May M. "Ossifying" hemangiomas of the temporal bone: Evaluation with CT. *Radiology* 1987; 164:831–835.
30. Lo WWM, Horn KL, Carberry JN, et al. Intratemporal vascular tumors: Evaluation with CT. *Radiology* 1986; 159:181–185.
31. Spagnoli MV, Goldberg HI, Grossman RI, et al. Intracranial meningiomas: High-field MR imaging. *Radiology* 1986; 161:369–375.
32. Brant-Zawadzki M, Kelly W. Brain tumors. In Brant-Zawadzki M, Norman D (Eds). *Magnetic Resonance Imaging of the Central Nervous System.* New York: Raven Press, 1987; 151–185.
33. Larson TC III, Reese DF, Baker HL Jr, McDonald TJ. Glomus tympanicum chemodectomas: Radiographic and clinical characteristics. *Radiology* 1987; 163:801–806.
34. Olsen WL, Dillon WP, Kelly WM, et al. MR imaging of paragangliomas. *AJNR* 1986; 7:1039–1042.
35. Bird CR, Hasso AN, Stewart CE, et al. Malignant primary neoplasms of the ear and temporal bone studied by high resolution computed tomography. *Radiology* 1983; 149:171–174.
36. Mafee MF, Hendrickson GC, Deitch RL, et al. Use of CT in stapedial otosclerosis. *Radiology* 1985; 156:709–714.
37. Mafee MF, Valvassori GE, Deitch RL, et al. Use of CT in the evaluation of cochlear otosclerosis. *Radiology* 1985; 156:703–708.
38. Swartz JD, Lansman AK, Berger AS, et al. Stapes prosthesis: Evaluation with CT. *Radiology* 1986; 158:179–182.
39. Harnsberger HR, Dart DJ, Parkin JL, et al. Cochlear implant candidates: Assessment with CT and MR imaging. *Radiology* 1987; 164:53–57.
40. Daniels DL, Czervionke LF, Millen SJ et. al. MR imaging of facial nerve enhancement in Bell palsy or after temporal bone surgery. *Radiology* 1989; 171:807–809.

13 The Skull, Face, Paranasal Sinuses, and Nasopharynx

PART ONE

The Skull

Introduction

This section provides a brief description of pediatric and adult skull base and calvarial CT anatomy and describes pathological conditions of the skull base and calvarium. MR plays a secondary role here with respect to anatomy, however, MR has a high detectability rate for pathological conditions such as metastasis and intracranial extension of osseous disease. For bone detail, obviously CT is the superior method. For detail within the soft tissues, MR is superior to contrast CT due to soft tissue intensity characteristics and to comparatively artifact-free orthogonal plane imagine. Techniques vary according to the indication for the examination. Often, abnormalities of the skull, face, and paranasal sinuses are incidentally discovered on an examination for an entirely different reason. There is, therefore, an added responsibility placed on the radiologist to detect these often unexpected abnormalities.

Our routine cranial CT technique includes bone window hard copy throughout the posterior fossa sections. Ideally, physician review of all CT scans for bone windows or bone window hard copy of all sections could be done. Careful attention to a localizer view, to scalp soft tissues, and to juxtaosseous areas is necessary on all scans. The variable echo orthogonal plane MR sections obtained routinely for cranial scanning provide considerable skull, face, paranasal sinus, and nasopharynx detail.

Normal Anatomy

The calvarium includes the outer and inner tables between which is the diploic space. Here, the CT and MR images are complementary under normal circumstances. CT demonstrates exquisite detail of the calvarial tables whereas MR detects the hyperintense diploic (marrow) signals between the signal-void tables.

The sagittal, coronal, lambdoid, and temporal squamosal sutures are easily identified by the CT technique in pediatric patients and often in young adults. The normal infantile cranial sutures are clearly demonstrated by CT (Fig. 13.1). Good sutural detail is important to distinguish between suture and fracture, to identify sutural dehiscence, and to diagnose sutural synostosis.

The upper surface of the skull base is the floor of the cranial cavity. The floor of the anterior fossa is formed by the orbital plates of the frontal bone, the cribriform plate of the ethmoid bone, and the lesser wing and frontal portion of the sphenoid bone (Fig. 13.2). The middle fossa is formed by the sphenoid wings anteriorly, the lateral sellar margin medially, the petrous pyramid posteriorly, and the temporal squamosa laterally. The foramina rotundum, ovale and spinosum, the internal carotid artery canal, and the superior orbital fissure are all middle fossa landmarks. The posterior fossa is the largest and deepest of the three fossae. It is formed by the petrous pyramids and clivus anteriorly, the parietal and occipital bones laterally, and the occipital bone inferiorly and posteriorly. Posterior fossa foramina include the foramen magnum, the internal auditory, jugular, and hypoglossal canals. The jugular tubercle is cephalad to the hypoglossal canal and is an important landmark not to be confused with a cerebellopontine angle (CPA) tumor (Fig. 13.3). Normal variants, such as biparietal foramina and digital impressions (Fig. 13.4), and dural calcific plaques and juxtafalx and tentorial calcifications are easily recognized (Fig. 13.5).

Congenital or Childhood-Onset Abnormalities

The Lückenschadel skull vault, petrous scalloping and large foramen magnum of the Chiari II malfor-

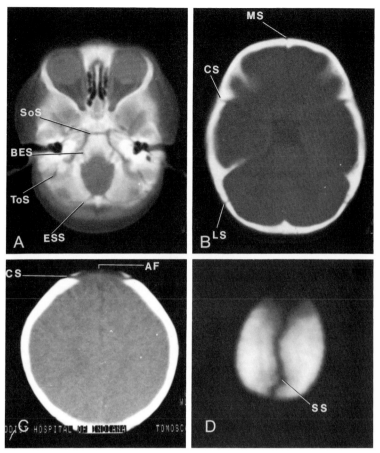

Figure 13.1. Normal infantile sutures. A–C is a 10-month-old infant; **D** is a 2-month-old. Axial soft tissue filter bone window CT scans. The occipital bone is seen divided by the basioccipital-exoccipital synchondrosis *(BES)* and the exoccipital-supraoccipital synchondrosis *(ESS)*. The occipital bone joins the sphenoid bone at the spheno-occipital synchondrosis *(SoS)* and the temporal bone at the temporo-occipital synchondrosis *(ToS)*. The coronal *(CS)*, lambdoid *(LS)*, and sagittal *(SS)* sutures are easily recognized. The metopic suture *(MS)* divides the frontal bone. The normal anterior fontanelle *(AF)* appears within the contour of the skull.

mation (Fig. 9.1) and the torcular-lambdoid inversion of Dandy-Walker malformation (Fig. 9.15) are discussed in Chapter 9.

Congenital or perinatal cerebral hemiatrophy [Dyke-Davidoff-Masson syndrome (Fig 6.25)] has been discussed in Chapter 6. Cephalohematoma (Fig. 7.1) and leptomeningeal cyst [the "growing fracture" (Fig. 7.2)] have already been discussed in Chapter 7. Congenital malformations such as C1-occipital fusion and the markedly large foramen magnum of Chiari II and III malformations are easily identified (Fig. 13.6).

CRANIOSYNOSTOSIS

The coronal, sagittal, and lambdoid sutures remain open until approximately 30 years of age and, occasionally, some sutures remain open throughout life. Craniosynostosis is the premature closure of one or more skull sutures. If the sutures close before 3 years of age, there is usually a resultant skull deformity and often, brain compression.[1] Males are far more likely to be affected.[1] Hereditary factors are not infrequently responsible such as acrocephalosyndactylism (Apert's syndrome) and craniofacial dyostosis (Crouzon's syndrome). Treatment of vitamin D-resistant rickets and chronic ventricular shunting may cause premature sutural synostosis.[2]

Dolichocephaly results from sagittal and brachycephaly results from coronal or lambdoidal sutural premature closure. Unilateral premature closure results in skull asymmetry (plagiocephaly) that can be distinguished from cerebral hemiatrophy by lack of brain atrophic changes. Concurrent premature closure of all sutures results in microcephaly, which can be distinguished from the more common dysplastic or atrophic microcephaly by lack of brain atrophy. Axial and coronal CT wide window technique is particularly effective for diagnosis of this condition (Fig. 13.7). Vertex and high convexity axial sections are particularly effective for sagittal, coronal, and lambdoidal premature sutural closure. Coronal sections demonstrate marginal hyperostosis associated with sagittal synostosis and both axial and coronal sections demonstrate skull and possible facial asymmetries and deformities. CT scans, including 3-D reformations, form a baseline for future surgical corrective procedures. MR in these conditions and in their sur-

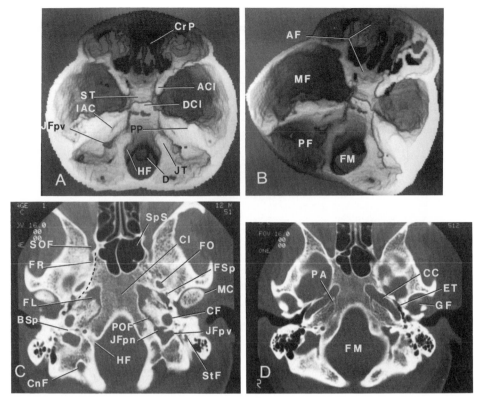

Figure 13.2. Normal skull base. Three-dimensional CT reformation of 3-mm sections **(A** and **B).** *Axial 1.5-mm thickness 16-cm FOV 600/4000 CT scans **(C** and **D). D** is 3-mm cephalad to **C.** The thin floor of the anterior fossa *(AF)* is evident by its perforated appearance on the 3-D reformatted images. The middle *(MF)* and posterior *(PF)* fossa floors are separated by the petrous pyramids *(PP).* The dens *(D)* is seen beneath the foramen magnum *(FM)* under the "basion" or inferior lip of the clivus *(Cl).* The jugular tubercle *(JT)* of the occipital bone forms the roof of the hypoglossal foramen *(HF).* Inferiorly, the jugular fossa is separated from the carotid foramen *(CF)* by a thin bone septum *(BSp).* More craniad, the thin petrosal spinous process separates the pars venosa *(JFpv)* from the more an-terior pars nervosa *(JFpn).* The parieto-occipital fissure *(POF)* and the foramen lacerum *(FL)* surround the petrous apex *(PA)* inferiorly.

C. The third segment of the facial nerve exits the styloid foramen *(StF).* The condyloid fossa *(Cnf),* located posterior to the occipital condyle, transmits only a minor vein. The foramen spinosum *(FSp)* for the middle meningeal artery, foramen ovale *(FO)* for the third division of the trigeminal nerve, the foramen rotundum *(FR)* for the second division of the trigeminal nerve, and the superior orbital fissure *(SOF)* lateral to the sphenoid sinus *(SpS)* transmitting the first division of the trigeminal nerve circumscribe a smooth arc *(dashes).* The eustachian tube *(ET)* is between the mandibular condyle glenoid fossa *(GF)* and the petrous carotid canal *(CC).*

Figure 13.3. The jugular tubercle. *Axial **(A)** and direct coronal **(B)** CT scans.* There is a very prominent right jugular tubercle *(closed arrow)* that can be mistaken for a hyperdense mass. Other sectioning artifact hyperdensities result from ridges of the middle fossa floor *(open arrows).* The jugular foramen is lateral to the jugular tubercle and the hypoglossal canal *(HC)* is beneath it. The occipital condyle *(OC)* articulates with the C1 superior articular surface *(C1); StP =* styloid process medial to the mastoid sinus.

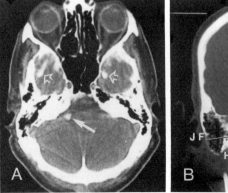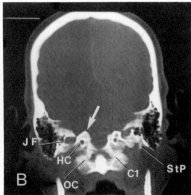

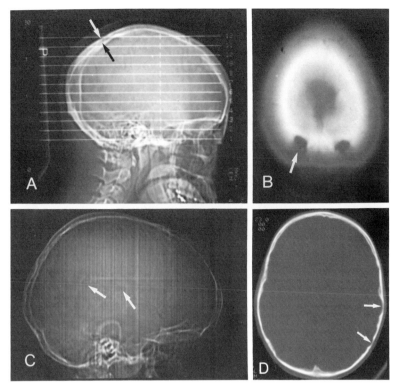

Figure 13.4. Normal variants. **B** and **C–D** are different cases. *Biparietal foramina: CT lateral localizer **(A)** and 10-mm thickness 346/3000 vertex CT scan **(B).*** There is marked thinning of the skull outer and inner tables *(arrows)* and virtual absence of the diploic space producing striking symmetrical CT homogeneous hypodense smoothly marginated lesions. *Digital impressions: CT lateral localizer view **(C)** and axial lateral ventricle-level 325/3000 CT scan **(D).*** Multiple left parietal inner table erosions are noted *(arrows)*. The CT scan was otherwise normal. There was no tumor, hydrocephalus, cyst, or brain asymmetry.

gical follow-up may be helpful by demonstrating the presence or absence of cerebral compression.[1,2]

MICROCEPHALY

Microcephalic infants usually have an abnormally small atrophic or dystrophic brain and a small and often thickened calvarium.[1] CT and MR of microcephaly demonstrate a uniformly small calvarium and evidence of cerebral atrophy or dystrophy.

HISTIOCYTOSIS X

Histiocytosis X is characterized by idiopathic histiocytic proliferation that causes lytic bone lesions in children and young adults. Three syndromes are included in this group of diseases: eosinophilic granu-

loma, Hand-Schüller-Christian syndrome and Letterer-Siwe's disease. They are listed here in order of increasing severity and decreasing age of onset.

Eosinophilic granuloma is the most common, is confined to bone and the majority of lesions are solitary. There is often a soft tissue component usually involving the scalp but the dura may be involved and, rarely, there may be extension into brain substance.[3] These lesions often present clinically as a "knot" or a palpable skull defect.

CT is the preferred method of investigation, however, MR may be a useful adjunct for evaluation of dural involvement. The scout view often demonstrates the lytic defect. Contrast injection CT with soft tissue and bone windows demonstrates a sharply

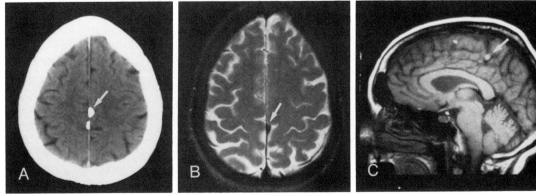

Figure 13.5. Falx calcifications. *Axial centrum semiovale-level 32/100 CT scan **(A)** and 2800/80 MR scan **(B).** Midsagittal 600/25 MR scan **(C).*** The CT hyperdense juxtafalx ossifications ("calcifications") are T1 centrally hyperintense with peripheral hypointensity. They are T2 hypointense with greater peripheral hypointensity. Peripheral dense ossification with central fatty marrow elements is the apparent explanation for these imaging findings.

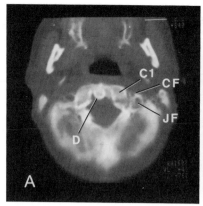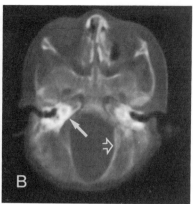

Figure 13.6. Congenital malformations affecting the skull base. **A:** Occipitalization of the atlas. *Axial 6-mm thickness 40/1600 CT scan.* The C1 *(C1)* lateral masses are fused to the occipital bone. The jugular *(JF)* and carotid *(CF)* foramina are seen within the com- bined bone mass. Although the dens *(D)* appears fused to the C1 anterior arch, it was not on complex motion sagittal tomograms. **B:** Chiari III malformation. There is a very large foramen magnum *(open arrow)* and there is posterior petrous "scalloping" *(closed arrow)*.

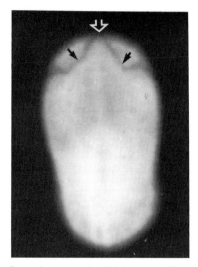

Figure 13.7. Sutural synostosis. *Axial vertex 133/400.* Five-month-old male infant with sagittal suture synostosis. The open coronal suture allows paracentral and lateral bone growth *(closed arrows)* producing an anterior midline parietal beak *(open arrow)*. There is marked dolichocephaly.

marginated lytic skull defect often involving the outer table more than the inner table (Fig. 13.8). The disproportion of table involvement produces a "beveled" appearance.[4] Coronal CT sections best demonstrate lesions parallel to the axial plane. Contrast enhancement of the soft tissue component may occur.[3]

ACHONDROPLASIA

Achondroplasia is a hereditary disorder of enchondral bone formation that affects the skull, the spine, and the skeleton in general. Because the skull base is enchondral bone and the calvarium is not, the skull base is primarily affected. The achondroplastic skull is brachiocephalic with a small base and a large calvarium. The foramen magnum is small. Hydrocephalus commonly occurs possibly due to fourth ventricle outlet compression. CT shows the characteristic small foramen magnum and demonstrates ventricular enlargement. The role of MR in this condition has not been established.

SICKLE CELL ANEMIA

Sickle cell anemia produces diploic expansion and outer table thinning, which results from erythroid hyperplasia and bone marrow expansion that is detectable by CT (Fig. 13.9). Because no skull bone marrow is found caudal to the internal occipital protuberance, no involvement is found below this landmark.[5]

FIBROUS DYSPLASIA

Fibrous dysplasia is a childhood-onset condition characterized by monostotic or polyostotic cancellous bone fibrous tissue replacement expansion and erosion. The two principal types of this disease demonstrated by CT are sclerotic and cystic. The sclerotic form is more common. It usually involves the face and adjacent skull base producing featureless dense bone thickening (Fig. 13.10). CT differential diagnosis includes Paget's disease, which will be discussed later in this chapter. The less common cystic or low density form produces a diploic expansile hypodense localized calvarial lesion. There is usually a sclerotic rim surrounding the cystic lesions. CT differential diagnosis for a solitary intradiploic expansile calvarial lesion includes epidermoid tumor, hemangioma, and histiocytosis X.[6] The epidermoid lesion also has a sclerotic margin.

OSTEOGENESIS IMPERFECTA

Osteogenesis imperfecta is a rare hereditary (autosomal dominant) bone disorder characterized by a deficiency of osteoblasts causing severe osteoporosis. There is an early onset form occurring at birth and a tarda form that may become manifest at puberty or adulthood. Clinically, the patients are markedly susceptible to fractures, which leads to marked deformities. Marked skull deformity with basilar invagination often develops (Fig. 13.11).

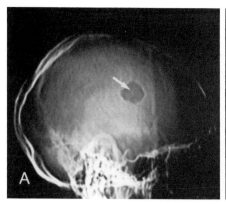
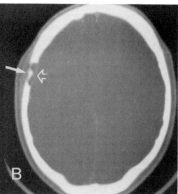
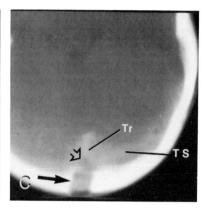

Figure 13.8.   Eosinophilic granuloma. A–B and **C** are different cases. **A** and **B:** *Lateral CT localizer view **(A)** and 30/1500 axial i.v. contrast CT scan **(B)**.* There is a "beveled edge" undulating sharply marginated anterior parietal bone osteolytic mass with a central localizer hyperintensity representing a partially sequestered portion *(closed arrow)*. There are subgaleal and epidural *(open arrow)* mass components. **C:** *Axial i.v. contrast 100/2000 10-mm thick CT scan at the fourth ventricle level.* An occipital bone undulating sharply marginated osteolytic *(closed arrow)* and epidural *(open arrow)* soft tissue mass without contrast enhancement displaces the contrast-enhanced torcula *(Tr); TS =* transverse sinus.

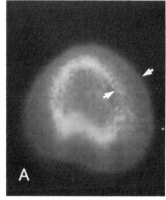
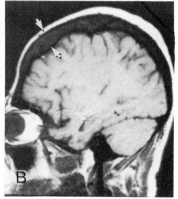

Figure 13.9.   Sickle cell disease. *Axial vertex 525/3000 CT scan **(A)**. Sagittal SE 600/25 5-mm thickness MR scan **(B)**.* There is marked CT density and MR intensity "salt and pepper" diploic space expansion with cortical thinning *(arrows)*. The occipital bone is not involved.

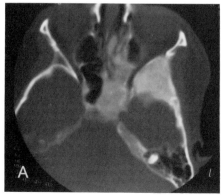
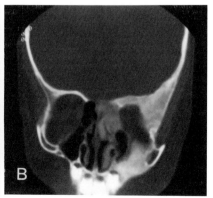

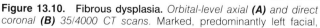
Figure 13.10.   Fibrous dysplasia. *Orbital-level axial **(A)** and direct coronal **(B)** 35/4000 CT scans.* Marked, predominantly left facial, smoothly homogeneous, expansile hyperostosis involves multiple facial bones and also includes the left petrous apex.

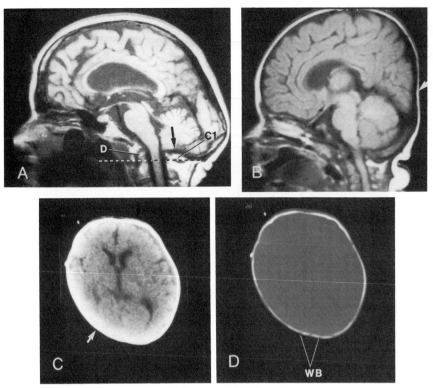

Figure 13.11. Osteogenesis imperfecta. **A** and **B–D** are different cases. **A:** Adult with marked basilar invagination. *Midsagittal SE 600/25 MR scan.* Dental artifact obscures detail of the palate, however, an estimated McGregor's line *(dashed line)* has been drawn. The dens *(D)* and C1 spinous process are well above the line and analysis of the skull base *(arrow)* shows an abnormally very high position.

B–D: Two-month-old infant with osteogenesis imperfecta. *Sagittal SE 600/25 MR scan **(B)**. Axial 35/100 **(C)** and 100/1000 **(D)** CT scans.* There are multiple occipital wormian bones *(WB)* within the deformed posterior skull *(arrow)*, which has assumed its shape due to supine recumbency. The brain is normal. (McGregor's line is from the hard palate to the posterior foramen magnum inferior margin.)

OSTEOPETROSIS

Osteopetrosis ("marble bone disease" or "Albers-Schönberg Disease") is a rare hereditary bone disorder caused by a persistence of calcified cartilage. The disease varies in clinical severity and includes a "tarda" or more benign form. In the more severe cases, there is extremely dense fragile bone leading to frequent fractures, hypoplastic anemia, and skull foraminal stenosis. Foraminal stenosis may cause visual and hearing impairment and subsequent blindness and deafness. Paranasal sinus hypoplasia also occurs (Fig. 13.12).[5]

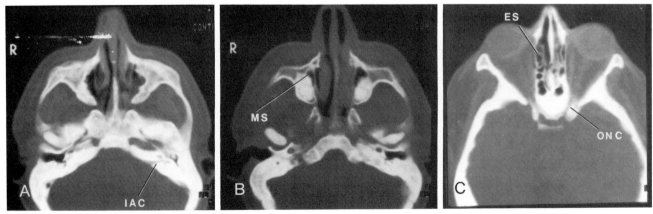

Figure 13.12. Osteopetrosis: A 22-year-old blind patient with sensorineural deafness. *Axial 38/3200 soft tissue filter CT scans.* There is marked stenosis of the internal auditory canals *(IAC)* and the optic nerve canal *(ONC)*. There is poor pneumatization of the ethmoid *(ES)* and maxillary *(MS)* sinuses. Surgical maxillary "windows" **(A)** are evident. There is virtual absence of mastoid pneumatization and all bones are extremely dense.

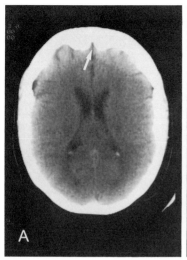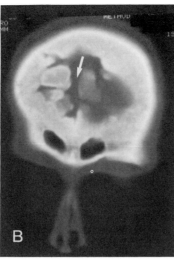

Figure 13.13. Hyperostosis frontalis interna. *Axial noncontrast lateral ventricle body-level 50/100 **(A)** and direct coronal frontal sinus-level 900/4000 **(B)** CT scans.* There is marked bifrontal inner table hyperostosis separated by a vertical cleft *(arrows).*

Adult-Onset Abnormalities

Skull fractures have already been discussed in Chapter 7. Other adult-onset skull base and calvarium abnormalities are categorized in this section.

HYPEROSTOSIS FRONTALIS INTERNA

Hyperostosis frontalis interna is characterized by bilateral and symmetrical osseous overgrowth of the inner table, which is separated by a midline cleft. It occurs predominantly in women over 35 years old. Axial bone window CT scans demonstrate the symmetrical undulating character of the frontal bone, exclusively inner table hyperostotic process with the characteristic sagittal plane straight midline cleft (Fig. 13.13).[2,4,6] Meningioma might be considered as a differential diagnostic consideration but the midline cleft excludes it.

PAGET'S DISEASE

Paget's disease (osteitis deformans) is a common bone disease of unknown cause that is characterized by osseous thickening, trabecular coarsening, and bone softening. The disease incidence increases with age and the skull is affected in the majority of Paget's patients. There are sclerotic, radiolucent (osteoporosis circumscripta), and mixed forms. The calvarial architecture is often distorted so severely that the tables and diploic space are no longer clearly defined. Basilar impression due to softening occurs in approximately one-third of skull Paget's disease patients. CSF dynamics may be impaired by basilar invagination leading to hydrocephalus. Stenosis of the foramen magnum and the optic and internal auditory canals may occur. Malignant transformation from Paget's disease to osteosarcoma occurs in less than 1% of patients.[7]

Often, if not the majority of time, the CT or MR scan has been ordered for indications other than Paget's disease. The diagnosis of Paget's disease and of basilar invagination can easily be made by CT and MR. CT demonstrates trabecular coarsening vault thickening and distortion of the normal architecture. MR demonstrates T1 and T2 heterogeneous signals of the abnormal thick calvarium (Fig. 13.14).[8] The MR sagittal image and also the MR and CT coronal sections demonstrate basilar impression more accurately than do the axial sections. CT scout view analysis of McGregor's line (hard palate posterior edge to lowest point of occipital bone) is recommended. Basilar invagination is diagnosed if the tip of the odontoid process is more than 4 mm above this line. It is difficult for the basilar invagination patient to hyperextend satisfactorily for CT coronal sections. As mentioned in Chapter 12, Paget's involvement of the temporal bone may cause deafness due to otospongiosis (otosclerosis) rather than due to stenosis of the internal auditory canal.

Fibrous dysplasia is probably the only serious practical differential diagnostic consideration. Fibrous dysplasia occurs in younger patients, most often involves the face, and does not produce the trabecular coarsening typical of Paget's disease.[2]

EPIDERMOID TUMORS

Epidermoid tumors or cysts can present on CT scans as a sharply marginated intradiploic expansile calvarial mass often having a sclerotic margin (Fig. 13.15). An associated intracranial mass typical of epidermoid tumor may be present. The CT differential diagnosis of a solitary intradiploic expansile mass includes cystic fibrous dysplasia and hemangioma. Hemangioma is likely to have a trabeculated internal appearance as compared to epidermoid waterdensity. Cystic fibrous dysplasia is usually homogeneously hypodense, lacking the trabeculated hemangioma matrix, and it typically has a smooth sclerotic border. Eosinophilic granuloma may be considered in the differential diagnosis in younger patients with solitary intradiploic calvarial lesions. An unusual solitary metastasis can present similar CT findings.

Figure 13.14. Paget's disease with basilar invagination. **A–B** and **C–D** are different cases. *CT lateral localizer view* **(A)** *and axial lateral ventricle atrial-level 100/2000* **(B)**. *Midsagittal SE 600/ 25* **(C)** *and coronal pons-level 2000/20* **(D)**. There is marked diploic thickening *(arrows)* and density/intensity heterogeneity "cotton-wool" with markedly increased cortical thickness. The dens *(D)* is well above McGregor's line *(dashes)* in both cases. (McGregor's line: hard palate to the posterior foramen magnum inferior edge. The normal dens should be less than 4 mm above the line.) Note the pontomedullary angulation demonstrated by MR. The petrous apices are upward angulated as evidenced by the downward course of the neurovascular bundle within the internal auditory canal *(n7–8)*.

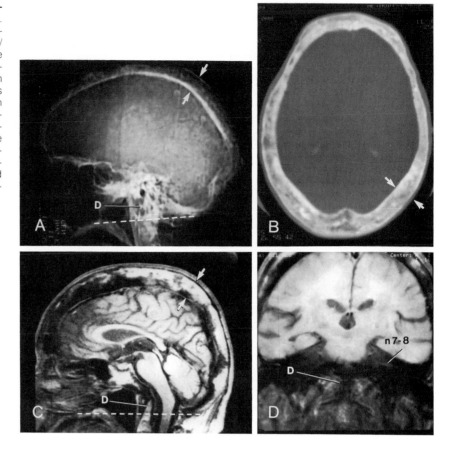

ARACHNOID CYSTS

Arachnoid cysts have been discussed in Chapter 5. They often produce ipsilateral middle fossa expansion and are easily recognized by CT and MR (Figs. 5.7 and 13.16).

Inner table erosion caused by supratentorial low grade astrocytomas is occasionally seen and can be detected by both CT and MR scanning (Fig. 13.17).

MENINGIOMA BONE CHANGES

Meningioma bone changes are usually hyperdense (Fig. 13.18). Rarely, associated osteolysis is present.[6] Meningioma bone changes are almost always associated with a detectable intracranial mass (Chapter 5).

OSTEOMAS

Skull osteomas are rare, benign, slow-growing, smoothly margined, high density neoplasms affecting the calvarium or skull base. They are sessile or nodular. They can arise from either the outer or inner table and grow away from the diploic space (Fig. 13.19). By CT, the inner table osteomas, particularly the sessile type, cannot be distinguished from a densely calcified meningioma.[6]

OSTEOCHONDROMAS

Osteochondromas are uncommon skull base tumors arising most often in the sphenoid bone. They are usually coarsely calcified and may be sessile much like skeletal osteochondromas elsewhere. They may resemble densely calcified meningiomas.[6]

OSTEOMYELITIS

Calvarial osteolysis may be caused by osteomyelitis, which usually results from direct extension of paranasal sinus disease, craniotomy, or penetrating injury. CT demonstrates a permeative osteolytic pattern contiguous with a fluid-containing facial sinus. There may be an epidural component or an adjacent brain abscess (Fig. 8.7). MR is useful to detect early evidence of intracranial disease. The major differential diagnostic points to exclude metastasis are adjacent sinus inflammation, pre-existing craniotomy or open trauma.[1,6]

METASTASIS

Skull metastasis is usually of breast or lung origin. One-third of these patients have intracranial metastasis. These lesions are usually osteolytic but may be osteoblastic or mixed. There may be contiguous soft tissue scalp or intracranial mass. Skull base metastasis can mimic glomus jugulare tumors (Fig. 12.26) and chordoma (Fig. 11.22).

CT often demonstrates scout view osteolytic defects as well as the characteristic multiple diploic origin osteolytic lesions with inner and outer table involvement. They usually lack sharp margination

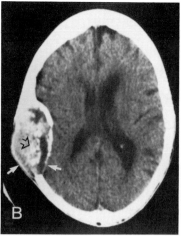

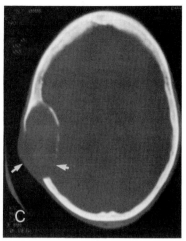

Figure 13.15.   Epidermoid tumor. *CT lateral localizer* **(A)** *and lateral ventricle atrial-level 36/100* **(B)** *and same level 36/3000* **(C)** *noncontrast CT scans.* There is a diploic markedly expansile parietal bone, smooth, thin, hyperdense undulating rimmed hypodense mass

containing calcified portions *(open arrows).* Some portions lack detectable cortication *(closed arrows).* Because of the large extradural mass effect, the septum pellucidum is shifted toward the left side.

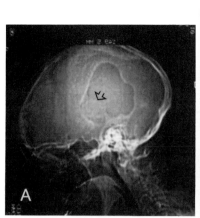

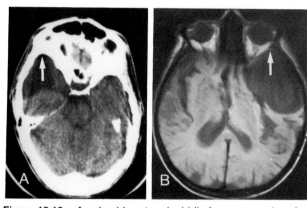

Figure 13.16.   Arachnoid cyst and middle fossa expansion. A and **B** are different cases. *Axial sella-level 36/150 CT scan* **(A)** *and SE 2000/20 orbit-level MR scan* **(B).** Note the middle fossa expansion by the water-density/intensity masses *(arrows).* There is a characteristic relatively horizontal posterior cyst margin.

and marginal sclerosis. Bone window hard copy images are necessary (Fig. 13.20). These cases have usually been studied with i.v. contrast CT to rule out cerebral metastasis. There is usually contrast enhancement of soft tissue components.[2,4,6]

It is important to analyze the calvarium or MR scans for evidence of metastasis. Interruption of the diploic hyperintense signal, loss of the cortical signal void, and contiguous abnormal soft tissue in orthogonal planes is very accurate for skull metastasis diagnosis.

MULTIPLE MYELOMA

Differential diagnosis of skull metastasis includes multiple myeloma from which it cannot be distinguished but which is usually clinically apparent before scanning.[2,6] An isolated plasmacytoma appears as a focal, often large, calvarial defect, which fre-

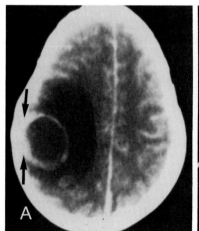

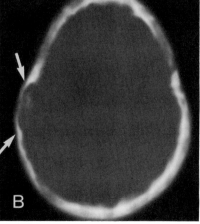

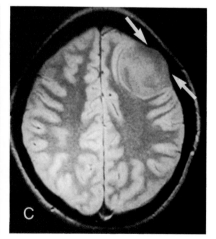

Figure 13.17.   Astrocytoma causing inner table erosion. A–B and **C** are different cases. *Axial low centrum semiovale-level i.v. contrast 36/100* **(A)** *and 36/3000* **(B)** *CT scans. Same level axial SE 2800/30 MR scan* **(C).** Both cases demonstrate low grade astrocytomas. The

CT case demonstrates an apparent predominantly cystic right parietal mass with an eccentric large "signet ring" solid portion eroding the skull inner table *(arrows).* The MR case demonstrates marked protrusion beyond the convexity of a left frontal mass *(arrows).*

Figure 13.18. Meningioma skull changes. **A–B, C–F,** and **G–H** are different cases. **A–B:** *Axial centrum semiovale-level i.v. contrast 60/ 150 (A) and 435/3200 (B) CT scans.* A smoothly marginated, homogeneously contrast-enhanced left convexity meningioma *(open arrow)* produces an anterior parietal bone erosive-like change within a large area of hyperostosis *(closed arrow).* **C–F:** *Left para-sagittal SE 600/25 noncontrast (C) and coronal SE 600/25 i.v. contrast MR scan (D). Vertex axial 327/3000 (E) and centrum 36/150 i.v. contrast (F) CT scans.* A convexity-parasagittal T1 gray matter-isointense i.v. contrast-enhancing, smoothly marginated epidural mass projects intracranially *(open arrows)* and has marked extracranial hyperostosis *(closed arrows).* Part of the hyperostotic portion contrast enhances **(D).** There is adjacent dural *(Du)* and falx *(F)* thickening and abnormal contrast enhancement. **G–H:** *Axial 250/600 (G) i.v. contrast CT scan and same orbital-level SE 2800/80 MR scan (H).* A markedly calcified partially contrast-enhanced sphenoid wing meningioma *(open arrow)* invades the posterior left orbit. There is marked sphenoid demineralized bone expansion *(closed arrow).*

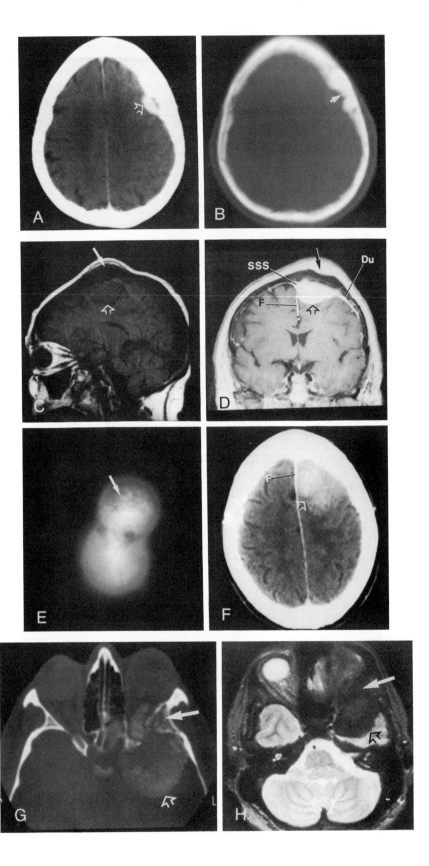

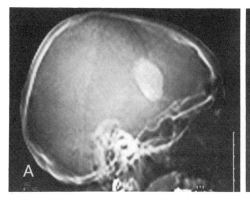
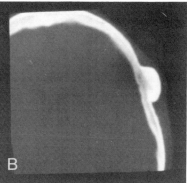

Figure 13.19. Skull osteoma. *Lateral CT localizer view* **(A)** *and axial 274/3200 CT scan* **(B)**. *A 39-mm diameter hyperdense outer table excrescence spares the diploic space and inner table.*

quently has an associated soft tissue component. Iodinated i.v. contrast (CT) should be withheld from these patients and given only if absolutely necessary and only if the patient is adequately hydrated.

BROWN TUMORS—HYPERPARATHYROIDISM

The differential diagnosis of multiple skull lytic defects in the adult also includes brown tumors of hyperparathyroidism. Brown tumors appear as lytic lesions within abnormal calvarial bone. The calvarium may be hypodense or hyperdense by CT. Lack of distinction of the tables, and presence of falx or tentorial calcification are additional clues.[4] The clinical history is almost always known before scanning.

PART TWO

Facial Structures, Paranasal Sinuses, and Nasopharynx

Introduction

CT remains the procedure of choice for paranasal sinus and nasal cavity imaging. MR is rapidly becoming the procedure of choice for imaging tissues deep to the sinuses such as the nasopharynx and parapharyngeal structures.[9] CT is particularly effective for paranasal sinus imaging because of the need to demonstrate high spatial resolution bone detail and due to bone-mucosa-air CT density resolution. The CT method is hindered, however, by metal-induced beam hardening dental artifacts, particularly with direct coronal scanning. MR is particularly effective for nasopharynx and neighboring structural detail because of MR detection of T1 and T2 soft tissue and blood flow characteristics and because of relatively artifact-free orthogonal plane imaging. CT technique for the nasopharynx requires i.v. contrast injection.

Often, the facial abnormality is incidental to the indication for the CT or MR study. Thus, careful scrutiny of the initial scan is very important so as not to miss evidence of an unsuspected serious condition. CT has no equal in facial trauma—a condition in which bone detail is of paramount importance. Three-dimensional reformation of contiguous

thin axial CT sections for facial bone fractures and congenital facial anomalies is playing an increasingly important role for surgical planning and follow-up.

CT of the face and paranasal sinus requires a thin section (1.5- or 3-mm) infraorbitomeatal plane axial and direct coronal plane, noncontrast, bone filter wide window technique. MR 5-mm axial and coronal, variable echo, small FOV technique for the paranasal sinuses and nasopharynx followed by coronal SE 600/25, 3-mm, small FOV scans in the area of interest is our current standard. The maxillary alveolar ridge should be included in these views. We do not use direct sagittal CT.

Normal Anatomy

FACIAL BONES

The facial bones containing air sinuses are discussed in the paranasal sinus section of this chapter. The role of the facial bone buttresses protecting the orbits and other facial structures from injury will be discussed in the trauma section of this chapter. Orbital anatomy will be discussed in Chapter 14.

PARANASAL SINUSES

The paranasal sinuses are mucosa-lined, air-filled cavities within the facial bones for which they are named (Fig. 13.21). The frontal sinuses are often asymmetric and vary in degree of development. The mucus drains through the frontal sinus ostium to the nasofrontal duct and/or directly to an adjacent ethmoid air cell via the nasofrontal recess to reach the middle meatus. A true "duct" is present only in a minority of patients. The ethmoid and maxillary sinuses are immediately lateral to the nasal cavity. The lateral margins of the ethmoid sinuses form the medial orbital walls.[10] The ethmoid sinuses have multiple septations. They may extend into the orbital roofs. A septum, the basal lamella, difficult to identify by CT, is the partition dividing the anterior and middle portions from the posterior portion. The anterior and middle portions drain to the middle meatus via the ethmoid infundibulum, which is continuous with the maxillary sinus ostium. The ethmoid

Figure 13.20. Skull metastasis. A–B and **C–H** are different cases. **A–B:** Metastatic lung carcinoma. *Axial skull base 100/600 9-mm thickness* **(A)** *and i.v. contrast direct coronal sella-level 5-mm thickness 90/300* **(B)** *CT scans.* A left skull base contrast-enhancing osteolytic tumor *(arrows)* has destroyed the petrous apex, the left sphenoid sinus lateral wall, and the floor of the middle fossa. Tumor invades the sphenoid sinus *(T-SpS)*, the cavernous sinus *(T-Cs)*, and the lateral recess of the nasopharynx *(T-LPR)*. Note that the formina ovale *(FO)* and spinosum *(FSp)* are not involved. **C–H:** *Midsagittal noncontrast* **(C)**, *coronal orbital-level i.v. contrast* **(D)**, *axial high-convexity noncontrast* **(E)**, *and same level i.v. contrast* **(F)** *SE 600/25 5-mm thickness MR scans. Same axial level 36/100 noncontrast* **(G)** *and 36/3200* **(H)** *CT scans.* There is CT osteolysis involving the diploic space and cortex and there is MR-increased T1 bone signal from the metastatic tumor *(closed arrows)*. Epidural mass effect with transdural pia-arachnoid and parenchymal invasion is demonstrated well by MR contrast enhancement with i.v. Gd-DTPA injection and suggested by CT due to sulcal displacement and obliteration *(open arrows)*.

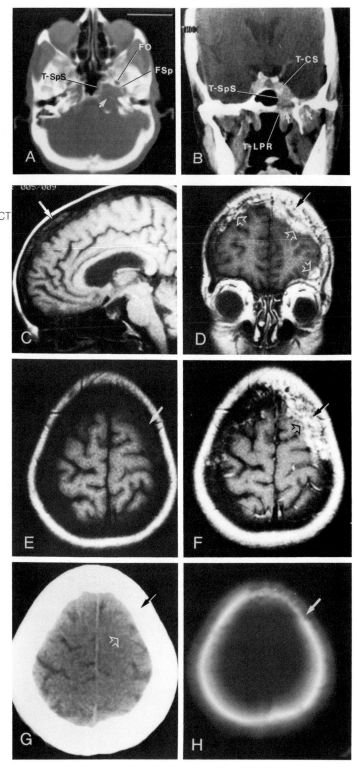

infundibulum is also often continuous with the nasofrontal duct or recess. The posterior portion of the ethmoid sinuses and the sphenoid sinus drain to the superior meatus via the sphenoethmoidal recess.[11–13] The sphenoid sinus has a major sagittal or parasagittal septum. The sphenoid sinus may extend laterally into the sphenoid wings.[14] Each side of the

sphenoid sinus drains via a small orifice (ostium) into the sphenoethmoidal recess, a mucosal-lined cleft that separates the superior turbinate from the sphenoid bone.[12] The maxillary sinuses drain via the maxillary ostium and ethmoid infundibulum into the hiatus semilunaris, which is a prominent curved cleft between the uncinate process and the ethmoidal bulla.

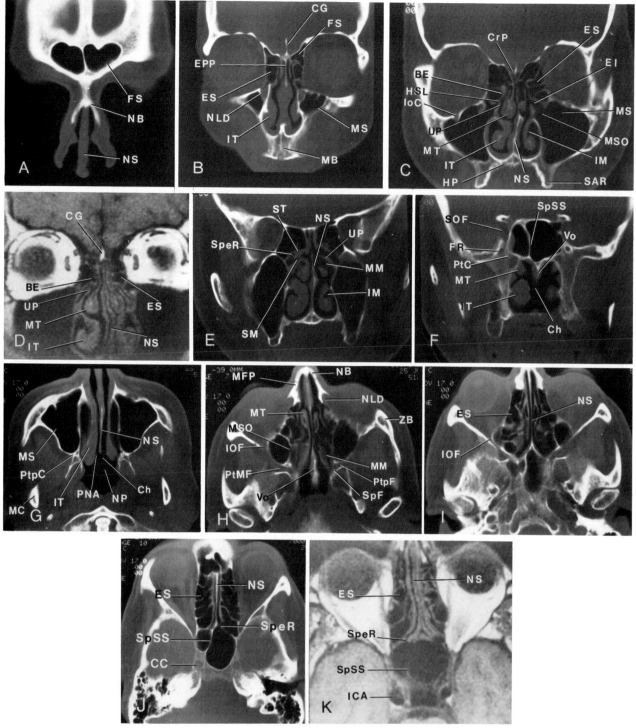

Figure 13.21. Normal paranasal sinus and nasal cavity. *Coronal (A–C and E–F) and axial (G–J) 3-mm thickness 375/4000 bone filter CT scans. Coronal (D) and axial (K) 3-mm thickness, 18-mm FOV, SE 600/25 MR scans.* (For sagittal MR and CT images, see Fig. 13.22.) All CT scans are of the same patient and the MR scans are of a different patient. The coronal scans are displayed from front to back and the axial scans are from caudal to cranial. The CT scans demonstrate right nasal turbinate hypertrophy, a small amount of fluid in the left maxillary sinus and slight right sphenoid sinus mucosal hypertrophy but are otherwise normal. A list of abbreviations used for structural labeling follows: *BE* = ethmoidal bulla; *CC* = carotid canal; *CG* = cristi galli; *Ch* = choanae; *CrP* = cribriform plate; *EI* = ethmoid infundibulum; *EPP* = ethmoid perpendicular plate; *ES* = ethmoid sinus; *FR* = foramen rotundum; *FS* = frontal sinus; *HP* = hard palate; *HSL* = hiatus semilunaris; *ICA* = internal carotid artery; *IM*

= inferior meatus; *IoC* = infraorbital canal; *IoF* = inferior orbital fissure; *IT* = inferior turbinate; *MB* = maxillary bone; *MC* = mandible condyle; *MFP* = maxillary frontal process; *MM* = middle meatus; *MS* = maxillary sinus; *MSO* = maxillary sinus ostium; *MT* = middle turbinate; *NB* = nasal bone; *NLD* = nasolacrimal duct; *NP* = nasopharynx; *NS* = nasal septum; *PNA* = posterior nasal aperture; *PtC* = pterygoid canal; *PtpC* = pterygopalatine canal; *PtpF* = pterygomaxillary fossa; *SAR* = superior alveolar ridge; *SM* = superior meatus; *SOF* = superior orbital fissure; *SpeR* = sphenoethmoidal recess; *SpF* = sphenopalatine foramen; *SpSS* = sphenoid sinus septum; *ST* = superior turbinate; *UP* = uncinate process; *Vo* = vomer; *ZB* = zygomatic bone. Note: A problem with the MR method for paranasal sinus diagnosis is the signal void of both bone and air as compared to the CT bone-air marked attenuation difference.

Drainage from the hiatus semilunaris is directed posteriorly along the middle meatus by ciliary action to the nasopharynx. Almost all mucus in the nasal cavity drains to the nasopharynx, under normal circumstances. Only the mucus that flows anterior to the middle turbinates drains forward to the nostrils (Fig. 13.22).[12] The middle meatus is the cleft formed between the uncinate process and the middle turbinate. The uncinate process is a prominent ridge anterior and inferior to the hiatus. The ethmoidal bulla is a prominent ethmoid sinus bulge at the hiatus superior margin. The ethmoid infundibulum is lateral to the hiatus and opens into its superior margin. Occasionally, an unusual maxillary sinus septation may be present and can play an important role with respect to pathophysiology and surgical planning.[11,12] The maxillary sinus ostium, the ethmoid infundibulum, and the middle meatus are collectively called the *ostiomeatal unit.* The ostiomeatal unit is an important physiological pathway for mucous flow from the maxillary, anterior ethmoidal, and the frontal sinuses and, therefore, an important CT landmark.[12]

The nasolacrimal ducts are located adjacent to the anteromedial corner of the maxillary sinuses and drain secretions that enter the lacrimal sac at the medial canthus. The duct courses the anteromedial orbital margin to the inferior meatus.[15,16]

NASAL CAVITY

Both CT and MR effectively image the nasal cavity. Because of their anatomic juxtaposition and their functional relationships, the study of paranasal sinuses and the nasal cavity requires the same technique and is essentially the same study.

The nasal cavity roof is formed by the nasal bones, the cribriform plate, and the sphenoid sinus. The hard palate forms the floor. The lateral nasal cavity wall is formed cranially by the ethmoid sinuses and caudally by the maxillary sinuses. The superior and middle conchae are ethmoid processes and the inferior concha is a separate bone. The middle concha is attached to the cribriform plate. The conchae are covered with mucosa forming the superior, middle, and inferior turbinates. Under and lateral to each turbinate is a corresponding nasal passage—the inferior, middle, and superior meatus. The nasolacrimal duct drains into the inferior meatus. The frontal, anterior ethmoid, and maxillary sinuses drain to the middle meatus. The sphenoid sinus and the posterior portion of the ethmoid sinus drains to the superior meatus. The anterior part of the nasal septum is cartilaginous. The posterior osseous part is formed by the perpendicular plate of the ethmoid bone superiorly and the vomer inferiorly.[13,15,16]

NASOPHARYNX

The nasopharynx is the most superior portion of the aerodigestive tract. Its inferior limit is the soft palate (Fig. 13.23). Nasopharyngeal functions include both nasal respiration and deglutition. Deep compartments of the nasopharynx are included here under the topic "nasopharynx." This is because the nasopharynx, itself, is simply a mucosa-lined facial cavity. Surrounding structures contribute to its support and function and are involved in pathological nasopharyngeal processes such as spread of tumor. Compartments of the nasopharynx are categorized as the superficial, which is the mucosal space, and deep compartments, which are the parapharyngeal space, carotid space, masticator space, retropharyngeal space, and prevertebral space.[9,16]

MR is already accepted as an important if not dominant method for investigation of nasopharyngeal lesions. The relatively artifact-free multiplanar

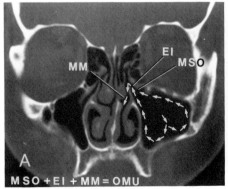 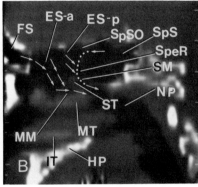 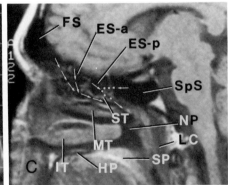

Figure 13.22. Sinus and nasal mucosal flow. **A, B,** and **C** are of different cases. *Direct coronal 3-mm thickness 375/4000 CT scan* **(A).** *(A is 3 mm anterior to Fig. 13.21C). Sagittal reformatted 3-mm axial CT sections* **(B).** *Parasagittal SE 600/25 5-mm MR scan* **(C).** The ostiomeatal unit is a functional unit directing mucous flow *(arrows)* to the nasopharynx. It is formed by the maxillary sinus ostium, the ethmoid infundibulum, and the middle meatus *(MSO + EI + MM = OMU).* Mucous secretions *(uninterrupted arrows)* from the maxillary *(MS),* frontal *(FS),* and anterior and middle portions of the ethmoid sinuses *(ES-a)* drain to the nasopharynx *(NP)* via the "OMU." Mucus drains from the sphenoid sinus *(SpS)* via the sphenoid sunus ostium *(SpSO). Drainage (dots and arrows)* of the sphenoid and posterior ethmoid sinuses *(ES-p)* is via the sphenoethmoidal recess *(SpeR)* between the anterior wall of the sphenoid sinus and the posterior wall of the ethmoid sinus. From the SpeR, the mucus flows through the superior meatus *(SM),* which is the space between the superior turbinate *(ST)* and the inferior walls of the ethmoid and sphenoid sinuses. From the SM, it flows to the NP. The sagittal MR definition is clearly superior to that on the CT sagittal reformatted image. The longus capitis *(LC),* hard *(HP),* and soft *(SP)* palates are clearly identified. Label abbreviations are the same as used for Figure 13.21.

high spatial and contrast resolution advantages of MR will likely overcome the greater cost of the examination. The images are obtained during quiet respiration. Variable echo (SE 2800/30 and 2800/80) 5-mm axial and coronal sections parallel and perpendicular to the hard palate, respectively, is a highly satisfactory technique.[9]

Intravenous contrast axial and direct coronal 5-mm thickness 17-cm FOV soft tissue filter technique is standard for CT of the nasopharynx.

Mucosal (Superficial) Space

The mucosal (superficial) space of the nasopharynx contains: *(a)* squamous mucosa; *(b)* adenoidal (lymphoid) tissue; *(c)* superior constrictor muscle; *(d)* levator palatini muscle; and *(e)* torus tubarius. The superior margin is formed by the adenoids and adjacent sphenoid and clivus mucosa. The anterior margin is formed by the choanae (posterior nasal apertures). The lateral and posterior margins are formed by the thick, structurally supportive pharyngobasilar fascia that functions as a barrier to the spread of disease into the deeper compartments. The mucosa, adenoid tissue, and lymph nodes are CT isodense and MR T1 muscle-isointense/T2 hyperintense.[9]

Although the pharyngobasilar fascia is not recognized by CT[15] and is only occasionally detected by MR,[9] the fascial limits can be determined indirectly. The pharyngobasilar fascia arises from the pharyngeal ligament (median raphe) posteriorly and runs laterally over the prevertebral muscles. It then courses anteriorly along its attachment at the skull base. The skull base attachment runs along a line drawn from the anterior margin of the carotid foramen posteriorly to the medial pterygoid plate anteriorly. The fascia is thick cranially and thin caudally (Fig. 13.23).[9]

Pasavant's ridge is a U-shaped muscular band formed by the coalescence of the levator and tensor palatini muscles[9] that inserts on the hard palate and acts as a sphincter during swallowing. The oropharynx and nasopharynx are closed during swallowing when the soft palate is tensed and elevated against Pasavant's ridge.[17,18] The ridge is partly responsible for the rounded appearance of the nasopharynx-oropharynx junction.

The torus tubarius is the mucosa-covered cartilagenous posterior edge of the eustachian tube orifice. It is CT isodense and MR T2 hyperintense. The eustachian tube is anterior to the torus and the nasopharyngeal lateral recess is posterior to it.[17]

Air extends only 3–4 mm into the eustachian tube with quiet breathing.[10] The lateral recesses appear to be larger in the adult probably because of adenoid involution. Lymphoid tissue may produce a corrugated appearance to CT and MR and hyperintense signal to T2-weighted MR.[9,15,16,18] MR can detect degenerative or cystic changes within the adenoidal tissue.[9] When a question arises whether a surface irregularity is a mass or normal lymphoid tissue, the Valsalva maneuver can be performed during CT scanning to change the shape and demonstrate plia-bility typical of lymphoid tissue.[19] This latter procedure is rarely performed, however. Minor physiological asymmetry of the lateral recesses is not uncommon.

The levator palatini can be identified by MR as an isointense muscular band lateral to the torus.[9] It is usually not clearly identifiable by CT because it produces a conglomerate image with the tensor palatini.[12,16] The pharyngobasilar fascia separates the levator from the tensor palatini until the tensor pierces the fascia in the lower nasopharynx to insert on the soft palate.

Parapharyngeal Spaces

The parapharyngeal spaces are bilateral, symetrical, fat-containing regions lateral to the nasopharynx. In addition to fat, this space also contains the: *(a)* ascending pharyngeal artery; *(b)* internal maxillary artery; *(c)* third division of the trigeminal nerve. It is characterized by fat CT density and MR signal intensities with an MR "speckled" appearance due to vascular signal-void effects. The medial wall of this space is the lateral margin of the tensor veli palatini and its lateral wall is the medial pterygoid fascia. The superior margin ends as a blind pouch. The deep lobe of the parotid gland protrudes into the posterior parapharyngeal space through the stylomandibular tunnel.[21] Lack of symmetry of the parapharyngeal space is significant and may indicate displacement by a mass.[9,16,20,21] Tumors arising in this space are usually of salivary gland origin.

Carotid Space

The carotid space extends from the skull base to the aortic arch, is enclosed by the carotid sheath, and is posterior to the parapharyngeal space. It receives fascial contributions from all layers of the deep cervical fascia. It contains the: *(a)* internal carotid artery; *(b)* internal jugular vein; *(c)* cranial nerves IX through XII; *(d)* cervical sympathetic nerve plexus; and *(e)* lymph nodes. The internal carotid artery is anteromedial to the internal jugular vein.[9,18] The nerves are located posterior to the internal carotid artery (Fig. 12.8). Contrast cranial CT and various MR techniques demonstrate the arteries and veins. CT demonstrates the styloid process posterolateral to the carotid foramen. MR may demonstrate the cranial nerves as foci of T1 slight hyperintensity adjacent to and posterior to the artery.[9,18,20] The retropharyngeal nodes are often detectable medial to the internal carotid artery. They are first-order drainage nodes from the nasopharynx and oropharynx and are often enlarged in patients with nasopharyngeal carcinoma or patients with prominent adenoidal tissue. Both reactive adenopathy and metastatic adenopathy are T2 signal hyperintense and cannot be distinguished by signal intensity alone.[9]

Masticator Space

The masticator space is the deep skull facial space lateral to the parapharyngeal space, which is named for the contained muscles of mastication. It is bor-

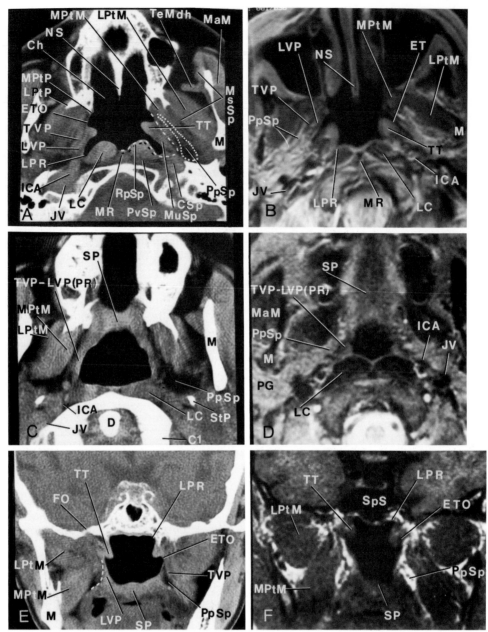

Figure 13.23. Normal nasopharynx. Axial 400/2000 **(A)** and 50/500 **(C)** and direct coronal 50/500 **(E)** 5-mm thickness, soft tissue filter CT scans. Matching level SE 3000/30 **(B)**, 2800/80 **(D)** 5-mm thickness, and 600/25 **(F)** 3-mm thickness MR scans. These CT images have been chosen for their unusual sharp detail. The sharp detail on ·these MR images is not unusual. MR images generally demonstrate superior nasopharyngeal detail compared to CT. The dashed white line represents the pharyngobasilar fascia that encloses the mucosal space (MuSp) and the dashed black line represents the anterior portion of the deep cervical fascia. The potential space between these two lines is the retropharyngeal space (RpSp). The dotted line encloses the parapharyngeal space (PpSp). The levator veli palatini (LVP) is enclosed by pharyngobasilar fascia and the tensor veli palatini (TVP) lies between the PpSp and the pharyngobasilar fascia **(A–B).** Note the characteristic indentations upon the airway caused by the torus tubarius (TT) and longus capitis muscle [**A–B** (LC)]. More inferiorly **(C–D),** Pasavant's muscle [TVP-LVP(PR)] and the combined longus capitis and longus coli muscles cause a characteristic airway appearance. The prevertebral space (PvSp) encloses the longus capitis and longus coli muscles. The masticator space is lateral, and the carotid space (CSp) is medial to the PpSp. Proton density flow-compensation effect partially obscures ICA and JV detail in **B** but not on the T2-weighted **D.** The MR fat signal is very bright on the heavily T1-weighted image **(F)** and tends to obscure other soft tissue detail. White dashes = pharyngobasilar fascia; black dashes = retropharyngeal fascia; dotted line encloses PPSp; C1 = first cervical vertebra; Ch = choanae; CSp = carotid space; D = dens; ET = eustachian tube; ETO = eustachian tube orifice; FO = foramen ovale; ICA = internal carotid artery; JV = jugular vein; LC = longus capitis muscle; LPR = lateral pharyngeal recess; LPtM = lateral pterygoid muscle; LPtP = lateral pterygoid plate; LVP = levator veli palatini; M = mandible; MaM = masseter muscle; MPtM = medial pterygoid muscle; MPtP = medial pterygoid plate; MR = median raphe; MsSP = masticator space; MuSp = mucosal space; NS = nasal septum; PG = parotid gland; PpSp = parapharyngeal space; PvSp = prevertebral space; RpSp = retropharyngeal space; SP = soft palate; SpS = sphenoid sinus; TeMdh = temporalis muscle (deep head); TT = torus tubarius; TVP = tensor veli palatini.

dered medially by the medial pterygoid fascia, laterally by the zygomatic arch, anteriorly by the maxillary sinus and pterygoid plates, and posteriorly by the mandible. It includes the: *(a)* ramus and posterior body of the mandible; *(b)* medial and lateral pterygoid muscles; *(c)* masseter muscle; *(d)* temporalis muscles; *(e)* inferior aveolar nerve; and *(f)* pterygoid venous plexus. The foramen ovale containing the third division of the trigeminal nerve is located at its apex.[21]

Retropharyngeal Space

The retropharyngeal space is a potential space between the pharyngobasilar fascia and the prevertebral fascia. It contains: *(a)* a lymphatic network and *(b)* fat. This space is normally not seen by CT or MR.[9,15,16,18]

Prevertebral Space

Posterior to the retropharyngeal space is the prevertebral space that contains the prevertebral muscles (longus colli and longus capitis) that are responsible for the characteristic posterior nasopharyngeal contour. This space can also be considered to contain the vertebral column.[9] The prevertebral muscles are virtually always symmetrical in the normal state. Benign lymphoid hypertrophy can blend with the prevertebral muscles to produce the appearance of a retropharyngeal mass.[15,16]

PTERYGOPALATINE FOSSA ("PTERYGOMAXILLARY FOSSA")

The pterygopalatine fossa is a fat-containing space below the orbital apex defined by the posterior wall of the maxillary antrum anteriorly and the pterygoid plates posteriorly. The perpendicular plate of the palatine bone contributes a large portion of the medial wall.[22] It is connected to other spaces by foramina and fissures. The fossa contains the sphenopalatine ganglion, the termination of the internal maxillary artery, and the palatine nerve. Because of

its strategic location and connections with other spaces, it is an important conduit for the spread of infection and tumor.[15,16,22,23] The foramen rotundum is located in the superoposterior wall. The sphenopalatine foramen in the medial wall connects the pterygopalatine fossa to the nasal cavity middle meatus. The pterygomaxillary fissure connects the pterygopalatine and the infratemporal fossae and the inferior orbital fissure connects the pterygopalatine fossa and the orbit (Fig. 13.21**H** and **I**). The pterygoid canal (vidian nerve canal) connecting the foramen lacerum with the pterygopalatine fossa is identified on coronal sections (13.21**F**) inferomedial to the foramen rotundum. It should not be confused with the pterygopalatine canal that is seen on axial sections (Fig. 13.21**G**). The vidian nerve is the combined greater superficial petrosal nerve and deep petrosal nerves. It enters the pterygopalatine fossa through the pterygoid canal. The maxillary division of the trigeminal nerve travels through the nearby foramen rotundum. The vidian nerve enters the splenopalatine ganglion from which nerves supply the lacrimal gland and mucous membranes of the nose and palate.[15,16,22,23] The pterygopalatine fossa is well visualized in the axial and sagittal planes.

Pathological Nasal and Sinus Conditions
CONGENITAL VARIATIONS AND ANOMALIES

There is a great variability in sinus development. Extensive pneumatization may occur. Four percent of all adult patients have aplastic or hypoplastic frontal sinuses. Aplastic or severely hypoplastic sphenoid sinuses occur in less than 1% of patients. CT and MR detect paranasal sinus development in infants and children earlier than does conventional x-ray. Conventional x-ray detects maxillary and ethmoid sinuses at age 2 years, the sphenoid sinus at age 4 years, and the frontal sinuses at age 6 years.[10,15,16] Almost 75% of CT scans of patients under 1 year of age have either nonidentifiable or opaque maxillary antra. In children between 2 and 6 years

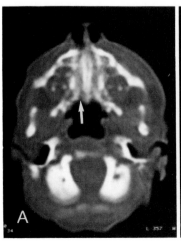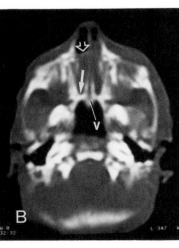

Figure 13.24.   Choanal atresia. *Axial 0.8 sec 350/1600 3 mm thickness CT scans. 13.24A is 3mm caudal to 13.24B.* The posterior nasal cavity is airless and there is an anterior air-fluid level *(open arrow)*. The vomer (V) is thickened and there is medial bowing and thickening of the lateral walls of the nasal cavity. There is an atretic plate *(closed arrow, 13.24B)* causing osseous choanal atresia above the membranous atretic portion *(closed arrow, 13.24A)*.

of age, sinus mucosal thickening and fluid are frequent and often unassociated with symptoms. These changes should be correlated with clinical findings before diagnosing sinusitis.[24]

Some of the more common facial congenital anomalies are paranasal sinus hypoplasia, cleft palate, nasal obstruction, and Crouzon's syndrome.

Nasal and paranasal sinus hypoplasia may be generalized or may be present in one vertical half of the face.

Cleft palate is the most common congenital malformation affecting the nose. It is the result of failure of fusion of the lateral palatine processes with each other, the nasal septum, or the primary palate. A complete cleft palate may be associated with a cleft lip and cleft anterior maxilla. CT can accurately demonstrate the osseous and soft tissue defect and possible associated additional facial fusion anomalies.[13]

Nasal airway obstruction can be a life-threatening emergency in the newborn and infant. Congenital nasal airway obstruction may occur as stenosis of the entire nasal cavity, the anterior cavity, or the choanae. Stenosis of the entire nasal cavity is usually osseous. Choanal obstruction is slightly more common in females and is usually caused by a bilateral combined osseous and membranous atretic plate. There are often associated (usually craniofacial) congenital anomalies.[27] Axial CT scanning parallel to the infraorbitomeatal line is recommended. Three-dimensional CT reformation of contiguous thin sections can aid surgical planning. Nasal suctioning before scanning is recommended to clear secretions in order to avoid mistaking mucus secretions for membranous stenosis. Osseous and membranous atresia can be distinguished by CT. CT of osseous choanal atresia demonstrates an abnormally broad vomer, medial bowed and thickened posterolateral nasal margins, thickened mucosa, and lack of an airway.[25] Membranous choanal atresia is associated with less osseous lateral nasal marginal changes and with a normal vomer. The distinction of the osseous and membranous type is important for surgical considerations.[25-27] (Fig. 13.24) The role of MR for diagnosis of neonatal and infantile nasal obstruction has yet to be established. Possible MR advantages over CT include sagittal images. CT has the definite advantage of bone discrimination.

Crouzon's syndrome (craniofacial dysostosis) is an inherited dysplasia characterized by sutural synostosis (particularly coronal), facial hypoplasia (particularly maxillary), high palatal arch (occasionally palatal cleft), hypertelorism, shallow orbits, and proptosis resulting in "frog-like" facies. Axial and coronal, thin section (5-mm), noncontrast CT accurately demonstrates this abnormality (Fig. 13.25).[15]

Since osseous abnormalities and sharply contrasting mucosal and air spaces characterize these facial congenital abnormalities, CT is preferred to MR as the investigative technique.[15,16] How much MR will contribute to the investigation of these conditions is not known. The superior MR soft tissue detail and true orthogonal plane imaging aids in the investigation of cleft deformities.

Figure 13.25. Crouzon's disease (craniofacial dysostosis). *Axial 1600/579 **(A–B)** and 641/1600 **(C)** and direct coronal 45/300 **(D)** CT scans.* There is maxillary bone hypoplasia, shallow orbits, proptosis, ocular hypertelorism, and sagittal and coronal craniostenosis. There are abnormal elongated orbital fissures *(arrow)*. (Courtesy of Mary K. Edwards, M.D., Indianapolis, IN.)

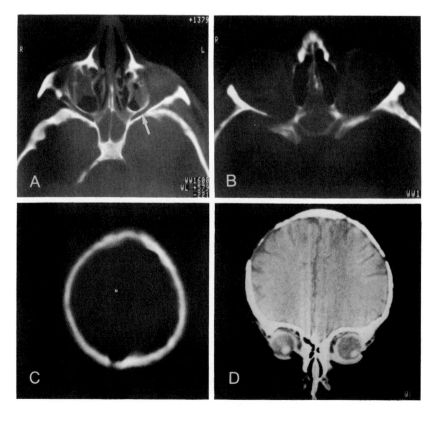

MR and CT combined play an important role in management of facial encephaloceles. CT best demonstrates the osseous defect and MR accurately detects brain versus CSF content, and accurately detects the margins of the dural sac.[29,30] MR, therefore, is often very helpful before surgery if encephalocele is considered in the differential diagnosis of nasal and nasopharyngeal masses.

TRAUMATIC CONDITIONS

CT is the method of choice for imaging facial fractures. Although MR soft tissue discrimination is superior, CT bone fragment identification is critical for patient management. Thin section (5-mm) axial and direct coronal edge enhancement, small FOV technique is preferred. The 3-D CT reformation technique of 3-mm axial sections is helpful for surgical planning of facial injuries.

The facial bones form protective struts, pillars, or buttresses.[31-35] The *struts* are formed by structurally strong and delicate facial bones or portions of facial bones oriented in the horizontal, sagittal, and coronal planes. These struts include the orbital roof and floor, the nasal septum, and the nasal bone.[33] The delicate struts are protected by the stronger externally palpable lateral and medial *pillars*. The lateral pillar is formed by the lateral superior alveolar ridge, the lateral maxillary sinus wall, the malar eminence, the lateral orbital wall, and the orbital process of the frontal bone. The medial pillar is formed by the medial superior alveolar ridge, medial maxillary antral wall, lacrimal bone, maxillary frontal process, and nasal process of the frontal bone.[32] Skeletal structures that resist backward and upward displacement of facial structures can be considered as *buttresses* of the face. Three buttresses resisting backward thrust or displacement include the temporal bone zygomatic process, the sphenoid bone pterygoid process, and greater wing. Three buttresses resisting upward thrust or displacement are the frontal bone zygomatic process and nasal process, and the roof of the mandibular fossa.[31]

The term "struts, pillars, and buttresses" has been used in this section in order to summarize part of the theoretical basis for facial fracture dynamics conveniently. This theoretical basis is useful for understanding, classifying, and reporting CT results. The facial fractures can be conveniently grouped into local facial fractures, trimalar fractures, and complex fractures.

Local fractures include fractures of the nasal arch (most common), nasoethmoid (Fig. 13.26), orbital floor, lower orbital rim, zygomatic arch, superior orbital rim, and frontal sinus. The usual orbital "blowout" fracture is an orbital floor fracture often associated with orbital tissue herniation possibly accompanied by the inferior rectus muscle. Medial blowout fractures through the thin lamina papyracea also occur and may be associated with severe orbital emphysema. Direct coronal CT, reformation coronal CT, or coronal MR is necessary for the surgical assessment of blowout fractures (Fig. 14.29 p. 368). CT images of most of the local-type fractures will be seen later in this section in combination with other fractures.[32,36]

The trimalar or "tripod" fractures include the lateral orbital wall (usually at the frontozygomatic suture), orbital floor, and zygomatic arch fractures. The lateral wall of the maxillary sinus is frequently involved. Posterior displacement and fragment rotation are common (Fig. 13.27).

More severe fractures include Le Fort I, II, and III; Le Fort variations; and "smash" fractures.[36-38] Posterior fragment displacement and rotation are common. Nasolacrimal duct and sac disruption may occur.[29,30]

The Le Fort fracture categorization is based upon three facial "planes of weakness." These fractures can also be considered as combined anterior pillar fractures with posterior fracture of thinner bones (struts) and fractures of buttresses that allow facial separation from the skull. The Le Fort fracture planes are illustrated in Figure 13.28. Separation of the fractured fragment can be detected clinically thus accounting for the term "facial separation" fractures. The higher Le Fort numbers indicate increased fracture severity and larger separated facial portions. With increasing fracture numbers (from I–III), the anterior planar intercept has a higher and more lat-

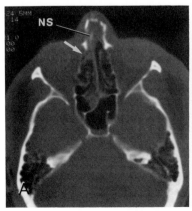
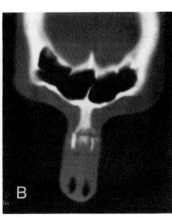

Figure 13.26. Nasoethmoid fracture. *Axial 400/3000* **(A)** *and direct coronal 300/3000* **(B)** *CT 5-mm thickness scans.* There is a horizontal comminuted nasal bone fracture with right-sided displacement of the nasal septum *(NS)*. There is a small fracture deformity of the right nasolacrimal duct wall with an adjacent lamina papyracea fracture and adjacent decreased ethmoid pneumatization *(arrow)*.

Figure 13.27. Trimalar fracture. **A–B** and **C–D** are different cases. *Axial (A) and coronal (B) 300/3000 5-mm thickness CT scans; 3-D CT reformations of 3-mm sections of another case (C–D).* Lateral orbital wall *(arrow-1)*, orbital floor *(arrow-2)*, and zygomatic arch *(arrow-3)* fractures are seen with fragment rotation. There is an associated lateral wall maxillary sinus fracture *(open arrow)*.

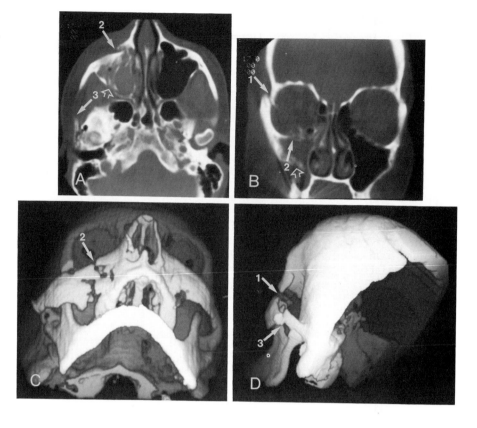

eral position. The posterior intercepts are closely approximated for the three Le Fort fractures. As might be expected, variations of these fracture types occur and it is not uncommon to have a lesser degree Le Fort fracture on one side than the other ["mixed Le Fort fracture" (Fig. 13.29)] or for a Le Fort II fracture to coexist with a trimalar fracture.[23,32,36]

The Le Fort I fracture horizontally traverses the inferior maxillary sinuses and follows the axial plane to interrupt the inferior pterygoid plates (Fig. 13.29).[32,36] This results in a mobile hard palate and superior alveolar ridge, "the floating palate."[32] It is also called the Gurein fracture.[38]

The Le Fort II fracture extends along a higher plane

involving the lateral maxillary sinuses, the anterior medial orbit, and the nasoethmoidal structures. These fracture lines describe a triangle or "pyramid" on the AP projection (Fig. 13.29). A larger posteriorly displaced separated facial fragment including the hard palate and nasal structures results.[23,32,38] Orbital emphysema may be present. Orbital bone fragments should be identified before fracture manipulation in order to prevent eye injury during fracture reduction.

The Le Fort III fracture (Fig. 13.30) plane has greater lateral extent than the Le Fort II fracture (Fig. 13.29). This fracture involves both the medial and lateral orbital walls and the cribriform plate.

Figure 13.28. Le Fort fractures. Skull phantom CT 3-D reformation AP **(A)** and lateral oblique **(B).** There is a higher and more lateral position of the fracture line with fractures I–III with posterior convergence to the pterygoid plates of all three fracture types.

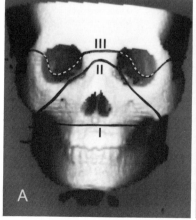
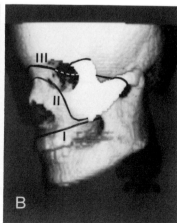

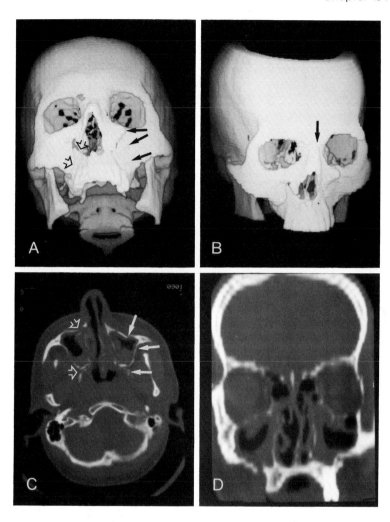

Figure 13.29.   Combined Le Fort I and II fractures. All scans of the same patient. *Frontal (A)* and frontal oblique *(B)* 3-D CT reformatted 3-mm axial images. Axial 400/3000 3-mm CT scan *(C)* and coronal CT reformation *(D).* The right side Le Fort I *(open arrows)* and the left side Le Fort II *(closed arrows)* classification of the fracture lines is an approximation. The more lateral fracture plane of the Le Fort II fracture is best seen on the conventional axial CT *(C).* On the 3-D image, this lateral fracture plane is adjacent to a more obvious medial maxillary fracture. There are bilateral pterygoid plate fractures. The 3-D image and the reformatted coronal image suggests an additional left frontozygomatic region fracture or disrupted suture. On the basis of the full series of conventional axial images, it was decided to classify this lesion as above.

Virtually the entire face becomes the major fragment. For this reason, the fracture is often called the "craniofacial disjunction" fracture.[18,38] The Le Fort III fracture is almost always associated with additional facial fractures within the major fragment. There is usually evidence of associated brain injury due to the massive trauma involved.[38] Attention should be directed to the cribriform plate due to the potential for development of CSF rhinorrhea. The CT investigation of CSF rhinorrhea will be discussed later in this chapter and has already been discussed in Chapter 7 (Fig. 7.26).

Facial "smash fracture" is a term applied to facial bone comminution of a given facial portion or of the entire face.[36] We prefer not to use this term. A case of facial fracture disrupting all buttresses, pillars, and struts is presented in Figure 13.31.

SINUSITIS

Sinus inflammation has long been categorized as acute, chronic, and recurrent. Recurrent sinusitis presents acutely and eventually produces chronic changes such as bone erosion and/or hyperostosis and mucosal hypertrophy and/or polyps. Acute sinusitis produces mucosal hypertrophy and retained secretions. Bone erosion and/or involvement of adjacent soft tissues (e.g., the orbit) with acute sinusitis should be considered a warning signal of a life-threatening condition such as mucormycosis, imminent meningitis, or intracranial abscess.

The principal causes of sinus inflammation are infectious and allergic—both of which processes may play a role in the same individual case. Tumors, benign and malignant, may obstruct the pathways of mucous drainage (Fig. 13.22), thus establishing a nidus for infection. It has been said that bacterial infection most often involves the maxillary sinuses asymmetrically and that allergy is more often the cause of pansinusitis. Despite the above etiological tendencies, it is difficult to distinguish infectious from allergic cases by CT or MR imaging in cases where imaging changes are confined to the mucosa and sinus cavity. To further complicate this distinction, the patient has usually been treated medically before the examination and the retained fluid and mucosal hypertrophy that may have been present might have remitted by the time of the study. First-episode acute sinusitis is usually simply medically treated without

Figure 13.30. Le Fort III fracture. *Axial maxillary sinus* **(A)** *and superior orbital* **(B)** *5-mm thickness 350/3000 and direct coronal orbital* **(C)** *and pterygoid plate-level* **(D)** *600/2000 CT scans.* The fracture planes extend from the superior alveolar ridge *(SAR)* inferiorly to the orbit *(O)* superiorly and from the nasion *(N)* anteriorly to the pterygoid plates *(PtPl)* posteriorly. The lateral fracture margins include the maxillary sinuses and orbital lateral walls.

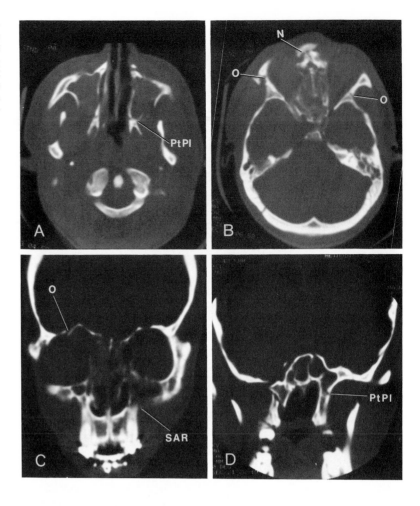

Figure 13.31. Facial fracture disrupting all buttresses, pillars, and struts. *Axial 445/4000 maxillary sinus-level* **(A)** *and orbital-level* **(B)** *and coronal 325/4000 orbital-* **(C)** *and pterygoid-* **(D)** *level 5-mm thickness CT scans.* Virtually all pillars and struts are fractured with resultant severe facial deformities. There are also bulbar and retrobulbar injuries. Ocular injuries will be discussed in Chapter 14.

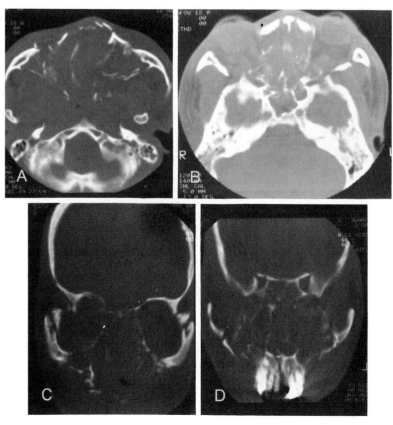

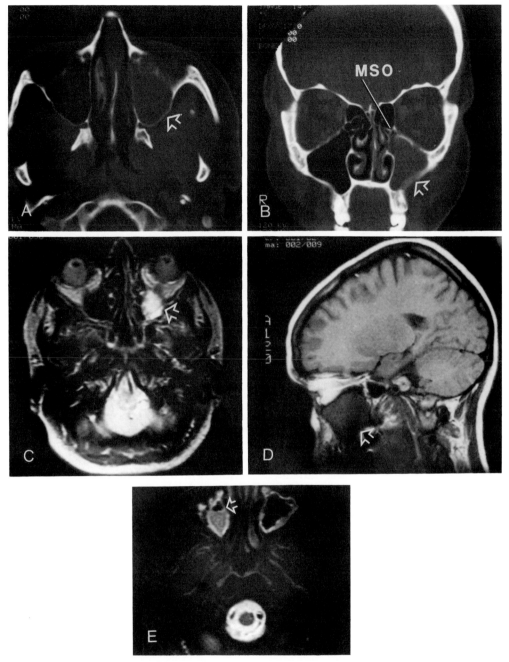

Figure 13.32. Acute maxillary sinusitis. **A–D** and **E** are different cases. *Axial 5-mm thickness* **(A)** *and direct coronal* **(B)** *3-mm thickness 565/3000 17-mm FOV CT scans. Axial SE 2800/30* **(C)** *and sagittal SE 600/25* **(D)** *5-mm thickness MR scans.* The left maxillary sinus is filled with water-density/intensity fluid *(open arrow).* The maxillary sinus ostium *(MSO)* is blocked by secretions and hypertrophied mucosa. There is no bone erosion. **E:** Acute maxillary sinusitis. *SE 2800/80 5-mm thickness.* The marked bilateral mucosal thickening is T2 signal hyperintense outlining the right maxillary contained secretions with an air-fluid level *(open arrow).*

a CT or MR examination. It is the recurrent "acute" episode (Fig. 13.32) that often is the indication for the (usually) CT examination.[10]

Thin section (3-mm) CT investigation of recurrent and chronic sinusitis has become a routine preoperative study before paranasal sinus endoscopic surgery.[12] CT and MR findings of paranasal abnormality is, however, often an unexpected finding on a brain scan. The presence of sinus fluid and/or mucosal thickening does not necessarily indicate symptomatic sinusitis. The unexpected diagnosis of sinusitis, however, occasionally explains a patient's symptoms. Examples include sinusitis as a cause of headache, frontal sinusitis with an adjacent brain abscess, and ethmoid sinusitis causing painful limitation of ocular motion. Careful analysis of the paranasal sinuses is necessary for all CT and MR head scans for these reasons. When paranasal sinus scans

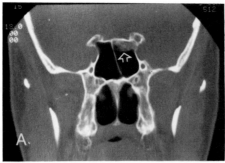

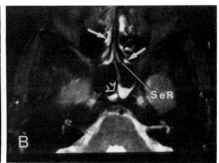

Figure 13.33.   Acute sinusitis—sphenoid. *Direct coronal 350/3000 3-mm thickness CT scan* **(A)** *and axial SE 2800/80 5-mm thickness MR scan* **(B).** Sphenoid sinus air-fluid levels *(open arrows).* There is ethmoid sinus mucosal thickening *(closed arrows)* that approximates the sphenoethmoidal recess *(SeR).* The SeR involvement probably is contributory to the retained secretions.

are specifically requested, CT is the method of choice because of superb CT bone detail and because of contrasting air, soft tissue, and bone structures. Thin section (3-mm) noncontrast bone filter axial and direct coronal noncontrast CT imaging is standard in our department for evaluation of sinusitis. Intravenous contrast CT with a soft tissue filter is necessary for detection of intracranial or extracranial soft tissue involvement. MR with i.v. contrast better demonstrates intracranial involvement because of the lack of adjacent bone obscuring juxtadural pathology.[32]

CT and MR of acute sinusitis (whether of bacterial, viral, or allergic etiology) demonstrates mucosal thickening and retained secretions. CT usually demonstrates lack of bone involvement.[32,38,39] The retained secretions and inflamed mucosa are typically water-CT density/MR intensity, often with an air-fluid level. The thickened mucosa is therefore strikingly prominent on T2-weighted images (Figs. 13.32 and 13.33). Occasionally, particularly with bacterial frontal sinusitis, there is an associated epidural abscess (Fig. 8.7).

Acute fungal paranasal sinus infections are usually caused by aspergillosis and mucormycosis and rarely by actimomycosis. They usually occur in diabetic and immunosuppressed patients. Mucormycosis

is more aggressive than aspergillosis and is often fatal if not treated early.[38] Aspergillosis and actinomycosis may produce sinus findings similar to mucormycosis but they are often of lesser degree and more localized. Maxillary sinus calcific small concretions may be seen in aspergillosis.[40] Mucormycosis infections tend to spread initially along vascular and neural channels and only later do they tend to invade bone. Direct invasion through bone, however, may occur. There is often evidence for severe sinusitis without bone involvement. Infection may spread from the maxillary sinus along the posterior alveolar artery into the infratemporal fossa and inferior orbital fissure. Extension can also occur from the superior orbital fissure to the middle cranial fossa and cavernous sinus. Intracranial extension through the cribriform plate is not uncommon. Brain abscesses and cerebral infarcts commonly complicate mucormycosis infection. The infarcts are secondary to arterial endothelial injury and also intraluminal invasions.[32,38,41]

Both CT and MR of mucormycosis can demonstrate the sinus air-fluid levels, the mucosal thickening and orbital, cerebral, and nasopharyngeal involvement. CT best demonstrates bone involvement (Fig. 13.34). It had formerly been observed that mu-

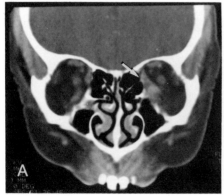

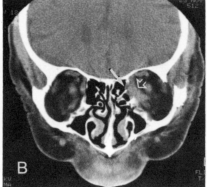

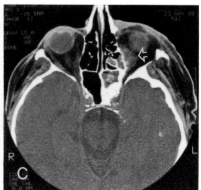

Figure 13.34.   Mucormycosis. *Direct coronal 30/500 5-mm thickness soft tissue filter noncontrast CT scan* **(A).** *Direct coronal* **(B)** *and axial* **(C)** *noncontrast bone filter CT scans 12 days later.* Interval lam-ina papyracea osteolysis *(closed arrow)* associated with the otherwise unchanged left medial orbital mass *(open arrow)* is seen. There is left ethmoid and sphenoid sinusitis.

cormycosis produced marked bone destruction and that osteolysis was a hallmark of this infection. The marked osteolysis is a late finding and now is less often seen due to earlier diagnosis and surgical debridement.[41] The radiologist must, therefore, be alert to fulminent paranasal sinusitis in a diabetic or immune-suppressed patient in order to diagnose this often fatal illness early. When bone erosion is seen, fungal infection, carcinoma, and chronic infection must be considered.

Chronic and/or recurrent paranasal sinusitis is a common sequella of acute sinusitis. Recently developed concepts of mucociliary activity and pathophysiology of paranasal sinus disease has led to the increasing popularity of endoscopic surgery for treatment of sinus obstructions. Sinus ostial obstruction blocks mucociliary clearance, which leads to sinus infection. The most common ostial obstruction is that of the ostiomeatal unit (Fig. 13.35). Surgical treatment is primarily directed to restoration of normal physiology by re-establishing normal mucociliary drainage and ventilation of the sinuses. This is accomplished by removal of localized disease obstructing the ethmoid pathways (Fig. 13.36). Although transnasal endoscopy can directly and accurately vi-

sualize the more anterior structures, the deeper structures beyond the anterior ostiomeatal region can only be nonsurgically visualized accurately by CT. The role of highly detailed CT scans is to evaluate these deeper structures, to add to endoscopic evidence of more proximal disease, to establish a baseline for future examinations, and to aid in surgical planning.[12] Mucosal thickening, indistinct bone margins and erosion of the mucoperiosteal line is followed by sclerotic bone reaction. CT shows mucosal thickening and obstruction of the ostiomeatal unit (Fig. 13.35). There is often a lack of an air-fluid level. Inflamed and hypertrophied mucosa has marked T2 MR hyperintensity. Mucoceles, osteolysis, and hyperostosis may develop. A small, thick-walled sinus often results from chronic infection.[42] Untreated acute and chronic sinusitis may extend to the brain, orbits, sella, nasopharynx, and other adjacent structures. CT evidence of bone erosion and adjacent epidural and parenchymal abnormalities should be looked for. Bone erosion in chronic paranasal sinusitis characteristically focally involves the semilunar hiatus, ethmoid bulla, or infraorbital canal often associated with adjacent bone thickening. When the consideration of brain or other soft tissue involvement arises, i.v.

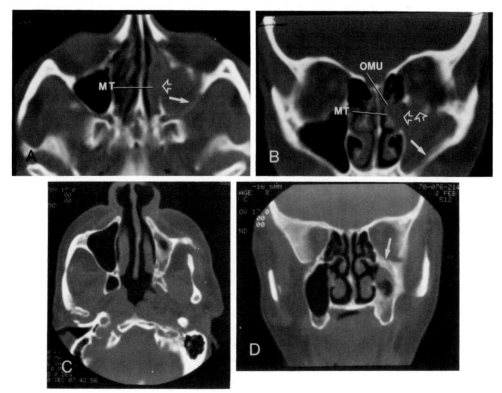

Figure 13.35.   Chronic sinusitis. A–B and **C–D** are different cases. *Axial (A) and direct coronal i.v. contrast (B) 280/3000 5-mm thickness CT scans. Axial (C) and direct coronal (D) noncontrast 5-mm thickness 500/3000 CT scans.* **A–B:** Inflammatory polyp. A left maxillary sinus soft tissue mass widens the infundibulum, obscures the ostiomeatal unit *(OMU)* and abuts the middle turbinate *(MT).* The left maxillary sinus is opaque and there is sinus wall erosion *(open ar-*

rows) and thickening (closed arrows). There was no abnormal contrast enhancement, even on narrower (soft tissue) windows. **C–D:** Chronic maxillary sinusitis with unilateral failure of sinus development. The left maxillary sinus is small, poorly pneumatized, and has thick osseous walls *(closed arrow). This condition developed during childhood.*

Figure 13.36. **Maxillary sinus windows.** *Axial **(A)** and direct coronal **(B)** 37/4000 5-mm thickness CT scans. Bilateral inferomedial maxillary sinus lateral wall defects are seen (arrows).*

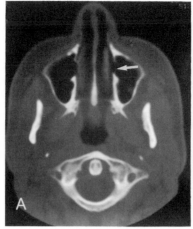
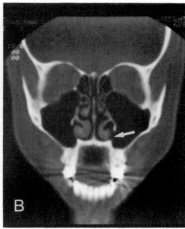

contrast MR is the diagnostic method of choice although i.v. contrast CT has long been shown to be effective. A mycetoma, usually aspergillosis, may develop and mimic a polyp.

RETENTION CYSTS

The retention cyst is also called a nonsecreting cyst, noninflammatory cyst, serous cyst, and mucous gland cyst. It is a collection of submucosal fluid producing a smooth, rounded mass usually found in the inferior portion of maxillary sinuses. They may also be found in the frontal and sphenoid sinuses. Retention cysts unassociated with generalized mucosal thickening are often considered to be without clinical significance. CT and MR demonstrate a CT nonenhancing smoothly marginated CT hypodense, MR T1/T2 water-isointense, thin-walled mass (Fig. 13.37) often associated with generalized sinus mucosal thickening. They may be mobile and pliable, which can be demonstrated by axial supine and direct coronal prone CT.[38]

MUCOCELES

A mucocele is a respiratory epithelial-lined fibrous sac within a sinus containing mucinous secretions. They usually result from sinus outflow obstruction by inflammation but may be the result of ostium obstruction by a neoplasm or from post-traumatic deformity[10] and are most common in the frontal and then the ethmoid sinuses.[38] An infected mucocele is called a "pyocele" and the clinical presentation is dominated by the infectious process.[10] Multiple mucoceles may develop in patients with aspirin intolerance. Chronic pressure erosion develops. Frontal sinus mucoceles may erode bone and displace the globe, brain, or produce a forehead bulge (the "Potts puffy tumor"). Sphenoid sinus mucoceles may erode the sinus lateral wall and expose the dura adjacent to the carotid artery or the optic nerve, thus producing a surgical hazard. Similar hazards may present in other locations, for example, ethmoid mucocele erosion may expose the cribriform plate dura.[32] The mucocele may become infected producing an additional hazard of intracranial extension and septicemia.

Both CT and MR demonstrate the mucocele. Bone erosion is best demonstrated by CT. MR may demonstrate either a water signal or a signal similar to subacute hemorrhage (Fig. 13.38). CT shows bone wall expansion, bone erosion, relatively smooth margination, and low or soft tissue density. Lack of bone destruction and reactive sclerosis favors mucocele over malignancy.[32,38] Rim contrast enhancement is not uncommon, but may be markedly prominent with pyoceles.[10] Nasal, frontal, and sphenoidal encephaloceles should also be included in the differential diagnosis. MR is far superior to CT for documenting herniated brain tissue in the encephalocele (Chapter 9).[30] The relationship of mucocele to vital structures and exclusion of an encephalocele must always be considered.

PNEUMOSINUS DILATANS

Pneumosinus dilatans is a rare condition of unknown etiology in which active remodeling with enlargement of a few air-cells of a particular sinus containing only air may occur without the presence of a mucocele, mass, or fluid. The dilated sinus may apply pressure to adjacent structures such as the optic nerves or chiasm and produce symptoms. The diagnosis can be made by both CT and MR. This rare entity should not be confused with generalized idiopathic large sinuses, sinus enlargement of acromegaly, unilateral sinus enlargement of Dyke-Davidoff-Masson syndrome, or sinus dilatation ("blistering") associated with meningioma.[10]

POLYPS

Polyps are serous- or mucin-containing masses that may fibrose. They may be nasal or within sinuses, or both, and are caused by allergy or inflammation. The maxillary sinus ostium is often involved. They are frequently associated with generalized mucosal thickening and are often multiple and bilateral. These lesions remodel bone but are not frankly osteolytic (Fig. 13.39). Ethmoid polyps may erode the medial orbital wall and cause proptosis. Antral choanal polyps originate within the maxillary sinus, expand the ostia, and present in the nasal cavity. They represent only approximately 5% of nasal polyps.[10,43] Se-

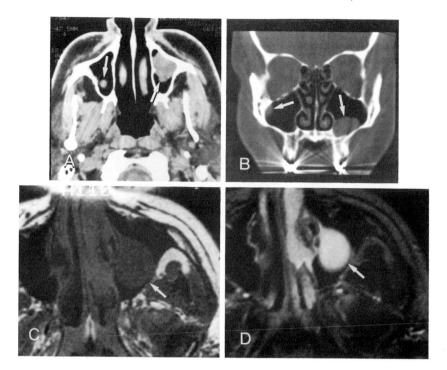

Figure 13.37.   Retention cysts. A–B and C–D are different cases. Case 1: *Axial 27/400 (A) and direct coronal 450/4000 (B) noncontrast 3-mm thickness 18-cm FOV soft tissue window CT scans.* Water-CT density cyst-like maxillary sinus masses are sharply marginated *(arrows)*. The sinuses are otherwise normal without evidence of generalized mucosal hypertrophy. Case 2: *Axial SE 600/25 (C) and 2800/80 (D) MR scans.* A maxillary sinus floor medial smoothly marginated water-isointense cyst *(arrow)* lies adjacent to swollen turbinates.

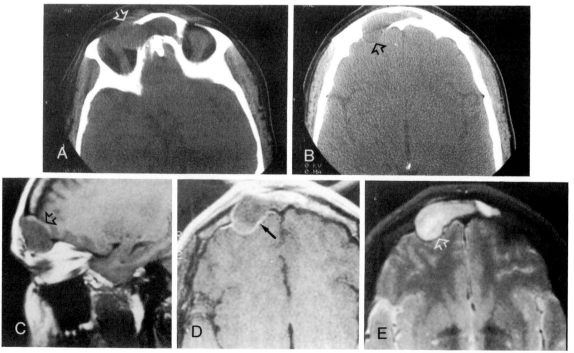

Figure 13.38.   Frontal sinus mucocele. *Axial superior orbital-level (A) and supraorbital-level (B) noncontrast 100/550 bone filter 3-mm thickness CT scans. Sagittal SE 600/25 MR scan (C), axial i.v. contrast SE 600/25 (D), and noncontrast SE 2800/80 (E) MR scans at same level.* A soft tissue-density/gray matter-T1 isointense/T2 water- isointense frontal sinus mass *(open arrows)* expands the frontal sinus, erodes the inner and outer frontal bone cortex, and displaces the globe downward. There is rim Gd-DTPA contrast enhancement of the mucocele and the immediately adjacent dura *(closed arrow)*.

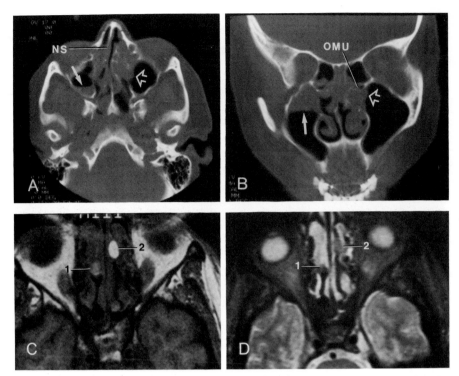

Figure 13.39. Nasal polyps. Cases **A–B** and **C–D** are different patients. **A–B:** *Axial (**A**) and direct coronal (**B**) i.v. contrast 287/4000 5-mm thickness bone filter CT scans.* There is a prominent polypoid soft tissue mass *(open arrow)* eroding the medial sinus wall, continuous with the middle turbinate, and effacing the ostiomeatal unit *(OMU).* There is a right maxillary sinus air-fluid level *(closed arrow).* Multiple other polypoid mucosal masses are seen bilaterally. Another polyp that is particularly prominent is continuous with the right inferior turbinate and is seen at the choanae **(A).** There was only slight abnormal contrast enhancement on soft tissue window images. **C–D:** Another case. *Axial SE 600/25 3-mm thickness, 18-cm FOV (**C**) and 2800/80 5-mm thickness, 20-cm FOV (**D**) MR scans.* There are two middle turbinate polyps *(1* and *2)* with different signal intensities.

vere polyposis occurs in children with cystic fibrosis and in adults with the triad of nasal polyposis, aspirin sensitivity, and bronchial asthma.[38].

Polyps demonstrate mucosal CT and MR signals and appear as nodular mucosal masses. The maxillary sinus ostium (Figs. 13.35 and 13.39) is a favored location, however, ethmoid and nasal turbinate involvement is also common. Those polyps involving the maxillary sinus ostium commonly obstruct the ostiomeatal complex, which often causes chronic sinusitis.

The markedly expansile polyp/polyps may have CT and MR characteristics similar to a mucocele. Polyps can usually be easily differentiated from retention cysts by the association of polyps with generalized sinus mucosal thickening and the inferior maxillary sinus location favored by the retention cyst.[15,38] Lack of frank bone destruction differentiates the polyp from sinus and nasal malignancies.

OTHER BENIGN SINUS AND NASAL CAVITY MASSES

Osteoma is probably the most common paranasal sinus tumor. It is a frequent incidental finding on cranial and facial CT and MR scans but may produce symptoms by blocking an ostium or causing bone pain due to direct pressure. They consist of compact and/or cancellous bone. The frontal sinus is the most common location followed by ethmoid, maxillary, and sphenoid sinus in decreasing order. They are most common in men. Multiple osteomas may occur associated with colonic polyps in Gardner's syndrome.

CT demonstrates these lesions better than MR due to the usual dense ossification MR signal void within an air-filled signal-void sinus. The osteoma may reach a very large size without blocking an ostium. By CT, they are round, very dense, smoothly marginated intrasinus masses (Fig. 13.40). Contrast injection is unnecessary. Differential diagnosis includes fibrous dysplasia from which it should be easily excluded by its focality and intrasinus location.[38]

Hemangiomas may occur in the paranasal sinuses as in other locations. Their usual origin is in the lateral ethmoid sinus wall. These pulsatile masses cause bone erosion. Intravenous contrast CT demonstrates tumor enhancement. As with other sinus masses, the biplanar delineation of lesion borders is important for surgical planning.[38]

Inverted papilloma is an uncommon benign epithelial neoplasm of the nasal fossa and paranasal sinus mucosa with a malignant potential. It usually presents as a lateral nasal wall mass that causes bone destruction and ipsilateral maxillary sinus opacification. It is locally invasive and may involve the ethmoid sinus, the orbit, and the anterior cranial fossa.

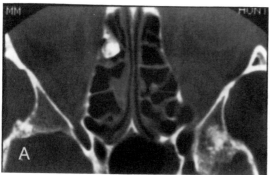 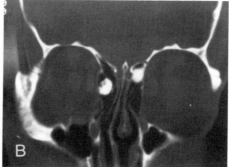

Figure 13.40. Ethmoid sinus osteomas. *Axial **(A)** bone filter 1.5-mm thickness and coronal **(B)** soft tissue filter, 5-mm thickness 28/ 450 CT scans. There are two bone density sharply marginated ethmoid sinus masses with expansion of the involved right ethmoid air* cell. With the exception of minimal degree mucosal hypertrophy, the ethmoid sinuses are otherwise normal. The nasal septum deviates to the right side.

CT demonstrates a bulky, infiltrating tissue-density, uncalcified mass that may contrastpenhance. There is associated sinus opacity due either to local invasion or blockage of ostia (Fig. 13.41). Secondary mucoceles may develop. Differential diagnostic considerations include ethesioneuroblastomas, polyps, and mucoceles. Whenever a nasal mass is associated with ipsilateral maxillary antrum opacity and bone destruction between the involved compartments, inverted papilloma must be considered.[38,44,45]

GRANULOMATOUS DISEASES

Granulomatous diseases of the paranasal sinuses and nasal fossa are uncommon and usually begin in the nasal fossa. This group of diseases includes Wegener's granulomatosis, midline granuloma, sarcoid, *Klebsiella* rhinoschleromatis, tuberculosis, syphilis, leprosy, and yaws.[38]

Wegener's granuloma is characterized by a triad including small vessel vasculitis, glomerulonephritis, and respiratory tract necrotizing granulomas. Nasal and paranasal sinus ulcerative granulomas are common. Midline granuloma is a condition characterized by similar nasal and paranasal sinus granulomas but lacking the Wegener's systemic manifestations.[10] Nasal septal and turbinate necrosis and ethmoid air cell destruction are often seen by CT.[38,45] Paranasal sinus obliteration commonly occurs probably due to combined granulomatous and chronic bacterial processes. CT demonstrates nasal septum and turbinate destruction, sinus opacity, and sinus wall obliterative hyperostosis (Fig. 13.42).[47] Nasal septum and turbinate destruction with sinus opacity are also seen with sarcoidosis.[45]

Nasal sarcoid occasionally occurs in patients with systemic sarcoidosis. Nasal mucosal polyps occasionally cause bone destruction.[10]

CSF RHINORRHEA

CSF rhinorrhea may result from trauma, may develop spontaneously, or may complicate surgery (particularly transsphenoidal hypophysectomy). A fracture involving the paranasal sinuses, particularly the cribriform plate and the sphenoid sinus, may result in CSF rhinorrhea and/or pneumocephalus. Spontaneous CSF rhinorrhea occurs in patients with pseudotumor cerebri, empty sella, and, occasionally, as an idiopathic occurrence. Chronic raised intracranial pressure can be associated with empty sella turcica and with skull base erosion (Fig. 13.43). Coronal (particularly) and axial CT thin (3-mm) sections using bone filtration may demonstrate sinus fluid levels and osseous defects. Thinner (1.5-mm) sections are sometimes required for small cribriform plate defects. Unusual sites of leakage may occur due to anatomic variations such as lateral extention of the sphenoid sinus. CT intrathecal contrast cisternography (Figs. 2.16 and 7.26) is the present method of choice for identification of the leakage site. This method demonstrates the leakage site and drainage through the appropriate meatus.

Malignant Paranasal Sinus and Nasal Tumors

Malignant tumors of the paranasal sinuses are far more common than those of the nasal cavity. Most of the malignant neoplasms of the paranasal sinuses and nasal cavity (80–90%) are squamous cell carcinomas. These tumors have a 2:1 male:female ratio of occurrence. Approximately 80% of all paranasal sinus carcinomas arise in the maxillary antra and most of the others arise in the ethmoid sinuses (Fig. 13.44).[10] Often, it is difficult to establish the sinus or nasal origin of tumors involving the medial sinus or lateral nasal wall. Bone destruction occurs in the vast majority of cases.[10] Sinus opacity frequently occurs due to blockage of ostia.[38] A secondary mucocele may develop that emphasizes the importance of identifying CT bone destruction.[38] Intravenous contrast, thin, CT axial and coronal sections best demonstrate the bone destruction, bone erosion, and soft tissue mass. Involvement of the infratemporal fossa by a malignant maxillary sinus tumor is common.[42] Contrast helps distinguish adenopathy from arteries and veins. Tumoral heterogeneous contrast enhancement usually occurs (Fig. 13.45).[39] MR tends to demonstrate lack of T2 hyperintensity in these masses as compared to homogeneous water-intensity of cysts and polyps.[10]

Early detection of sinus malignancy is perhaps the most important sinus and nasal imaging consideration. Bone destruction particularly of the infratemporal maxillary sinus surface should be considered suspicious of malignancy. Benign masses can cause focal erosions but do not produce frank destruction and they spare the infratemporal maxillary surface.[42] Sinus wall expansion associated with bone destruction frequently occurs in malignancy.[10] Sinus expansion alone is, therefore, not a sign of benignity.[10] By comparison, mucocele expansion is smooth and lacks destruction.[10,42] Chronic sinusitis is usually associated with smaller, thick-walled sinuses.[42] Tumoral contrast enhancement is found in malignancy although it may also be seen with polyps, papillomas, and mucocele margins.[32,48] Paranasal sinus malignant tumors tend to spread to the infratemporal fossa, pterygomaxillary fossa, nasopharyngeal mucosa, brain, or orbit. Evidence of spread has critical importance for treatment planning.[32]

Approximately 6% of nasal cavity and paranasal sinus malignant tumors arise from mucosal glandular elements. The majority of these tumors are adenoid cystic carcinomas (cylindromas) and the next most common are adenocarcinomas. Approximately half of adenoid cystic carcinomas arise in the palate and the maxillary sinus is the next most frequent site. Adenocarcinomas are more likely found in the ethmoid sinus.[10]

The ethesioneuroblastoma is a rare neurogenic tumor of the olfactory epithelium that clinically presents as a nasal mass. The tumor has two occurrence peaks: one in the sixth decade and another in the second decade.[38] Some of these superior ethmoid sinus polypoid tumors are slow growing but others are markedly aggressive. Intracranial extension is common because the tumor tends to spread along the olfactory nerves through the cribriform plate into the anterior cranial cavity (Fig. 13.46).[32] Distant metastases, primarily to the nodes and lungs, occur in approximately 20% of patients.[10] Ethesioneuroblastomas appear as a combined ethmoid sinus, intracranial contrast-enhancing mass that can be mistaken for a meningioma due to the often sharp margination of the convex upward intracranial portion.[32]

Paranasal sinus melanomas, lymphomas, primary plasmocytomas, and chondrosarcomas may also occur. Matrix calcification may be detected by CT in chondrosarcomas. Chondrosarcomas have a predilection for the ethmoid sinus.[40] In the pediatric population, rhabdomyosarcoma is probably most frequent. Metastatic paranasal sinus and nasal tumors are rare.[38] Secondary tumors of the paranasal sinuses and nasal cavity usually occur by direct extension of tumors of adjacent structures such as the nasopharynx, oral cavity, alveolar ridge, orbit, and pituitary gland.[38,48]

Nasopharynx Lesions

CT and MR examination of the nasopharynx region is usually performed to exclude a neoplasm, however, most images obtained by MR and by CT of the nasopharynx are coincidental to a study of the brain, sinuses, or orbits. It is, therefore, necessary that the radiologist be familiar with nasopharyngeal anatomy and pathology for analysis of suspected and unexpected nasopharyngeal region abnormalities. The method of approach to this brief review of nasopharyngeal pathological imaging will be regional after Dillon.[9] Benign conditions will precede malignant conditions for each of the six groups: mucosal space, parapharyngeal space, carotid space, retropharyngeal space, masticator space, and prevertebral space.

MUCOSAL SPACE

Infection and hypertrophy of the abundant lymphoid tissue of the nasopharynx commonly occurs (adenoiditis). Although adenoiditis may produce a mucosal space mass, the tissues remain pliable, which can be demonstrated by CT with blowing against pinched nares filling the lateral recesses with air.[19] Adenoidal tissue has isointense T1 and hyperintense T2 tissue characteristics (Fig. 13.47). Prominent adenoid tissue is a normal infancy and childhood finding and its presence may be of no clinical significance. Degenerative cysts within chronically inflamed adenoid tissue will have an even higher T2 signal.[9] Most carcinomas are invasive by the time they clinically present, however, the MR distinction of superficial noninvasive carcinoma from adenoid hypertrophy by MR is difficult due to the signal similarity.[9]

Juvenile angiofibroma is an uncommon, very vascular, benign tumor of mesenchymal origin arising in the nasopharynx. It occurs almost exclusively in young or adolescent boys. The tumor characteristically fills the nasopharynx and extends into and expands the pterygomaxillary fossa and infratemporal fossa. The posterior wall of the maxillary sinus is characteristically bowed forward. Contrast CT demonstrates these tumors sufficiently in order to establish the diagnosis. Contrast CT 3-mm axial and direct coronal sections are recommended (Fig. 13.48). Because of the marked vascularity of these tumors, the MR signal may resemble that of the "salt and pepper" glomus tumors. More experience is necessary in order to determine the MR juvenile angiofibroma intensity characteristics. The rarer lymphangioma may have similar CT characteristics but will not demonstrate marked contrast enhancement.

Thornwaldt's cyst is a 1- to 5-mm diameter midline nasopharyngeal cystic notocordal remnant that is occasionally found between the longus capitus muscles. It has water-density and T1 and T2 hyperintensity (Fig. 13.49).[9,49] It may occasionally become infected.

Almost all adult nasopharyngeal malignancies (98%)[9] are carcinomas. The vast majority (approxi-

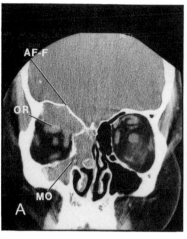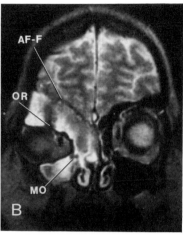

Figure 13.41. Inverted papilloma. *Coronal noncontrast 51/500 CT scan (13.41A) and SE 2000/80 MR scan (13.41B). There is an ethmoid infundibulum epicenter CT-isodense, T2 mixed muscle-isointense/hyperintense expansile mass. The mass obliterates the right middle turbinate, expands and erodes the maxillary ostium (MO), the ethmoid and frontal sinuse and erodes the downward displaced right orbital roof (OR). The right orbit is compressed by the expanded sinuses and the floor of the anterior fossa (AF·F) is elevated.*

mately 80%)[9] are squamous cell carcinomas. Approximately 18% of nasopharyngeal malignancies are of glandular cell origin (adenocarcinoma, cylindroma, and mucoepidermoid carcinoma). Non-Hodgkin's lymphoma is the next most common nasopharyngeal malignancy (<2%). Rhabdomyosarcoma is the most common nasopharyngeal tumor of children. Rarely, chordomas or sarcomas of the skull base may present as nasopharyngeal masses.[9,50]

Nasopharyngeal carcinoma has an occurrence rate of 1/100,000 people in Caucasian populations and as high as 20/100,000 in southern China. American-born Chinese are also highly susceptible.[9,38] Alcohol and tobacco use are also associated with a higher incidence of this cancer. Seventy to eighty percent occur in men and it favors the middle-aged and older patient.[9,38]

Squamous carcinoma most often develops in the nasopharyngeal lateral recess. At first, the lesion is superficial but usually, by the time of diagnosis, deep extension has occurred. Deep musculofacial plane invasion most often involves the levator and tensor muscles. Eustachian tube dysfunction occurs leading rapidly to the development of serous otitis media. Parapharyngeal space, soft palate, nasal cavity, and intracranial extension may occur.[9] Intracranial extension is usually extradural through the foramen lacerum, ovale, or through the superior orbital fissure. Cavernous sinus involvement results from foramen lacerum invasion. Because of the location of the trigeminal nerve third division just below the foramen ovale, pain and anesthesia in the n.V$_3$ distribution may be an early sign of nasopharyngeal carcinoma.[51] Trismus frequently develops due to pterygoid muscle involvement and nasal obstruction and epistaxis may result from anterior extension.[9]

Both CT and MR are extremely valuable for detection of nasopharyngeal carcinoma. There is usually CT tumor contrast enhancement. MR, because of its T1 and T2 tissue sensitivity, vascular flow detection, and virtually artifact-free orthogonal imaging is su-

perior to CT for detection of nasopharyngeal lesions. The role of Gd-DTPA has, so far, not improved the early MR detection of these lesions in our experience. T1-weighted images demonstrate fatty tissue tumor invasion and T2-weighted images demonstrate tumor hyperintensity (Fig. 13.50). Contrast axial and coronal CT is superior to MR for detection of bone destruction, however, the CT artifact at the skull base and the CT inferior tissue discrimination favors the MR method. More experience with MR is necessary to standardize MR technique for the nasopharynx and to determine the need for MR i.v. contrast.

CT and MR differential diagnosis of nasopharyngeal squamous carcinoma includes adenoid cystic carcinoma and chordoma. Adenoid cystic carcinomas, lymphomas, and sarcomas may, at first, spare the lateral recess,[51] however, they are generally indistinguishable from squamous carcinomas.[49] Chordomas present primarily as clivus destructive masses and are discussed in the prevertebral space group.

PARAPHARYNGEAL SPACE

Masses arising within parapharyngeal space are uncommon and are almost always tumors of salivary gland origin.[9,21] Lesions here are more likely an extension or invasion by other processes, such as squamous cell carcinoma. Both benign and malignant parapharyngeal space origin masses do occur, however. Benign lesions include mixed tumors of minor salivary glands, lipomas, branchial cleft cysts, n.V$_3$ schwannomas, hemangiopericytomas, tonsillar abscesses, and leiomyomas. Parapharyngeal space malignant lesions include adenoid cystic carcinoma, mucoepidermoid carcinoma, liposarcoma metastatic nodal deposits, and neurogenic sarcomas.[9]

Both CT and MR demonstrate inward bulging of the intact nasopharyngeal mucosa. These lesions must be differentiated from lesions of the deep lobe of the parotid gland for consideration of surgical approach.

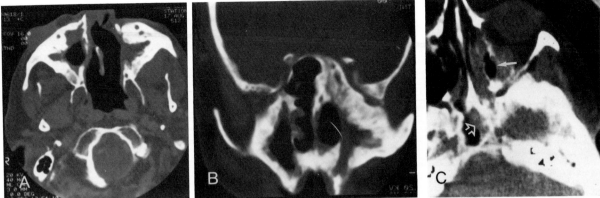

Figure 13.42. **Wegener's granulomatosis. A–B** and **C** are different cases. *Axial (A) and direct modified coronal (B) 575/2000 and axial 100/400 (C) i.v. contrast CT scans.* **A–B:** There is marked bilateral maxillary and left sphenoid sinus wall hyperostosis. Marked right-sided turbinate erosion and destruction is seen. (There has been left-sided surgical biopsy and debidement. This case is shown principally for the hyperostotic "filling in" of the maxillary antra.) **C:** A left ethmoid and orbital "isodense" mass has eroded portions of the lamina papyracea *(closed arrow)* and infiltrates the ethmoid sinus medially and orbit laterally. There is probable mass within the sphenoid sinus *(open arrow)*.

CAROTID SPACE

A variety of lesions, mostly benign, arise in the carotid space due to the presence of the carotid artery, jugular vein, cranial nerves IX–XII, sympathetic chain, and retropharyngeal nodes. These lesions include paragangliomas, glomus tumors, schwannomas, extracranial meningiomas, adenopathy, lymphoma, cellulitis, and abscess. The close approximation of this space to the jugular and carotid foramina and the petrous pyramid accounts for the inclusion of certain lesions under both headings. The paragangliomas and schwannomas have been discussed in detail in Chapter 12. How these lesions affect the carotid space will be described here. Jugular foramen masses, extracranial meningiomas, skull base metastatic disease, and chordomas may extend caudally into the upper nasopharynx and may present

as carotid space masses. Chordomas (Fig. 11.22) and skull base metastases have already been discussed in Chapter 11. Most nasopharyngeal paragangliomas also have a jugular fossa component. CT contrast enhancement, MR T1- and T2-flow-void and heterogeneous T2 intensities are characteristic of paragangliomas seen in the nasopharynx and elsewhere.[9,49]

Schwannomas that appear in the carotid space may also involve the jugular foramen in a dumbbell configuration. Both lesions uniformly contrast enhance by CT but the glomus tumor demonstrates typical jugular foramen erosion. MR T1 characteristics include isointensity with occasional cystic components in larger tumors. The T2 relatively homogeneous hyperintensity demonstrated by the schwannoma differentiates it from the paraganglioma (glomus tumor).

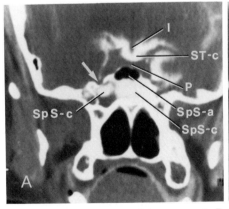
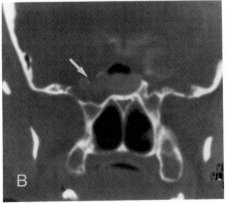
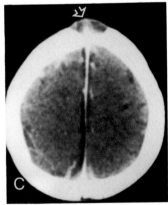

Figure 13.43. **Raised intracranial pressure. A–B** and **C** are different cases. **A–B:** Adult with pseudotumor cerebri. CSF rhinorrhea with empty sella. *Direct coronal 78/600 (A) and 426/3200 (B) CT cisternogram same level 3-mm thickness sections.* Intrathecal contrast fills the intrasellar cistern *(ST-c)* and enters the sphenoid sinus *(SpS-c)* through a middle fossa floor defect *(closed arrow)*. The pituitary infundibulum *(I)* and pituitary gland *(P)* are outlined with contrast. Air *(SpS-a)* is seen in the superior portion of the sphenoid sinus in this prone patient. **C:** Infant with *H. influenza* meningitis (same case as Fig. 8.6). *Axial high convexity 37/100 i.v. contrast 10-mm thickness CT scan.* Bulging anterior fontanel *(open arrow)*.

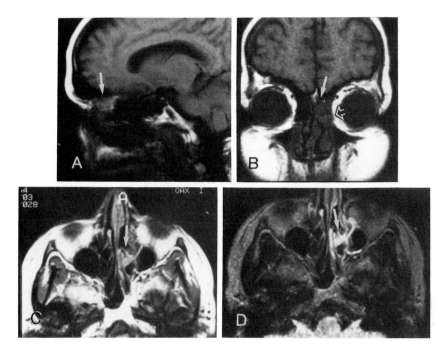

Figure 13.44. Ethmoid sinus squamous carcinoma. *Left parasagittal (A) and coronal (B) SE 600/25 and axial SE 2000/20 (C) and 2000/80 (D) 5-mm thickness MR scans.* An ethmoid T1 gray matter-isointense and T2 water-isointense mass *(closed arrows)* infiltrates the left ethmoid sinus, abuts the cribriform plate, and invades the orbit *(open arrow).*

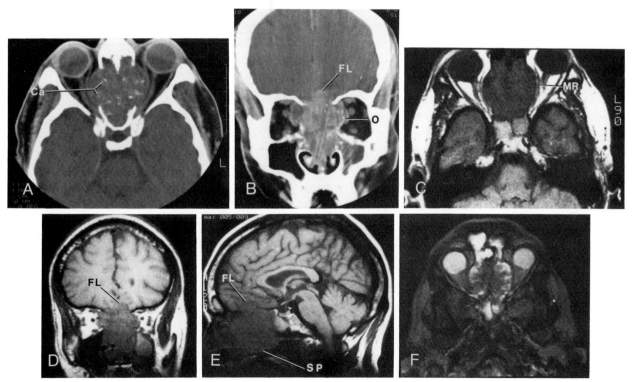

Figure 13.45. Nasal squamous carcinoma. *Axial (A) and direct coronal (B) 45/400 i.v. contrast CT scans. Axial (C), coronal (D), and midsagittal (E) SE 600/25; and axial (F) 2000/80 MR scans.* A partially calcified *(Ca)* diffusely enhanced destructive nasal mass destroys most of the nasal tissues, anterior fossa floor, and orbital me-dial margins. The tumor invades the left frontal lobe *(FL)* and the orbit *(O).* It invades the soft palate *(SP)* and medial rectus *(MR)* muscles. It demonstrates T1 homogeneous gray matter-hypointense and T2 heterogeneous signals.

Figure 13.46.   Esthesioneuroblastoma. *Axial i.v. contrast 50/250 10-mm thickness CT scan* **(A).** *Same level axial SE 2000/100* **(B)** *and SE 700/25 coronal* **(C)** *and sagittal* **(D)** *MR scans.* There is a very large destructive mass with CT heterogeneous enhancement. It has T1 and T2 partial hyperintensity (extracellular methemoglobin) and areas of serpentine signal void (marked vascularity) **(B).** The mass has a nasoethmoid epicenter and invades the brain, orbits, nasal cavity, and nasopharynx. The tumor hemorrhagic and vascular characteristics and the extent of tumor invasion are most clearly demonstrated by the MR method.

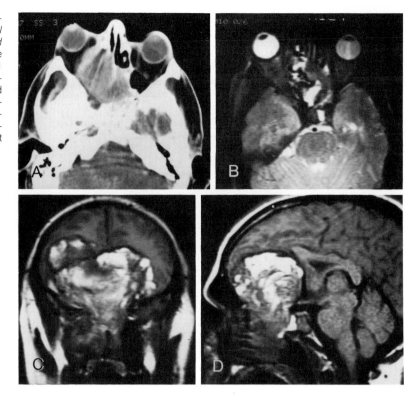

Figure 13.47.   Adenoid hypertrophy. Three-year-old normal boy. *Lateral CT localizer* **(A).** *Midsagittal SE 600/25* **(B)** *and axial 2000/30* **(C)** *and 2000/80* **(D)** *MR scans.* There is T1 nasal mucosa-isointense and T2 water-isointense hypertrophied adenoidal tissue *(closed arrow).* There is markedly T2 hyperintense maxillary sinus mucosal thickening *(open arrow).* The prevertebral space longus colli and capitis muscles *(LC)* produce a characteristic posterior symmetrical contour. The sphenoid sinus *(SpS)* lacks pneumatization.

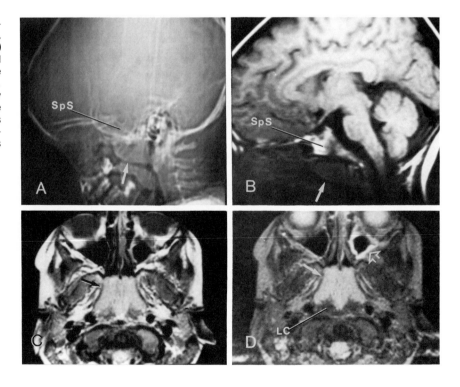

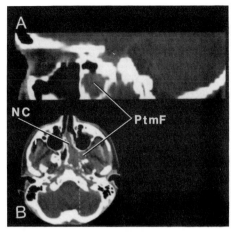

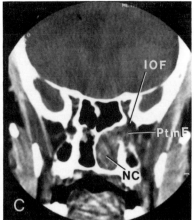

Figure 13.48.   Juvenile angiofibroma. *CT sagittal reformation **(A)** of a series of 3-mm i.v. contrast axial sections **(B)** in the plane of the interrupted vertical line. Direct coronal 38/300 section **(C)**. There is* a homogeneous moderately contrast-enhancing mass expanding the pterygomaxillary fossa *(PtmF)*, extending into the nasal cavity *(NC)* and inferior orbital fissure *(IOF)*.

RETROPHARYNEAL SPACE

Retropharyngeal adenopathy may present as a carotid space mass and may be caused by metastatic disease, lymph proliferative disorders, or recurrent adenoid infection in children. Normal retropharyngeal lymph nodes are CT isodense and they are MR T1 muscle-isointense and T2 moderately hyperintense.[9] Signs of abnormal retropharyngeal lymph nodes are cross-sectional diameters greater than 1.5 cm, CT hypodense, and MR T1 muscle-hypointense/ T2 hyperintense foci irrespective of node size, associated obliteration of facial planes, and presence of three or more contiguous 8–15 mm or greater diameter ill-defined nodes. CT rim-contrast enhancement of metastatic nodes tends to be uniformly thick. The pattern of enhancement in inflammatory disease, usually tuberculosis, is usually thick and irregular.[42] Necrotic nodal areas demonstrate marked T2 hyperintensity.[9] CT contrast enhancement and MR signal-void identify principal vascular structures such as the internal carotid artery and jugular vein.[9,52] By these techniques, vessels are distinguished from other structures including nodes.

The retropharyngeal nodes receive lymphatic drainage from the nasal fossa, soft palate, paranasal sinuses, middle ear, nasopharynx, and oropharynx. Nasopharyngeal carcinoma commonly spreads to the retropharyngeal lymph nodes. This results in lymph node enlargement, obliteration of carotid space soft tissue planes, and nodal necrosis, and infiltrative CT and MR changes.[9,52] Since lymph nodes and schwannomas both have T1 muscle-isointense and T2 hyperintense characteristics, a schwannoma and a retropharyngeal node may be difficult to distinguish by the MR technique.[9,52]

MASTICATOR SPACE

Masticator space masses are usually of odontogenic origin; most often, from dental infections and mandibular neoplasms. These masses deviate the parapharyngeal space medially. Adjacent carcinomas frequently spread to the masticator space. The foramen ovale at its apex provides a pathway for spread to the intracranial space of tumor and infection.[9,21]

PREVERTEBRAL SPACE

The principal pathological considerations of the prevertebral space masses include chordoma, meta-

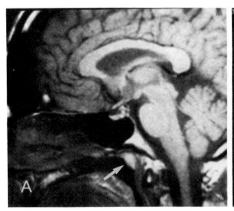

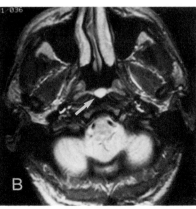

Figure 13.49.   Thornwaldt's cyst. *Midsagittal 600/25 and axial SE 2800/30 5-mm section MR scans. There is a central T1 **(A)**, proton density **(B)**, and T2-weighted image (not shown) hyperintense, smooth, sharply marginated mass in the mucosal space cleft between the longus muscles (arrows).*

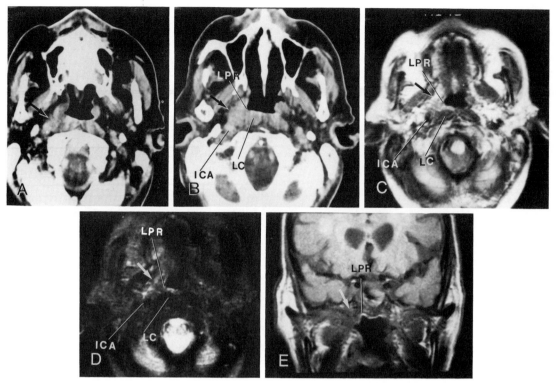

Figure 13.50. Nasopharyngeal carcinoma. *Axial i.v. contrast 10-mm thickness CT scan **A** is 10 mm caudal to **B**. Level A axial SE 2000/25 **(C)** and 2000/100 **(D)** 10-mm thickness and coronal 2000/25 5-mm thickness **(E)** nonflow-compensated MR scans. A para-pharyngeal epicenter mass (arrows) effaces the CT fat planes of the* carotid space *(ICA)* and prevertebral *(LC)* spaces. The right torus tubarius CT and MR definition is obscured and there is T2 tumor hyperintensity. There is subtle effacement of the right lateral pharyngeal recess *(LPR)* not evident on the coronal section. Only slight CT tumor contrast enhancement occurred.

static disease to the spine, and osteomyelitis, abscess and cellulitis.

References

1. Williams AL. Congenital anomalies. In Williams AL, Haughton VM (Eds). *Cranial Computed Tomography.* St. Louis: CV Mosby Co, 1985; 316–349.
2. DuBoulay GH. *Principles of X-ray Diagnosis of the Skull.* London: Butterworth's, 1965.
3. McGahan. CT of eosinophilic adenoma of the skull. *AJNR* 1980; 1:576–577.
4. Williams AL. Tumors. In *Cranial Computed Tomography.* St. Louis: CV Mosby Co, 1985; 148–239.
5. Ethier R. Thickness and texture. In Newton TH, Potts DG (Eds). *Radiology of the Skull and Brain.* St. Louis: CV Mosby Co, 1971; 179–204.
6. Grossman CB. The skull base. In Gonzalez CF, Grossman CB, Masdeu CF (Eds). *Head and Spine Imaging.* New York: John Wiley & Sons, 1985; 693–714.
7. Steinbach HL. Paget's disease. In Newton TH, Potts DG (Eds). *Radiology of the Skull and Brain.* St. Louis: CV Mosby Co, 1971; 755–762.
8. Tjon-A-Tham RTO, Bloem JL, Falke THM, et al. Magnetic resonance imaging in Paget's disease of the skull. *AJNR* 1985; 6:879–881.
9. Dillon WP. The nasopharynx. In Brant-Zawadski M, Norman D (Eds). *Magnetic Resonance Imaging of the Central Nervous System.* New York: Raven Press, 1987; 329–358.
10. Som PM. The paranasal sinuses. In Bergeron RT, Osborn A, Som PM (Eds). *Head and Neck Imaging Excluding the Brain.* St. Louis: CV Mosby Co, 1984; 1–143.
11. Terrier F, Weber W, Ruefenacht D, Porcellini B. Anatomy of the ethmoid: CT, endoscopic and macroscopic. *AJNR* 1985; 6:77–84.
12. Zinreich SJ, Kennedy DW, Rosenbaum AE, et al. Paranasal sinuses: CT imaging requirements for endoscopic surgery. *Radiology* 1987; 163:769–775.
13. Osborn A. The nose. In Bergeron RT, Osborn A, Som PM (Eds). *Head and Neck Imaging Excluding the Brain.* St. Louis: CV Mosby Co, 1984; 143–171.
14. Reicher MA, Bentson JR, Halbach VV, et al. Pneumosinus dilatans of the sphenoid sinus. *AJNR* 1986; 7:865–868.
15. Sataloff RT, Grossman CB, Naheedy MH, Gonzalez CF. Paranasal sinuses and nasopharynx. In Gonzalez CF, Grossman CB, Masdeu JC (Eds). *Head and Spine Imaging.* New York: John Wiley & Sons, 1985; 715–740.
16. Sataloff RT, Grossman CB, Gonzalez CF, Naheedy MH. Computed tomography of the face and paranasal sinuses: Part I. Normal anatomy. *Head Neck Surg* 1984; 7:110–122.
17. Silver AJ, Mawad ME, Hilal SK, et al. Computed tomography of the nasopharynx and related spaces. Part I: Anatomy. *Radiology* 1983; 147:725–731.
18. Mancuso AA, Bohman L, Hanafee W, Maxwell D. Computed tomography of the nasopharynx: normal and variants of normal. *Radiology* 1980; 137:113–121.
19. Bohman L, Mancuso A, Thompson J, Hanafee W. CT approach to benign nasopharyngeal masses. *AJR* 1981; 136:173–180.
20. Bergeron RT, Osborn AG. Abnormalities of the base of the skull and neck. *Syllabus: A Categorical Course in Neuroradiology.* 73rd Scientific Assembly and Annual Meeting of the RSNA, Chicago, 1987; 81–90.
21. Curtin HD. Separation of the masticator space from the parapharyngeal space. *Radiology* 1987; 163:195–204.
22. Curtin HD, Williams R. Computed tomographic anatomy of the pterygopalatine fossa. *Radiographics* 1985; 5:429–440.
23. Daniels DL, Rausching W, Lovas J, et al. Pterygopalatine fossa: Computed tomographic studies. *Radiology* 1983; 149:511–516.
24. Glasier CM, Ascher DP, Williams KD. Incidental paranasal sinus abnormalities on CT of children: clinical correlation. *AJNR* 1986; 7:861–864.
25. Chinwuba C, Wallman J, Strand R. Nasal airway obstruction: CT assessment. *Radiology* 1986; 159:503–506.

26. Slovis TL, Renfro B, Watts FB, et al. Choanal atresia: Precise CT evaluation. *Radiology* 1985; 155:345–348.
27. Tadmor R, Ravid M, Millet D, Leventon G. Computed tomographic demonstration of choanal atresia. *AJNR* 1984; 5:743–745.
28. Blaschke DP, Osborn AG. The mandible and teeth. In Bergeron RT, Osborn A, Som P (Eds). *Head and Neck Imaging Excluding the Brain*. St. Louis: CV Mosby Co, 1984; 279–341.
29. Whelan MA, Reede DL, Lin JP, Edwards JH. The base of the skull. In Bergeron RT, Osborn A, Som P (Eds). *Head and Neck Imaging Excluding the Brain*. St. Louis: CV Mosby Co, 1984; 531–574.
30. Naidich TP, Zimmerman RA. Common congenital malformations of the brain. In Brant-Zawadzki M, Norman D (Eds). *Magnetic Resonance Imaging of the Central Nervous System*. New York: Raven Press, 1987; 131–150.
31. Anderson JE. *Grant's Atlas of Anatomy*, 7th Edition. Baltimore: Williams & Wilkins, 1978; 7–8.
32. Mancuso AA, Hanafee WN. In *Computed Tomography of the Head and Neck. Facial Trauma*, 2nd Edition. Baltimore: Williams & Wilkins, 1985; 43–60.
33. Gentry LR, Manor WF, Turski PA, Strother CM. High resolution CT analysis of facial struts in trauma: Normal anatomy. *AJR* 1983; 40:523–532.
34. Jend H-H, Jend-Rossmann I. Sphenotemporal buttress fracture: A report of five cases. *Neuroradiology* 1984; 26:411–413.
35. Gentry LR, Manor WF, Turski PA, Strother CM. High resolution CT analysis of facial struts in trauma: Osseous and soft-tissue complications. *AJR* 1983; 140:533–541.
36. Dolan KD, Jacoby CB, Smoker WRK. The radiology of facial fractures. *Radiographics* 1984; 4:577–663.
37. Harris L, Marano GD, McCorkle D. Nasofrontal duct: CT in frontal sinus trauma. *Radiology* 1987; 165:195–198.
38. Sataloff RT, Grossman CB, Gonzalez C, Naheedy N. Computed tomography of the face and paranasal sinuses: Part II. Abnormal anatomy and pathologic conditions. *Head Neck Surg* 1985; 7:369–389.
39. Som PM, Lawson W, Biller HF, Lanzieri CF. Ethmoid sinus disease: CT evaluation in 400 cases. Part 1. Non-surgical patients. *Radiology* 1986; 159:591–597.
40. Kopp W, Fotter R, Steiner H, et al. Aspergillosis of the paranasal sinuses. *Radiology* 1985; 156:715–716.
41. Gamba JL, Woodruff WW, Djang WT, Yeats AE. Craniofacial mucormycosis: Assessment with CT. *Radiology* 1986; 160:207–212.
42. Silver AJ, Baredes S, Bello JA, et al. The opacified maxillary sinus: CT findings in chronic sinusitis and malignant tumors. *Radiology* 1987; 163:205–210.
43. Nino-Murcia M, Rao VM, Mikaelian DO, Som P. Acute sinusitis mimicking antrochoanal polyp. *AJNR* 1986; 7:513–516.
44. Momose KJ, Weber AL, Goodman M, et al. Radiological aspects of inverted papilloma. *Radiology* 1980; 134:73–79.
45. Mancuso AA, Hanafee WN. Benign Sinus. In Mancuso AA, Hanafee WN (Eds). *Computed Tomography and Magnetic Resonance Imaging of the Head and Neck*, 2nd Edition. Baltimore: Williams & Wilkins, 1985, 20–41.
46. Som PM, Lawson W, Cohen BA. Giant-cell lesions of the facial bones. *Radiology* 1983; 147:129–134.
47. Paling MR, Roberts RL, Fauci AS. Paranasal sinus obliteration in Wegener granulomatosis. *Radiology* 1982; 144:539–543.
48. Mancuso AA, Hanafee WN. Malignant sinus. In Mancuso AA, Hanafee WN (Eds). *Computed Tomography and Magnetic Resonance Imaging of the Head and Neck*, 2nd Edition. Baltimore: Williams & Wilkins, 1985; 1–19.
49. Mancuso AA, Som PM. The upper aerodigestive tract (nasopharynx, oropharynx, and floor of the mouth). In Bergeron RT, Osborn AG, Som PM (Eds). *Head and Neck Imaging Excluding the Brain*. St. Louis: CV Mosby Co, 1984; 374–401.
50. Bass IS, Haller JO, Berdon WE. Nasopharyngeal carcinoma: Clinical and radiographic findings in children. *Radiology* 1985; 156:651–654.
51. Silver AJ, Mawad ME, Hilal SK, et al. Computed tomography of the nasopharynx and related spaces. Part II: Pathology. *Radiology* 1983; 147:733–738.
52. Reede DL, Bergeron RT, Osborn AG. CT of the soft tissues of the neck. In Bergeron RT, Osborn AG, Som PM (Eds). *Head and Neck Imaging Excluding the Brain*. St. Louis: CV Mosby Co, 1984; 491–530.

CHAPTER

14

The Orbit

Introduction

CT and MR are the principal imaging methods for investigation of orbital disease beyond the globe examination by fundoscopy and ultrasound and beyond a plain film x-ray, which might be helpful for evaluation of trauma. CT is superior to MR for identification of calcification and bone abnormalities and for investigating most cases of orbital trauma. MR more effectively examines fat tissue characteristics, has greater imaging plane capability, and does not have known harmful dosage effects. MR vascular flow detection can identify venous vascular occlusion and

vascular patency. The comparison of the CT and MR techniques for examination of the optic foramen is shown in Figure 14.1. The far superior CT detection of bone and calcium helps identify osseous abnormalities and calcified abnormalities such as retinoblastoma, hamartoma, choroid osteoma, and optic disk drusen. MR, exclusively, can identify the entire visual pathways (Fig. 14.2).

MR is contraindicated in the presence of ferromagnetic ocular foreign bodies,[1] in patients with ferromagnetic cerebral aneurysm clips, in patients with cardiac pacemakers and with other ferromagnetic materials and implanted electronic programmed devices. Eye make-up should be removed before the MR scan.

An etiological format of presentation has been cho-

Figure 14.1. The optic nerve canal. *Direct coronal 16-cm FOV 3-mm thickness soft tissue filter 300/4000 CT scan* **(A).** *Coronal SE 600/25 18-cm FOV 3-mm thickness MR scan* **(B).** *Axial i.v. contrast 16-cm FOV 3-mm thickness 50/550 CT scan* **(C).** *Same level SE 600/25 18-cm FOV 3-mm thickness MR scan* **(D).** The intracanalicular segment of the optic nerve *(ON-c)* lies above the ophthalmic artery *(OA)* in the optic canal *(OC)*. Clockwise, the optic canal is surrounded by the planum sphenoidale *(PSp)*, the anterior clinoid process *(ACP)*, the optic strut *(OSt)*, and the wall of the sphenoid sinus *(SpS)*. The optic strut separates the optic canal from the superior orbital fissure *(SOF)* and the contrast-enhanced cavernous sinus *(CS)*; the inferior orbital fissure *(IOF)*.

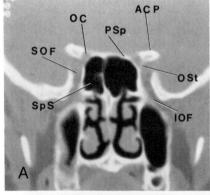

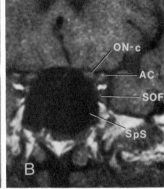

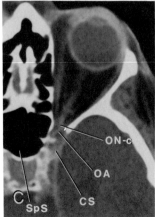

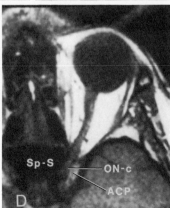

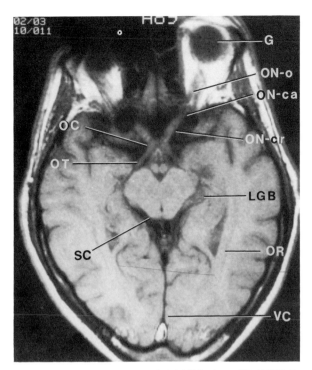

Figure 14.2. Visual pathways. *Axial IOM plane SE 600/25 3-mm thickness MR scan.* Abbreviations: *G*, globe; *LGB*, lateral geniculate body; *OC*, optic chiasm; *ON-ca*, optic nerve—intracanalicular portion; *ON-cr*, optic nerve—intracranial portion; *ON-o*, optic nerve—intraorbital portion; *OR*, optic radiation; *OT*, optic tract; *VC*, visual cortex. The superior colliculus *(SC)* is labeled for reference.

sen. The last category ("other conditions") includes conditions that did not fit well into the etiological categorization. At the end of the chapter is a gamut list designed to help categorize orbital abnormalities and aid in their differentiation.

Imaging Technique

CT TECHNIQUE

CT orbital imaging technique has long been established. Noncontrast 3-mm sections in the infraorbitomeatal (IOM) plane are followed by i.v. contrast 3-mm sections in both the axial and coronal planes. The basis for this technique is the usual parallel course of the optic nerve in the IOM plane, the need to establish a baseline for detection of calcium and for density change after contrast injection, and the need to evaluate detailed structural relationships in at least two orthogonal planes.[2] The supine hanging head technique is our standard method for direct coronal imaging. With head hyperextension and maximum gantry tilt, a good approximation of a plane perpendicular to the IOM can usually be obtained. Occasionally, when dental work causes unacceptable artifact, prone direct coronal sections are attempted. Marked spondylosis and cervical fractures are contraindications for head hyperextension. Orbital coronal and sagittal reformations of 3-mm sections are occasionally necessary for patients unable to assume

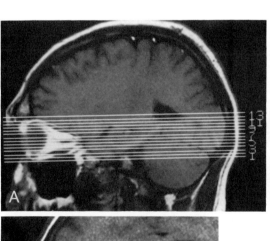

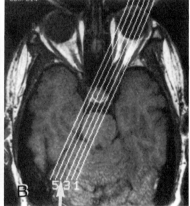

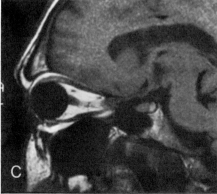

Figure 14.3. MR orbit technique. Axial IOM plane 3-mm section localizer parallel to the optic nerve **(A).** Sagittal oblique 3-mm section localizer parallel to the optic nerve **(B)** and section 4 *(arrow, B)* **(C).** Note the partial volume averaging of fat and optic nerve in **C** due to the undulating course of the nerve.

a hyperextended position. Direct sagittal scans are rarely done due to the cumbersome technique.[3] CT imaging factors include a moderately wide window width (400–500) to allow for bone detail without significantly compromising the orbital muscle, fat, water, and contrast resolution.[2,3] Bone window (WW = 4000) films are also standard.

MR TECHNIQUE

Orbital MR technique has not yet been standardized and varies according to the MR equipment, the availability of convenient surface coils, the choice of *three* orthogonal imaging planes (Fig. 14.3), the choice of T1-, proton density-, and T2-weighted images, the need for i.v. contrast and patient throughput requirements. Most of the images in this chapter were obtained using the standard head coil with a 1.5 Tesla unit. Orbital MR technique requires greater patient cooperation than does CT due to the longer scan time (usually minutes versus seconds). Patients should keep their open eyes fixed on a point throughout the scan. Closed eyes tend to wander.

The T1 hyperintense signal of fat can obscure paramagnetic contrast enhancement. Methods that cause fat to be less T1 signal-intense are called fat suppression techniques. Two fat suppression methods currently receiving attention are chemical presaturation and short-TI inversion recovery ("STIR") techniques. The inversion recovery technique has been disappointing because all tissue signals are altered and a relatively long TR is required. With chemical presaturation, the fat (or water) within a particular imaging volume can be selectively presaturated immediately before the excitation pulse by applying an additional pulse at fat (or water) frequency. This destroys the longitudinal magnetization of the fat (or water). This method can be used with short TR/short TE SE or with GRE techniques. It is more effective for smaller volume and is more selective than STIR. A useful application is a chemical presaturation i.v. Gd-DTPA optic nerve meningioma investigation. With chemical presaturation, the contrast enhanced tumor is more easily distinguished from the adjacent suppressed relatively hypointense retrobulbar fat.[4a]

Surface coils provide excellent detail of superficial structures close to the applied coil (i.e., the globe) but experience a significant loss of signal intensity from more distant structures (i.e., the orbital apex). Spin echo (SE) surface-coil technique is usually limited to T1-weighted pulse sequences because of the shorter scan time in order to limit motion artifact.[4]

Lens detail, which is seen clearly by heavily T1-weighted surface coil technique (SE 600/25) is not seen clearly on our 1.5 T scanner using the head coil technique. A major limiting factor for head coil orbital scanning is wraparound artifact, which increases as field of view (FOV) is decreased.

Normal Orbit Anatomy

Orbital anatomy will be described under the following topics: the orbital bones, the lacrimal gland, the globe, the extraocular muscles and muscle cone, the optic nerve and sheath, the ophthalmic artery,

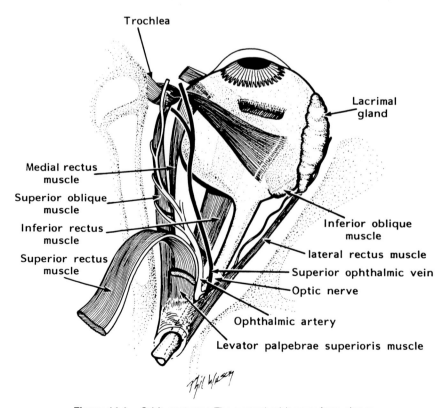

Figure 14.4. Orbit anatomy. The normal orbit seen from above.

the superior ophthalmic vein, and the retrobulbar tissue (Figs. 14.4 and 14.5).

ORBITAL BONES

The orbit can be considered a pyramidal structure that has a floor and roof, medial and lateral walls, and an apex. The floor is formed principally by the maxillary sinus roof (thin) with a major thick anterolateral zygomatic contribution. The roof is mainly formed by the frontal bone (floor of the anterior fossa). The medial wall is principally formed by the lamina papyracea of the ethmoid bone. The lateral orbital margin is formed mainly by the zygomatic bone anteriorly and the greater wing of the sphenoid bone posteriorly. The lacrimal fossa is a small shallow concavity of the zygomatic process of the frontal bone.[5] The orbital apex approaches the optic foramen, which is in the lesser wing of the sphenoid bone. The optic foramen is separated from the superior orbital fissure by the optic strut, a bone spur extending from the anterior clinoid process to the lateral wall of the sphenoid sinus (Fig. 14.1).[6]

The superior orbital fissure is just lateral to the optic canal and separated from it by the optic strut. The annulus of Zinn is an orbital apex tendinous ring from which the four rectus muscles originate. It encircles the optic foramen and the medial portion of the superior orbital fissure. The superior and inferior divisions of the oculomotor nerve (n.III), the abducens nerve (n.VI), and the nasociliary nerve (branch of n.V$_1$) course through the annulus of Zinn. Superolateral to the annulus within the superior orbital fissure are the trochlear nerve (n.IV), the lacrimal and frontal nerves (branches of n.V$_1$), and the superior ophthalmic vein. The inferior ophthalmic vein courses beneath the annulus. The reader is referred to Chapter 11 for detail of the cavernous sinus (Fig. 11.5A).[7]

LACRIMAL GLAND

The lacrimal gland position partially depends upon the orbital shape. The lacrimal gland rests in the frontal bone lacrimal fossa and, often, the anterior portion of the gland extends beyond the osseous orbital confines. Shallow orbits tend to have superficial lacrimal glands that appear mostly outside of the orbit. The externally positioned lacrimal gland may be confused with lacrimal glandular enlargement and the appearance of the shallow orbit may give the false impression of proptosis (Fig. 14.6).[5,8]

GLOBE

The MR technique provides much more detail of globe structures than does CT. The three layers of the globe, from outside to inside, are the sclera, uvea, and retina. The middle layer (the uvea) includes the choroid, ciliary body, and iris from posterior to anterior. It is a highly vascular pigmented layer. CT cannot identify these three separate layers in the normal state and, instead, identifies an isodense contrast-enhancing single layer. MR identifies the sclera and a combined retina-choroid layer. The sclera is hypointense to all sequences. The retina and the choroid cannot be distinguished from each other on any sequence and together appear hyperintense on T1-weighted and proton images (Fig. 14.5).[9,10] The lens is homogeneously CT hyperdense. MR demonstrates lens cortex water-T1 hyperintensity. The nucleus is water-T1 isointense/T2 hypointense.[10] The lens divides the globe into an anterior portion (the anterior and posterior chambers) and a posterior portion (vitreous body). The iris separates the anterior from the posterior chamber. Both the anterior and posterior chambers are filled with aqueous humor. The aqueous and vitreous humors have water-CT and MR density and intensity characteristics, respectively. The orbital septum is a continuation of the anterior orbital periosteum which inserts on the tarsal plates of the eyelids. This septum is important for containment of inflammatory processes. The lacrimal gland is a postseptal structure. The cornea is continuous with the sclera and is the anterior margin of the anterior chamber. The cornea has three layers that can be detected by careful scrutiny (not seen on our cases) of surface coil T1-weighted and proton MR images by virtue of a central hypointense layer between two comparatively hyperintense layers. The innermost layer is not distinguished from the aqueous on T2 technique.[10] The eyelids may trap a small amount of air, which should not be confused with orbital emphysema. The ciliary body, the iris, and the zonules (suspensory ligament from lens to ciliary body) are well identified on T1-weighted and proton images (Figs. 14.5 and 14.7).[10] Gadolinium i.v. contrast MR technique enhances the ciliary body and iris (Fig. 14.7). Fat suppression STIR with i.v. gadolinium contrast may prove useful for detailed globe imaging. The hyaloid canal is a canal-like remnant of the posterior chamber hyaloid artery between the lens and optic disk. It is not detected in the normal adult.[6,10]

EXTRAOCULAR MUSCLES AND THE MUSCLE CONE

The muscle cone is a conal sheath formed by the superior, medial, inferior, and lateral rectus muscles, and intermuscular fascia. These muscles have an orbital apex attachment at the fibrous annulus of Zinn and insert on the sclera of the anterior globe. In addition to the four rectus extraocular muscles forming the muscle cone, the superior oblique and inferior oblique muscles are well demonstrated by both CT and MR technique. The superior oblique muscle courses from the orbital apex, superomedial to the medial rectus through the medially positioned trochlea to insert on the sclera of the superolateral globe surface beneath the superior rectus. The inferior oblique is the only muscle arising in the anterior orbit. It has its osseous insertion at the anteromedial orbital floor and courses caudal to the inferior rectus along the orbital floor to insert on the inferolateral sclera.[6,9] A useful mnemonic "RO-RU" stands for rectus over oblique and rectus under oblique from cranial to caudal.

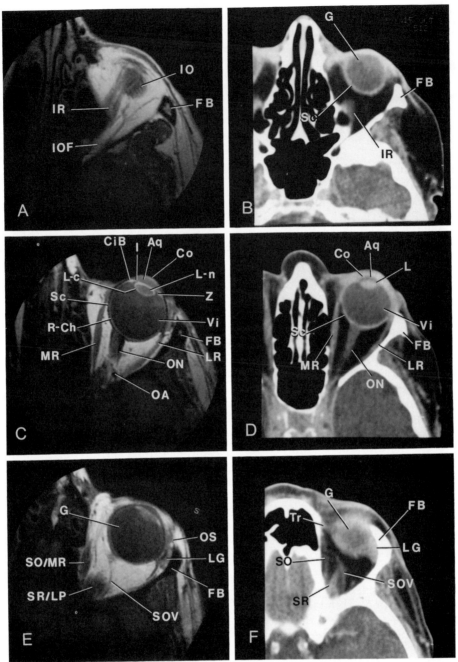

Figure 14.5. The normal orbit. *A, C, and E are axial surface coil SE 800/20 MR scans and **B, D,** and **F** are axial 30/400 i.v. contrast CT scans.* The lens *(L)* separates the vitreous *(Vi)* from the aqueous *(Aq)* humors. The hyperintense lens capsule *(L-c)* encloses the relatively hypointense lens nucleus *(L-n)*. The hypointense sclera *(Sc)* surrounds the hyperintense combined retina and choroid *(R-Ch)* layers. Lateral to the lens is the ciliary body *(CiB)*. The zonule *(Z)*, vitreous-iosintense, is lateral to the lens and is located between the lens and the ciliary body. The iris *(I)* extends from the ciliary body anterior to the lens. The superior ophthalmic vein *(SOV)* posterolateral to the annulus of Zinn *(AZ)* courses posterolaterally under the superior rectus muscle *(SR)*. The ophthalmic artery *(OA)* is inferolateral to the optic nerve *(ON)* at the orbital apex and then courses over the optic nerve. It is responsible for a flow artifact in **C.** The superior oblique muscle *(SO)* is seen superomedial to the medial rectus muscle *(MR)* coursing anteriorly to the trochlea [*Tr* (Figs. 14.2 and 14.5 **E** and **F**)] where it abruptly angles greater than 90° to insert on the superolateral sclera. The inferior oblique muscle *(IO)* anterior origin and posterolateral course is best seen on coronal sections as is the close relationship of the superior rectus and levator palpebrae muscles **(K** and **L).** The orbital septum *(OS)* between frontal bone periosteum and the tarsal plates can be identified on axial sections. The orbital septum can also be identified on sagittal sections. The lacrimal gland *(LG)* is seen in the frontal bone *(FB)* lacrimal fossa. It is extraconal and postseptal. Abbreviations: *Aq,* aqueous humor; *Az,* annulus of Zinn; *CiB,* ciliary body; *Co,* cornea; *FB,* frontal bone; *G,* globe; *I,* iris; *IO,* inferior oblique muscle; *IR,* inferior rectus muscle; *L,* lens; *LG,* lacrimal gland; *L-c,* lens cortex; *LEl,* lower eyelid; *L-n,* lens nucleus; *LP,* levator palpebrae muscle; *LR,* lateral rectus muscle; *MR,* medial rectus muscle; *OA,* ophthalmic artery; *OS,* orbital septum; *R-Ch,* retina-choroid, *Sc,* sclera; *SO,* superior oblique muscle; *SO/MR,* superior oblique/medial rectus; *SOV,* superior ophthalmic vein; *SR,* superior rectus muscle; *SR/LP,* superior rectus/levator palpebrae; *Tr,* trochlea; *UEl,* upper eyelid, *Vi,* vitreous; *Z,* zonule.

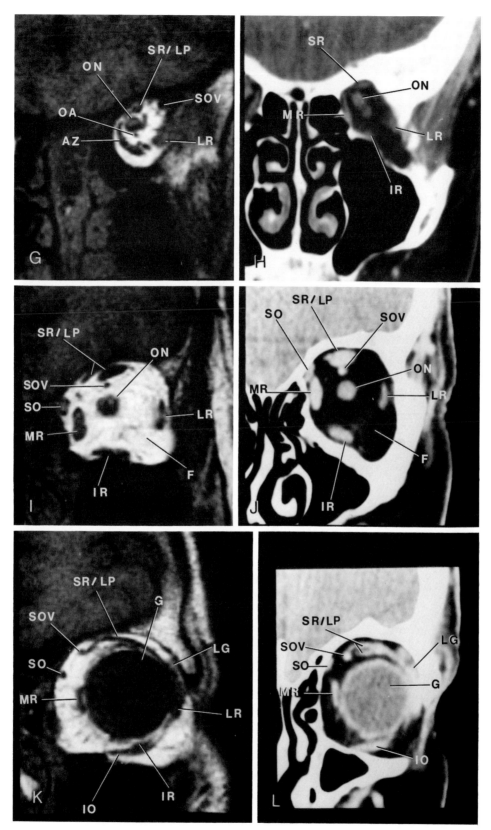

Figure 14.5. (continued). G, I, and **K** are coronal head coil SE 600/ 25 MR scans and **H, J,** and **L** are direct coronal 30/450 i.v. contrast CT scans.

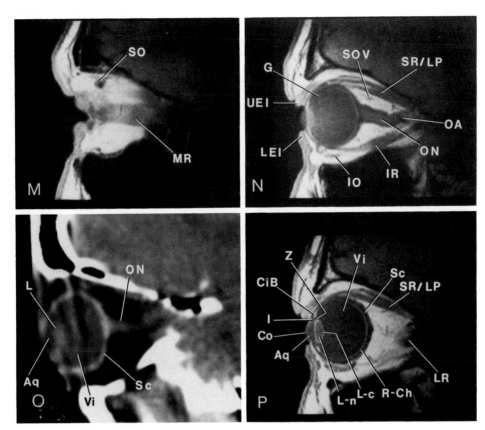

Figure 14.5. (continued). *M, N,* and *P* *are sagittal surface coil SE 800/20 MR scans and **O** is a direct sagittal 25/250 CT scan.*

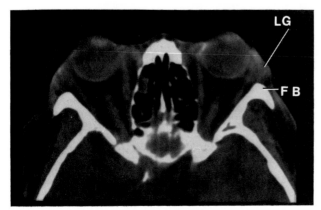

Figure 14.6. **Shallow orbit with extraorbital lacrimal glands.** *Axial IOM plane 30/400 3-mm thickness CT scan.* The lacrimal glands *(LG)* are anterior to the lateral orbital margins *(FB).*

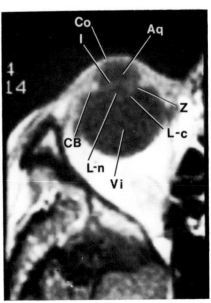

Figure 14.7. **MR globe contrast enhancement.** *Axial i.v. contrast SE 600/25 3-mm thickness 18-cm FOV MR scan.* There is ciliary body *(CB)* and iris *(I)* contrast enhancement. *Aq,* aqueous humor; *CB,* ciliary body; *Co,* cornea; *L-c,* lens cortex; *L-n,* lens nucleus; *Vi,* vitreous; *Z,* zonule.

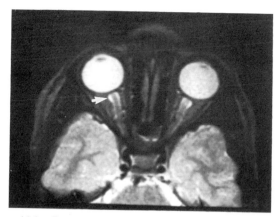

Figure 14.8. Prominent perioptic nerve subarachnoid space. *Axial SE 2800/80 MR scan. The optic nerves are surrounded by a CSF-filled arachnoid membrane. The CSF causes the T2 signal-hyperintensity (arrow).*

The levator palpebrae is so closely approximated to the superior rectus that the two muscles usually present as a combined image. The extraocular muscles are CT isodense, MR muscle-isointense, and slightly enhance with i.v. contrast. The confines of the muscle cone provide a pathologically significant and clinically useful barrier for limitation of and identification of disease processes, respectively. Retrobulbar lesions may therefore be described as "intraconal" or "extraconal."

OPTIC NERVE AND SHEATH

The optic nerve extends from the optic disk through the muscle cone and optic canal to join the contralateral optic nerve at the optic chiasm. The optic nerve sheath is a continuation of the pia-arachnoid-dura intracranial membranes. The subarachoid space surrounding the nerve can be seen with positive contrast cisternography.[6] T2-weighted MR technique demonstrates CSF surrounding the optic nerves that, in some normal cases, may be quite prominent (Fig. 14.8). The intracanalicular portion of the nerve measures 4–9 mm in diameter.[9] The optic nerve undulates slightly along its course and is subject to partial volume averaging by both CT and MR. Fat-nerve MR chemical shift misregistration artifact can cause erroneous optic nerve lateral margin signals.[2,4,5,11]

OPHTHALMIC ARTERY

The ophthalmic artery accompanies the optic nerve into the optic canal where it is initially caudal and lateral to the nerve. It then turns cranial and courses medial to the nerve. After it emerges from the canal, it has a characteristic appearance on axial CT and MR scans. Intravenous contrast enhancement improves its CT detail.[5]

SUPERIOR OPHTHALMIC VEIN

The superior ophthalmic vein is the most prominent orbital blood vessel virtually always seen on scans. It has a lateral diagonal intraconal course under the superior rectus muscle from the anterome-

dial orbit past the orbital apex to exit through the superior orbital fissure. Its characteristic appearance is easily detected on axial CT and MR scans and its location beneath the superior rectus muscle makes it easy to detect in all orthogonal views.[5,11] Intravenous contrast improves its detail for CT.

RETROBULBAR TISSUE

The large amount of retrobulbar intra- and extraconal fat (−65 to −100 H) provides excellent CT structural contrast. It also provides excellent MR structural contrast but is responsible for chemical shift artifacts. Fat suppression techniques help correct this source of error.[12,13]

Pathological Orbital Conditions

Pathological orbital conditions have been divided into the following categories: congenital and childhood abnormalities; tumors, inflammatory conditions; trauma, and other ocular and optic nerve conditions that do not fit well into an etiological classification.

CONGENITAL AND CHILDHOOD ORBITAL CONDITIONS

Congenital and childhood orbital abnormalities will be discussed according to the regional focus of the abnormality. The three main categories are abnormalities of the orbit, abnormalities of the globe, and abnormalities of the optic nerve.

Abnormalities of the Osseous Orbit

Orbital abnormalities include a very large number of rare anomalies that may involve hypotelorism (abnormally small interorbital distance) and hypertelorism (abnormally large interorbital distance). Measurement of normal distance and lists of abnormal conditions have been described[14,15] but only a few of these conditions will be described. Hypotelorism is usually seen in conjunction with ethmoid hypoplasia. Holoprosencephaly is often associated with severe facial dysmorphism and hypotelorism, the most extreme example being cyclopia. A much greater number of congenital anomalies occur together with hypertelorism. Included in this group are anomalies featuring premature sutural synostosis such as Apert's syndrome (acrocephalosyndactyly), Crouzon's syndrome [craniofacial dysostosis (Fig. 13.25)], cleft lip, and facial cleft abnormalities.[14,16] Small or large orbits are often the result of abnormally small (microphthalmos) and large globes. Neurofibromatosis can be associated with orbital enlargement for several reasons that include osseous dysplasia, buphthalmos, plexiform neurofibroma, and other orbital neoplasms. Sphenoid osseous dysplasia associated with neurofibromatosis can be associated with an orbital encephalocele.[16,17]

Abnormalities of the Globe

A wide spectrum of globe abnormalities ranging in severity from anophthalmos (absent eye) and cyclopia to coloboma and buphthalmos occur.

Ocular colobomas and associated orbital cysts are

relatively common malformations that result from lack of fusion of the fetal optic fissure with resultant retina, choroid, and sclera deformity. The lack of fusion typically results in a characteristic posterior globe conical deformity, notch, or cyst and is frequently associated with microphthalmos (Fig. 14.9A).[18,19] The notch or cyst may extend into the optic nerve. The cyst may be quite large. They are bilateral in approximately 60% of cases. Colobomas may occur in any portion of the globe including the iris and lens.[18,19] Other microphthalmic disorders may be associated with anomalies of the digits, teeth, and palate.[19]

Posterior staphylomas occur in the adult but are included here because they have an imaging appearance resembling colobomas. Staphylomas are associated with highly myopic eyes that are characterized by an increased AP diameter. This abnormality is associated with CT detectable posterior ocular scleral-uveal rim thinning and bulging at the involved site. Retinal detachment is a common occurrence with this condition (Fig. 14.9B–C).[20]

Buphthalmos (congenital glaucoma) is a hereditary disorder of the anterior ocular chamber drainage system resulting in increased tension and enlargement of the immature globe. Orbital enlargement detectable by both CT and MR may occur with a characteristically increased anteroposterior orbital diameter.[14,19]

Another cause for an enlarged globe is plexiform neurofibromatosis that may be manifest at birth (severe form) or adolescence. These lesions are not encapsulated and grow along the nerve of origin. There may be involvement of the choroid, sclera, posterior ciliary nerves, and small intraconal nerves. CT abnormalities include orbital enlargement, periorbital and eyelid soft tissue swelling, extensive orbital soft tissue infiltration, and buphthalmos (Fig. 14.10). Uveal and scleral thickening associated with this form of buphthalmos is common.[17] An enlarged globe in all dimensions without glaucoma characterizes macrophthalmos.[19] MR usually demonstrates T1 hypointensity and T2 hyperintensity.[9]

Persistent hyperplastic primary vitreous (PHPV)

results from unilateral or bilateral failure of regression of the ocular primary vitreous.[21] PHPV is important, not only as a cause of blindness but as the third most common cause of childhood leukoria (white or off-white pupillary light reflex).[21] As such, it must be differentiated from retinoblastoma.[22] CT findings of PHPV include vitreous body hyperdensity, retrolental soft tissue along the hyaloid (Cloquet) canal, microphthalmos, vitreous layered blood, and vitreous soft tissue contrast enhancement. Lateral decubitus scanning will confirm the layering of hemorrhage that emanates from the very vascular primitive vitreous tissue. Unlike retinoblastoma, there is no calcification and there is associated microphthalmos.[21]

Coats' disease is another cause of leukoria. It is a primary vascular retinal anomaly characterized by telangiectasis. The telangiectatic vessels leak lipoproteinaceous exudate into the subretinal space resulting in massive retinal detachment.[23] Like primary hyperplastic primary vitreous, it lacks calcium and is associated with microphthalmos. CT demonstrates a small globe, hyperdense subretinal exudate, and lack of calcification.[23]

Abnormalities of the Optic Nerve

Septo-optic dysplasia (deMorsier's syndrome) includes optic disk and nerve hypoplasia associated with absence of the septum pellucidum, pointing of the inferior frontal horns of the lateral ventricles, flattening of the frontal horn roofs, and growth retardation (Fig. 14.11).[24] Optic nerve hypoplasia may also occur in other conditions including lobar and alobar holoprosencephaly.

TUMORS

The two principal optic nerve tumors, optic nerve glioma and optic nerve meningioma, are discussed separately here along with metastasis to the optic nerve. Other orbital tumors conveniently fit into an histological classification. It will be seen that, although MR has orbital imaging advantages that have already been discussed, the CT detection of calcium

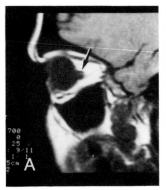
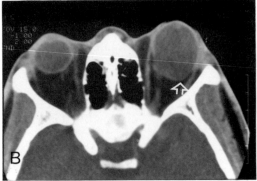
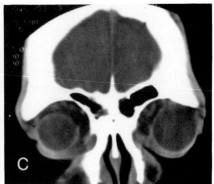

Figure 14.9. Ocular coloboma and staphyloma. Figures A and B-C are different cases. First case: ocular coloboma sagittal SE 700/25 MR scan. There is a vitreous-filled "notch" extending into the optic nerve *(closed arrow)*. Second case: Staphyloma. Axial **(B)** 57/550 and direct coronal **(C)** 83/550 CT scan. Note the sagittally elongated left globe with posterolateral scleral thinning *(open arrow)* and proptosis.

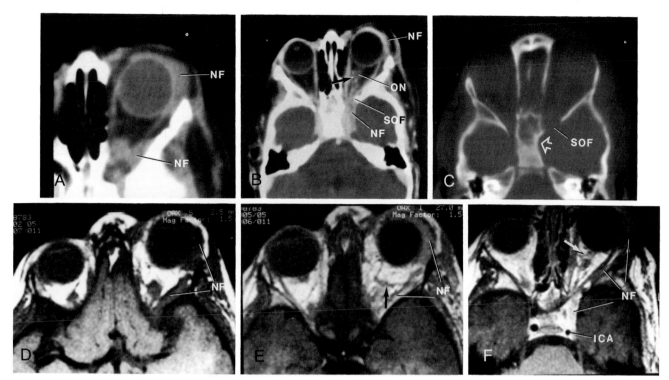

Figure 14.10. Plexiform neurofibroma buphthalmos and sphenoid dysplasia. Two-year-old neurofibromatosis patient. Same patient as shown in Figures 6.21 and 9.20. *Axial noncontrast (A) and i.v. contrast (B) 50/350 and 342/1712 (C) CT scans. Axial noncontrast (D) and i.v. contrast (E and F) SE 600/25 MR scans.* There is a lateral left orbital preseptal and postseptal extraconal mass *(NF)* that displaces the globe and the lateral rectus muscle. It is CT muscle-isodense, MR T1 muscle-isointense/T2 muscle-slightly hyperintense and .it moderately con trast enhances by both CT and MR tech-

niques. In addition to the plexiform neurofibroma, this patient has an enlarged left globe (buphthalmos), an enlarged superior orbital fissure *(SOF)*, a stenosed or atretic left internal carotid artery *(ICA)*, and many abnormally enlarged small signal-void orbital blood vessels *(closed arrows)*. The mass appears interposed between the medial wall of the cavernous sinus and the sphenoid bone. There is no evidence for tumor encasement of the left internal carotid artery. Note the inward curve of the left sphenoid medial cavernous sinus wall *(open arrow)*.

in retinoblastoma, bone erosion in dermoids, and bone destruction in metastasis represents at least a limited advantage of the older method. The CT method of orbital tumor investigation remains credible with a greater than 95% detection rate of surgically proven orbital tumors.[11] Major reasons to favor MR, however, are lack of harmful radiation effects and artifact-free images in other than the axial plane. The CT and MR differential diagnosis of orbital lesions will, for the most part, be discussed in gamut form at the end of this chapter.

Optic Nerve Tumors

Enlargement of the optic nerve is usually caused by neoplasms. The types of enlargements are tubular (most common), fusiform, and excrescent.[25] The most common tumors of the optic nerve are optic gliomas and optic nerve sheath meningiomas. Because optic nerve involvement by either glioma or meningioma could be the orbital manifestation of an intracranial process, it is necessary to obtain images of sufficient quality to exclude extraorbital involvement. This is a major reason why surface coil imaging (lacking depth) alone is not sufficient for a complete study.

Optic Nerve Glioma. An optic nerve glioma is a common childhood neoplasm that usually presents in

the first decade of life but it may occur at any age. There is an increased incidence, particularly with bilateral lesions, in patients with neurofibromatosis.[26,27] They are usually low grade gliomas. They may produce tubular, fusiform, or excrescent tumors. There is considerable variation in tumor extent. These tumors may involve the optic nerves, optic chiasm, optic tracts, lateral geniculate bodies, and even the optic radiations. In some cases, the tumor is confined to the retrochiasmal structures sparing the optic nerves. Bulky intraorbital tumors cause proptosis. CT demonstrates a homogeneous isodense usually noncalcified minimally contrast-enhancing mass. There is usually lack of clear distinction between tumor and nerve (Fig. 14.12). The optic canal is usually enlarged.[11,25–28] Optic gliomas have been reported to have T1 and T2 intensities approximating gray matter.[9] Figure 14.12 demonstrates T1 gray matter-isointensity and T2 hyperintensity. A large series of MR cases will be necessary to draw conclusions concerning MR characteristics of optic nerve gliomas.

Meningiomas of the Optic Nerve. True meningiomas of the optic nerve (1–2% of intracranial meningiomas) are far less common than greater sphenoid wing meningiomas (15% of intracranial meningiomas).[11] Approximately one-third of greater sphenoid wing meningiomas involve the orbit. Ap-

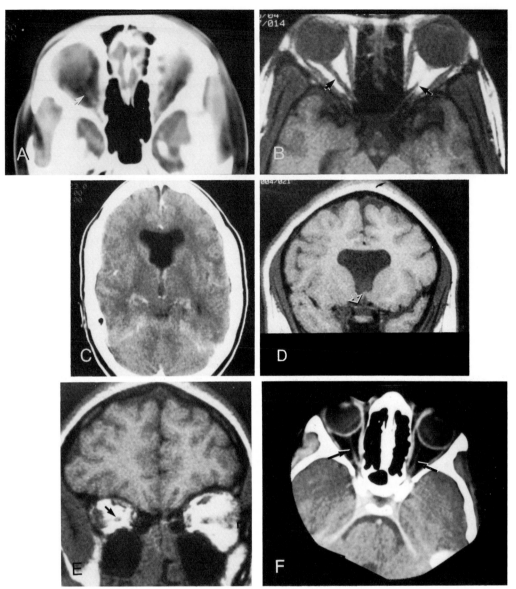

Figure 14.11. Septo-optic dysplasia. De Morsier's syndrome. A–E and **F** are different cases. *Axial SOM plane 32/400 10-mm thickness CT scan* **(A)** *and IOM SE 600/25 3-mm thickness MR scan* **(B)**. *Frontal horn-level axial SOM plane 36/100 i.v. contrast CT scan* **(C)** *and coronal SE 600/25 head coil 18-cm FOV MR scans* **(D and E)**. Another case (same case as Fig. 9.10). *Axial IOM i.v. contrast CT scan* **(F)**. Case 1 **(A–E):** Bilateral optic nerve dysgenesis *(closed arrows)* is best demonstrated by coronal MR **(E)** where comparison to rectus muscle size is dramatic. There is also optic chiasm—dysgenesis *(open arrow)*. There is axial CT and coronal MR evidence for agenesis of the septum pellucidum. Case 2 **(F):** Same case as Figure 9.10. There is marked hypoplasia of the optic nerves *(arrows)*.

proximately 5% of primary orbital tumors and 33% of primary tumors of the optic nerve or sheath are meningiomas.[9] Meningiomas arising within the orbit, however, are almost always optic nerve meningiomas.[27] The radiologist must make every effort to exclude extraorbital involvement in order to make the diagnosis of true meningioma of the optic nerve sheath (see Chapter 5). True optic nerve sheath meningiomas most commonly present in middle-aged patients. There is a female predominance (80%).[9] If seen in the third decade or younger, the patient usually has neurofibromatosis. It usually is tubular in form

around the optic nerve and does not usually extend to the optic foramen. It may present as a bulky perineural mass and may be eccentric in its relationship to the nerve.[25] If it does extend beyond the optic canal, however, foraminal hyperostosis often occurs (Fig. 14.13).[9,27]

The CT demonstration of bone involvement is better than MR. CT shows hyperdensity, usually homogeneous marked contrast enhancement and, frequently, calcification.[27] The pattern of i.v. contrast enhancement of optic nerve sheath meningiomas may be very specific. Immediately adjacent to the optic

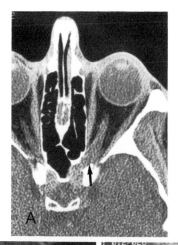

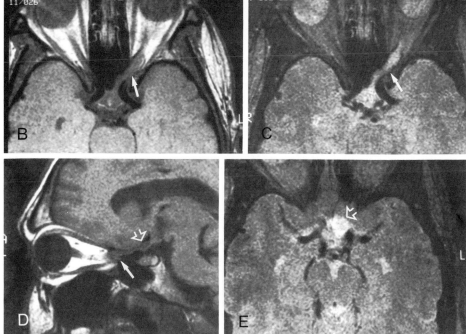

Figure 14.12.   Optic nerve glioma. *Axial 1.5-mm IOM bone filter i.v. contrast injection 100/550 CT scan **(A).** Same plane head coil SE 2000/20 **(B)** and SE 2000/80 **(C)** 5-mm thickness MR scans. Sagittal SE 600/25 MR scan in the plane of the optic nerve **(D).** Axial SE 2000/80 chiasmatic cistern-level MR scan **(E)**. A slightly contrast-* enhanced diffusely swollen optic nerve and enlarged optic canal *(arrow)* are seen by CT. It is T1 hypointense and T2 hyperintense compared to fat. The optic chiasm *(open arrow)* is involved with tumor and is equally T1 hypointense/T2 hyperintense.

nerve there may be marked parallel linear enhancement surrounded by the less markedly enhanced tumor mass. Thus, the noncontrast-enhanced nerve may be outlined by a thin, markedly enhanced rim and then by the less markedly enhanced, thicker perineural mass.[28] This pattern can be seen on both axial and coronal sections. Many lesions demonstrate the nerve within a tumor mass (the so-called "tram-track sign"), however, the thin linear band of bright enhancement adjacent to the nerve appears specific for meningioma (Fig. 14.14).[28]

Our initial MR experience with optic nerve meningiomas is similar to that of other meningiomas with tumor optic nerve-isointensity to both T1 and T2 technique (Fig. 14.14). MR i.v. contrast agents using fat suppression technique may play a significant role in the investigation of this tumor. The advantages of MR over CT for investigation of optic nerve tumors include direct identification of the optic nerve in orthogonal planes, more accurate demonstration of intracanalicular involvement free of bone-induced artifacts and more accurate identification of the optic chiasm and visual pathways.[29] CT, however, may be more specific due to identification of calcification and the specific perineural contrast-enhancement pattern. Both MR and i.v. contrast CT can distinguish

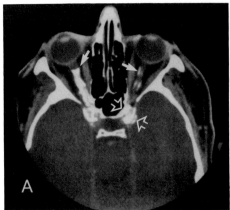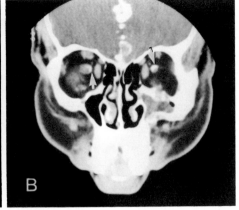

Figure 14.13. Optic nerve sheath meningioma—tubular type. *Axial (A) and direct coronal (B) i.v. contrast 50/400 3-mm thickness CT scans.* There is marked partially eccentric bilateral perineural calcification *(closed arrows).* There is only slight detectable contrast en-hancement of already calcified portions. The tumors extend into the optic canals and there is hyperostotic canal narrowing and adjacent dural-tumoral calcification *(open arrows)* (compare to Fig. 14.1).

nerve sheath lesions from intrinsic optic nerve lesions by presence or absence or the intact optic nerve within or adjacent to the mass.[9]

Subarachnoid Spread. The subarachnoid spread of tumor, may involve the optic tracts, chiasm, and nerves. MR i.v. contrast technique is the method of choice (Fig. 14.15).

Malignant Orbital Tumors (Childhood)

The three most common malignant orbital tumors (excluding optic nerve glioma) of childhood are retinoblastoma, rhabdomyosarcoma, and neuroblastoma.[11,26]

Retinoblastoma. Retinoblastoma is the most common intraocular malignant lesion of infancy and

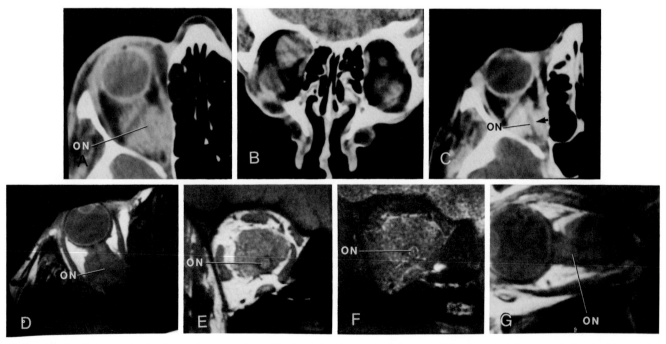

Figure 14.14. Optic nerve sheath meningioma. *Noncontrast axial (A) and coronal (B) 30/400 CT scans. Axial i.v. contrast same level CT scan (C) and SE 700/25 surface coil MR scan (D). Coronal SE 2000/25 (E) and 2000/100 (F) surface coil MR scans. Sagittal SE 700/25 MR scan (G).* An eccentric fusiform mass surrounds the optic nerve *(ON).* It extends posteriorly into the orbital apex but does not extend into the optic canal. It is noncalcified, CT muscle-isodense, markedly contrast enhancing, and demonstrates the surrounded optic nerve with a barely perceptible perineural band of increased en-hancement *(arrow).* MR characteristics are similar to intracranial meningiomas. The tumor is MR T1 fat-hypointense and T2 fat-isointense. The optic nerve and its tumor interface is well identified by MR. From 4 o'clock to 7 o'clock, only a thin sheath of tumor en-compasses the nerve. Note the loss of orbital structural differentiation in **F** due to T2 signal-isointensities. Optic canal involvement would be better studied by head coil rather than by surface coil technique due to signal drop-off of deeper structures.

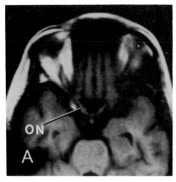
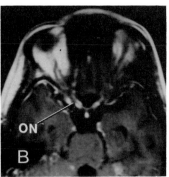
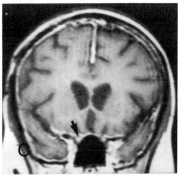

Figure 14.15.   Optic nerve sheath metastasis. Glioblastoma subarachnoid deposits. *Axial SE 600/25 noncontrast **(A)** and i.v. gadolinium-DTPA **(B)** and coronal i.v. contrast **(C)** MR scans.* Diffuse contrast-enhancing subarachnoid tumor deposits include those surrounding the optic nerve *(ON)* producing a "tramtrack" sign. Contrast-enhancing tumor is seen within the optic nerve canal on coronal section *(arrow).* Thinner sections and smaller FOV would have yielded more detail of the optic nerves and chiasm.

childhood. It occurs in one or both retinas with an incidence of approximately one in 20,000 live births. The presenting clinical findings include leukoria, strabismus, poor vision, and orbital inflammation. The vast majority of cases (90%) occur de novo. It is also inherited as an autosomal dominant of high penetrance. The offspring of a victim with a family history of retinoblastoma or with bilateral lesions has a 50% chance of having the disease. The offspring of a victim without a family history with unilateral reinoblastoma has a 10–15% chance of having the disease.[27,30] The lesions are bilateral in approximately 30% of cases.[9,30]

These retinal tumors are usually entirely intraocular at time of discovery. They can, however, perforate the sclera. Orbital soft tissue and intracranial extension along the optic nerve may occur. Treatment includes enucleation and/or radiation.[27] The most important role of CT or MR in the investigation of retinoblastoma is to search for contralateral disease and extraocular spread of tumor in order to plan the therapeutic approach.

CT demonstrates single or bilateral posterior smoothly contoured, calcified, hyperdense, intraocular contrast-enhancing masses (Fig. 14.16).[11,27,31,32] The MR signal of retinoblastoma may vary according to the amount of calcification and hemorrhage. Hemorrhage within the tumor or associated intraocular hemorrhage may demonstrate appropriate T1- and T2-weighted signal intensities. Those lesions without hemorrhage are likely to be T1 optic nerve-isointense.[32] Both CT and MR can accurately detect extraocular extension. CT is the better method for characterizing the intraocular mass (calcification) and MR is superior for visualization of extraocular extension.[9]

Rhabdomyosarcoma. Intraorbital rhabdomyosarcoma is an uncommon highly malignant extraocular muscle tumor of childhood. It is more common in boys who may present with rapidly progressive exophthalmos, subconjunctival mass, chemosis, or lid nodules. It may invade the periorbital soft tissues, paranasal sinuses, nasopharynx, and brain.[27,31]

CT demonstrates a retrobulbar noncalcified contrast-enhancing mass often with bone destruction and proptosis.[27,31] There is often preseptal involvement.[26]

Neuroblastoma. Intraorbital metastasis is relatively common in patients with neuroblastoma. Intracranial and facial tumor extension is common and preseptal extension is rare. CT, as described in a small series, demonstrates a hyperdense, often partially calcified, contrast-enhancing orbital mass highly invasive of neighboring structures with permeative osteolysis.[26] Because of the common calcification and characteristic osteolysis, CT has some theoretical advantages over MR for tumor characterization. MR has greater soft tissue discrimination, however.

Malignant Orbital Tumors (Adult)

Malignant orbital tumors of the adult may be classified as primary and secondary. The secondary group includes local invasive as well as distant metastatic. Most primary and metastatic ocular neoplasms involve the choroid.[33]

Malignant Uveal Melanoma. The most common primary intraocular malignancy in white adults is malignant uveal melanoma. The tumor is unusual in blacks. The white:black ratio is 15:1.[33] These lesions and retinoblastoma are easily diagnosed by ophthalmoscopy. The malignant uveal melanoma is almost always a unilateral lesion that commonly presents with loss of visual acuity and may have as-

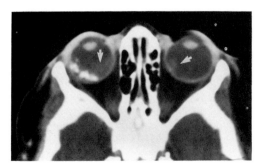

Figure 14.16.   Retinoblastoma—bilateral. *Axial noncontrast 60/400 orbital CT scan.* There is extensive calcification of the right globe tumor. Bilateral noncalcified portions are also present *(arrows).*

sociated glaucoma, retinal destruction, and vitreous hemorrhage.[27] Intraorbital extraocular melanomas are rare and are usually metastatic deposits or local extension from facial or ocular melanomas.[27]

CT demonstrates an intraocular slightly hyperdense sharply marginated moderately contrast-enhancing mass within the globe involving any portion of the uvea (Fig. 14.17). Associated retinal detachment is common and the subretinal exudate may have a moderately high density, which is difficult to distinguish from tumor by the noncontrast CT technique. Tumor contrast enhancement is helpful for this distinction.[9,33,34]

The MR detection specificity for melanin (high T1/low T2 signal intensity) is virtually diagnostic for choroidal melanoma, however, hemorrhagic tumors and subretinal hemorrhages that contain intracellular methemoglobin may be mistaken by MR for melanoma due to signal similarity. These tumors commonly lack melanin signal and the absence of the characteristic T1 hyperintense and T2 hypointense signal is not evidence against the diagnosis.[34,35]

Lymphoma. Seventy-five percent of patients with orbital lymphoma either have the systemic disease or will develop it. Reactive lymphoid hyperplasia and well-differentiated lymphocytic lymphoma have a similar histological appearance and clinical presentation. They both tend to occur in the elderly as proptosis or a palpable mass. They are extraocular and most often occur in the anterior orbit, the retrobulbar region, or superior orbital compartment. They usually do not destroy or erode bone or enlarge the orbits.[27] There is often associated periorbital edema.[35]

CT of orbital lymphoma demonstrates a moderately high density, moderately contrast-enhancing mass without bone destruction or erosion, which is often irregularly marginated in the locations already mentioned (Fig. 14.18).[31]

MR of orbital lymphoma may demonstrate T1 optic nerve and T2 fat-isointense characteristics.[9]

Sinus Carcinoma. Orbital extension of paranasal sinus carcinoma usually invades the orbit by bone destruction. Most are squamous cell carcinomas. CT demonstrates contiguous orbital bone destruction and orbital tumor invasion (Figs. 13.44 and 13.45). There is usually a moderate degree of contrast enhancement. MR has the advantage of superior soft tissue resolution and true direct orthogonal plane imaging. CT detects bone erosion and destruction. Both methods do a credible job defining these lesions.

Metastatic Carcinoma. Lung and breast metastatic carcinomas are the most common primary cancers metastasizing to the orbit. Gastrointestinal, genitourinary, and thyroid origins are also common. The anterior superior orbit and the orbital apex are common sites of metastasis. In the pediatric population, neuroblastoma, Ewing's sarcoma, and Wilms' tumor are the most common origin. Leukemic chloroma is also a common cause in children. Symptoms include the sudden onset of pain, swelling, and diplopia.[27]

CT demonstrates metastatic tumor that may involve any orbital structure (Fig. 14.19). It often demonstrates bone destruction associated with a contrast-enhancing mass. Ocular metastases may occur, most often to the choroid. The intraocular metastasis lacks melanin signal.

Angiomas, Varices, and Vascular Malformations

This group of orbital vascular lesions includes cavernous hemangioma, capillary hemangioma, lymphangioma, venous varix, and dural arteriovenous malformations.

Cavernous Hemangioma. Cavernous heman-

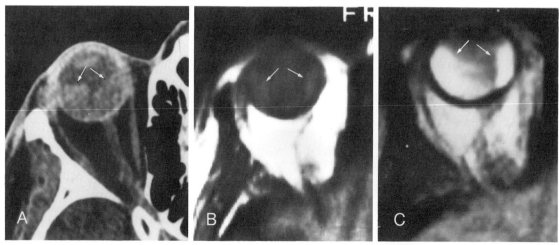

Figure 14.17. Uveal melanoma. *Axial i.v. contrast 60/300 CT scan (A) and SE 500/17 (B) and 2500/35 (C) MR scans.* There is slight CT contrast enhancement of fat-T1 hypointense/T2 hyperintense uveal mass *(arrows).* There is absence of melanin signal and there is no evidence of hemorrhage. (Courtesy of Solomon Batnitzky, M.D., Kansas City, Kansas.)

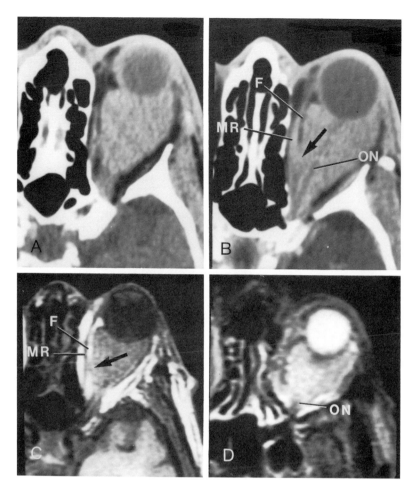

Figure 14.18. Orbital lymphoma. *Axial 21/300 non-contrast* **(A)** *and i.v. contrast* **(B)** *CT scans and same level 600/25 3-mm thickness* **(C)** *and 2000/80* **(D)** *MR scans. A large, mostly intraconal mass slightly and uniformly contrast enhances demonstrating the encased optic nerve (ON) "tramtrack sign." A portion of the mass (arrow) effaces the fat margin between the medial rectus (MR) and thin strip of remaining intraconal fat (F). MR identifies the optic nerve at the orbital apex. The mass is fat-T1 hypointense/T2 isointense.*

gioma is the most common benign orbital neoplasm. It has a predilection for middle-aged females and may occur anywhere in the orbit. It is slow growing and, most commonly, is retrobulbar and produces proptosis.

CT usually demonstrates a smoothly marginated intraconal homogeneous high-density mass with marked contrast enhancement. Occasionally, pheboliths are found; however, the lesions are usually not calcified. There is frequent sparing of the orbital apex.[11,31] It is usually found lateral to the optic nerve (Fig. 14.20).[27]

MR usually demonstrates fat-T1 hypointensity and T2 hyperintensity.[9,11] MR vascular flow effects may predominate, resulting in a degree of unpredictability with respect to the T2-weighted signal.[11]

Capillary Hemangiomas. Orbital capillary hemangiomas are tumors of early childhood that grow for less than 1 year and then involute. They clinically appear as a "strawberry nevus" preseptally on

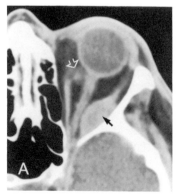
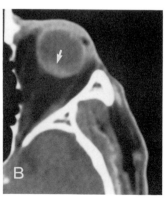

Figure 14.19. Orbital metastatic tumor. **A** and **B** are different cases. **A:** Orbital lung carcinoma metastasis. *Axial 50/100 i.v. contrast CT scan. The lateral rectus muscle (closed arrow) is infiltrated with tumor and diffusely enlarged with peripheral contrast enhancement surrounding an irregular central isodense portion. Another smaller metastasis is interposed between the medial rectus muscle, the optic nerve, and the globe (open arrow).* **B:** Ocular breast carcinoma metastasis. *Axial i.v. contrast 100/450 CT scan. There is a contrast-enhanced choroidal mass (closed arrow).*

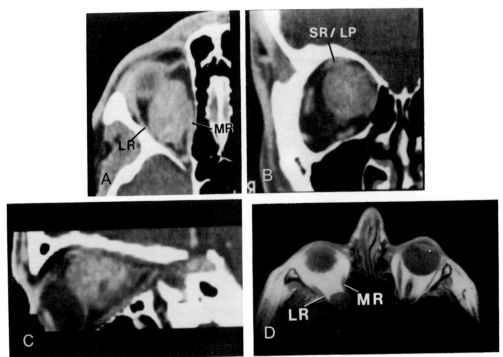

Figure 14.20. Orbital cavernous hemangioma. **A–C** and **D** are different cases. Case 1: *Axial 31/550 16-cm FOV 1.5-mm thickness (A), direct coronal 31/400 13-cm FOV 3-mm thickness (B), and* parasagittal reformation of 1.5-mm images parallel to the optic nerve **(C)** i.v. contrast CT scans. Case 2: Axial heavily T1-weighted MR scan **(D).** A sharply marginated intraconal mass displaces the medial *(MR)* and lateral *(LR)* rectus muscles. The larger first case shows homogeneous moderate degree contrast enhancement and displacement upward of the superior rectus/levator palpebrae *(SR/LP)* muscles. The second case demonstrates hemangioma T1 optic nerve-isointensity. (Courtesy of Richard R. Smith, M.D., Indianapolis, IN.)

an eyelid or they occur in the retrobulbar space and produce proptosis. CT demonstrates a well-marginated contrast-enhancing usually extraconal masses. Progress scans demonstrate regression.[27]

Lymphangioma. Orbital lymphangiomas occur in children and young adults. They are composed of lymphoid follicles and channels. Unlike capillary hemangiomas, they tend to increase in size. They tend to be infiltrative, lack a capsule, and may be intraconal or extraconal. There is a tendency to hemorrhage. CT characteristically demonstrates a heterogeneous mixed attenuation ill-defined intraconal or extraconal mass. They may minimally contrast enhance. When intraconal, they are usually medial to the optic nerve. MR demonstrates T1 fat-isointensity or hypointensity and T2 fat-hyperintensity.[9,27]

Venous Varix. An orbital venous varix is a congenital malformation that presents in childhood or early adulthood and becomes increasingly symptomatic with age. Intermittent proptosis and pain are the common presenting complaints. Symptoms commonly occur upon waking after the patient has been recumbent for a long period.[27]

CT demonstrates a sharply marginated, intraconal, possibly lobulated hyperdense mass that markedly contrast enhances and markedly enlarges with the Valsalva maneuver or with jugular venous compression.[27,36] MR demonstration of flow effects and orthogonal (particularly sagittal) imaging is very ef-

fective. Thrombosis of a varix can be documented; however, careful attention to chemical shift artifact is necessary to avoid misinterpreting erroneous signals suggesting flow phenomenon.[4]

Dural AVM Orbital dural AVMs presumably develop in a previously thrombosed cavernous sinus. Enlargement of the superior ophthalmic vein and uniform enlargement of the extraocular muscles and the presence of abnormal enlarged blood vessels are characteristic (Fig. 14.21) resembling a carotid-cavernous fistula.[9]

Other Tumors

Meningiomas. Meningiomas other than optic nerve meningiomas commonly involve the orbit. These are usually sphenoid wing meningiomas principally involving the middle fossa.

CT characteristics include sphenoid greater and lesser wing hyperplasia and hyperostosis. The tumor is smoothly marginated, hyperdense, calcified, and homogeneous contrast enhancing. There is usually middle fossa and often orbital involvement (Fig. 14.22). MR characteristics include gray matter-T1 and T2 isointensity. Extensively calcified tumors are more T1 and T2 hypointense. Without i.v. contrast, the intracranial portion may be difficult to detect by MR (Fig. 14.22**D**). CT is far superior to MR for bone detail. MR demonstrates superior orbital soft tissue de-

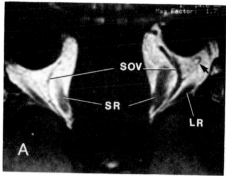
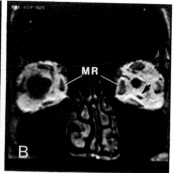

Figure 14.21. Dural AVM. *Axial superior orbital-level **(A)** and coronal **(B)** SE 600/25 3-mm thickness MR scans. The left superior ophthalmic vein (SOV) is markedly enlarged. The left extraocular muscles (SR, MR, and LR) are uniformly moderately enlarged. The* muscular enlargement is limited to the muscle "belly" and not the tendonous insertions *(LR).* Multiple enlarged abnormal blood vessels are seen throughout the left retrobulbar fat *(arrows).*

tail as seen in Figure 14.22**D.** MR i.v. contrast is often necessary for accurate demonstration of the intracranial portion, however, it may mask the intraorbital tumor-fat interface.[9,27]

Neurofibroma. A neurofibroma can occur anywhere in the orbit. CT demonstrates isodense or hyperdense, usually sharply marginated, moderately contrast-enhancing, round or oval masses. Plexiform neurofibromas involving the orbital apex can be easily confused with optic gliomas and meningiomas.

Sphenoid dysplasia[9,11,27] and, occasionally, macrophthalmos occur with neurofibromatosis (Fig. 14.10).[9] In patients with neurofibromatosis, as already explained, an intraorbital tumor is more likely to be a meningioma or optic glioma than a neurofibroma.[11] MR demonstrates fat-T1 hypointensity/T2 hyperintensity similar to that for neurofibromas in other locations.[9,11]

Dermoid. Orbital dermoid tumors present differently in children and adults. In young children, they

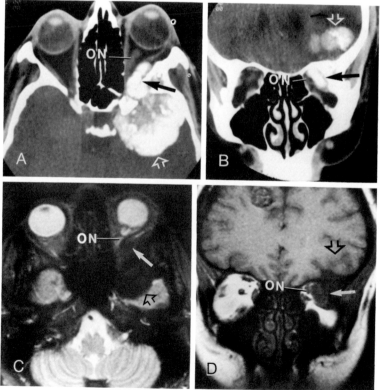

Figure 14.22. Sphenoid wing meningioma invading orbit. *Axial **(A)** and direct coronal **(B)** noncontrast CT scans and analogous axial SE 2000/80 **(C)** and coronal 600/25 **(D)** noncontrast MR scans. Two major calcified tumor components are seen on either side of the thickened hyperostotic sphenoid bone. The larger, intracranial com-*ponent *(open arrows)* displaces the temporal lobe and the smaller intraorbital portion *(closed arrow)* displaces the optic nerve *(ON)* and lateral rectus muscle. Bone detail is far superior by CT. The MR coronal soft tissue detail is superior to that shown by CT. Note the additional falx meningioma **(D).**

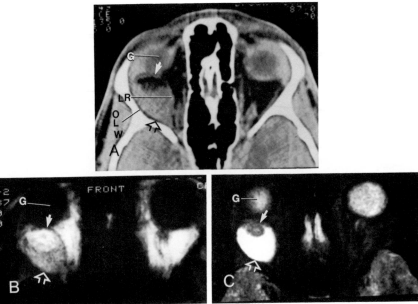

Figure 14.23. Orbital dermoid tumor. *Axial 82/600 CT scan* **(A).** *Axial SE 500/17* **(B)** *and 2500/120* **(C)** *MR scans.* There is an intraorbital extraconal mass behind the globe *(G)* remodeling the orbital lateral wall *(OLW)* and medially displacing the lateral rectus muscle *(LR)*. It contains fat signals anteriorly *(closed arrows)* and water signals posteriorly *(open arrows)*. (Courtesy of Solomon Batnitzky, M.D., Kansas City, KS.)

often present as small orbital rim superficial masses, usually superotemporal in the lacrimal fossa. They often have erosive or diploic expansile bone involvement. In older children and adults, the dermoid tumor may present as a deep orbital mass.[37]

CT demonstrates a low-density (often fat density), sharply marginated orbital extraconal mass often with osseous involvement. The associated bone involvement and fat density is virtually pathognomonic for dermoid (Fig. 14.23).[5,37] There is CT lack of contrast enhancement although the rim may enhance.[27] CT has an advantage over MR for diagnosis of dermoid due to CT bone detail. MR of fat-containing dermoid tumors demonstrates fat intensity characteristics and may demonstrate fat-fluid levels.[9]

Lacrimal Gland Tumors. Half of lacrimal gland tumors are epithelial in origin. The most common type is benign mixed adenoma. It carries an excellent prognosis, provided it is totally excised at first surgery. It is, therefore, very important to document its entire extent.[38] Adenocystic carcinoma and malignant mixed tumor follow in decreasing incidence. Dermoid tumors, as already discussed, arise from epithelial rests and are most often located in the lacrimal fossa.[11,27,38] The other 50% of lacrimal gland masses include idiopathic pseudotumor, dacryoadenitis, sarcoidosis, Sjögren's syndrome, leukemia, and lymphoma.[27,38]

CT of benign mixed tumors demonstrates a smooth, sharply marginated, hyperdense contrast-enhancing lacrimal fossa mass, often displacing the orbital contents and indenting the globe (Fig. 14.24). Malignant tumors are often invasive, irregularly margin-

ated, and destructive of bone.[11,27,38] Lacrimal gland involvement caused by systemic diseases is often bilateral. CT of inflammatory and lymphoid lesions demonstrates diffuse glandular enlargement with contrast enhancement.[38]

MR for lacrimal fossa masses defines soft tissue detail better than CT but cannot document bone invasion with equal accuracy. A large series of lacrimal gland masses will need to be studied in order to determine whether MR signal intensity patterns will be specific for different conditions and to establish the role of MR i.v. contrast.[4]

INFLAMMATORY AND INFILTRATIVE CONDITIONS

"Inflammatory and infiltrative orbital conditions" is a term used here to include a group of non-neoplastic conditions that can, at times, produce imaging characteristics that are hard to distinguish from neoplasms. The most common conditions, orbital pseudotumor, orbital infection, and Graves' orbitopathy will be discussed first.

Orbital Pseudotumor

Orbital pseudotumor is the most common cause of intraorbital mass in the adult.[9] It is, essentially, an exclusionary diagnosis characterized by idiopathic orbital inflammation caused by non-neoplastic, predominantly lymphocytic tissue infiltration. The pathological spectrum varies from diffuse orbital inflammation to inflammatory tumefaction. Exclusively focal areas may be involved such as the lacrimal gland (adenitis), sclera (scleritis), or a region of the muscle cone (myositis). Pseudotumor is almost

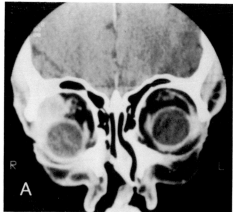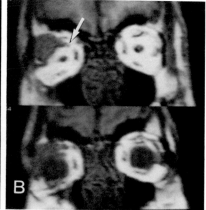

Figure 14.24. Lacrimal gland benign mixed cell tumor. Direct coronal i.v. contrast CT scan **(A)** and coronal T1-weighted MR scans **(B)**. There is a contrast-enhancing T1 muscle-isointense mass centered at the lacrimal fossa displacing the globe downward and extending into the intraconal fat *(arrow).* The lateral rectus muscle is not identifiable. (Courtesy of Richard R. Smith, M.D., Indianapolis, IN.)

always the cause of localized myositis—a rare condition. Uveal-scleral thickening is common. The onset of symptoms is usually rapid and includes pain, marked proptosis, soft tissue swelling, and impaired muscle motility.[39,40] It is usually highly sensitive to steroid therapy and the final diagnosis is often based on the steroid response.[5,9,11,27]

CT and MR characteristically demonstrate an ill-defined retrobulbar mass often associated with proptosis, enlargement of one or more extraocular muscles, scleral thickening, and thickening of the optic nerve sheath. Lacrimal gland infiltration commonly occurs. Preseptal infiltration is not uncommon.[11] The thickened optic nerve joining the thickened sclera has been called the "T-sign." Unfortunately, the T-sign can be seen with any infiltrative process and is not specific for pseudotumor.[5] There is often contrast enhancement of the inflammatory mass and of the thickened sclera and optic nerve (Fig. 14.25).[39] MR signal intensity of orbital pseudotumor is T1 fat-hypointense and T2 fat-isointense. This signal pattern is not specific for pseudotumor, however, and can be seen with Graves' orbitopathy, lymphoma, abscess, and sarcoidosis.[4,9,41]

Orbital Infection

This is usually secondary to adjacent sinus disease or to orbital foreign body. Forms of orbital infections include preseptal and postseptal cellulitis, myositis,

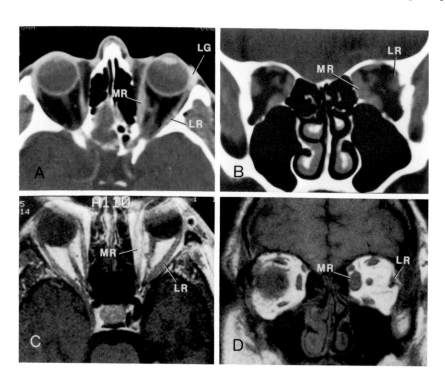

Figure 14.25. Orbital pseudotumor. *Intravenous contrast axial **(A)** and coronal **(B)** 16-cm FOV 60/450 CT scans. Intravenous contrast axial **(C)** and noncontrast coronal **(D)** SE 600/25 18 cm FOV MR scans.* There is moderate-to-marked left medial rectus *(MR)* thickening with moderate degree contrast enhancement. There is moderate degree lateral rectus *(LR)* thickening. A band of inflammatory tissue bridges the medial rectus and optic nerve on axial sections. The orbital apex is involved and muscular thickening is not confined only to the muscle belly. The *MR* muscle signal is optic nerve-isointense.

Figure 14.26. Orbital inflammation. **A–B** and **C–D** are different cases. Case 1: Orbital abscess. *Direct coronal 95/350 globe-level (A) and 600/4000 optic nerve-level (B) i.v. contrast CT scans.* A pre- and postseptal, intra- and extraconal multilocular *(closed arrows)* mass causes marked proptosis and chemosis. There is contrast enhancement surrounding the loculations. Mucosal thickening obstructs the ostiomeatal unit and there is opacity of ethmoid air cells and maxillary sinus mucosal thickening adjacent to the inferior orbit *(open arrow)*. Case 2: Orbital preseptal cellulitis. *Axial SE 600/25 (C) and 2800/80 (D) MR scans.* There is a T1 fat-hypointense/T2 fat-hyperintense eyelid-conjunctival mass *(closed arrows)* contained by the orbital septum *(open arrows)*. There is involvement of the left nasal tissues.

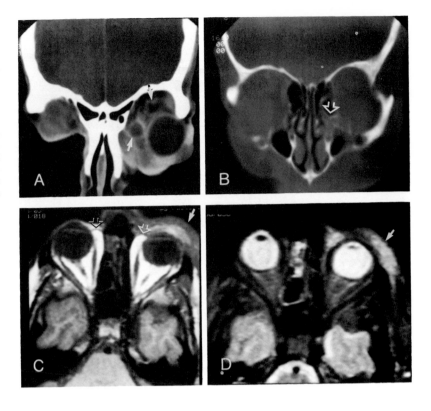

scleritis, endophthalmitis, and encapsulated abscess.[42,43]

CT, and probably MR, pre- and postseptal orbital findings can be similar to those of orbital pseudotumor. Evidence of adjacent sinusitis and orbital foreign bodies should be carefully excluded (Fig. 14.26).[9,43]

An unusual infection, ocular toxocariasis, is caused by visceral larva migrans. The ocular lesions of *Toxocara canis* occur months or years after the initial infection and after larval death as a result of inflammatory reaction. Ocular granuloma, choroidal lesions, and diffuse endophthalmitis with retinal detachment may occur. CT may demonstrate an ocular mass, retinal detachment, and intracranial disease.[44]

Graves' Orbitopathy

This condition is characterized by bilateral (90% of cases) proptosis caused by extraocular muscle lymphocytic infiltration and edema. It is often, although not always, associated with hyperthyroidism and treated hyperthyroidism and can be seen with Hashimoto's disease, hypothyroidism, and in euthyroid patients. Pain is usually not a typical feature of this condition.[9] There may be an increase in orbital fat content further aggravating the degree of proptosis.[9,45] Any or all muscles may be involved although the medial and inferior rectus muscles are most often affected. The muscular enlargement is often not uniform with some muscles far more affected than others. Individual muscular enlargement is maximum in the middle and the ends usually taper to a fine

point not involving the tendons ("spindle-like enlargement").[9]

CT demonstrates proptosis with sharply marginated, enlarged, slightly hyperdense extraocular muscles. There is usually homogeneous, moderate degree contrast enhancement (Fig. 14.27). Even slight muscle swelling at the orbital apex may obscure orbital apical detail mimicking other conditions such as orbital pseudotumor. More severe swelling may cause significant compression of the optic nerve at the apex ("dysthyroid optic neuropathy"). There is sparing of the retro-orbital fat and lack of involvement of the sclera. The optic nerve may appear enlarged.[11,31] Increased orbital fat and proptosis may also be found in Cushing's disease and in patients with generalized obesity without associated endocrinopathy.[45]

MR demonstrates T1 muscle-isointensity and T2 fat-isointensity of the involved muscles.[4,9,11] The typical CT evidence of muscle involvement and sparing of other tissues is also seen with MR. Both CT and MR appear equally accurate for diagnosis of this condition.

Sarcoid and Other Granulomatous Diseases

The eye is affected in approximately one-quarter of sarcoid patients and the optic nerve is involved in 1–5% of sarcoid patients. Sarcoidosis can affect the conjunctiva, uvea, cornea, sclera, retina, extraocular muscles, and lens. The lacrimal gland is commonly involved. Both CT[5,46] and MR[4] changes may be identical to those of pseudotumor. These changes include optic nerve and scleral thickening, the tramtrack sign,

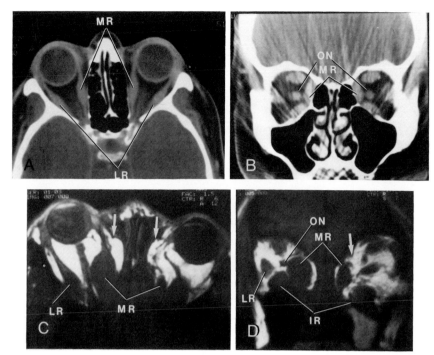

Figure 14.27. Graves' orbitopathy. A–B and **C–D** are different cases. *Axial 100/550* **(A)** *and direct coronal 75/550* **(B)** *i.v. contrast CT scans. Axial* **(C)** *and coronal* **(D)** *600/25 MR scans.* There is "spindle-type" extraocular muscle enlargement affecting the muscle bellies and sparing the tendon insertions. The normal optic nerves *(ON)* are surrounded by sharply marginated slightly contrast-en- hanced T1 optic nerve-isointense enlarged extraocular muscle bellies *(MR, LR, IR)*. There is bilateral proptosis. Bilateral ethmoidectomies *(arrows on* **C–D)** have been done for orbital decompression in the second case. Muscular enlargement is uniform in the first case **(A–B)** and asymmetrical in the second case **(C–D)**. (**C–D** courtesy of Benjamin B. Kuzma, M.D., Indianapolis, IN.)

muscular irregular thickening, and contrast-enhancing masses (Fig. 4.28).[4,5,9,46] Tuberculosis and Wegener's granulomatosis can also affect the orbit.[5] Wegener's orbital changes are often (if not usually) accompanied by adjacent sinus disease.[11]

TRAUMA

Complex facial fractures have already been discussed in Chapter 13. Orbital involvement associated with these fractures will be discussed in this section. This section also includes the effects of blunt force upon the orbital contents and orbital penetrating missiles and foreign bodies.

"Blow-out" Fractures

The orbital blow-out fracture occurs at the orbital floor or the medial wall with orbital fragment displacement into the maxillary or ethmoid sinus, respectively. This fracture is the result of the transmitted force of an object such as a fist to the orbital tissues with a resultant fracture relieving the increased orbital pressure. Severe orbital emphysema may develop. There may be an accompanying orbital rim fracture. Entrapment of muscle or orbital fat frequently results in an ocular motility problem. Endophthalmos due to protrusion of contents into sinuses, tissue entrapment holding back the globe, or posttraumatic atrophy may result. These factors must be taken into consideration when the image is interpreted because of their surgical importance.[47]

Although CT provides excellent images of blow-out fractures and associated orbital rim and soft tissue changes,[47,48] MR better demonstrates soft tissue detail and can identify entrapped muscles within the herniated tissue (Fig. 14.29).[49] What role each method will routinely play will have to be decided after clinical trials. Noncontrast CT, 3-mm axial and direct coronal small FOV sections with soft tissue filtration are routinely obtained. Image reformation with a series of very thin (1.5-mm) sections is less useful than the direct coronal images.[50] If direct coronal images cannot be obtained, however, we feel that it is necessary to resort to image reformation. MR technique includes T1-weighted, small FOV head coil images.[49] Although surface coils may be used, they are often (usually, in our experience) not necessary.

Orbital Fracture Fragments

The position and relationship of orbital fragments, particularly with complex fractures, is important surgical information. The role of 3-D CT reformation after the accumulation of contiguous thin (1.5-mm) sections can be useful for planning facial reconstruction surgery (Fig. 13.27). Thin-section, 3-mm thickness axial and direct coronal images, however, have a proven utility and is our standard technique. Identification of intraorbital bone fragments before sur-

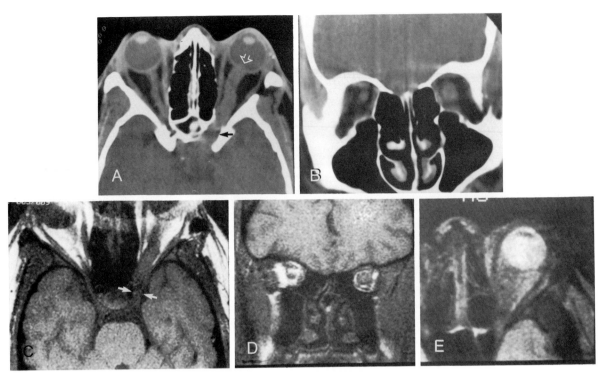

Figure 14.28. Optic nerve sarcoid. *Axial (A) and direct coronal (B) 100/500 noncontrast CT scans. Axial (C) and coronal (D) 600/25 MR scans. Axial 2000/80 MR scan (E).* Marked uniform thickening of the left optic nerve erodes the optic canal *(closed arrows).* There is papillary involvement *(open arrow).* The lesion is MR fat-T1 hypointense/ T2 isointense and the enlarged optic nerve cannot be identified on the T2-weighted image. Technical note: Wraparound artifact obscures orbital detail on the MR axial study due to the head coil and small FOV. The orbital apices are better seen, however, than they would be with surface coil imaging.

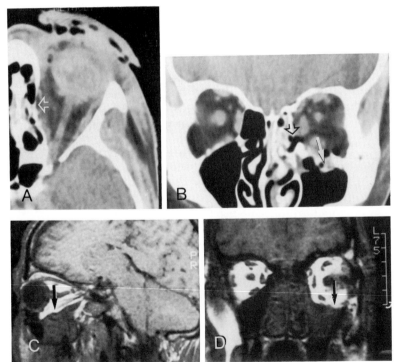

Figure 14.29. "Blow-out" fractures. *A–B* and *C–D* are different cases. *A–B: Noncontrast axial (A) and direct coronal (B) 19/450 CT scans.* There is a downward displacement, "downward blow-out," of the orbital floor fragment through which there is soft tissue herniation *(closed arrow).* There is also a lamina papyracea fracture, "medial blow-out" *(open arrows).* Orbital emphysema is well seen on the coronal image. The globe is ruptured, contains vitreous hemorrhage, and the eyelids are severely contused. This is an unusual case that is chosen because of the combined medial and inferior fracture components. The globe usually remains intact with blow-out fractures. *C–D: Sagittal (C) and coronal (D) SE 600/25 MR scans.* A downward blow-out fracture *(closed arrows)* is unaccompanied by muscular entrapment. There is blood in the fractured left maxillary sinus. Note: This scan was performed because the patient was unable to hyperextend for a direct coronal CT scan and coronal reformations were unsatisfactory.

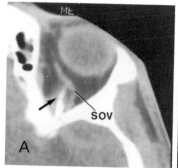
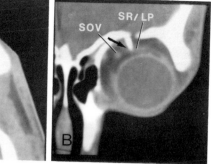

Figure 14.30. Intraorbital fracture fragment. *Axial **(A)** and direct coronal **(B)** 37/550 noncontrast CT scans.* An angular orbital roof fragment *(closed arrows)* projects downward abutting the superior rectus/levator palpebrae muscles *(SR/LP)* and displacing the midportion of the superior ophthalmic vein *(SOV).*

gical manipulation is important in order to prevent further soft tissue structural damage, particularly to the optic nerve, by a sharp fragment (Fig. 14.30).

Orbital Apex Fracture

The most significant clinical consideration of orbital apex fracture is optic nerve injury.[51] There is some controversy considering the effectiveness of decompressive surgery in the event of an optic canal fracture, however. Optic nerve injury does not have to be associated with a fracture.[52] Carotid-cavernous fistula not uncommonly is associated with orbital apex fracture. Very thin (1.5-mm) axial and coronal sections of the orbital apex using bone filter noncontrast CT technique has been recommended.[52] Because these fractures usually occur in association with severe facial injuries, we first review our routine (3-mm axial and coronal) sections and order appropriate additional sections if clinically necessary. Inasmuch as MR better identifies orbital apical soft tissues, it will likely prove to be a superior method for evaluating the integrity of the optic nerve and optic nerve canal and may provide clues of a carotid cavernous fistula due to MR flow effects.

Foreign Body

CT localization of opaque foreign bodies has been highly successful. An object such as glass or wood may not be detected if its attenuation is close to that of orbital soft tissues. Scan technique includes direct axial and coronal overlapping (to account for eye motion) 5-mm sections. Usually the axial and coronal images will determine if a peripheral foreign body is intra- or extraocular. If there is still confusion, scanning with the patient in a fixed lateral gaze should help.[31]

Retinal and Choroidal Detachment

Fluid or hemorrhage can collect beneath the retina and choroid under different clinical circumstances including trauma.[29,53,54] These topics will be discussed under "Other ocular conditions."

Vitreous Body Hemorrhage

Vitreous hemorrhage is commonly seen in diabetics, hypertensives, trauma victims, ocular tumor patients, and infants with persistent hyperplastic primary vitreous. Acute hemorrhage is diagnosed by CT (Fig. 14.29) and by MR.

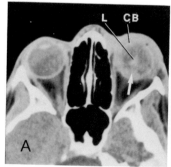
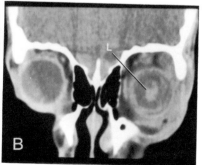

Figure 14.31. Dislocated lens and choroidal hematoma trauma. *Axial 56/400 3-mm thickness 15-cm FOV **(A)** and direct coronal 86/400 5-mm thickness 16-cm FOV **(B)** noncontrast CT scans.* The left lens *(L)* is posteriorly displaced and is seen in the center of the vitreous humor. A density that probably represents the ciliary body *(CB)* is adjacent to the void formerly occupied by the lens. There is a biconvex hyperdense choroid hematoma *(arrow)* that does not shift with postural change.

Figure 14.32. Carotid-cavernous fistula (same case as Fig. 11.26). *Axial (A) and direct coronal (B) i.v. contrast −5/ 400 CT scans.* There is a markedly enlarged contrast-enhanced superior ophthalmic vein *(SOV)*. This case also has an enlarged cavernous sinus which is seen in Figure 11.26.

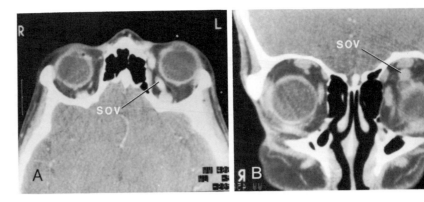

Globe Disruption

This is caused by penetrating injury. The deformed and usually hemorrhagic globe is well demonstrated by CT, occasionally containing intraocular air.[31] Lens dislocation may occur and can be diagnosed by CT (Fig. 14.31).

Carotid-Cavernous Fistula

Carotid-cavernous fistulae are discussed in Chapter 11 (Fig. 11.26). These lesions are usually the result of severe facial trauma or of rupture of a cavernous carotid aneurysm. Both CT and MR identify enlarged superior ophthalmic veins and cavernous sinuses by means of CT i.v. contrast enhancement and MR flow effects, respectively (Fig. 14.32). There is usually uniform enlargement of the extraocular muscles similar to that seen in dural AVMs.

Subperiosteal Hematoma

Orbital subperiosteal hematoma is a rare entity usually in the subfrontal location (orbital roof). It is usually caused by blunt trauma and its presentation may be delayed. CT and MR in coronal planes, and sagittal MR demonstrate a smoothly marginated orbital roof mass having blood CT density or MR intensity. The orbital contents are appropriately displaced.[55]

OTHER OCULAR CONDITIONS

Different ocular and optic nerve conditions that did not fit into the etiological classification will be discussed in this section. Retinal and choroidal detachment can result from a variety of conditions and are discussed within this generalized category rather than under one single etiological category. Other conditions to be discussed within this section are optic disk drusen, choroidal osteoma, scleral calcification, and phthisis bulbi—all four of which are characterized by calcification.

Retinal and Choroidal Detachment

Retinal detachment most frequently occurs in diabetics and hypertensives but may also occur in

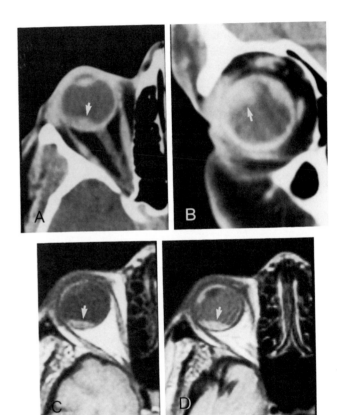

Figure 14.33. Retinal detachment with hemorrhage. **A–B** and **C–D** are different cases. **A–B:** *Axial (A) and direct hanging head coronal (B) i.v. contrast 18/300 CT scans.* There is a biconvex gravity-dependent hyperdense fluid collection *(arrows).* **C–D:** *Axial SE 600/ 25 (C) and 2000/25 (D) MR scan.* There is a T1-/proton density, and T2-(not shown) weighted image hyperintense fluid collection *(arrows).*

trauma-related vitreous hemorrhage (Fig. 14.33). Severe myopia, surgical aphakia, and a history of contralateral retinal detachment are additional predisposing factors for the development of this condition.[9] Retinal detachment also occurs with tumor, such as ocular melanoma,[29,33] and with Coats' disease, persistent hyperplastic vitreous, and retrolental fibroplasia in infants.[22] The retinal traction applied by tightening of organized membranes may partially or totally detach the retina.[53]

Choroidal detachment occurs due to intraocular surgery, penetrating ocular trauma, and inflammatory choroidal disorders.[54] Ocular hypotony, developing from these conditions, is considered to be the causative factor.[54]

Certain CT and MR characteristics also help distinguish retinal from choroidal detachment. The subretinal fluid usually shifts beneath the thin pliable retina as can be demonstrated by changing the head position during scanning. Also, the usually crescentric subretinal collection stops at the optic disk posteriorly and the ora serrata (behind the ciliary body) anteriorly. The choroid is thicker than the retina and does not allow for fluid shifting. The subchoroid fluid is less mobile and has a more pronounced lenticular shape. In choroidal detachment, the entire uveal tract may be involved including detachment of the ciliary body.[54]

These changes are seen by ultrasonography, CT, and MR (Figs. 14.31 and 14.33).[9,29,54] CT density and MR intensity depend upon the presence of effusion or blood and the chronicity of hemorrhage. High protein effusions produce an MR T1 signal-hyperintensity.[9,54] MR T1- and T2-weighted techniques can help distinguish ocular melanotic melanoma from associated retinal detachment due to melanin paramagnetic properties.[9,54]

Optic Disk Drusen

Drusen are hyalin-like concretions of unknown etiology located within ("buried") or on the optic nerve head. They are usually visible in the adult. They are commonly calcified and are frequently (75%) bilateral. They may resemble papilledema ("pseudopapilledema") fundoscopically. Axial noncontrast CT demonstrates punctate papilla calcification (Fig. 14.34). The CT picture is pathognomic for optic disk drusen.[31,56,57]

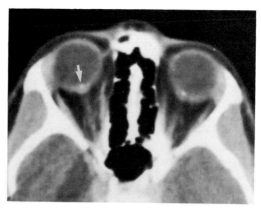

Figure 14.34.   Optic disk drusen. *Axial 400/36 i.v. contrast CT scan.* There are bilateral papillary punctate calcifications *(arrow)*. A small posterior globe deformity leading to the optic nerve resembling the defect of coloboma is more prominent on the right side.

Choroidal Osteoma

These are rare juxtapapillary, choroidal benign masses of mature bone that occur predominantly (90%) in young women (average age, 20 years).[31,58] CT demonstrates a small bone-density juxtapapillary choroidal mass.

Scleral Calcification (Scleral Plaques)

Scleral calcifications may occur in systemic hypercalcemic states. They also occur at the extraocular muscle scleral insertion in elderly patients.[31]

Phthisis Bulbi

Phthisis bulbi is a nonfunctioning contracted and calcified globe usually secondary to trauma or infection. The calcification usually begins posteriorly. CT and MR demonstrate a small contracted and deformed calcified globe. There is occasionally adjacent abundant fibrotic soft tissue (Fig. 14.35).[57]

Treatment of Retinal Detachment

A scleral "buckle" is often used to produce apposition of the choroid to the retina in cases of retinal

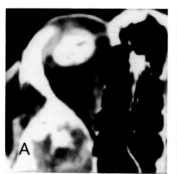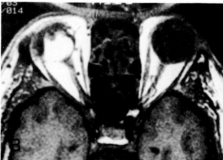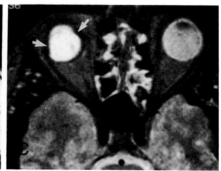

Figure 14.35.   Phthisis bulbi. A and **B–C** are different cases. **A:** *Axial noncontrast 33/150 CT scan.* The right globe is shrunken, misshapen, and calcified. **B–C:** *Axial 600/25* **(B)** *and 2800/80* **(C)** *MR scans.* The right globe is shrunken and misshapen. It contains central abnormal T1/T2 signal-hyperintensity representing hemorrhagic products and/or high protein content. Bilateral hypointensity *(arrows)* represents calcification.

detachment. Retinal tears are treated with laser or cryotherapy, however, when subretinal fluid is present and when there is persistent traction on the retina by vitreous organized membranes, the buckling procedure is used.

In order to create sclera-choroid apposition to the retina, a small piece of material, such as silicone rubber, is used either within a surgical scleral "pocket" or placed on the sclera at the point of maximum detachment. A coronal band of similar material is then tightened around the globe like a belt to increase the depth of the indent ("buckle") and to maintain apposition of the sclera-choroid to the retina. This creates an increase of the globe sagittal dimension.[59]

CT demonstrates the implant, band, deformity, and persistent retinal detachment, if present (Fig. 14.36). The various materials used have different densities. MR provides greater retina-choroid detail compared to CT and may become the procedure of choice. Ultrasound is quite effective, however, and probably will remain the initial investigative tool for retinal detachment.

Surgical Aphakia

Absence of the lens (surgical aphakia) is almost always due to cataract surgery. Absence of the lens is easily detected by both CT and MR (Fig. 14.37).

Cosmetic Globe Replacement

Cosmetic globe replacement requires an orbital spherical implant. The tenon capsule is the fascia surrounding the globe from the optic nerve posteriorly to the ciliary bodies anteriorly. It therefore invests the attachments of the rectus muscles.[6] The implant is placed within the tenon capsule. A removable cosmetic prosthesis then is applied by the patient to the implant surface.[60]

The implant CT densities and MR intensities vary with the material used. Silicon and glass appear denser than methylmethacrylate. The glass usually is hollow with a central glass hypodensity. Air is often

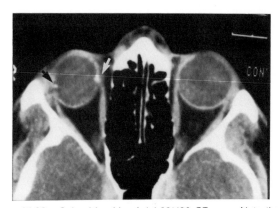

Figure 14.36. Scleral buckle. *Axial 38/400 CT scan.* Note the hyperdense scleral band *(arrows)* narrowing the ocular coronal diameter. The "buckle" producing the focal indent under the band is not seen. No retinal detachment is demonstrated.

seen trapped between the implant and removable prosthesis (Fig. 14.38).[60]

OTHER OPTIC NERVE CONDITIONS

Three conditions involving the optic nerve will be described in this section. These conditions are optic hydrops, optic foramen stenosis, and optic neuritis.

With papilledema, the optic nerve perineural CSF spaces are distended and there is axonal edema and congestion.[25,61] MR, intrathecal contrast CT, and occasionally coronal noncontrast CT can demonstrate the perineural subarachnoid space dilatation and optic disk flattening in patients with papilledema caused by raised intracranial pressure (Fig. 14.39) as well as by other conditions.[25,61,62] CSF CT cisternography is seldom performed now that MR scanners are available.

Optic Hydrops

This is a term used for isolated optic nerve sheath dilation. It occurs in the absence of raised intracranial pressure and may be caused by a variety of focal diseases such as sellar and suprasellar masses, optic nerve and orbital tumors, and by bony proliferative diseases such as osteopetrosis.[61] The nerve sheath dilation is the result of enlargement of the optic nerve subarachnoid space. In the absence of generalized raised intracranial pressure, such as occurs with pseudotumor cerebri and obstructive hydrocephalus, the mechanism is thought to be isolated increased nerve sheath subarachnoid space pressure caused by the offending lesions (so-called optic CSF "block").[61,62] MR demonstrates a distended optic nerve sheath surrounding the optic nerve.

Optic Foraminal Stenosis

This can result from bony proliferative conditions such as osteopetrosis (Fig. 13.12). Intrathecal CT cisternography with positive contrast agents such as iopamidol and iohexol demonstrate the optic nerve subarachnoid space. The appearance of a normal size optic nerve within the optic canal with an obliterated subarachnoid space is evidence of stenosis. This technique, the "optic neurogram," has been used for evaluating the need of surgical optic canal decompression.[63] We have not used this procedure.

Optic Neuritis

Optic neuritis is an acute inflammation of the optic nerve usually caused by multiple sclerosis. Although not usually detectable by CT, nerve enlargement (edema) and contrast enhancement may be seen.[64] With continuing MR technique refinements, optic neuritis may become reliably detectable.

Imaging Gamuts/ Differential Diagnosis

This section consists of four tables characterizing orbital lesions. Tables 14.1–14.4 hopefully will serve the reader as a useful guide for image diagnosis.

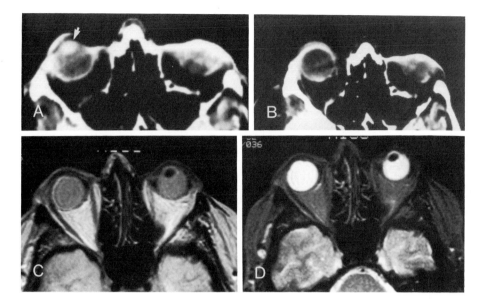

Figure 14.37. Surgical aphakia. *Axial 37/ 100 preoperative* **(A)** *and postoperative* **(B)** *CT scans. SE 2800/30* **(C)** *and 2800/80* **(D)** *postoperative MR scans.* The right hyperdense lens *(arrow)* present on the preoperative exam is absent on the postoperative studies.

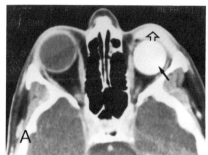

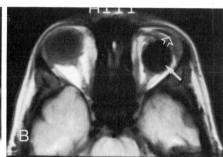

Figure 14.38. Orbital prosthesis. *Axial i.v. contrast 30/400 CT scan* **(A)** *and SE 2000/ 25 MR scan* **(B).** A removable cosmetic prosthesis *(open arrows)* is mounted on the orbital spherical implant *(closed arrows).*

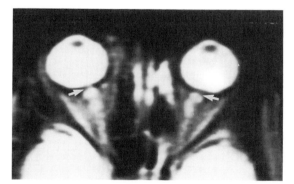

Figure 14.39. Pseudotumor cerebri. *Axial SE 2000/100 MR scan.* There is marked undulating dilatation of the T2 water-isointense optic nerve sheaths with flattening of the posterior globes at the papilla. The normal-sized optic nerves are seen only close to the optic nerve head *(arrows)* probably due to the relatively poor resolution of this thick-section, large FOV scan. Presence of a lesser degree of nerve sheath dilatation is commonly encountered and has been interpreted as a normal finding as seen in Figure 14.8.

Table 14.1. CT Classification of "Optic Nerve Enlargement"* (Optic nerve and perineural lesions)**

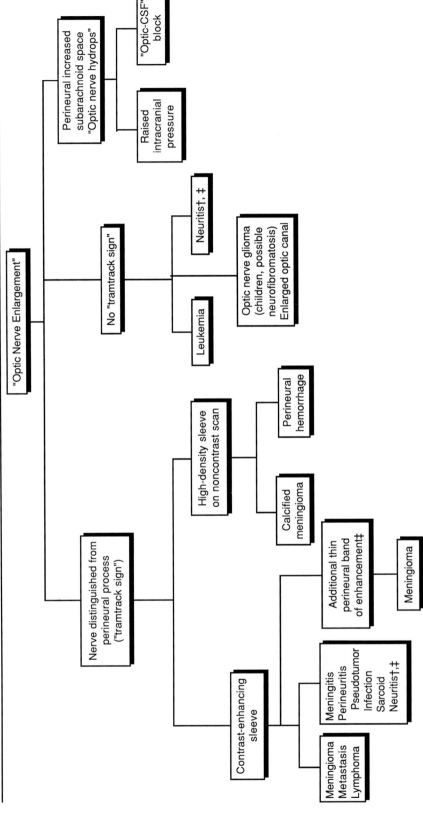

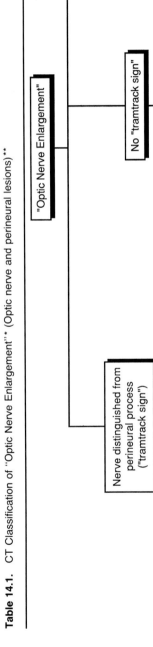

*Modified from Rothfus WE, Curtin HD, Slamovits TL, Kennerdell JS. Optic nerve/sheath enlargement: A differential approach based on high-resolution CT morphology. *Radiology* 1984; 150:409–415.

**This table does not imply that the absence of the "tramtrack" sign excludes those conditions under the tramtrack heading.

†A case of optic neuritis is reported with a tramtrack sign.

‡Data from Johns TT, Citrin CM, Black J, Sherman JL. CT evaluation of perineural orbital lesions: Evaluation of the "tram-track" sign. *AJNR* 1984; 5:589–590.

Table 14.2. Globe Abnormalities Classified According to Globe Size*

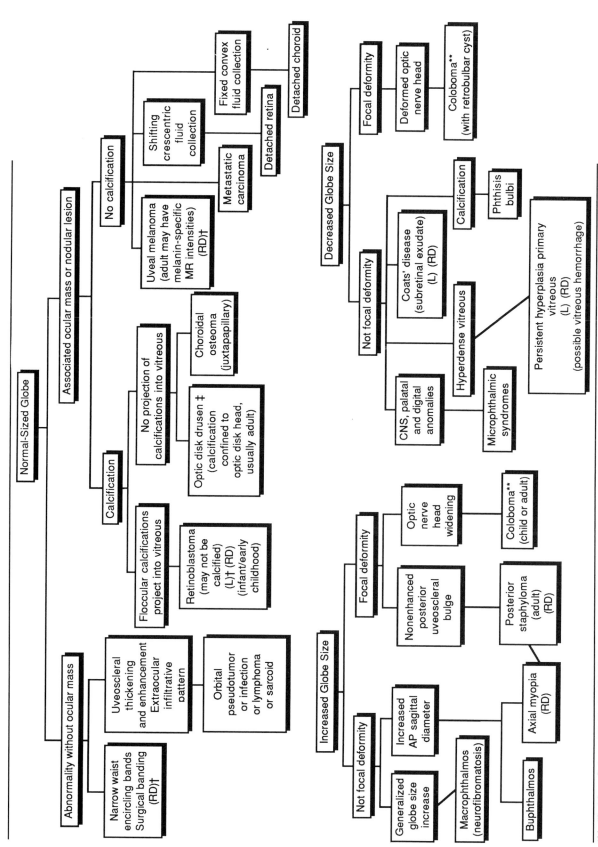

*Modified from Osborne DR, Foulks GN. Computed tomographic analysis of deformity and dimensional changes in the eyeball. *Radiology* 1984; 153:669–674.

** Coloboma may have normal globe size.

†(RD) = Conditions associated with retinal detachment. May mask lesion. (L) = leukoria.

‡Astrocytic hamartomas of the optic nerve; "giant drusen" can occur with tuberous sclerosis. May resemble retinoblastoma. From Turner RM, Gutman I, Hilal SK, et al. CT of drusen bodies and other calcific lesions of the optic nerve: Case report and differential diagnosis. *AJNR* 1983; 4:175–178.

Table 14.3. Features of Orbital Masses*

Lesion	Clinical Data and Features	CT and MR Features†
Cavernous hemangioma	Most common benign orbital tumor	Large smoothly marginated, usually intraconal and lateral to the optic nerve, marked contrast enhancement (CT), possible phleboliths, possible flow effects (MR), hyperdense, T1 ↓ / T2 ↑ (vs. fat)
Lymphangioma	Children and young adults	High attenuation, intra- or extraconal mass, tendency to hemorrhage, minimal contrast enhancement, intraconal masses are usually medial to the optic nerve, ill-defined heterogeneous density mass, T1 ↓ ↔/T2 ↑ (vs. fat)
Venous varix	Children or young adults, intermittent proptosis and pain	Intraconal, marked CT contrast enhancement, enlarges with Valsalva maneuver, may thrombose, MR flow effects.
Meningioma	5% of primary orbital tumors, 33% of primary tumors optic nerve, extension into orbit, primarily extraorbital meningioma is common; 80% are females	See optic nerve gamut, calcification, marked contrast enhancement, CT hyperdense, T1 ↓/T2↔ (vs. fat); tramtrack sign with additional perineural band of CT enhancement
Neurofibroma	May be associated with neurofibromatosis	Usually smoothly marginated tumor anywhere in orbit, plexiform neurofibromas can be confused with gliomas, contrast enhancement, CT isodense or hyperdense T1 ↓/T2 ↑ (vs. fat)
Lacrimal		
Benign mixed tumor	Most common epithelial lacrimal tumor	Sharply marginated lacrimal fossa mass, hyperdense (CT), contrast enhancement
Malignant tumor	Includes adenocystic carcinoma and malignant mixed tumor	Invasive, irregular, and destructive of bone
Inflammatory	Includes pseudotumor, dacryoadenitis and sarcoid	Diffuse glandular enlargement with contrast enhancement
Lymphoid	Includes Sjögren's syndrome, leukemia, and lymphoma	Diffuse glandular enlargement with contrast enhancement, involvement by systemic diseases is often bilateral
Dermoid		Water- or fat-density/intensity may have osseous erosion, no CT contrast enhancement
Dermoid	Children—superotemporal, older children and adults—deep orbital mass often with bone erosion	Often associated bone erosion, extraconal, lacks contrast enhancement although rim may enhance;‡ may have fat density/intensity but often water density and intensity T1↔ ↓ / T2↔ ↑ (vs. fat)
Pseudotumor	Sensitive to steroid therapy; most common intraorbital mass	Diffuse involvement of extraocular muscles, fat, optic nerve, sclera and often preseptal tissues; T-sign, inflamed tissue may contrast enhance, T1 ↓/T2↔ (vs. fat)
Orbital infections	Often adjacent sinus infection or foreign bodies	May have adjacent paranasal sinusitis or associated foreign body, pre- and/or postseptal involvement similar to pseudotumor, T1 ↓/T2↔ (vs. fat)
Sarcoidosis	Eye involved in ¼ of sarcoid patients; may affect conjunctiva, uvea, cornea, sclera, retina, lens, and extraocular muscles; lacrimal gland commonly involved	Similar to pseudotumor, T1 ↓/T2↔ (vs. fat)
Lymphoma	Most patients have systemic lymphoma, usually elderly, usually extraocular; pre- or postseptal	Pre- or postseptal, T-sign, extra- or intraconal, high density and moderate contrast enhancement (often no tramtrack) (CT), usually not bone destructive, T1 ↓/T2↔ (vs. fat)
Graves' orbitopathy	Usually history and/or features of thyroid disease; usually bilateral	Usually asymmetrical and exclusively confined to extraocular muscles with a sharply defined "spindle-shaped" infiltration; may have increased retrobulbar fat; proptosis; moderate degree contrast enhancement; T1 ↓/T2↔ (vs. fat)

Lesion	Clinical Data and Features	CT and MR Features†
Metastatic tumor	Primary, usually adenocarcinoma in the adult; neuroblastoma, Ewing's, Wilms', and leukemia in children	Bone destruction; often extraconal or combined extra/intraconal; contrast enhancement T1 ↓/T2 ↑ (vs. fat)
Neuroblastoma	Children, intracranial and facial extension, common; preseptal extension is rare	Calcification is common; osteolysis is characteristic
Paranasal sinus carcinoma		Sinus disease with contiguous bone destruction; moderate degree contrast enhancement
Rhabdomyosarcoma	Children, highly malignant; preseptal extension common; paranasal sinus, nasopharynx, and brain extension common	Noncalcified; bone destruction; extensive contrast-enhancing soft tissue mass
Ocular tumors		
Retinoblastoma	Neonate and infants; often bilateral; 10% familial; leukoria; retinal detachment; intraocular but may invade sclera and extend along optic nerve	Smoothly contoured intraocular posterior hyperdense contrast-enhancing mass; characteristically calcified; T1 muscle-isointense; T2 not predictable due to calcifications; may have tumoral or intraocular hemorrhage
Uveal melanoma	Adult; may be associated with vitreous hemorrhage; unusual in blacks	Intraocular hyperdense, moderately contrast-enhancing, sharply marginated, unilateral mass within any part of the uvea; may have associated retinal detachment; may have vitreous hemorrhage; melanotic tumors have T1↔/T2 ↑ (vs. fat).
Metastasis	Adult; known primary; often other metastases	Choroid mass; lacks melanin MR signal

*Adapted from Forbes G. Radiology of the orbit. In Harwood-Nash DC, Hackman MS, Lukin RR (Eds). *Syllabus: A Categorical Course in Radiology.* Oak Brook, IL: Radiological Society of North America, 1986; 91–105.
†MR symbols: ↑ = hyperintensity; ↔ = isointensity; ↓ = hypointensity.
‡Data from Ruchman MC, Stefanyszyn MA, Flanagan JC, et al. Orbital tumors. In Gonzalez CF, Becker MH, Flanagan JC (Eds). *Diagnostic Imaging in Ophthalmology.* New York: Springer-Verlag, 1986; 201–238.

Table 14.4. Causes of and MR Characteristics of Extraocular Muscle Enlargement*

	Signal Intensity vs. Fat	
	Short TR/TE "T1"	Long TR/TE "T2"
Thyroid orbitopathy ("spindle-shaped" enlargement, usually bilateral and not uniform)	↓	↔
Myositis	↓	↔
Idiopathic pseudotumor	↓	↔
Bacterial (adjacent sinus infection)	↓	↔
Sarcoid	↓	
Carotid-cavernous fistula and dural AVM (unilateral uniform enlargement, enlarged veins)	↓	↔
Malignancy		
Metastasis (breast, lung)	↓	↑
Lymphoma	↓	↔
Leukemia		
Rhabdomyosarcoma		
Lymphangioma	↔↓	
Hematoma (intensity varies with stage of hemorrhage)		
Trauma (edema, hemorrhage)		
Acromegaly		
Orbital apex mass		
Trichinosis		
Amyloidosis		

*Adapted from Atlas SW, Bilaniuk LT, Zimmerman RA. Orbit. In Stark DD, Bradley WG Jr (Eds). *Magnetic Resonance Imaging.* St. Louis: CV Mosby Co, 1988; 570–613.

References

1. Kelly WM, Paglen PG, Pearson JA, et al. Ferromagnetism of intraocular foreign body causes unilateral blindness after MR study. *AJNR* 1986; 7:243–245.
2. Unsold R, DeGroot J, Newton TH. Images of the optic nerve: Anatomic-CT correlation. *AJR* 1980; 135:767–773.
3. Ball JB Jr. Direct oblique sagittal CT of orbital wall fractures. *AJNR* 1987; 8:147–154.
4. Atlas ST, Grossman RI, Hackney DB, et al. STIR MR imaging of the orbit. *AJNR* 1988; 9:969–974.
4a. Prorok, RJ, Signa applications guide. Vol II 3rd Ed. 4/90. GE medical systems, 21–23.
5. Benes SC. Computed tomography of the orbit. In Gonzalez CF, Masdeu JC, Grossman CT (Eds). *Head and Spine Imaging.* New York: John Wiley & Sons, 1985; 577–635.
6. Goss CM (Ed). *Anatomy of the Human Body by Henry Gray.* Philadelphia: Lea & Febiger, 1959; 1093–1122.
7. Daniels DL, Pech P, Kay MC et al. Orbital apex: Correlative anatomic and CT study. *AJNR* 1985; 6:705–710.
8. Russell EJ, Czervionke L, Huckman M et al. CT of the inferomedial orbit and the lacrimal drainage apparatus: normal and pathologic anatomy. *AJNR* 1985; 6:759–766.
9. Atlas SW, Bilaniuk LT, Zimmerman RA. Orbit. In Stark DD, Bradley WG Jr (Eds). *Magnetic Resonance Imaging.* St Louis: CV Mosby Co, 1988; 570–613.
10. Gomori JM, Grossman RI, Shields JA, et al. Ocular MR imaging and spectroscopy: An ex vivo study. *Radiology* 1986; 160:201–205.
11. Forbes G. Radiology of the orbit. In Harwood-Nash DC, Hackman MS, Lukin RR (Eds). *Syllabus: A Categorical Course in Radiology.* Oak Brook, IL: Radiological Society of North America, 1986; 91–105.
12. Daniels DL, Kneeland JB, Shimakawa A et al. MR imaging of the optic nerve and sheath: Correcting the chemical shift misregistration effect. *AJNR* 1986; 7:249–253.
13. Atlas SW, Grossman RI, Axel L. Orbital lesions: Proton spectroscopic phase-dependent contrast MR imaging. *Radiology* 1987; 164:510–514.
14. Becker MH, McCarthy JG. Congenital abnormalities. In Gonzalez

CF, Becker MH, Flanagan JC (Eds). *Diagnostic Imaging in Ophthalmology.* New York: Springer-Verlag, 1986; 115–188.
15. Mafee MF, Pruzansky S, Corrales MM, et al. CT in the evaluation of the orbit and the bony interorbital distance. *AJNR* 1983; 4:1049–1052.
16. Linder B, Campo SM, Schafer M. CT and MRI of orbital abnormalities in neurofibromatosis and selected craniofacial anomalies. *Radiol Clin North Am* 1987; 25:787–802.
17. Reed D, Robertson WD, Rootman J, Douglas G. Plexiform neurofibromatosis of the orbit: CT evaluation. *AJNR* 1986; 7:259–263.
18. Simmons JD, LaMasters D, Char D. Computed tomography of ocular colobomas. *AJNR* 1983; 4:1049–1052.
19. Osborne Dr, Foulks GN. Computed tomographic analysis of deformity and dimensional changes in the eyeball. *Radiology* 1984; 153:669–674.
20. Anderson RL, Epstein GA, Daver EA. Computed tomographic diagnosis of posterior ocular staphyloma. *AJNR* 1983; 4:90–91.
21. Mafee MF, Goldberg MF, Valvassori GE, Capek V. Computed tomography in the evaluation of patients with persistent hyperplastic primary vitreous (PHPV). *Radiology* 1982; 145:713–717.
22. Hoppen KD, Katz NNK, Dorwart RH, et al. Childhood leukoria: Computed tomographic appearance and differential diagnosis with histopathologic correlation. *Radiographics* 1985; 5:377–394.
23. Sherman JL, McLean IN, Brallier DR. Coat's disease: CT-pathologic correlation in two cases. *Radiology* 1983; 146:77–78.
24. Barkovich AJ, Norman D. Absence of the septum pellucidum: A useful sign in the diagnosis of congenital brain abnormalities. *AJNR* 1989; 152;353–360.
25. Rothfus WE, Curtin HD, Slamovits TL, Kennerdell JS. Optic nerve/sheath enlargement: A differential approach based on high-resolution CT morphology. *Radiology* 1984; 150:409–415.
26. Lallemand DP, Brasch RC, Char DH, Norman D. Orbital tumors in children. Characterization by computed tomography. *Radiology* 1984; 151:85–88.
27. Ruchman MC, Stefanyszyn MA, Flanagan JC, et al. Orbital tumors. In Gonzalez CF, Becker MH, Flanagan JC (Eds). *Diagnostic Imaging in Ophthalmology.* New York: Springer-Verlag, 1986; 201–238.
28. Johns TT, Citrin CM, Black J, Sherman JL. CT evaluation of perineural orbital lesions: evaluation of the "tram-track" sign. *AJNR* 1984; 5:587–590.
29. Bilaniuk LT, Schenck JF, Zimmerman RA, et al. Ocular and orbital lesions: Surface coil MR imaging. *Radiology* 1985; 156:669–674.
30. Price HI, Batnitzky S, Danzinger A, et al. The neuroradiology of retinoblastoma. *Radiographics* 1982; 2:7–24.
31. Grogan JP, Daniels DL. The orbit. In Williams AL, Haughton VM (Eds). *Cranial Computed Tomography. A Comprehensive Text.* St. Louis: CV Mosby, 1985; 555–598.
32. Sullivan JA, Harms SE. Surface-coil MR imaging of orbital neoplasms. *AJNR* 1986; 7:29–34.
33. Mafee MF, Peyman GA, McKusick MA. Malignant uveal melanoma and similar lesions studied by computed tomography. *Radiology* 1985; 156:403–408.
34. Mafee MF, Peyman GA, Grosolano JE, et al. Malignant uveal melanoma and simulating lesions: MR imaging evaluation. *Radiology* 1986; 100:773–780.
35. Peyster RG, Augsburger JJ, Shields JA. Intraocular tumors: Evaluation with MR imaging. *Radiology* 1988; 168:773–779.
36. Winter J, Centeno RS, Bentson JR. Maneuver to aid diagnosis of orbital varix by computed tomography. *AJNR* 1982; 3:39–40.
37. Nugent RA, Lapointe JS, Rootman J, et al. Orbital dermoids: Features on CT. *Radiology* 1987; 165:475–478.
38. Mafee MF, Haik BG. Lacrimal gland and fossa lesions: Role of computed tomography. *Radiol Clin North Am* 1987; 25:767–779.
39. Rothfus WE, Curtin HD. Extraocular muscle enlargement: A CT review. *Radiology* 1984; 151:677–681.
40. Dresner SC, Rothfus WE, Slamovits TL, et al. Computed tomography of orbital myositis. *AJR* 1984; 143:671–674.
41. Atlas SW, Grossman RI, Savino PJ. Surface-coil MR of orbital pseudotumor. *AJNR* 1987; 8:141–146.
42. Towbin R, Han BK, Kaufman RA, Burke M. Postseptal cellulitis: CT in diagnosis and management. *Radiology* 1986; 158:735–737.
43. Zimmerman RA, Bilaniuk LT. CT of orbital infection and its cerebral complications. *AJR* 1980; 134:45–50.
44. Edwards MG, Pordell GR Ocular toxocariasis studied by CT scanning. *Radiology* 1985; 157:685–686.
45. Peyster RG, Ginsberg F, Silber JH, Adler LP. Exophthalmos caused by excessive fat: CT volumetric analysis and differential diagnosis. *AJNR* 1986; 7:35–40.
46. Post MJD, Quencer RM, Tabei SZ. CT demonstration of sarcoidosis of the optic nerve, frontal lobes, and falx cerebri: Case report and literature review. *AJNR* 1982; 3:523–526.
47. Mauriello JA Jr, Gonzalez CF, Grossman CB, Flanagan JC. Orbital trauma. In *Diagnostic Imaging in Ophthalmology.* New York: Springer-Verlag, 1986; 323–341.
48. Zilkha A. Computed tomography of blow-out fracture of the medial orbital wall. *AJNR* 1981; 2:427–429.
49. Tonami H, Nakagawa T, Ohguchi M, et al. Surface coil MR imaging of orbital blow-out fractures: A comparison with reformatted CT. *AJNR* 1987; 8:445–449.
50. Mancuso AA, Hanafee WN. Facial trauma. In Mancuso AA, Hanafee WN (Eds). *Computed Tomography and Magnetic Resonance Imaging of the Head and Neck,* 2nd Edition. Baltimore: Williams & Wilkins, 1985; 42–60.
51. Unger JM. Orbital apex fractures: the contribution of computed tomography. *Radiology* 1984; 150:713–717.
52. Guyon JJ, Brant-Zawadzki M, Seiff SR. CT demonstration of optic canal fractures. *AJNR* 1984; 5:575–578.
53. Mauriello JA Jr, Gonzalez CF, Grossman CB, Flanagan JC. Orbital trauma. In *Diagnostic Imaging in Ophthalmology.* New York: Springer-Verlag, 1986; 323–341.
54. Mafee MF, Linder B, Peyman GA, et al. Choroidal hematoma and effusion: Evaluation with MR imaging. *Radiology* 1988; 168:781–786.
55. Seigel RS, Williams AG, Hutchinson JW, et al. Subperiosteal hematomas of the orbit: Angiographic and computed tomographic diagnosis. *Radiology* 1982; 143:711–714.
56. Ramirez H, Blatt ES, Hibri N. Computed tomographic identification of calcified optic nerve drusen. *Radiology* 1983; 148:137–139.
57. Turner RM, Gutman I, Hilal SK, et al. CT of drusen bodies and other calcific lesions of the optic nerve: Case report and differential diagnosis. *AJNR* 1983; 4:175–178.
58. Bryan RN, Lewis RA, Miller SL. Choroidal osteoma. *AJNR* 1983; 4:491–494.
59. Johnson MH, Smyser GS, DeFilipp GS, Wong SW. Silicone implants for treatment of retinal detachment: Computed tomographic appearance. *AJNR* 1984; 5:59–60.
60. Gale ME, Vincent ME, Sutula FC. Orbital implants and prostheses: Postoperative computed tomographic appearance. *AJNR* 1985; 6:403–407.
61. Jinkins JR. "Papilledema": Neuroradiologic evaluation of optic disk protrusion with dynamic orbital CT. *AJNR* 1987; 8:681–690.
62. Jinkins JR. Optic hydrops: Isolated nerve sheath dilation demonstrated by CT. *AJNR* 1987; 8:867–870.
63. Jinkins JR. The optic neurogram evaluation of CSF "block" caused by compressive lesions at the optic canal. *AJNR* 1987; 8:135–139.
64. Peyster RG, Hoover ED, Hershey BL, Haskin ME. High resolution CT of lesions of the optic nerve. *AJR* 1983; 140:869–874.

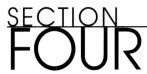

SECTION
FOUR

The Spine

CHAPTER

15

The Spine

Normal Spine

This chapter begins with a MR and CT anatomy atlas-style section (Figs. 15.1–15.11). The anatomical atlas is accompanied by a descriptive text that refers to specific points of the atlas figures. The customary text-format then discusses technique and pathological conditions.

As a general rule, CT produces superior spinal bone detail and MR produces superior soft tissue detail. MR has the additional advantage of direct orthogonal plane (particularly sagittal) imaging. The role of CT versus MR for the investigation of different pathological processes will be discussed in the appropriate sections of this chapter. MR has become our imaging investigative method of choice for examination of the spine soft tissues. Examples include degenerative disk disease, tumors of the spinal soft tissues, and spinal inflammatory processes. CT remains the favored investigative method for fine bone detail. Examples include spinal fractures and dislocations and spinal bone tumors.

ADULT SPINE NORMAL ANATOMY

Bone Anatomy and the Spinal Canal (Figs. 15.1–15.11)

Each vertebra consists of a body and posterior elements. The posterior elements include the neural ring, articular facets, and transverse processes. The neural ring includes the posterior margin of the vertebral body, pedicles and laminae. (Figs. 15.1–15.4). Details of the vertebral body, dense cortex, and cancellous matrix are accurately identified by CT (Fig. 15.2). The cortex is MR signal-void and the cancellous matrix is T1/T2 muscle-isointense or slightly hyperintense in young patients (Figs. 15.4–15.6).[1,2] The cancellous bone signal increases with the patient's age due to replacement of bone matrix by fat.[3] Focal fat replacement of hematopoietic bone marrow commonly occurs and will be discussed under the topic "degenerative diseases of the spine."[4] Chemical shift artifact may produce T1-weighted hypointense lines at the interface between disk and vertebral body.[1] The lumbar superior articular facet is lateral and anterior to the inferior facet of the vertebra above it (Figs. 15.2 and 15.3). The cervical superior and inferior facets are the cranial and caudal articular surfaces of the block-like lateral masses. The lateral C3–7 superior vertebral endplate lip-like articular surfaces (uncinate processes) and the cervical vertebral artery transverse foramina are a unique characteristic of the cervical spine (Fig. 15.9).[5] The collagenous meniscus and the often prominent fat pad contribute to the MR signal of the cervical facet joint (Fig. 15.8).[6,7]

The lateral recess is formed by the superior articular facet posteriorly, the pedicle laterally, and the posterior surface of the vertebral body anteriorly.[8] The basivertebral veins have a characteristic lumbar and thoracic midvertebral body axial and sagittal appearance (Figs. 15.1, 15.5, 15.7).[3,9] The axial appearance is a "Y"-shaped groove that can be identified by both CT and MR. On MR sagittal images it appears as a posterior central vertebral body groove having high signal intensity due to fat content and flow enhancement effects (Figs. 15.5 and 15.7).[1] The communicating epidural veins of the retrovertebral venous plexus are located in the anterior epidural space (Figs. 15.4 and 15.5).[3] A posterior central vertebral osseous protuberance is often identified by CT at the junction of the basivertebral vein and the retrovertebral venous plexus. The central osseous protuberance can be confused with an osteophyte (Fig. 15.5). Unlike the disk-level osteophyte the protuberance is at the midvertebral level.[2,3,10]

The spinal canal has a characteristic shape at each level. It is round at C1, triangular from C2 to C7 (Fig. 15.10), and ovoid in the thoracic and upper lumbar region (Figs. 15.6 and 15.7). It becomes triangular or trefoil at the lower lumbar region (Fig. 15.5). Lumbar spinal canal AP diameters less than 11.5 mm and interpedicular diameters less than 16 mm, are small.[11] Cross-sectional area measurements are less useful. The normal C3–7 cervical spinal canal sagittal diameter should be greater than 10 mm. A C3–7 cervical spinal canal sagittal diameter of 9 mm or less can be considered stenotic; a canal 7 mm or

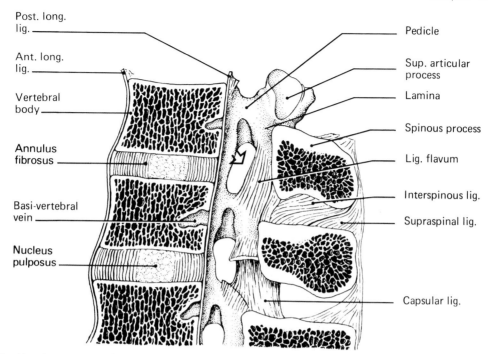

Figure 15.1.   **L3–5 midsagittal section diagram.** *Open arrow* points into the neural foramen. (With permission of Churchill Livingstone. From Grossman CB, Post MJD. The adult spine. In: Gonzalez CF, Grossman CB, Masdeu JC (Eds). *Head and Spine Imaging.* New York, John Wiley & Sons, 1985; 782.)

less is markedly stenotic and very often associated with clinical spinal cord compression. Spinal canal CT measurements should be obtained with axial sections perpendicular to the canal long axis using bone windows.[11] The interfacet and interpedicular distances increase and the height of the pedicles decreases from the upper lumbar to the lower lumbar levels.

Disk Anatomy

The intervertebral disk has a posterocentral nucleus pulposus of notocordal origin surrounded by the annulus fibrosus. The nucleus pulposus is particularly well developed in the cervical and lumbar regions. The 23 disks vary in size, shape, and thickness at the different vertebral levels. They occupy

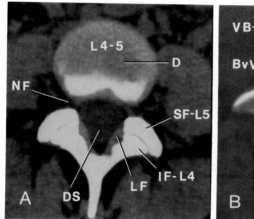
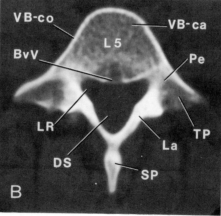
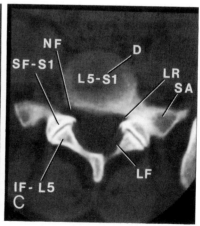

Figure 15.2.   **Normal lumbar spine CT anatomy.** *Axial L4–5 level 24/150 **(A)**, L5-level 350/2000 **(B)**, L5–S1 level 390/2000 **(C)** CT scans. The normal L4–5 disk (D) has a slight convex-anterior curve or is flat at the spinal canal. The disk and the ligamentum flavum (LF) are homogeneously dural sac (DS)-hyperdense. The L5–S1 disk is flat or may have a slight convex posterior curve. There is partial volume averaging of the hyperdense posterior endplate of L4 upon the L4–5 disk in **A** and of either the S1 endplate or the annulus fibrosis upon the L5–S1 disk in **C**. The hyperintense smoothly marginated vertebral body cortex (VB–co) encloses the evenly mottled L5 cancellous bone VB–ca. The basivertebral vein (BvV) is seen at the midvertebral body level. **B** is at the L5 "osseous level" demonstrating the L5 body, pedicles (Pe), transverse process (TP), laminae (La), and spinous process (SP). The wide L5 lateral recess (LR) extends laterally. **A** and **C** are at both intervertebral disk and "articular" levels. The normal inferior facet (IF) posterior medial relationship to the superior facet (SF) is well demonstrated. The S1 medial superior facet hypertrophy slightly narrows the left lateral recess. The neural foramen (NF) is well seen at disk and articular levels; sacral ala (SA).

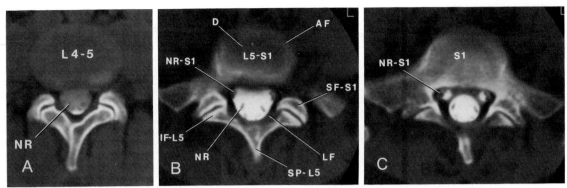

Figure 15.3. **Normal lumbar CT myelogram.** *Axial L4–5 level 577/ 2000* **(A)**, *L5–S1 level 250/1825* **(B)**, *and S1-level 250/1825* **(C)** *CT myelogram.* In addition to the already described plain lumbar CT findings in **A–C**, the CSF is now contrast enhanced demonstrating normal nerve roots *(NR)*. The L5–S1 nerve root sleeve *(NR–S1)* at the L5–S1 level appears as an outward dural sac protruberance and appears separated from the sac at the S1 level due to the root sleeve downward course. The annulus fibrosus *(AF)* is slightly disk-hyperdense. The superior facet *(SF)* is anterolateral to the inferior facet *(IF)*.

proportionately more height in the lumbar and cervical regions than in the thoracic spine. They are thicker anteriorly in the lumbar and cervical regions contributing to the lordotic curvatures (Figs. 15.4 and 15.10). On axial sections, the thoracic and upper four lumbar disks have a posterior marginal concavity and the posterior margin of the lumbosacral disk is flat or slightly convex posteriorly (Figs. 15.2 and 15.7). The posterior concavity may be caused by posterior longitudinal ligament reinforcement.[10] The normal CT disk density varies from +60 to +120 H (Fig. 15.2). This results in excellent contrast compared to the thecal sac (0–30 H).[2] The disk periphery has a higher CT density than the central portion. This may be caused by partial volume averaging with the vertebral body cortex and/or by a denser annulus fibrosus. The collagenous peripheral annulus fibers (Sharpey's fibers) have a tendency to calcify. The MR disk signal demonstrates slight T1 cancellous bone-hypointensity (hypointensity compared to cancellous bone) and T2 cancellous bone-hyperintensity (Fig. 15.4). Progressive loss of disk T2 hyperintensity with age is due to disk desiccation.[3] On MR T2-weighted sagittal images, the normal hydrated disk of patients over 30 years old has a central lower signal "cleft." The cleft may represent invagination of annulus pulposus lamellae into the nucleus (Figs. 15.4 and 15.7).[12]

Ligament Anatomy

The ligamentum flavum attaches to the laminae (Fig. 15.1). It is thickest in the lumbar region (Figs. 15.2 and 15.4) and thinnest in the cervical (Fig. 15.8). The ligamentum flavum is CT tissue isodense and has a T1-weighted intermediate signal intensity and T2 signal hypointensity whereas other ligaments have T1 and T2 hypointensity (Fig. 15.4).[6] The thin posterior longitudinal ligament which runs the length of the spinal canal is rarely recognized on CT or MR images except, perhaps, on MR scans where it is posteriorly displaced by a herniated or bulging disk. MR does not distinguish the low T1 and T2 signal intensity ligaments from bone cortex. The annulus, ligaments, and dura have similar MR signals and are thus not readily distinguishable if adjacent to each other such as in the sagittal view.[3] The transverse

Figure 15.4. **Normal lumbar MR scan.** **A–C:** *Midsagittal SE 1500/ 25* **(A)**, *2000/80* **(B)**, *and coronal 600/25* **(C)** *MR scans.* The conus medullaris *(CM)* is sharply contrasted against CSF on the T1/proton density-weighted **(A)** and the T2-weighted image **(B)** but is not seen on the heavily T1-weighted image **(C)**; sacral ala *(SA)*. **D–F:** *Lateral sagittal SE 2000/30* **(D)**, *axial 2000/20 L4–5 disk-level* **(E)**, *and L5 articular-level* **(F)** *MR scans.* The nerve roots *(NR)* course under the pedicle *(Pe)* for which they are named and are located in the cranial portion of the proximal intervertebral neural foramen *(NF)*. Nerve roots and the dorsal root ganglia *(NR/G)* are well-contrasted against the T1-weighted neural foraminal fat hyperintensity. The facet joints *(arrows)* between the superior *(SF)* and inferior *(IF)* facets are hypertense compared to cortex and often demonstrate a fat pad *(FP in **F**)*. The annulus fibrosus *(AF)* is hypointense compared to the nucleus pulposus. The intranuclear cleft *(InC)* is well seen in **G**. Epidural veins *(EdV)* are clearly identified due to signal-void on the presaturation axial images. The T1 CSF-hyperintense ligamentum flavum *(LF)* is seen best on axial images but is also well identified on the lateral sagittal image. The pars interarticularis *(PI)* connects the superior and inferior facets. Note how the nerve root sleeves at the L4–5 level are continuous with the dural sac *(DS)* and are separated at the L5 level. **G–I:** *SE 2000/80 lateral sagittal* **(G)**, *axial L1–2 level* **(H)**, *and L3–4 level* **(I)** *MR scans.* The T2 hypointense nerve roots *(NR)* of the cauda equina *(CE)* are sharply contrasted against the T2 hyperintense CSF. The roots typically group posteriorly in the upper lumbar region **(H)**. The annulus fibrosus *(AF)* is T2 hypointense compared to the normal hyperintense nucleus pulposus *(NP)*.

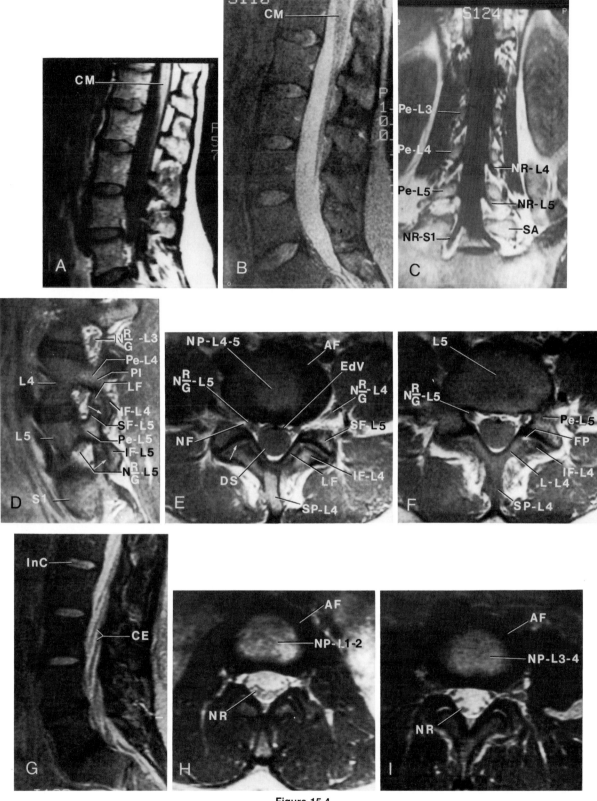

Figure 15.4

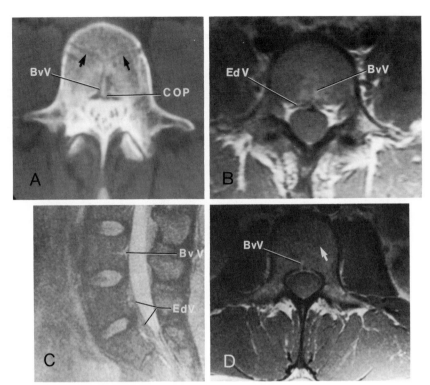

Figure 15.5. Normal basivertebral and epidural veins. A-D are different patients. *Axial L5-level CT myelogram (A) and SE 2000/20 MR scans (B and D). Midsagittal 2000/80 MR scan (C).* CT demonstrates a central osseous protruberance (COP) central to the bas-ivertebral vein (BvV). Note the "Y-shaped" venous tributaries (arrows). MR demonstrates additional epidural veins (EdV) anterior to the dural sac.

ligament of the atlas inserts upon the C1 lateral masses to maintain apposition of the odontoid peg to the transverse arch of the atlas.[3,13]

Thecal Sac and Epidural Space

The thecal sac is surrounded by epidural fat.The lumbar posterior epidural fat is recognized on sagittal MR section as the posterior medial fatty window.[6] The sac is contained by the arachnoid membrane which surrounds the subarachnoid space. Nerve root sleeves are dura-arachnoid prolongations investing nerve roots. The cervical epidural space is small. The size of the thoracic epidural space may be large or small and the epidural space is generally large in the lumbar region.[2] The thecal sac CT density measurement is from 0 to +30 H and it is MR water-isointense. The lumbar thecal sac should be greater than 10 mm sagittal diameter in the normal patient.[2]

The epidural veins are demonstrated by both CT and MR by virtue of their density and intensity difference with fat. MR, therefore, best demonstrates them on T1-weighted images (Fig. 15.5).[2,3,10] They are most pronounced in the lumbar region especially when associated with a herniated lumbar disk.[3]

Spinal Cord and Nerve Roots

The cephalic end of the spinal cord is continuous with the medulla oblongata. The cervical spinal cord is elliptical and flattest at C4–5. It is round at T1. The average spinal cord sagittal diameter at C4-T1 is approximately 7 mm and it is almost 8 mm at C2–4. The average transverse diameter at C3–6 is 13.5 mm and it is smaller above and below.[14] At T5, it is much smaller, averaging 8 mm coronal and 6 mm sagittal diameter.[2,10] The lumbar enlargement begins at T9 and reaches its maximum size at T12. The spinal cord tapers rapidly caudal to T12 and terminates in adults at L1–2. The normal conus medullaris has a distinctive oval appearance. The average conus measures less than 8 mm sagittal diameter and 11 mm transverse diameter (Fig. 15.6).[15] The filum terminale extends from the conus medullaris to the first coccygeal segment. The spinal cord is positioned centrally in the cervical (Fig. 15.10) and lower thoracic spine and anteriorly in the midthoracic spine (Fig. 15.7).[2] The cauda equina has a characteristic posterior location (Fig. 15.6).[16]

The spinal cord can occasionally be visualized by noncontrast CT (without intrathecal contrast) when the subarachnoid space is large. It is routinely iden-

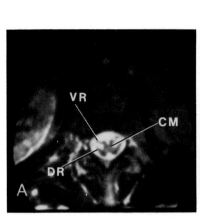
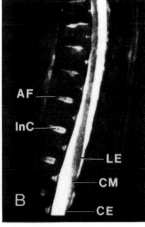
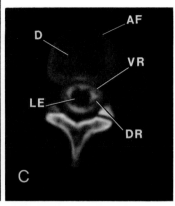

Figure 15.6. Normal conus and lumbar enlargement. **A, B,** and **C** are different patients. *Axial L1-level GRE 50/13 10° tip-angle (A) and midsagittal SE 2000/100 (B) MR scans. Axial 506/2000 CT myelogram (C).* The conus medullaris *(CM)* begins at the caudal tapering of the lumbar enlargement *(LE).* The dorsal *(DR)* and ventral *(VR)* nerve roots, and the cauda equina *(CE)* are well demonstrated by both the MR and the CT myelographic methods. The cauda equina position is characteristically posterior. The T2 hypointense intranuclear cleft *(InC)* within the T2 hyperintense nucleus pulposus is surrounded by the hypointense annulus fibrosus *(AF)* on the MR scans. The CT hyperdense annulus is seen surrounding the isodense disk *(D).*

tified from the foramen magnum to C2 (Fig. 15.10). It can occasionally be identified at lower levels of the cervical spine and in the thoracic spine.[2,10] A major advantage of the MR spine method is the identification and characterization of the spinal cord (Fig. 15.10), nerve roots, and ganglia (Fig. 15.4). New MR techniques are used that eliminate CSF and blood flow artifacts, produce hyperintense CSF signal that contrasts with isointense neural tissue, and can identify the central gray matter.[3,17] MR images can routinely identify nerve roots in the lumbar and cervical subarachnoid space (Figs. 15.4 and 15.10).[1,3,18,19] CT without intrathecal contrast can routinely identify lumbar nerve root sleeves and can occasionally identify lumbar nerve roots within the subarachnoid space.[1,2,10,20] The cervical nerve roots are posterior to the epidural veins in the neural foramen.[18,19] The cervical ventral root is anterior and caudal to the dorsal root and therefore the ventral root abuts the uncinate process and the dorsal root and ganglion abut the superior facet (Fig. 15.10).[19]

Paraspinal Muscles

Both CT and MR demonstrate excellent paraspinal muscle detail. The cervical paravertebral musculature is the most complex. The paraspinal muscles are least prominent in the thoracic region. Figure 15.11 demonstrates both CT and MR muscle detail.[21,22]

Vascular Structures

The spinal epidural veins have been referred to earlier in this chapter with respect to the basiverte-bral veins and retrovertebral venous plexus. They have characteristic CT and MR appearances.

Intravenous Contrast Enhancement

Intravenous Gd-DTPA, a paramagnetic metal ion chelate, prominently enhances all neural foraminal soft tissues except nerve roots.[23,24] The dorsal root ganglion and the periradicular nerve sheath contrast enhance.

Intravenous contrast spinal CT using standard iodinated x-ray contrast material has been proposed as a method to demonstrate herniated intervertebral disks, both preoperative and recurrent. We do not routinely use the contrast technique. High dose i.v. contrast cervical CT has been proposed as a means to enhance the epidural and intervertebral foraminal veins (Fig. 15.10). Venous displacement and venous dural edge enhancement are then used as markers indirectly indicating presence of a herniated disk.[25]

Intrathecal Contrast Enhancement

This CT method almost always follows a conventional myelographic exam in which there is sufficient diagnostic doubt to warrant further investigation. Intrathecal CT myelography is only occasionally performed for CT examination alone. One such indication for the use of CT myelography only is a cervical examination on an equipment-monitored and equipment-life-supported patient with a halo frame

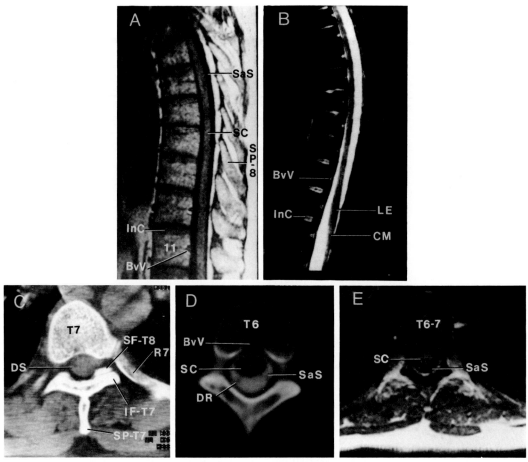

Figure 15.7. Normal thoracic spine. A–E are five different patients. *Thoracic midsagittal SE 600/25* **(A)** *and 2000/100* **(B)** *MR scans. Axial T7-level 61/600 CT scan* **(C)**, *T6-level 506/2000 CT myelogram* **(D)**, *and T6–7 SE 600/25 MR scan* **(E).** The spinal cord *(SC)* maintains a T1/T2 midrange intensity compared to the CSF of the subarachnoid space *(SaS)* which changes from hypointense to hyperintense. It has an anterior position in the midthoracic spine and a posterior position at the thoracolumbar junction. The physiological spinal cord lumbar enlargement *(LE)* and conus medullaris *(CM)* is best demonstrated by MR with the T2 technique. The CT method requires intrathecal contrast for spinal cord and nerve root *(DR)* identification but still lacks the MR discrimination of intrinsic spinal cord signals. The MR identification of intervertebral disk detail, such as normal T1 and T2 signals and the intranuclear cleft *(InC)*, is well demonstrated. The basivertebral veins *(BvV)* are directly seen by MR and the basivertebral groove is identified by CT. The midthoracic spinous processes are sharply downward angulated *(SP-8)* and have a lumbar-type horizontal position in the lower thoracic spine. There is a coronal plane facet articulation in the midthoracic spine *(SF/IF)*. Note the rib *(R7)* articulation in **C. C** is in the "articular plane" and **D** is in the "osseous plane." (**B** courtesy of Douglas H. Yock, Jr., M.D., Minneapolis MN, and the Siemen's Corporation.)

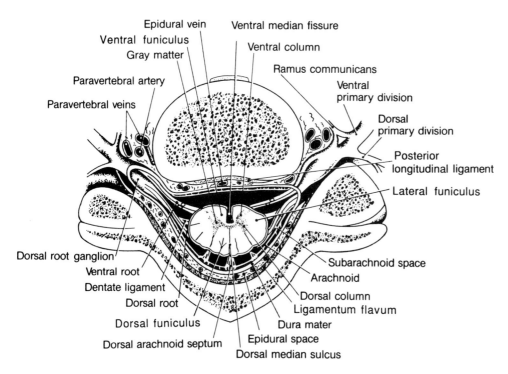

Epidural vein
Ventral funiculus
Gray matter
Paravertebral artery
Paravertebral veins

Ventral median fissure
Ventral column
Ramus communicans
Ventral primary division
Dorsal primary division
Posterior longitudinal ligament
Lateral funiculus

Dorsal root ganglion
Ventral root
Dentate ligament
Dorsal root
Dorsal funiculus
Dorsal arachnoid septum

Subarachnoid space
Arachnoid
Dorsal column
Ligamentum flavum
Dura mater
Epidural space
Dorsal median sulcus

Figure 15.8. Normal midcervical spine axial diagram. Articular level schematic diagram. (With permission of Churchill Livingstone. From Grossman CB, Post MJD. The adult spine. In Gonzalez CF, Grossman CB, Masdeu JC (Eds). *Head and Spine Imaging.* New York, John Wiley & Sons, 1985; 784.)

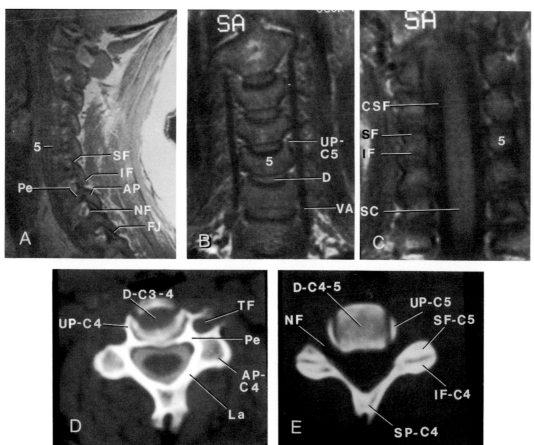

Figure 15.9. Normal cervical spine. Uncinate processes, facets, and neural foramina. **A, B–C, D,** and **E** are different cases. *Sagittal facet-level* **(A)** *and coronal vertebral body-level* **(B)** *and spinal canal-level* **(C)** *SE 2000/30 MR scans. Axial C3–4 353/2000 CT myelogram* **(D)** *and C4–5 415/1500 CT scan* **(E).** The intervertebral neural foramen *(NF)* is formed anteriorly by the vertebral body posterior inferior edge above, the disk *(D)* in the middle, and the uncinate process *(UP)* below. The pedicles *(Pe)* form the superior and inferior margins and the facets *(SF* and *IF)* form the posterior margins. The superior and inferior facets are fused to form an articular pillar *(AP)* which projects laterally from the junction of the pedicle and lamina *(La).* The facet joints *(FJ)* have a diagonal sagittal **(A)** and a horizontal coronal **(E)** orientation. The vertebral artery *(VA)* courses the transverse foramen *(TF)* in the transverse processes of C1–6; spinal cord *(SC).*

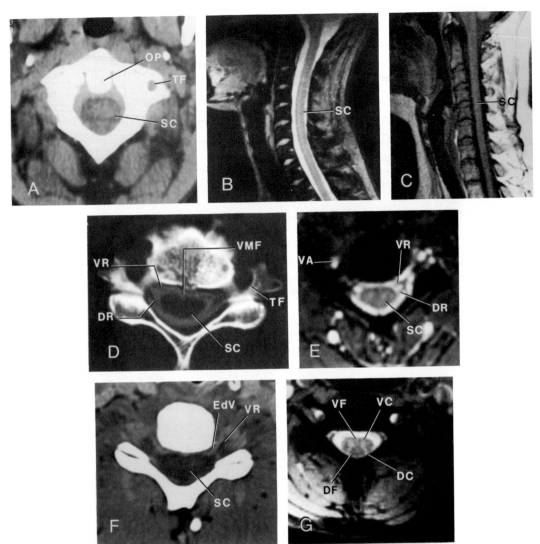

Figure 15.10. Normal cervical spine anatomy. All illustrations from different cases. *Axial 50/500 C1-level CT scan* **(A)**. *Midsagittal SE 2000/90* **(B)** *and 600/25* **(C)** *MR scans. Axial C4–5 353/2000 CT myelogram* **(D)**. *Axial C5–6 300/25 60° tip-angle MR scan* **(E),** *axial 30/450 i.v. contrast CT scan* **(F),** *and 30/11 partial tip-angle MR scan* **(G)**. The spinal cord *(SC)*, ventral *(VC)* and dorsal *(DC)* columns, the ventral *(VF)* and dorsal *(DF)* funiculus, and the ventral *(VR)* and dorsal *(DR)* nerve roots are clearly identified by gradient recalled echo (GRE) partial flip-angle technique. The T1/T2 intermediate intensity spinal cord contrasts with the T1 hypointense and the T2 hyperin- tense CSF. CT myelography and i.v. contrast CT scanning also demonstrate nerve roots, however, CT myelography is the only CT technique that reliably and accurately demonstrates spinal cord outline. Ventral median fissure *(VMF)*. Intravenous contrast enhancement of the more anterior epidural veins *(EdV)* outlines the posterior nerve roots within the intervertebral neural foramen. The vertebral artery *(VA)* is within the transverse foramen *(TF)*; odontoid peg *(OP)*. (**B** and **G** courtesy of Douglas H. Yock, Jr., M.D., Minneapolis, MN, and the Siemen's Corporation.)

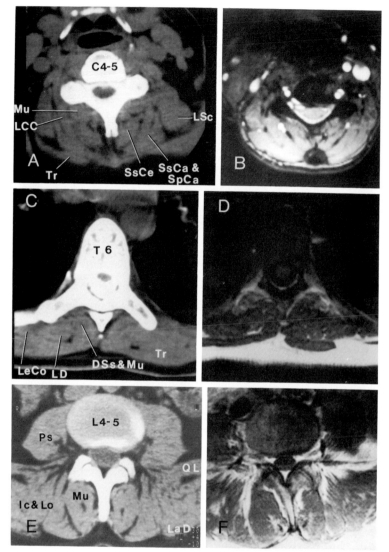

Figure 15.11. Normal paraspinal muscles. *The left column of labeled CT scans 62/550 (A), 3/400 (C), 40/300 (E) should be compared to the right column MR scans GRE 50/17/30° (B), 600/25 (D), SE 2000/20 (F).* Abbreviations: *DSs,* dorsal semispinalis; *Ic,* iliocostalis; *LaD,* latissimus dorsi; *LCC,* longissimus capitis and cervicis; *LD,* longissimus dorsi; *LSc,* levator scapulae; *LeCo,* levator costae; *Lo,* longissimus; *Mu,* multifidus; *Ps,* psoas; *QL,* quadratus lumborum; *SpCa,* splenius capitis; *SsCa,* semispinalis capitis; *SsCe,* semispinalis cervicis; *Tr,* trapezius.

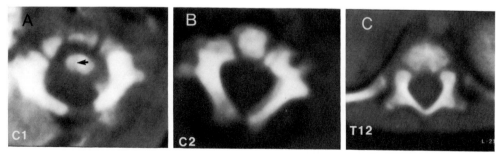

Figure 15.12. Normal pediatric spine findings at 4 months age. *Axial C1-level (A), C2-level (B), and T12-level (C) 210/2000 CT scans.* **A** demonstrates incomplete ossification and lack of fusion of the anterior and posterior arches. There is a small vertical odontoid synchondrosis *(arrow).* **B** demonstrates open C2 neurocentric junctions and lack of posterior laminar fusion. **C** demonstrates open neurocentric junctions.

device that cannot be studied by MR. The method has been discussed in Chapter 2.

CT myelography enhances CSF density identifying the spinal cord, nerve roots, and filum terminale. Fine detail such as the cervical cord ventral median fissure and ventral and dorsal nerve roots can be seen on thin section-targeted scans (Fig. 15.10).[2,10] There is less need for CT myelography with continued MR developments such as very thin sections improved surface coil technique and more rapid sequences and improved artifact suppression.

PEDIATRIC NORMAL SPINE CONSIDERATIONS

This small section will discuss easily recognized pediatric spinal developmental features. The infant spine is relatively straight lacking the adult curvatures. Therefore, varying the axial plane section angle is often unnecessary. The newborn vertebral canal is large in proportion to the vertebral body. A wide cartilagenous neurocentral junction separates the vertebral bodies and pedicles in the newborn, may be seen as a notch at age 2, and may be seen as a dense band at age 18. The newborn C1 anterior arch is usually cartilagenous. Behind the cartilagenous C1 anterior arch are the usually bifid odontoid ossification centers (Fig. 15.12).[26] The spinous process cartilagenous centers ossify by age 2 except for C1, the sacrum, and occasionally L5. The normal conus at birth is no lower than L2-3 and by age 12, it is no lower than mid-L2.

CT and MR Technique

CT SPINE TECHNIQUE

The principal considerations that influence the choice of spine CT technique (Fig. 15.13) are pathological disease category, location, and need for multiplanar image reformation. Thin-section (3 mm cervical and 5 mm lumbar) small-FOV soft tissue and bone windows with a soft tissue filter are routine.

Pathological Disease Category

The CT investigation of lumbar spondylosis and degenerative disk disease, in most institutions, requires five or six 5-mm thick sections parallel to the L3-S1 interspaces (Figs. 15.13C). The CT investigation of spine trauma, tumors, congenital anomalies, and inflammatory disease often includes CT myelography and is often supplemented by sagittal and coronal reformations (Fig. 15.13G).[2] These studies can document the condition and position of the spinal cord. Sagittal and modified axial reformations have been promoted as the routine CT method of choice for the investigation of lumbar spondylosis.[27] This latter technique requires a large series of parallel images[28] and is not, generally, the accepted method of investigation. Unique problems in the investigation of truama may develop such as investigation of cervical

facet fracture and/or subluxation. Axial sections parallel to the facet joints best demonstrate this condition by CT as will be demonstrated later in this chapter. Rotatory subluxation requires a unique thick section investigative technique which also will be later discussed.[2]

Location

The location of spine investigation also influences the technique used. For example, the CT examination of a relatively straight segment of spine such as L1-3, T2-5, or C1-4 can be formed at one gantry angle and still be relatively parallel to most interspaces. The images thus obtained can also be reformatted in other planes. Investigation of the sacral foramina is very effective with sections parallel to the sacrum (Fig. 15.13D),[2] whereas imaging requirements for the sciatic nerve requires serial axial sections.[29]

Multiplanar Reformation

Multiplanar reformation requires multiple parallel thin sections which are all obtained at the same gantry tilt (Fig. 15.13E–G). Ideally, a very fast scanner such as the scanning beam "cine" CT system can produce a rapid sequence of quality thin sections for reformation in order to reduce motion artifact.

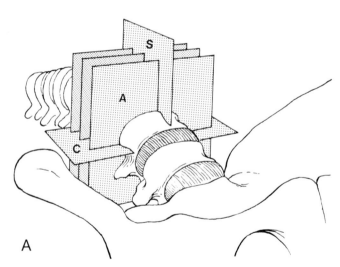

Figure 15.13. CT spine technique. Orthogonal planar anatomic diagram of the lower spine **(A).** Diagram demonstrating the effect of axial plane of section on imaging of the disk **(B).** Localizer view showing sections parallel to the interspaces **(C).** Localizer demonstrating reverse angulation for coronal sacral imaging **(D).** Sagittal reformation of a "file" of contiguous axial sections **(E).** Paraxial reformation of a file of axial 5-mm thickness sections to obtain a tangential disk section **(F).** Curved plane reformation of a file of contiguous axial CT myelogram sections for scoliosis **(G).** Three-dimensional cervical spine reformation of a file of contiguous sections **(H).** Axial lumbar post-i.v. contrast injection CT scan **(I).**

A: Line diagram demonstrating axial *(A),* sagittal *(S),* and coronal *(C)* sections. (From Grossman CB, Post MJD. The adult spine. In Gonzalez CF, Grossman CB, Masdeu JM (Eds). *Head and Spine Imaging.* New York, John Wiley & Sons, 1985; 794, Fig. 25.15**A.** Courtesy of Churchill Livingstone Company, New York.)

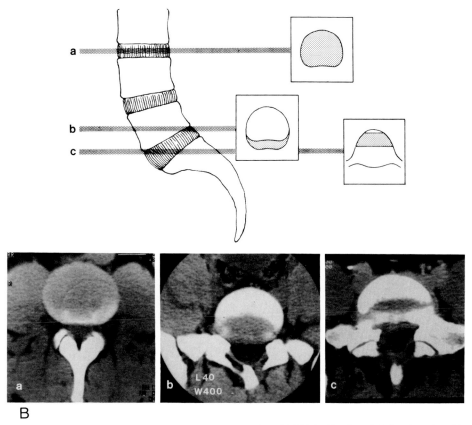

B

Figure 15.13. **B:** *Top*—Annotated line diagram. *Bottom*—Annotated 5-mm thickness, 15-cm FOV, axial CT sections matching top section planes. Note soft tissue window 40/400. (From Grossman CB, Post MJD. The adult spine. In Gonzalez CF, Grossman CB, Masdeu JM (Eds). *Head and Spine Imaging.* New York, John Wiley & Sons, 1985; 789, Fig. 25.9**A.** Courtesy of Churchill Livingstone Company, New York.)

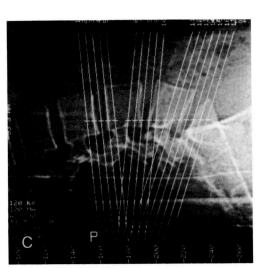

Figure 15.13 **C:** Annotated lateral L3–S1 localizer image with chosen sections paralleling the disk interspaces. The sections converge posteriorly so as not to leave unscanned levels of the spinal canal.

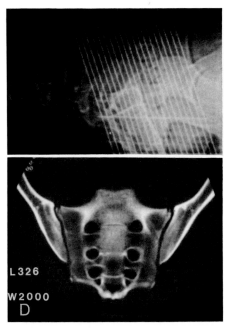

Figure 15.13. **D:** Reverse gantry angulation localizer *(top)* demonstrating proper angle (–20° maximum) for sacral direct coronal imaging *(bottom).* Note: bone window 326/2000.

Figure 15.13.   **E:** Sagittal reformation of sacral agenesis. *Top:* mid-sagittal plane line *1* is superimposed upon a modified direct coronal sacral image of a contiguous section file. Midsagittal reformation *(below).*

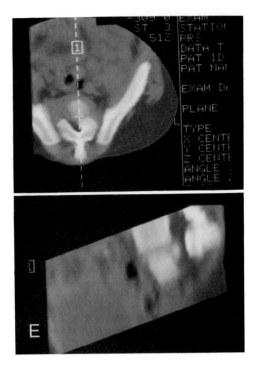

Figure 15.13.   **F:** *Top*—localizer view for oblique axial scanning demonstrating 0° section *31. Middle*—section *31* axial scan receives an axial 47.7° oblique axial section command *(line 1). Bottom*—new oblique reformatted section *1* at 45.7° through the L5–S1 interspace.

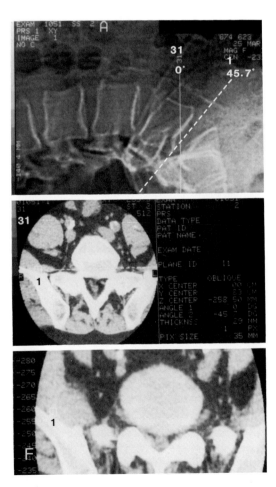

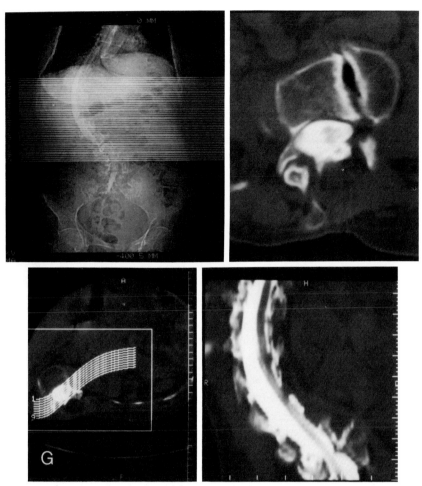

Figure 15.13.   G: Scoliosis. *Top left*—AP localizer annotated with contiguous axial sections. *Top right*—a single section demonstrating a portion of a "vacuum" disk and portions of the apposing vertebral bodies. *Bottom left*—curved plane localizer for coronal reformation *(bottom right)*.

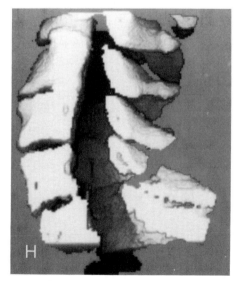

Figure 15.13.   H: Cervical trauma 3–D reformation image of a contiguous 3-mm thickness axial section file.

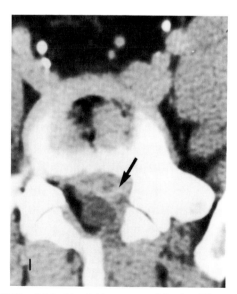

Figure 15.13.   I: L5–S1 axial i.v. contrast injection CT scan for evaluation of recurrent herniated disk demonstrating contrast enhanced epidural scar *(arrow)* surrounding the herniated disk.

Three-dimensional CT Reformation

Three-dimensional CT reformation method has proven helpful in the preoperative planning for correction of congenital malformations, reduction of spinal fractures (Fig. 15.13H), and relief of spinal stenoses. It remains to be seen for what conditions and in what situations the method is cost effective. The collection of data is similar to that of multiplanar reformation. Several equipment manufacturers now provide equipment to perform 3-D CT reformation.

Intravenous Contrast

Intravenous contrast techniques (same injection technique as for i.v. contrast cranial exam) has been used with limited success for detection of postoperative recurrent herniated pulposis (Fig. 15.13I) and cervical herniated disk (Fig. 15.10).

MR SPINE TECHNIQUE

MR technique changes frequently due to the rapid pace of MR technological development and clinical research reporting. For this reason, a review of technical principles (Fig. 15.14) rather than a strict MR imaging protocol will be presented.

Surface coil techniques improve image quality and reduce imaging time by preferentially receiving signal from a limited tissue volume such as the cervical spine (Fig. 15.10B). The greater (signal-to-noise) S/N ratio that results requires fewer excitations and, therefore, scan time is decreased. New developments in surface coil technology will enable larger fields to be examined concurrently using multiple surface coils.[30]

Changes in MR spine techniques frequently follow improved software programs and hardware innovations. Certain MR imaging goals have not changed despite many improvements. These goals include sagittal and axial T1 and T2 or T2* imaging of each patient. The T2 spin echo technique utilizes flow compensation, variable band width, and cardiac or pulse gating. Both the T2 spin echo and the T2* gradient refocused echo technique produce the so-called "myelographic effect" (Fig. 15.10B) and often demonstrate spinal cord gray-white matter structural detail (Fig. 15.10G).[30] The spin echo T2-weighted technique is superior to the T2* technique for evaluation of spinal cord edema, contusion, and MS plaque, and also for the state of disk hydration. Comparison of the T1- and the T2-weighted images is necessary for anatomical and pathological structural and chemical (e.g., blood, edema) analysis. The sagittal sequence precedes the axial for longitudinal localization and determination of the obliquity of the axial angle (Fig. 15.14E).

Goals of spine imaging such as thin sections, high detail of small parts, fast scans, and artifact suppression often require methods that satisfy some goals while compromising others. For example, gradient refocused echo sequences with partial flip (tip) angle technique (GRASS, FLASH, FAST, FISP) produces excellent S/N fast scans but are more susceptible to artifacts caused by field inhomogeneities. The shortest TE possible helps prevent enlarged bone contours caused by these artifacts.[31] Thin sections are necessary for high detail of small parts but have reduced signal. Increased acquisition time (number of excitations—NEXs) improves thin section detail but increases motion artifact. Strip scanning (rectangular FOVs) decreases scan time with the minor penalty of a smaller FOV. Matrix reduction in one parameter (e.g., 256×128) proportionally reduces scan time by 50% with slight detail compromise but with in-

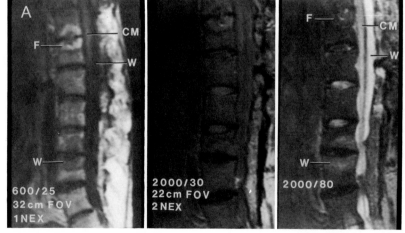

Figure 15.14. MR technique. A: Sequence changes influencing image quality. Midsagittal T1 heavily-weighted image *(left)*, proton-density image *(middle)* and T2 heavily-weighted image *(right)*. The conus medullaris *(CM)* is not identified on the proton density (2000/ 30) image. There is fat *(F)* and water *(W)* intensity inversion on T1- and T2-weighted images. Resolution is diminished on the T1-weighted image due to the larger FOV and diminished signal due to only 1 NEX.

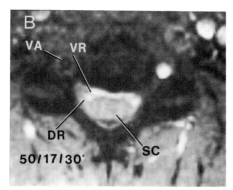

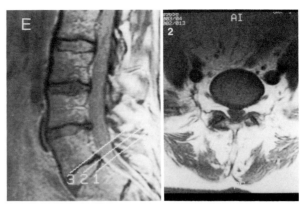

Figure 15.14. **B:** Gradient reversal "myelographic" and flow effects. The muscle isointense spinal cord *(SC)* and nerve roots *(DR, VR)* are well outlined by the hyperintense CSF. The occluded right vertebral artery *(VA)* is devoid of signal.

Figure 15.14. **E:** Oblique imaging. Lumbar oblique axial images are obtained by setting cursors on the localizer image *(left)*. Section 2 *(right)* is in the plane of the intervertebral disk.

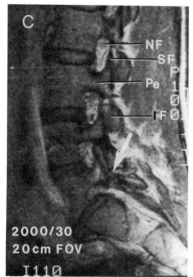

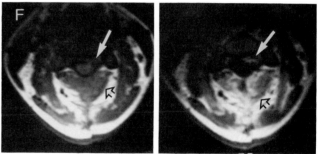

Figure 15.14. **F:** MR i.v. contrast. Cervical epidural abscess. Post-laminectomy. *Noncontrast (left) and i.v. Gd-DTPA contrast (right) SE 600/25 MR scans.* The anterior epidural abscess *(closed arrow)*, the posterior soft tissue abscess *(open arrow)*, and the vertebral body contrast enhance.

Figure 15.14. **C:** Bone detail. Proton-density, small FOV 256 × 256 matrix flow-compensation 1 NEX MR scan. L5 spondylolytic defect *(arrow)*. Other evidence of fine bone detail includes the neural foramina *(NF)*, pedicles *(Pe)*, and superior *(SF)* and inferior *(IF)* facets.

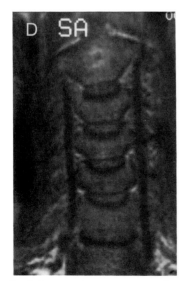

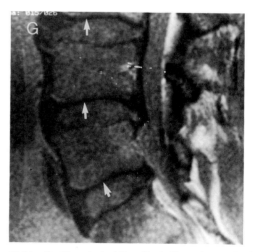

Figure 15.14. **D:** Orthogonal imaging planes. *SE 600/25 coronal plane cervical spine image.*

Figure 15.14. **G:** Chemical shift artifact. There is greater hypointensity of the inferior vertebral margins *(arrows)*. Changing the frequency-encoding axis will redirect the chemical shift phenomenon.

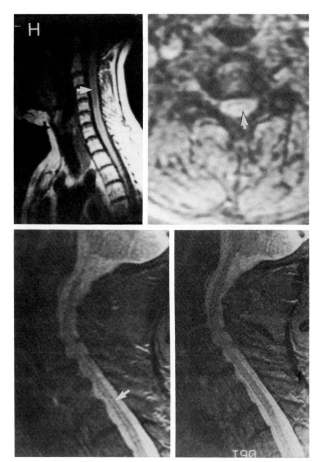

Figure 15.14. **H:** Gibb's phenomenon. *Top left and right and bottom left* images are with a 256/128 matrix. The *bottom right* image is the same case as the bottom left but with a 256 × 256 matrix and 1 NEX instead of 256 × 128 and 2 NEX so that scan time (8 min) is the same. A pseudosyrinx is seen at top left *(arrow)*. Hypointense spinal cord rimming is seen at *top right and bottom left*. The finer matrix *(bottom right)* markedly reduces the artifact. Although the *bottom right image* is more grainy due to decreased signal, structures are generally sharper.

creased truncation artifact. Reduction of truncation artifact requires a finer matrix (256 × 256) thus increasing acquisition time unless the NEX is decreased (Fig. 15.14**G**). Cardiac or pulse-gating reduces the artifacts and signal loss due to CSF motion but also increases acquisition times.[32] Surface coil technique images smaller FOVs but is limited to relatively superficial structures. Higher field magnets produce increased signal but also increase the effect of chemical shift artifact such as the T1 hypointense line at the disk-vertebral endplate junction (Fig. 15.14**G**). By changing the frequency-encoding direction, this artifact can be eliminated from its initial location but will appear perpendicular to the new frequency-encoding direction.[1] Fat suppression techniques have been developed to suppress chemical shift artifacts.

Flow-motion artifact can also be suppressed with gradient motion nulling (flow compensation), spatial presaturation methods, and cardiac or pulse-gating. Flow-compensation technique may actually make a hydromyelia less conspicuous by causing an increase

of the cystic fluid intensity due to its pulsation effect. For this reason, when investigating a spinal cord cyst, we obtain high detail scans without flow-motion suppression. Phase "wrap-around" artifact can also be suppressed with special acquisition techniques. Some of these methods to suppress artifact are mutually exclusive and no doubt new techniques for artifact suppression will be developed. These methods, and others, are explained in Chapters 1 and 3.

The MR ability to image in any plane is particularly advantageous for studying the lumbosacral disk, which often is at an angle greater than 20° and, therefore, beyond the CT tilt limit (Fig. 15.14**E**). Three-dimensional acquisition technique offers advantages such as very thin sections and oblique plane imaging of structures (oblique sagittal cervical and lumbar neural foramen images).

Gd-DTPA and other paramagnetic MR i.v. contrast agents improve MR sensitivity for intramedullary and intradural[23] neoplasms, for inflammatory processes (Fig. 15.14**F**), and for postoperative scars.[33,34]

New magnetic configurations such as the "hybrid" magnet (resistive coils in combination with a permanent magnet core) have a midfield strength, less fringe field effect, and allow scanning that does not interfere with life support and monitoring equipment. This type of scanner can greatly increase the use of MR for acute spinal injuries and for acutely ill patients. Halo vests made with MR-compatible material and ventilatory and monitoring equipment that can function in a strong magnetic field have been developed.[35]

Pediatric Pathological Considerations

These abnormalities have been divided into three categories: minor osseous spinal abnormalities, abnormalities that include dysraphism and/or low conus, and other pathological conditions. Since the neural tube influences bone growth, bone abnormalities frequently are associated with neurological abnormalities.[36] MR is the most sensitive imaging technique for neural tissue and for this reason and for orthogonal plane imaging capability, it is the procedure of choice for initial examination of congenital spinal anomalies.[3] CT myelography is also very effective, however, it requires intrathecal contrast and lacks the direct orthogonal plane capability.

MINOR OSSEOUS SPINAL ANOMALIES

Minor osseous spinal anomalies commonly occur in the cervical spine. These anomalies include atlanto-occipital fusion (Fig. 15.15), unfused cervical laminae, block vertebral bodies, hypoplastic pedicles, and os odontoideum. Occult spinal bifida at L5 and/or S1 is often seen (Fig. 15.16). Lack of a vertebral arch, a cleft vertebral arch and a hemivertebra may occur as isolated phenomena and may be of minor consequence and not associated with neurological abnormalities.[36]

Chiari I malformation, although usually present-

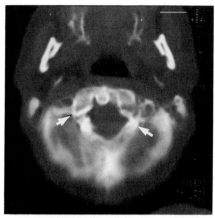

Figure 15.15.   Atlanto-occipital fusion. *Axial 42/1600 CT scan.* C1 and the occiput are fused *(arrows).*

ing in young adults, is included in this section for convenience. This malformation is characterized by caudal elongation, greater than 2 mm, of pointed cerebellar tonsils into the spinal canal and a small "tight" cisterna magna.[37] As many as 50% of cases have hydromyelia—long segment smooth dilatation of the central canal.[3] It is very rarely associated with myelomeningocele or tethered cord.[36] Naidich describes a case of lipomyelomeningocele associated with Chiari I malformation.[38] Hydrocephalus and Klippel-Feil anomaly may occur.[37] These patients may present with ataxia suggesting the diagnosis of a posterior fossa mass or of multiple sclerosis. Commonly associated craniovertebral abnormalities include occipitalization of the atlas, basilar impression, platybasia, small foramen magnum, and block C2-3 vertebral body.[2] MR is the method of choice for examination of this anomaly (Fig. 15.17). CT myelography with sagittal reformation is a far less satisfactory alternative. Lateral cervical puncture intrathecal contrast introduction should be avoided in these patients. The CT technique requires, in addition to immediate scanning after intrathecal contrast injection, 4-, 8-, and 12-hour delayed scans in order to diagnose associated hydromyelia (see Chapter 2). Even with the delayed scans, hydromyelia may not be detected.

ABNORMALITIES INCLUDING DYSRAPHISM AND/OR A LOW CONUS

Dysraphism is the incomplete or absent fusion of spine parts that normally unite. Although technically inaccurate, it is convenient to think of dysraphic conditions as a continuum with the tethered conus as the most minor and myelomeningocele as the most severe.[36]

The terms used to describe these conditions include "spina bifida occulta" and "spina bifida aperta." Spina bifida occulta indicates a minor defect in fusion of the laminae and lack of protrusion of spinal contents. Spina bifida aperta "cystica" indicates herniation of spinal contents and implies the presence of a myelomeningocele. The plaque-like open (not skin-covered) neural tube of myelomeningocele is called a

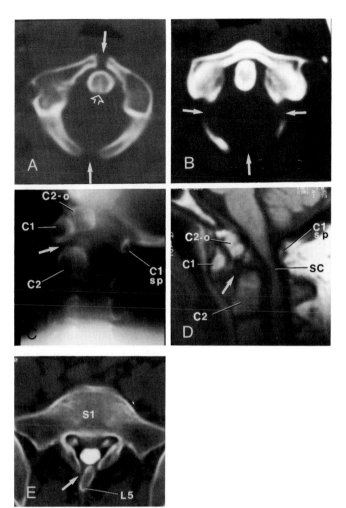

Figure 15.16   Minor fusion abnormalities. Case 1: Sagittal cleft of C1, 7-year-old male. *Axial 400/2500 CT scan* **(A).** There are clefts of the anterior and posterior C1 arch *(closed arrows).* Note the dens vertical synostosis *(open arrow)* Case 2: *Hypoplastic C1 neural arch axial 660/2000 CT scan* **(B).** There is marked lamina hypoplasia with lack of posterior fusion or of fusion to the pillars *(arrows).*
Case 3: *Midsaggital polyspiral tomogram* **(C)** *and SE 600/25 MR scan* **(D).** There is a detached *(arrows)* unstable odontoid peg (os odontoideum, *C2-o*) closely approximated to the anterior arch of the atlas *(C1).* The C1 spinous process *(C1-sp)* is hypoplastic. Note how the os-C1 complex subluxes over the C2 body on flexion during the MR scan compressing the spinal cord *(SC).* Lack of a trauma history and the associated anomaly—C1 posterior arch hypoplasia—is evidence for os odontoideum and against type-2 fracture. The dens hyperintensity, on the other hand, suggests fat-marrow replacement after a fracture. Regardless of etiology, the instability and spinal cord compression is the most important finding.
Case 4: Spina bifida occulta S1 **(E).** *Axial 577/2000 CT myelogram.* The L5 spinous process *(L5)* lies partially in S1 posterior laminar defect. The thecal sac is normal.

"placode." A skin-covered dorsal mass may be associated with spina bifida occulta and is usually a lipoma.[39]

Tethered Conus

Tethered conus is a common congenital spinal abnormality. Patients present in childhood often with muscle weakness, minor foot deformities, abnormal reflexes, pain, and bladder dysfunction. Scoliosis is common. Approximately half of these patients have

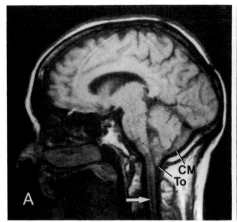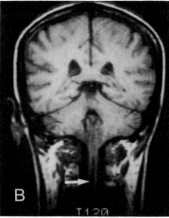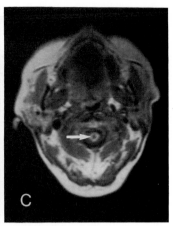

Figure 15.17. Chiari I malformation. *Sagittal* **(A)** *and coronal* **(B)** *SE 600/25 cranial and axial* **(C)** *2000/20 cervical MR scans. The pointed tonsils (To) are more than 2 mm below the foramen magnum* inferior margin. The cisterna magna *(CM)* is small and barely detectable. There is a prominent hydromyelic cavity *(closed arrows)*.

a low-back skin abnormality such as a hairy patch or subcutaneous masses.[36]

Tethered conus cases can be divided into three groups, all of which are associated with spina bifida occulta, low conus, thickened filum terminale, and enlarged thecal sac.[36,37]

The conus tip of the mildest form of the three groups is one-half to one and one-half vertebral bodies below normal and has a slightly widened filum (greater than 1.5 mm diameter).[36] The moderate degree form has a conus ending at the same level but the filum measures approximately 5 mm diameter and may contain a focal or diffuse fatty or fibrous tumor.[36]

The most severe type is associated with lack of the normal lumbar cord enlargement. Instead, the spinal cord may gradually taper into a very thick filum at about L5 or below. Alternatively the conus-filum may not taper at all remaining from 6–12 mm in diameter. A subgroup of this latter severe type of tethered conus may end in a lipoma. The lipoma almost always has a dorsal location.[36,39] Distinction of this variety and lipomyelomeningocele is difficult. The occult rather than overt spina bifida is a helpful clue.[36] An MR scan is sufficient for diagnosis and CT myelography is unnecessary. The tethered conus will be shown in this text with examples of lipomyelomeningocele and diastematomyelia (tethered "hemicords") rather than as an isolated finding.

Lipomatous Lesions (Lipoma, Lipomeningocele, and Lipomyelomeningocele)

The term "lipomyeloschisis" (dorsal dysraphism with lipoma) includes intradural lipoma, lipomeningocele (rare), and lipomyelomeningocele.[38] Lipomas of the cervical and thoracic spinal cord are rare and are usually only discovered in the adult. They are more common in males.[36]

Lipoma occurring with the tethered conus has already been discussed. Lipomeningoceles are very rare due to the usual presence of neural elements within the fatty portion.

Lipomyelomeningoceles almost always involve the lumbar spine. The patients usually have a skin-covered focal spina bifida, focal clefting of the dorsal spinal cord, and deep extension of a subcutaneous lipoma into the cleft of the tethered spinal cord. There is an associated meningocele. A cutaneous stigmata such as lipoma, dimple, dermal sinus, hypertrichosis, and hemangioma is usually present.[38,40] Lipomyelomeningocele is usually accompanied by lesser neurological symptoms than myelomeningocele. Surgery is usually aimed at release of the tethered spinal cord. MR is superior to CT although CT and CT myelography are quite accurate (Fig. 15.18).

Meningocele and Myelomeningocele

Meningocele, an enlargement of the thecal sac without inclusion of neural elements, is uncommon. Most meningoceles are midline and skin-covered. They protrude dorsally and occur in the lumbosacral region associated with spina bifida. Anterior and lateral meningoceles may also occur. Anterior meningoceles are associated with sacrococcygeal dysplasia agenesis or erosion and are more common in females. The rare anterior and lateral meningoceles usually present in the adult due to pelvic mass pressure effects. Lateral meningoceles usually protrude through enlarged midthoracic spine intervertebral neural foramina and most often occur in patients with neurofibromatosis. They may become so large as to occupy much of the thoracic cavity. Simple meningocele is not associated with the Chiari II malformations.[36] MR is the procedure of choice for meningocele investigation although CT myelography is very accurate.[36,39]

Meningomyelocele, like lipomyelomeningocele, is associated with widely spread lumbosacral laminae. Neural tissue is usually visibly exposed through a midline bone, soft tissue, and cutaneous defect.[41] The flat placode may be considered as a sagittally cleft spinal cord, the edges of which merge with the dorsal cutaneous tissue of the skin defect. Meningomyelo-

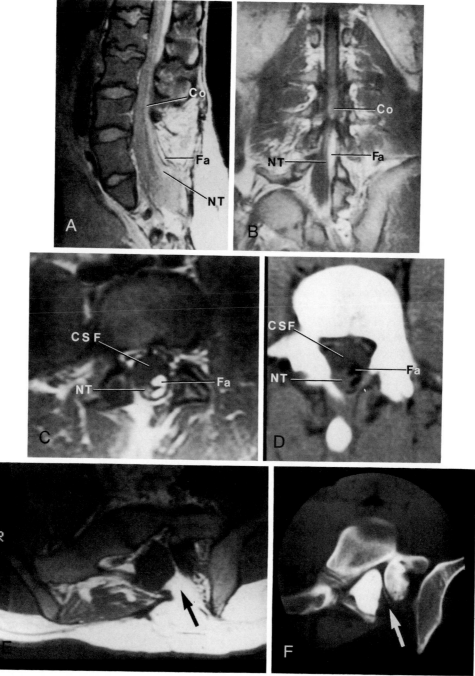

Figure 15.18.   Lipomyelomeningocele. *Sagittal SE 2000/30 **(A)** and coronal 600/25 **(B)** MR scans. Axial L5-level SE 600/25 MR **(C)** and 39/550 CT **(D)** scans. Axial top S1-level SE 600/25 MR **(E)** and same level 383/2000 CT myelogram **(F)**. A large spina bifida from L4 through the sacrum is noted. The subcutaneous lipoma is continuous (arrow)* with the intramedullary fat *(Fa)* that merges with the neural tissue *(NT)* of the lipomyelomeningocele. The conus *(Co)* is tethered. The enlarged thecal sac contains CSF. The intrathecal water, fat, and neural tissues are identifiable on all CT and MR sections of this figure.

cele is almost always associated with diverse brain anomalies, typically the Chiari II deformity.[41] The low spinal cord usually ends as a placode on the skin surface. The bifida and placode may be more cephalic, however, with a relatively normal appearing conus caudally. The dorsal nerve roots exit at the lateral edges of the placode and the ventral roots exit from the central undersurface. Due to the placode low position (tethered), the nerve roots often run horizontally or upward. Scoliosis and kyphosis are common. There is frequently associated hydromyelia and diastematomyelia.[36,39]

The imaging investigation of meningomyeloceles usually follows neonatal emergency surgery to close the defect in order to prevent infection. Imaging then documents the baseline for evaluation of associated

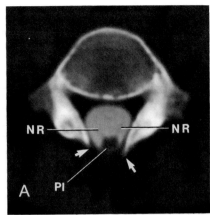
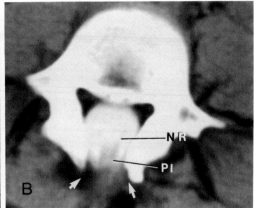

Figure 15.19. Repaired myelomeningocele. *Axial 350/1500* **(A)** *and 30/500* **(B)** *CT myelogram sections at inferior L5. The placode (PI) is attached to the surgically closed "dura" posteriorly* **(B)** *and is no longer exposed to the surface. Note the tethered ventral nerve roots (NR) arising from the placode anterior margin coursing horizontally anteriorly toward the lateral recesses. There is a moderately large spina bifida (arrows).*

malformations, tethering, hydromyelia, and hydrocephalus.[39] The initial surgery may have released the tether and thus "floated" the placode. The placode location and possible "retethering" can be evaluated on the postoperative exam (Fig. 15.19). MR is the procedure of choice due to the lack of need for intrathecal contrast, the tremendous value of orthogonal plane imaging, superior tissue discrimination, and the possible presence of additional spine and cranial anomalies amenable to MR investigation. CT myelography is very accurate, however. Postoperative follow-up will demonstrate the free placode within the repaired (closed) thecal sac (Fig. 15.19).[36,41]

Chiari II Abnormality

This subject was discussed in Chapter 9. The reader is referred to that discussion.

Diastematomyelia

Diastematomyelia is a form of spinal dysraphism characterized by a partial or complete sagittal spinal cord cleft which produces two usually asymmetrical hemicords in the lower thoracic and upper lumbar region.[36,42,43] There are two principal types of this anomaly. The first type (better known but less common) has an osseous spur separating the cord into two parts that each have their own arachnoid and dural sheath. The second type (more common) has no spur and has a split cord that lies within a single arachnoid and dural sheath.[36,39] The spur variety often has a rejoined conus caudal to the spur while the nonspur variety often does not. Tethered conus is usually found[42] and lipoma, hydromyelia,[44] and myelomeningocele, usually lipomyelomeningocele,[36] is common. Approximately 50% of cases have scoliosis. An external marker such as hypertrichosis is often present.

MR is the imaging system of choice except, perhaps, for identification of the osseous spicule. The spicule may have marrow fat and be identified by its combined bone cortex signal-void and medullary fat

MR signals. CT myelography accurately detects the lesion but lacks the "longitudinality" of the MR sagittal and coronal sections (Fig. 15.20).[39,45]

The hemicords of diastematomyelia should not be confused with diplomyelia—an extremely rare condition. Diplomyelia is a true spinal cord duplication with each duplicated cord having a central canal and two dorsal and two ventral horns with corresponding nerve root pairs. Each hemicord of diastematomyelia also has a central canal but only one dorsal and ventral horn.

Hydrosyringomyelia

The combined term hydrosyringomyelia may be used to include two somewhat unclearly differentiated conditions—hydromyelia and syringomyelia. Hydromyelia refers to the long smooth dilatation of the central canal[3] and syringomyelia refers to the more irregular often short segment cord cavity that may communicate with the central canal.[3,36] Hydromyelia is usually congenital in origin. It is characterized by cystic dilatation of the ependymal-lined central canal. It is most common in the cervical area frequently extending into the thoracic cord. It can extend along the entire cord length.[36] The usually glial-lined syringomyelia cavity may develop de novo, after trauma, and may coexist with a spinal cord tumor.[2] Hydromyelia is associated with Chiari malformations and myelomeningocele,[36] and can also be seen in diastematomyelia[44] and lipomyelomeningocele.[38] It may develop or enlarge with ventriculoperitoneal shunt malfunction.[36] The distinction between hydromyelia and syringomyelia, however, is often unclear. For example, a post-traumatic "syringomyelia," at least in large part, is a cystic dilatation of the central canal.[3]

MR is the procedure of choice for investigation of spinal cord cavities. It is more accurate than CT myelography, does not require intrathecal contrast injection, does not require repetitive delayed scans, and lacks ionizing radiation.

Heavily T1-weighted MR sagittal and coronal im-

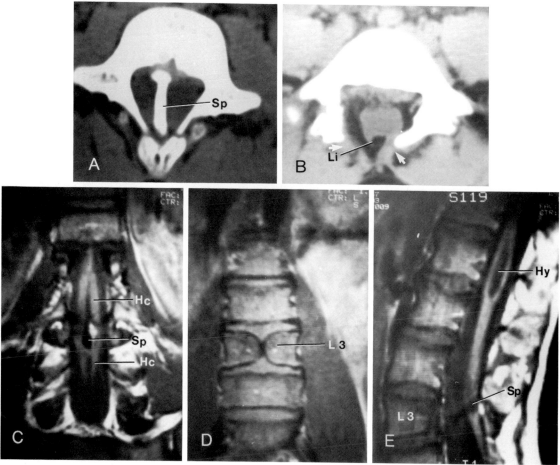

Figure 15.20.   **Diastematomyelia.** *Axial 37/450 L3-level **(A)** and L5-level **(B)** CT scans. Coronal SE 1500/25 spinal canal **(C)** and vertebral body-**(D)** level and 600/25 midsagittal **(E)** MR scans.* A CT hyperdense/MR hypointense osseous spur *(Sp)* divides the tethered spinal cord into two hemicords *(Hc)* of approximately equal size. The spur extends dorsally from the *(L3)* butterfly vertebral body to the deformed L3 spinous process. There is an MR T1 hyperintense signal adjacent to the spur probably representing fat marrow. There is hydromyelia *(Hy)*, L5 spina bifida *(arrows)*, and a lipoma *(Li)*. CT demonstrates the dorsal skin "dimple."

ages are particularly useful.[39] The characteristic MR appearance of hydromyelia is that of a central, smoothly marginated T1/T2 water-isointense tubular cavity (Figs. 15.17 and 15.21). Although myelomalacia may exhibit water-T1/T2 isointensity, it is likely that the T2 signal will be somewhat water-hypointense and heterogeneous. The clinical history and associated imaging abnormalities usually strongly suggest the correct diagnosis. It is important not to exclusively use flow-compensation sequences for spinal cord cavity investigation due to the need for the cavity CSF to contrast adequately with the surrounding cord parenchyma. Flow-compensation methods often increase CSF signal. Comparing T1-weighted MR sequences with and without flow-compensation may help confirm the cystic nature of a lesion. MR truncation artifact producing a "pseudo-syrinx" should be avoided (Fig. 15.14**H**).

Lateral cervical puncture CT intrathecal contrast injection should be avoided. CT myelography is not as accurate as MR and is more inconvenient due to dependence upon contrast entering the cavity, usually on delayed films obtained at 4, 8, and 12 hours after myelography (Fig. 15.21**B**). Central cord enhancement of myelomalacia with CT myelography is not an uncommon cause for misdiagnosis.[39] CT signs of hydromyelia include a collapsed ribbon-like spinal cord containing contrast, an enlarged cord with dilated central canal contrast, and an enlarged cord without contrast with evidence of Chiari malformation or other associated conditions.

Sacral Agenesis (Sacral Dysgenesis)

Sacral agenesis is a rare condition that falls within the category of caudal regression.[46] It occurs more frequently in children of diabetic mothers. Tethered conus and myelomeningocele are common. CT myelography (and MR) demonstrate both the dysplastic sacrum and the tethered cord (Fig. 15.22).

Teratoma

These rare tumors may be sacrococcygeal or intraspinal (intradural or intramedullary). The sacrococcygeal variety presents as a bone and soft tissue mass. The intraspinal lesion is usually associated with spina bifida occulta, has varying CT density, and usually extends over several vertebral segments.[36]

Figure 15.21. Hydromyelia. *Sagittal 40/500 cervical MR scan (A) and axial T10 CT myelogram 8-hour delay 40/500 CT (B).* There is a T1 water-intensity "stack of coins" appearance of the spinal cord cavity (A). Contrast is identified in the lower extent of the cavity in this same patient by CT (B).

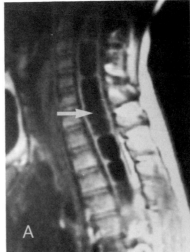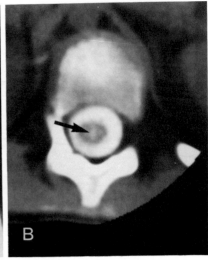

Dermoid Tumor and Dermal Sinus and Epidermoid Tumors

These tumors constitute 14% of pediatric intraspinal tumors.[36] They are also associated with spina bifida occulta. Dermoid tumors are more common in the lumbosacral spine whereas epidermoid tumors are more evenly distributed throughout the spinal canal. Dermal sinuses are seen almost exclusively with dermoid tumors in 40–50% of cases.[36] An occasional spinal epidermoid tumor results from introduction of epidermal cells into the subarachnoid space during lumbar puncture, discography, or surgery. The dermal sinus appears as a midline skin dimple that may discharge cyst contents or CSF. Dermal sinus infection may result in absence of meningitis. Chemical meningitis from dermoid cyst rupture may also oc-

cur. Masses below the conus tend to be small and those at or above the conus may be large enough to block the CSF pathways. MR and CT myelography can accurately detect the dermoid and can trace the sinus tract to the spinal cord.[36]

Neurenteric Cyst

The neurenteric cyst results from coexistence of an intestinal duplication and a cleft vertebral body with connection of the cyst through the cleft to the dura or cord. CT myelography can demonstrate the cyst, cleft, and the intradural cystic components.[36] MR should be at least as accurate.

OTHER PATHOLOGICAL CONDITIONS

The lesions under this category are neurofibromatosis, achondroplasia, osteopetrosis, osteogenesis imperfecta, and macopolysaccharidosis.

Neurofibromatosis

Neurofibromatosis or von Recklinghausen's disease is an uncommon autosomal dominant hereditary condition which often involves the spine. Spontaneous mutation may account for 50% of the cases. Resultant abnormalities include scoliosis, cervical or lumbar kyphosis, posterior vertebral body scalloping and spinal canal expansion with dural ectasia, cystic dilatation of nerve root sleeves, lateral thoracic meningoceles, schwannomas, and neurofibromas. Many of these latter abnormalities present in the young adult or later in adulthood. The neurofibromas and schwannomas are often of the "dumbbell" type—a combined intradural and extradural mass extending through the intervertebral neural foramen.[2,36]

We prefer MR as the technique for investigation of neurofibromatosis because of its tissue sensitivity, orthogonal plane imaging capability, and lack of dependence on intrathecal contrast. CT myelography is quite accurate, however. The general topic, "neurofibromatosis" is discussed in Chapter 9. Differential diagnostic considerations include Marfan's disease for

Figure 15.22. Sacral dysgenesis. Figures A and B are different cases. *Midsagittal (scoliotic patient) SE 600/20 MR scan (A). CT midsagittal reformation (B-top) of a direct coronal sacral scan (B-bottom).* The sacrum is markedly hypoplastic *(arrows).*

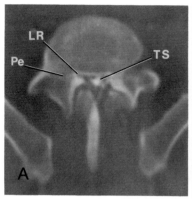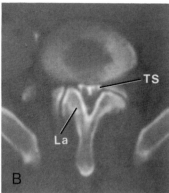

Figure 15.23. Achondroplasia. *Axial 446/4000 CT myelogram (lumbar injection) at the L5 level* **(A)** *and L5–S1 level* **(B)**. The thecal sac *(TS)* is almost obliterated with crowded nerve roots due to short thick pedicles *(Pe)* and thick laminae *(La)*. The lateral recesses *(LR)* are severely stenotic.

scoliosis and dural ectasia, idiopathic root sleeve dilatation for enlarged nerve root sleeves alone, spine nerofibroma or meningioma unassociated with neurofibromatosis and lateral meningocele unassociated with neurofibromatosis. Multiplicity of neurofibromas and plexiform neurofibromatosis confirms the diagnosis and the presence of a dumbbell intradural mass and dural ectasia is also virtual confirmation of the diagnosis. The imaging appearance of some of these conditions is discussed under the separate heading ("neurofibroma") later in this chapter.

Achondroplasia

Achondroplasia, although rare, is the most common form of dwarfism. Neurological symptoms result from compression caused by the narrow spinal canal and small foramen magnum. The stenosis is most marked in the AP diameter and is most prominent in the lumbar region. The stenosis is probably due to premature fusion of the neurocentral synchondrosis and overgrowth of periosteal bone. There may be thoracolumbar kyphosis. Disk bulges and atlantoaxial subluxation often further compromise the already stenotic condition.[2,47]

MR is the procedure of choice for initial work-up of neurologically symptomatic achondroplasia. CT may be necessary for more accurate bone detail and to distinguish bone from ligament for surgical plan-

ning.[47,48] CT myelography accurately diagnoses achondroplastic conditions but requires intrathecal contrast and lacks direct orthogonal plane imaging (Fig. 15.23).[48] If CT myelography proves to be a necessary means of investigation, caution during contrast injection is necessary due to the stenotic spinal canal and the danger of intramedullary injection if the lateral cervical approach is chosen.[48]

Osteopetrosis. Osteopetrosis may also cause severe spinal stenosis. Extreme bone hyperdensity is characteristic of this rare disorder (Fig. 15.24).

Osteogenesis Imperfecta. Osteogeneis imperfecta (Figs. 13.11 and 15.25) is associated with basilar invagination. It has already been discussed in Chapter 13.

Mucopolysaccharidosis

Mucopolysaccharidosis (MPS) is a rare group of metabolic diseases in which the patient lacks various lysosomal enzymes needed to metabolize mucopolysaccharides and their breakdown products. The mucopolysaccharides are then deposited in bone, dura, leptomeninges, cartilage, and ligaments. There are six major groups within this disease category including Hurler's syndrome (MPS-I) and Sanfillipo's syndrome (MPS-III), which are associated with severe mental retardation. Morquio's syndrome (MPS-IV) is usually not associated with mental retardation. Communicating hydrocephalus may develop due to dural and leptomeningeal thickening interfering with CSF absorption.[36,49–51]

Several of these syndromes are associated with severe vertebral abnormalities. Morquio's syndrome has the most severe vertebral abnormalities. The vertebral abnormalities of Hurler's syndrome and Maroteaux-Lamy syndrome [MPS-VI spondyloepiphyseal dysplasia (Fig. 15.26)] are less severe.

Morquio's syndrome is characterized by severe dwarfism with platyspondly. Most cases have odontoid hypoplasia, transverse ligament laxity, and atlantoaxial subluxation. Ligmental laxity contributes to the characteristic thoracolumbar kyphosis (gibbus). The already narrow spinal canal caused by pedical shortening, thick lamina, and dural thickening is further compromised by C1-2 subluxation and

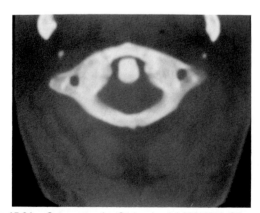

Figure 15.24. **Osteopetrosis.** *C1-level axial 393/4000 CT scan.* The atlas and odontoid peg are markedly hyperdense and the C1 spinal canal and transverse foramina are small.

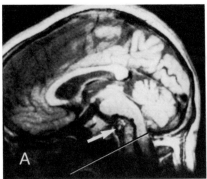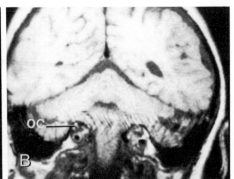

Figure 15.25. Osteogenesis imperfecta tarda. *Sagittal (A) and coronal (B) SE 700/25 MR scans.* The soft skull base is indented by the occipital condyles *(OC)* such that the odontoid peg and anterior arch of the atlas *(arrow)* markedly invaginate cephalad to (McGregor's line). Note the markedly curved medulla and intracranial uppermost cervical spinal cord.

thoracolumbar gibbus deformity with frequent development of spinal cord compression. The foramen magnum is characteristically constricted.[2,49–51]

If the purpose of imaging these patients is to evaluate spinal cord compromise, MR is the method of choice. If the purpose is to plan for a surgical procedure, CT or CT myelography may be helpful.[49,50]

LEPTOMENINGEAL AND DURAL VARIANTS OR ABNORMALITIES

Conjoined Nerve Roots

Conjoined nerve roots are nerves of adjacent levels that emerge from a common root sleeve. They commonly occur in the lower lumbar region (usually at L5-S1) and should not be confused with a herniated disk.[52] They usually separate after a short course and exit from their respective foramina but they may remain together and separate after exiting a common foramen. This latter situation has significant surgical implications.[53] Conjoined roots are more susceptible to the compressive effects of a herniated disk or lateral recess stenosis.[53]

The characteristic imaging feature is the enlarged nerve root sleeve containing two nerve pairs. There may be an enlarged lateral recess to accommodate the abnormally large root sleeve.[54]

The nonmyelographic CT findings include an enlarged water-density nerve root sleeve in a larger lateral recess of a lower lumbar interspace (Fig. 15.27). The major differential diagnostic consideration is a herniated lumbar disk, which should be disk-density (+60 to +120 H), clearly extra-axial, and unassociated with lateral recess enlargement. The presence of a unilateral enlarged combined nerve root sleeve with contralateral epidural fat and nondisplaced epidural veins by CT or MR methods establishes the diagnosis beyond a reasonable doubt. MR gradient echo or T2-weighted spin-echo techniques may demonstrate the two pairs of nerve roots within the conjoined nerve root sleeve. Myelography and CT myelography are rarely necessary.

The differential diagnosis other than herniated disk includes synovial cyst, dural ectasia, neurofibromatosis, Marfan's disease, and fat density/intensity contralateral mass producing a confusing asymmetry.

Arachnoid Cyst

Congenital spinal canal arachnoid cysts are rare lesions that may clinically present in the young and middle-aged adult with progressive spastic paraparesis. They are thin-walled CSF-filled intradural structures. Multiple cysts may be present. Arachnoid cysts are usually posterior to the spinal cord in the thoracic region. They are not associated with spina bifida.[10,36]

Although CT myelography with a 6-hour delay series can identify this lesion due to cyst content contrast, MR variable echo sequences differentiate the thin wall water-isointense cyst from the displaced spinal cord (Fig. 15.28).

Dural Ectasia

Dural ectasia may be idiopathic (Fig. 15.29) and may occur with Marfan's disease, neurofibromatosis, and with ankylosing spondylitis. Marfan's disease is

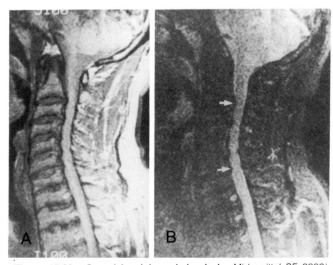

Figure 15.26. Spondyloepiphyseal dysplasia. *Midsagittal SE 2000/30 (A) and 2000/80 MR scans (B).* There is prominent platyspondyly with C2–3 *(top arrow)* to C6–7 *(bottom arrow)* stensois associated with dorsal disk bulging. There is no basilar invagination.

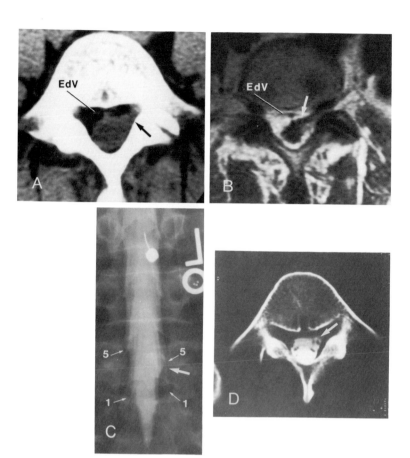

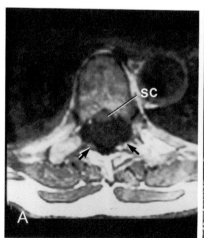

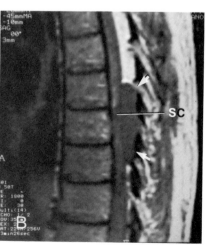

Figure 15.27.   Conjoined nerve roots. A–C and **D** are different patients. *Axial 28/350 L5-level CT scan* **(A).** *Axial L5-level* **(B)** *SE 600/25 MR scan.* AP film of conventional myelogram, same patient **(C).** Different patient, *L5-level 243/600 CT myelogram* **(D).** The L5 *(5)* and S1 *(1)* nerve roots are labeled. A large nerve root sleeve *(arrow)* at the L5 level represents combined sleeves of the L5 and S1 nerves. Instead of a right-sided corresponding nerve root sleeve, epidural fat is seen. The presence of a unilateral enlarged nerve root sleeve and of contralateral epidural fat abutting a normal smooth dural sac and of nondisplaced epidural veins *(EdV)* is definite evidence against a herniated disk. Note the two nerve root pairs in the CT myelogram of the other similar case **(D).**

an autosomal dominant hereditary condition with ocular, cardiovascular soft tissue, and skeletal manifestations. Vertebral manifestations include kyphoscoliosis, dural ectasia (Fig. 15.29), and atlantoaxial subluxation.[2,36] MR is the procedure of choice for Marfan's disease due to the combined cardiovascular (dissecting aneurysm), ocular, and skeletal manifestations. CT is quite adequate for diagnosis of dural ectasia and atlantoaxial subluxation, however.[2,36]

Pathological Conditions of the Adult Spine

Pathological conditions of the adult spine are categorized etiologically in this section. With the exception of primarily osseous abnormalities such as fractures, dislocations, Paget's disease, osteopetrosis, and sickle cell disease, MR is clearly the procedure of choice for investigation of these conditions.[3] The MR orthogonal plane imaging (particularly the sagittal

Figure 15.28.   Arachnoid cyst. *Axial T8-level* **(A)** *and sagittal* **(B)** *SE 1800/30 MR scans.* A dorsal expansile water-intensity intradural mass *(arrows)* compresses the spinal cord *(SC).*

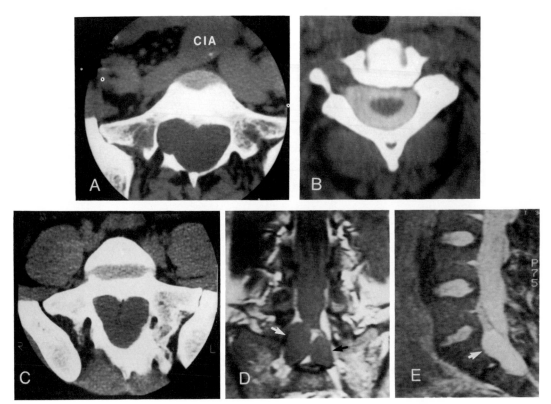

Figure 15.29. Dural ectasia. **A, B,** and **C–E** are three different patients. Case 1: *Axial L5–S1 72/300 CT scan of a patient with Marfan's disease* **(A).** Note the common iliac artery aneurysm *(CIA).* Case 2: *Axial 80/450 CT myelogram at C2–3 of a patient with idiopathic cervical dural ectasia* **(B).** There is marked enlargement of the right neural foramen. Case 3: *Axial 66/450 L5–S1 CT scan* **(C),** and co-ronal SE 1500/25 **(D)** and sagittal 1500/75 **(E)** MR scans of a patient with idiopathic dural ectasia and nerve root sleeve "cysts." CSF density/intensity and positive contrast-enhanced thecal sac and nerve root sleeve dilatation with corresponding bone erosion is present. Bone erosion is detectable by both the MR and CT method. S1 root sleeve enlargement is particularly striking *(arrows).*

image) and the accurate tissue characterization are the reasons for the MR advantage over CT. MR, as distinct from CT, directly visualizes the spinal cord and nerve roots without need for intrathecal contrast.

BULGING AND HERNIATED DISK

Bulging Lumbar Disk

A disk bulge is often encountered during the work-up of low back pain. It results from disk degeneration, subsequent diffuse perimeter bulging, and resultant annulus fibrosus stretching. A dorsal disk bulge indicates posterior bulging of the posterior longitudinal ligament. The bulge is usually symmetrical but is occasionally greater on one side.[55] The basic difference between bulging disk and herniated disk is the intact but generally stretched annulus of the bulging disk. The disk bulge is part of spondylotic process (degenerative spine disease).[55] The bulging lumbar disk narrows the spinal canal and may compress the thecal sac. Disk bulging is common past the age of 40 and it is, therefore, difficult to distinguish normal aging from symptomatic spondylosis by imaging alone in cases without markedly abnormal findings.[55] It may compromise an already stenotic canal or lateral recess.[2] It does not usually cause the discrete nerve root compression and radicular pain that results from a herniated disk.[10]

Sagittal section MR has the unique ability to image all lumbar and lower thoracic intervertebral disks. T2-weighted images demonstrate the state of disk hydration. A desiccated disk has a relatively hypointense T2 signal compared to the normal disk due to its decreased water content. The circumferential disk bulge is easily detected by sagittal and axial T1- and T2-weighted images. Due to intensity differences of CSF, disk, and neural tissue, excellent contrast is obtained (Fig. 15.30). T2-weighted images clearly identify the thecal sac displacement due to ligament, calcium, and bone cortex hypointensity compared to the T2 CSF hyperintensity. The T2-weighted image, however, lacks definition between the moderately hyperintense posterior epidural fat and thecal sac CSF. The "proton density" (long TR/short TE) image is useful because both the anterior and posterior thecal sac margins are clearly identifiable. Axial sections demonstrate the smooth posterior bulge symmetry, although sometimes with a moderate degree of eccentricity. Vacuum disk phenomenon can be identified by MR as a characteristic linear signal void that can be distinguished from the more nodular disk calcification. There is little clinical usefulness of vacuum disk phenomenon, other than an indicator of degenerative disk disease.[56] The fact that MR routinely demonstrates the conus medullaris is a distinct advantage over CT investigation of low back

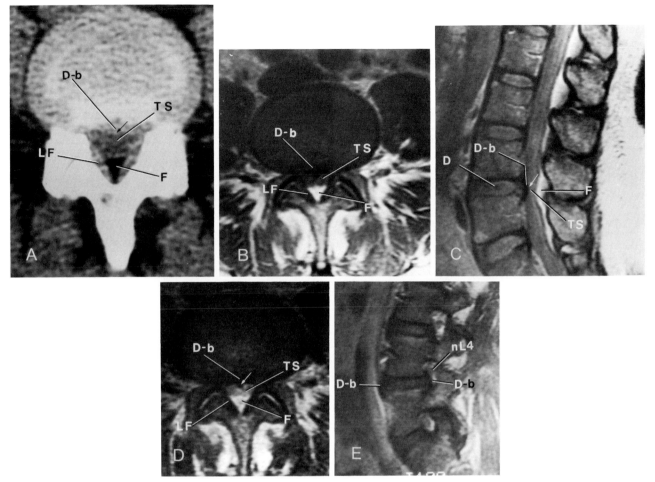

Figure 15.30. Bulging lumbar disk. *Axial 39/450 L4–5-level CT scan* **(A).** *Same level SE 2000/20 MR scan* **(B).** *Midsagittal SE 2000/20* **(C)** *and axial L4–5-level 2000/80* **(D)** *MR scans. Lateral sagittal SE 2000/ 20 MR scan* **(E).** The circumferential disk bulge *(D–b)* posterior edge is CT disk-isodense and MR disk-hypointense probably due to posterior longitudinal ligament and dural hypointensity. It has a smooth convex-posterior appearance. The thecal sac *(TS)* is symmetrically compressed by the bulging disk causing stenosis. There is a small dorsal osteophyte *(arrow)*. The posterior epidural fat window *(F)* pre-sents an unyielding barrier to the thecal sac and produces an indentation upon it **(C).** There is hypertrophy of the ligamentum flavum *(LF)*. The proton density sagittal image most clearly defines the degree of stenoses because of epidural fat and thecal sac contrasting intensities. There is L4–5 disk proton density and T2 MR signal hypointensity *(D)* caused by disk degeneration, however, the interspace height is still preserved. The L4–5 lateral disk bulge abuts the L4 nerve and dorsal root ganglion *(nL4)*.

pain. Conus compression or tumor can mimic clinical findings of herniated disk and spondylosis. Intrathecal contrast is necessary for CT conus imaging.

The CT appearance of the bulging disk is a disk-density (+60 to +120 H) smooth symmetric perimeter bulge with occasional minor eccentricity. Since the thecal sac density usually measures less than +12 H, contrast is sufficient for sharp detail. The disk bulge periphery may be markedly CT hyperdense due to calcification of Sharpey's fibers (annulus fibrosus peripheral collagenous fibers) and osteophyte formation.[2,10] The peripheral hyperdensity may also be caused by partial volume averaging of the vertebral body anterior edge. These well-contrasted structures are, in turn, sharply contrasted against the CT hypodense thecal sac CSF. Sagittal reformation and paraxial reformation (to parallel the interspace) can be very useful adjuncts to the direct axial CT scan.

CT myelography is usually unnecessary after a diagnosis of disk bulge on a quality CT scan.[2]

The major differential diagnostic consideration for bulging disk is the herniated disk. This topic will be covered next. Other diagnostic considerations include epidural metastatic tumor and abscess. A central subligamental (posterior longitudinal ligament) herniated nucleus pulposus often cannot be differentiated from a diffuse disk bulge by CT.[2]

Herniated Lumbar Disk

Herniated disks differ from disk bulges by a focal (rather than diffuse) bulging[10,55] and an annulus fibrosus tear through which the disk material herniates.[10] The extruded disk portion or fragment is almost always CT disk-density (+60 to +120 H)[2] and MR disk-isointensity.[57] The sagittal MR documentation of the dorsally extruded disk material [the

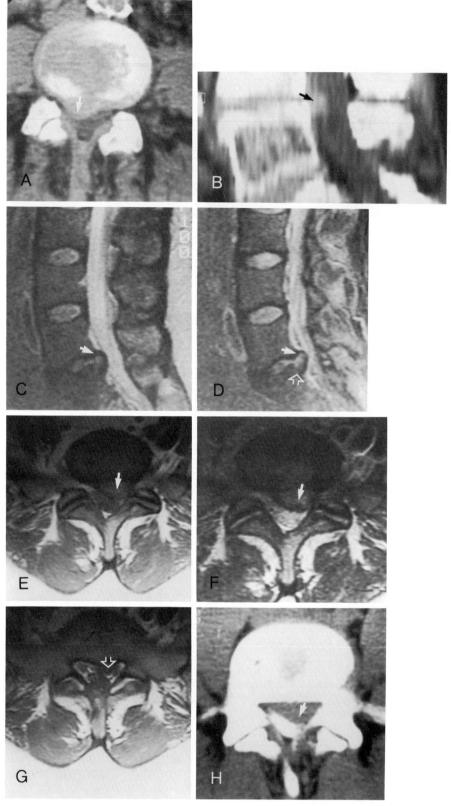

Figure 15.31. Herniated nucleus pulposus—paracentral. A–B, C–G, and **H** are different cases. Case 1: *Axial L4–5 33/400 CT scan (A) with paracentral sagittal reformation (B).* Case 2: *Midsagittal (C) and parasagittal (D) SE 2000/80 MR scans. L5–S1 level 2000/20 (E) and 2000/60 (F) and top S1-level 2000/20 (G) MR scans.* Case 3: *L4–5-level 21/450 CT myelogram (H).* The paracentral herniated disks *(closed arrows)* are disk density/intensity focal protrusions. A tooth-paste sign is seen in **C** and **D** where disk intensity material extrudes beyond the disk margins displacing nerve roots. The T2-weighted image shows better definition between the herniated disk and the thecal sac **(F).** The caudal portion of the herniated disk in case 2 *(open arrow)* is seen at the top S1 level **(G).** Although the CT myelogram demonstrates thecal sac marked edge enhancement, it offers no particular advantage over the noncontrast CT scan.

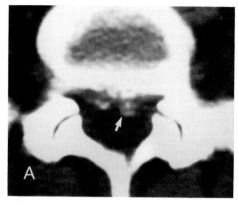

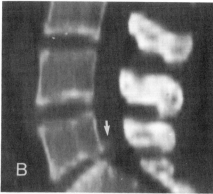

Figure 15.32. Calcified herniated nucleus pulposus. L5–S1-level axial 50/550 CT scan **(A)** and sagittal reformation **(B)**. There is a calcified central herniated nucleus pulposus *(arrows)*.

toothpaste sign (Fig. 15.31)] further adds to the MR advantage over CT for investigation of lumbar herniated disk.[57] It should be remembered, however, that CT does an accurate and credible job. CT better demonstrates calcium (Fig. 15.32) or gas [vacuum phenomenon (Fig. 15.33)].[2,10] The herniated disk portion may be continuous with the parent disk (simple herniated disk), may be separated from it (free fragment disk herniation), or may be a combination of both. The herniated disk may be contained by the strong central posterior longitudinal ligament (subligamentous herniated disk).[58] There are three major locations of clinical herniated disks: central (Fig. 15.34), paracentral "posterolateral" (Fig. 15.31), and lateral "foraminal" (Fig. 15.35). Further-lateral herniated disks are called "far-lateral." These resemble disk bulges but are discretely focal compared to the diffusely circumferential bulges. The posterior longitudinal ligament is thinner and weaker laterally, which explains the common occurrence of herniation through the ligament at the posterolateral and foraminal location.[2] The subligamentous herniated disk appears as a smoothly marginated focal bulge (Fig. 15.34).

The simple paracentral or "posterolateral" herniated disk remains attached to the parent disk and may or may not have ruptured through the posterior longitudinal ligament.[10] The subligamentous herniated disk appears as a smoothly marginated prominent bulge which is usually in a posterolateral location but may be central. The "toothpaste sign," lesion size, and focal character help distinguish the subligamentous herniated disk from a disk bulge. The free fragment herniated disk is completely separate from the parent disk and is extraligamentous (Fig. 15.36). It can migrate upward or downward usually stopping at the pedicle level[59] and produce nerve root compression above or below the parent disk level. A far distant herniated fragment is called a sequestered herniated disk. It may be associated with fibrosis and can mimic an intradural tumor. Both the extraligamentous simple and free fragment disks often have an irregular polypoid or angular contour as compared to the smooth contour of the subligamentous variety. Compressed nerve roots often become enlarged or swollen.[2]

Paracentral "posterolateral" disk herniation usu-

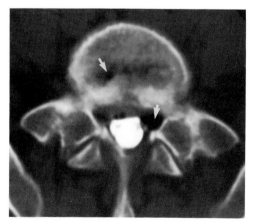

Figure 15.33. Gas-containing "vacuum" herniated nucleus pulposus. Top S1-level axial 421/2000 CT myelogram. There is gas-density in the desiccated intervertebral disk and in the S1 left lateral recess *(arrows)*. There is a corresponding thecal sac deformity.

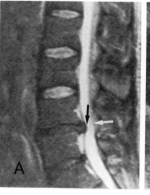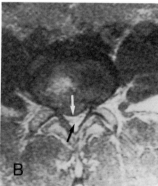

Figure 15.34. Central L4–5 and L5–S1 herniated nucleus pulposus. *Midsagittal (A) and axial L4–5-level (B) SE 2000/100 MR scans.* The L4–5 and L5–S1 interspaces are narrowed and the T2 disk signal is hypointense. There is a moderately large toothpaste sign L4–5 herniated disk and a smaller disk herniation at L5–S1. The herniated disks appear to abut a thin hypointense line probably representing the displaced dura. There is L4–5 stenosis demonstrated best on the axial section where the herniated disk anteriorly and the posterior fat identify the markedly compressed dural sac *(arrows)*. The brighter axial posterior fat signal is due to its proximity to the surface coil. The L4–5 herniated disk was subligamentous at surgery.

Figure 15.35. Lateral and far-lateral herniated nucleus pulposus. **A** and **B–D** are different cases. *Axial L4–5-level 60/450 CT myelogram* **(A)**. *Axial L4–5* **(B)** *and right-sided sagittal 2000/30* **(C** *and* **D)** *MR scans.* **D** is lateral to **C**. A lateral and far-lateral herniated disk in each case is present, characterized by a focal bulge of disk density/intensity *(arrows),* which compromises the intervertebral neural foramina *(NF).* Note that the herniated disk abuts the fourth lumbar nerve *(nL4)* in **D**. A paracentral herniated disk at L4–5 would displace the fifth lumbar nerve. These two cases demonstrate the difficulty of classifying the lateral and far-lateral types. A combination of both types is present in each case.

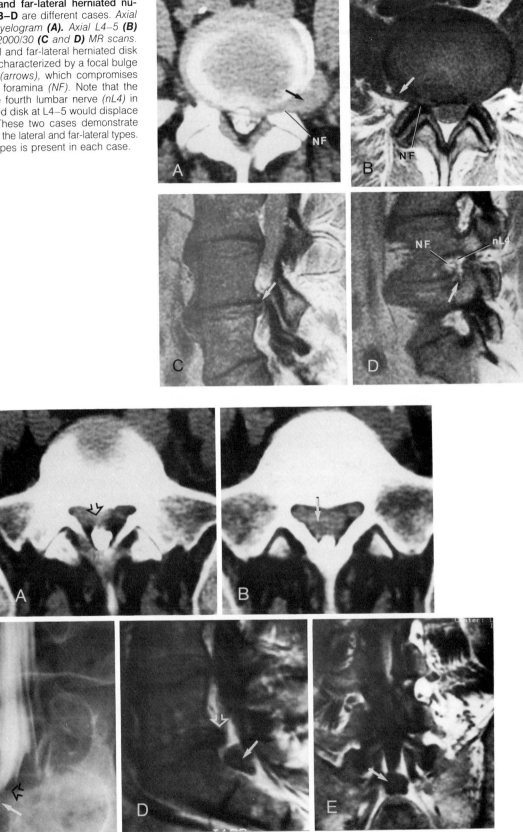

Figure 15.36. **Migrated herniated disk fragment.** *Axial L5–S1-level* **(A)** *and top-S1-level* **(B)** *49/500 CT myelogram. Oblique conventional lumbar myelogram* **(C)**. *Sagittal* **(D)** *and coronal* **(E)** *SE 1500/ 25 MR scans.* A right paracentral herniated disk *(open arrow)* appears separate **(D)** from a large disk-CT density/MR intensity inferior fragment *(closed arrows).*

ally protrudes into the lateral recess and compresses the thecal sac and nerve root sleeves. The lateral "foraminal" herniated disk protrudes into the intervertebral neural foramen. Lateral lumbar disk herniation may not produce a myelographic defect because the nerve root sleeve ends close to the dorsal root ganglion and the disk extrusion is remote from the thecal sac.[60] Although the lateral herniated disk may not compress the nerve root sleeve or thecal sac, it is likely to compress the intraforaminal nerves. For this reason, the lateral herniated disk produces the same radicular symptoms that a paracentral herniated disk would at the adjacent interspace above.[15] Both CT and MR accurately demonstrate lateral disk herniation.

The most common location for lumbar disk herniation is paracentral. Lateral and central herniations are less common.[2] Greater than 90% of lumbar herniated disks occur at L4–5 or L5-S1. L3–4 is the next most common level. L2–3 and L1–2 herniated disks are quite rare.[55] Rarely, an intradural disk herniation may occur.[61,62] Herniation of nuclear material through a vertebral endplate produces a radiological "Schmorl's node." This "internal herniation" causes a characteristic CT smoothly marginated hypodensity with a sclerotic rim (Fig. 15.37). MR findings are often revealing of the pathological process. The sagittal sequence demonstrates the herniated nuclear materal eroding through the endplate into the cancellous bone.

MR demonstrates three types of vertebral endplate changes associated with lumbar herniated disks. These changes are characterized by abnormal T1 and T2 superior or inferior vertebral body water, fat, or calcium intensities. This topic will be discussed later in this chapter with spondylotic disease.[63]

Recurrence of low back pain after laminectomy and diskectomy ("failed back surgery syndrome") can be caused by recurrent herniated disk and/or extradural scar. Other causes include spondylosis, spondylitis, arachnoiditis, and spondylolisthesis. Since reoperation and removal of scar tissue often leads to a poor clinical result and removal of recurrent herniated disk often leads to a good result, the imaging goal is to distinguish recurrent herniated disk from epidural fibrosis.[64] Myelography is inaccurate in making this distinction. High-dose i.v. contrast injection lumbar CT may demonstrate rim-contrast enhancement surrounding a recurrent herniated disk (Fig. 15.38A and B) and homogeneous contrast enhancement of epidural fibrosis ("scar").[55,65] Unfortunately, results of contrast-enhanced studies can be equivocal and may not be reliable.[30,59,66] MR may be more effective than CT for distinguishing recurrent herniated disk from epidural scar, particularly with i.v. MR contrast injection.[30,64] Scanning should commence immediately after i.v. injection of MR contrast material due to the rapid scar and slow herniated disk contrast uptake.[64] Recurrent herniated disk and epidural scar frequently coexist (Fig. 15.38E and F). Early homogeneous uptake is typical of scar (Fig. 15.38G and H) and lack of early uptake is typ-

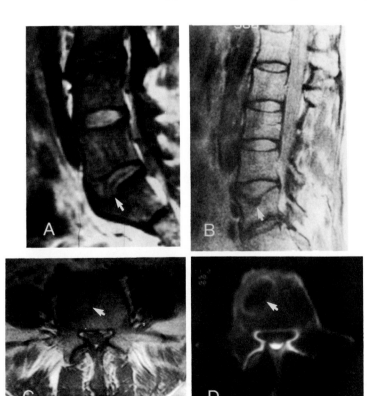

Figure 15.37. Schmorl's nodes. A and **B–D** are different cases. Case 1: *Sagittal SE 1500/40 MR scan.* Case 2: *Sagittal SE 2000/30* **(B)** *and axial 2000/20* **(C)** *MR scans. Axial 723/2000 CT myelogram.* Herniated disk material erodes into or through the vertebral endplate producing a smoothly marginated disk MR-isointense/CT-isodense lesion with an MR T1-hypointense/CT-hyperdense rim *(arrows).*

Figure 15.38. Investigation for recurrent herniated lumbar disk. A–B and **C–H** are different cases. Both are recurrent left paracentral herniated disks with associated epidural scars. *L5–S1 level 50/400 CT myelogram **(A)** and i.v. contrast **(B)** CT scan. Left-sided sagittal SE 2000/ 30 **(C)** and 2000/80 **(D)** flow-compensation MR scans. Axial L5–S1 level SE 600/25 precontrast **(E)** and post-i.v. Gd-DTPA **(F)** MR scans. Same axial techniques, respectively, at top S1 level **(G–H)**.* Contrast-enhanced scar *(closed arrow)* and herniated L5–S1 noncontrast-enhanced herniated disks *(open arrows)* are identified. Herniated disk mass effect is evidenced by left S1 nerve *(nS1)* and dural sac *(DS)* displacement **(B** and **F)**. Note how the enhanced scar in **H** has the appearance of normal fat-surrounding nondisplaced structures. There is a prominent toothpaste sign with extrusion of disk-intensity material **(C–D)**. Laminectomy defects are seen in both cases and there is obvious left gluteal atrophy in case 2.

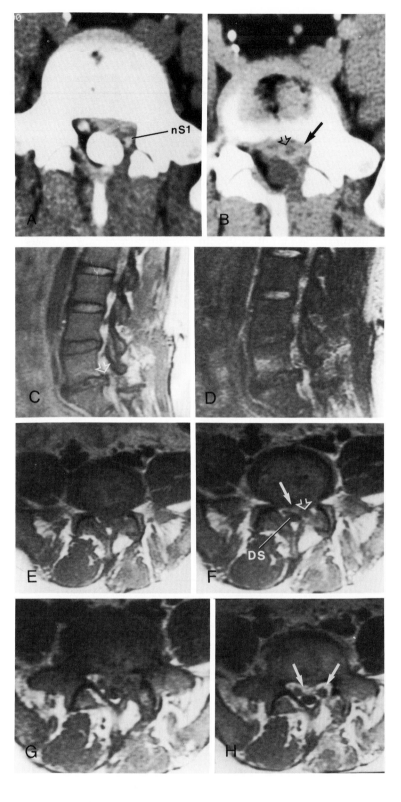

ical of a herniated disk. The MR sagittal image is particularly helpful to identify the toothpaste sign (Fig. 15.28C and **D**). If on sagittal and axial sections disk intensity material extrudes from the disk and displaces the dura, nerve roots, or epidural veins, it represents evidence of a herniated disk rather than

epidural scar formation. Epidural scar is not usually associated with mass effect and it is usually T1 hypointense.[64]

A herniated disk may spontaneously regress. It has been suggested that after conservative therapy for herniated lumbar disk, patients whose symptoms have ameliorated or totally remitted may no longer have a detectable herniation.

After a very brief initial period of enthusiasm, the use of chymopapain chemonucleolysis has markedly decreased. CT on long-term follow-up (5–6 months) often shows decreased size of the herniation and may show vacuum disk phenomenon.[67] Follow-up MR shows decreased disk height, decreased size of the herniated disk, and decreased T2 disk signal.[68] Chemical nucleolysis has lost popularity due to the higher than expected frequency of complications including anaphylaxis, subarachnoid hemorrhage, infection, and transverse myelitis.[69] Currently, much attention has been focused on percutaneous diskectomy as an alternative to open surgery.[69]

The major differential diagnostic consideration for herniated lumbar disk is a bulging disk. The focal character of the herniated disk and the contour irregularity of the free-fragment type are CT and MR distinguishing features. The MR toothpaste sign[57] is very reliable. The lack of diffuse disk bulge of the particular disk involved further supports the impression of herniated disk versus asymmetric disk bulge. Other diagnostic considerations include conjoined nerve roots, diskitis, intradural-extradural dumbbell tumors, metastasis, and synovial cyst. Conjoined nerve roots demonstrate preserved lateral recess epidural fat, low-density/water-intensity CSF of the conjoined root sleeve and root sleeve asymmetry of the thecal sac. MR and CT myelography demonstrate two root pairs within the conjoined nerve root sleeve.[2,10,55]

There is lack of epidural vein displacement with conjoined nerve roots.

Herniated Thoracic Disk

Thoracic herniated disks occur uncommonly. They may be more common than had originally been thought now that MR imaging is available. Most thoracic herniated disks occur in the mid and lower thoracic spine. The spinal canal is smallest in the midthoracic region and the thoracic kyphosis apposes the thoracic spinal cord anteriorly (Fig. 15.7). These two characteristics (narrow canal and anterior cord) contribute to thoracic herniated disk symptomatology caused by even small disk protrusions.[2,10,55]

Conventional myelography, often with lateral complex motion conventional tomography, followed by CT myelography at the appropriate spine level, was the previous method that we had used before MR for identification of a thoracic herniated disk or other thoracic level abnormality. The spinal cord cannot, as a rule, be identified by CT without intrathecal contrast. Either MR or myelography followed by CT myelography is necessary to identify small nonobstructing ventral lesions in the thoracic spine.[2,55,70] MR has become our preferred standard approach to thoracic spine investigation. Both MR and CT myelography can identify compression, displacement, and deformity of the spinal cord (Fig. 15.39).[2,10,55,70] The usual thoracic herniated disk is central or paracentral. Herniated thoracic disk MR and CT characteristics parallel those of lumbar disk herniation with

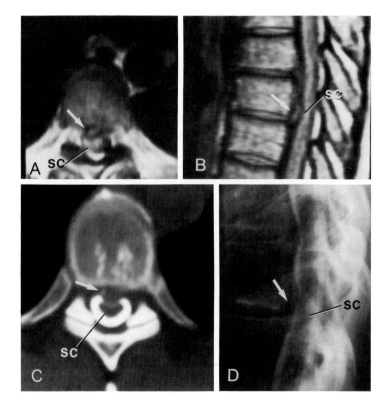

Figure 15.39.   Thoracic herniated disk T8–9. *Axial **(A)** and sagittal **(B)** SE 1500/25 MR scans. Axial 348/2000 CT myelogram **(C)** and lateral conventional myelogram **(D).** A partially calcified T8–9 extruded disk (arrows) compresses the dural sac and deforms the spinal cord (SC). The herniated disk is MR proton density-isointense and CT disk-hypodense. Note the disk calcification.*

the exception that the spinal canal is of smaller caliber, the involved structure is the spinal cord rather than the cauda equina and there is a less apparent toothpaste sign. Thoracic disks and thoracic disk herniations are frequently calcified.[2,10,70] Noncontrast CT may be required to identify a heavily calcified ("hard") extruded thoracic disk in order to plan the surgical approach. Differential diagnosis includes thoracic osteophyte, which is contiguous with the posterior vertebral body periosteum.[2] More laterally positioned extradural-type masses include dumbbell neurofibromas. Metastasis and diskitis can also be considered.

Herniated Cervical Disk

Most cervical herniated disks occur at the C5–6 and C6–7 levels. Cervical disk herniation above C4–5 is very unusual. As with lumbar herniated disks, most cervical herniated disks are degenerative. Some, however, are the result of acute trauma. There is a paucity of cervical epidural fat and the cervical thecal sac occupies most of the spinal canal. There is considerable variability concerning "normal" average sagittal diameter measurements of the cervical spinal canal. Figures vary from 11.7–14.8 mm.[71,72] There is fairly good agreement, however, that a cervical spinal canal less than 10 mm wide in the sagittal diameter is narrow. The canal can be considered to be stenotic if it measures 9 mm or less in the sagittal diameter and it is severely stenotic if the measurement is 7 mm or less.[2,72] The average spinal cord sagittal diameter at C4-T1 measures approximately 7 mm.[14] Minor degrees of disk protrusion and herniation in patients with narrow canals may, therefore, produce symptomatic nerve root and/or spinal cord compression.[55,71] The presence of anteroposterior spinal cord compression with spinal cord flattening in a relatively wide canal in the coronal dimension may be asymptomatic, however, these patients are more susceptible to traumatic spinal cord injury.[71,72] Nerve root swelling and displacement and intervertebral neural foraminal occlusion reliably correlate to patient symptoms.[72] MR evidence of cervical disk degeneration, disk herniation, spinal cord compression or nerve root compression may or may not be clinically symptomatic, however.[30,73]

CT, MR, and myelography with CT myelography (Figs. 15.40 and 15.41) are all accepted methods of cervical investigation. Plain, thin (1.5-mm) cervical CT and i.v. contrast CT scans may reliably demonstrate a herniated cervical disk, on occasion, but is not a sensitive method compared to MR.

Intravenous contrast injection CT enhances the foraminal epidural and intervertebral foraminal veins (Fig. 15.10). Venous displacement helps document disk herniation and nerve root compression.[25] We have not found the noncontrast or the i.v. contrast method reliable or cost-effective. We still perform water-soluble contrast cervical myelography followed by CT myelography at the level of interest for selected patients that do not have definite MR findings. Thinner

sections (as thin as 1 mm) and oblique imaging planes are necessary to produce the degree of reliability necessary to match that of myelography and CT myelography.[55] Improvements in 3-D imaging, surface coil technology, and sequences are now available. We currently use 3-D technique to obtain T2-weighted 1-mm thickness axial and sagittal sections and our early results are very promising. Paramagnetic i.v. MR contrast increases the conspicuity of extradural cervical masses and may prove to be an accepted technique for cervical herniated disk investigation.[30,74] Noncontrast CT may still be required for surgical planning in order to distinguish "hard" from "soft" disks and for improved bone detail.

Differential diagnostic considerations for cervical herniated disk or disk bulge includes hypertrophic facet and uncinate process spurs, dumbbell neurofibroma, and metastasis.

DEGENERATIVE DISEASES OF THE SPINE, "SPONDYLOSIS," AND ACQUIRED STENOSIS

Degenerative disk disease contributes to segmental instability, disk degeneration and resorption, loss of intervertebral height, marginal vertebral body osteophyte formation, and annulus fibrosus and ligamental laxity. Facet joint degenerative changes result from, and add to, joint capsular weakness, laxity, and instability. Facet osteophyte formation and laminar and ligamental hypertrophy develop. Forward (spondylolisthesis) and backward (retrolisthesis) subluxation, vacuum disk and facet phenomenon, spinal canal and lateral recess stenosis (acquired stenosis) result. These various processes interplay in the development of progressive degenerative changes and are often responsible for back pain.[2,5,6,10,74,75]

Both CT and MR demonstrate this group of degenerative abnormalities (Fig. 15.42). We feel that MR is more versatile but that CT is certainly adequate. MR advantages include direct sagittal[6] and sagittal oblique (foraminal)[74] imaging and superior soft tissue analysis.

MR directly detects abnormal disk signal on the T2-weighted image and can detect vacuum disk phenomenon. CT detects vacuum disk phenomenon and disk calcification better, however, this latter information is of questionable clinical value. Both the CT and MR methods accurately detect bulging disk and osteophyte formation. Disk calcification is most frequently seen associated with degenerative spine disease. It can rarely be seen in hypervitaminosis D and ochronosis.[2]

Although CT cortical bone detail is clearly superior to MR, both CT and MR can accurately detect foraminal compromise and facet hypertrophy. MR has the advantage of direct sagittal visualization of foraminal nerve compression and displacement.[6] CT reliably demonstrates vacuum facet phenomenon while MR does not. Laminar and ligamentum flavum hypertrophy are well documented by both CT and MR. Recognition of the ligamentum flavum is aided by T1-weighted intermediate signal intensity.[6] Liga-

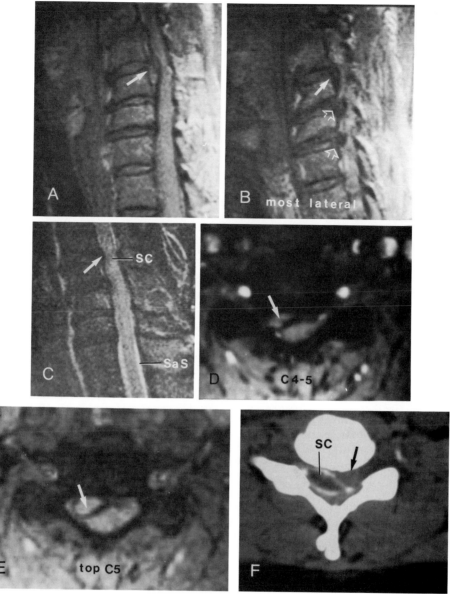

Figure 15.40. C4–5 HNP with spondylosis and spinal stenosis. A–E and **F** are different cases. *Right-sided sagittal SE 2000/30 (A and B) and midsagittal 2000/100 (C) MR scans. Axial C4–5 (D) and top C5 (E) gradient recalled echo 50/17 30° tip-angle MR scans. Different case, axial C5–6 28/350 CT myelogram (F).* The herniated C4–5 disk protrudes posteriorly and caudally *(closed arrows)* with a toothpaste sign **(A)**. It overlaps the C5 vertebral body and fills the C5 lateral recess. There is C5–7 interspace narrowing and generalized cervical disk T2 hypointensity. C5–6 and C6–7 osteophytes project into the intervertebral neural foramina *(open arrows)* on the

most lateral sagittal section. Spinal stenosis is seen as evidenced by the herniated hypointense disk midsagittal component obliterating the subarachnoid space *(SaS)* on the midsagittal T2-weighted image. The GRE axial images demonstrate extruded disk hyperintensity within a hypointense rim differing from the proton density sagittal image **(A)** demonstrating extruded disk isointensity. The spinal cord *(SC)* is displaced in the second case. Although the CT myelogram has excellent edge definition, the same information is clear on the MR scan.

mentum flavum calcification (reliably detected by CT and not MR) may be normal unless adjacent laterally to the apophyseal joint.[10]

Lumbar degenerative spondylolisthesis usually occurs at L4–5, and is usually grade I ($< -25\%$ slippage of L4 over L5). Retrolisthesis occurs commonly in the cervical and lumbar regions.[5] The MR direct sagittal image and the third generation CT localizer image demonstrate the degree of spondylolisthesis.

Axial sections demonstrate apophyseal joint overriding. Spondylolysis is not caused by degenerative disease and will be discussed later in this section.

Acquired spinal stenosis can affect the spinal canal, lateral recesses, or neural foramina. Spinal canal stenosis is caused by disk bulging and also by laminar, ligamentum flavum, and facet hypertrophy. Even a minor degree of acquired stenotic change in a patient with a congenitally narrow spinal canal can

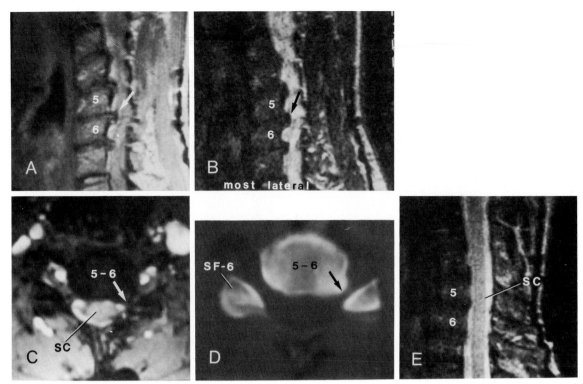

Figure 15.41. Cervical spondylosis with C5–6 disk herniation and foraminal stenosis. *Left sagittal 2000/30* **(A)** *and further lateral 2000/80* **(B)**. *MR scans. Axial C5–6 50/17 30° tip-angle GRE MR scan* **(C)** *and 300/1500 CT scan* **(D)**. *Midsagittal SE 2000/80 MR scan* **(E)**. There is a herniated C5–6 disk **(A)** with associated uncinate process hyperostosis producing foraminal stenosis *(arrows)*. Except for **A**, which demonstrates a toothpaste sign, the disk herniation and osteophytosis is difficult to differentiate. Foraminal stenosis is seen in **B–D**. There is no spinal cord *(SC)* compression and no spinal canal stenosis although a slight central C5–6 bulge is noted on the midsagittal section; the C6 superior facet *(SF–6)*.

produce severe stenosis. The stenotic lumbar spinal canal axial section assumes a characteristic exaggerated trefoil appearance (Fig. 15.42). There is a basic impracticality using the sagittal lumbar spinal canal measurement of 11.5 mm[11] as evidence of stenosis because of the inclusion of the posterior interlaminar fat pad. Since the fat paid is unyielding and varies in size, direct sagittal measurement of the thecal sac is more practical. Sacs smaller than 10 mm sagittal diameter are considered stenotic.

Since the average sagittal diameter of the C4-T1 spinal cord is approximately 7 mm and from C2 to C4 it is approximately 8 mm, a cervical spinal canal sagittal diameter of 7 mm or less is severely stenotic often resulting in cord compression and deformity.[14,72] The above statement seems particularly evident due to the fact that the ligamentum flavum and epidural soft tissues occupy some of this scarce space. The degree of cross-sectional cervical spinal cord deformity usually correlates with clinical symptomatology.[14] Other measurements have been described but we do not find them useful for evaluation of acquired stenosis. In general, crowded lumbar nerve roots or cervical spinal cord compression and deformity within a markedly narrowed spinal canal with a locally obliterated subarachnoid space is sufficient for diagnosis.[2,5,6,10] Lumbar lateral recess and foraminal stenosis is caused in large part by superior facet hypertrophy with a significant contribution from posterior disk bulging.

Pathological changes in cervical spondylosis, like lumbar spondylosis, include facet, laminar, and ligamental hypertrophy associated with degenerative disk disease and osteophytosis (Fig. 15.43). In addition, uncinate joint degenerative changes and osteophytosis add to the cervical spondylotic neural foraminal compromise. These spondylotic changes often superimpose upon a pre-existing congenitally narrow cervical spinal canal similar to spondylotic lumbar changes. Cervical spondylosis occurs at all levels but is most prevalent from C4 through C7. Sometimes a distinction of terms refers to "cervical spondylosis" as disk-vertebral body degenerative changes and "osteoarthritis" as apophyseal joint changes. The latter distinction will not be used here. Coexistence of cervical herniated disk disease with spinal stenosis and of cervical spondylosis with spondylolisthesis and retrolisthesis frequently occurs. MR distinction of "soft" disk herniation from osteophyte (Figs. 15.40, 15.41, and 15.43) can be difficult on the basis of calcific or "soft tissue" signal alone due to fat marrow content of some osteophytes.

The cervical toothpaste sign is as important to cervical herniated disk diagnosis as it is to diagnosis of

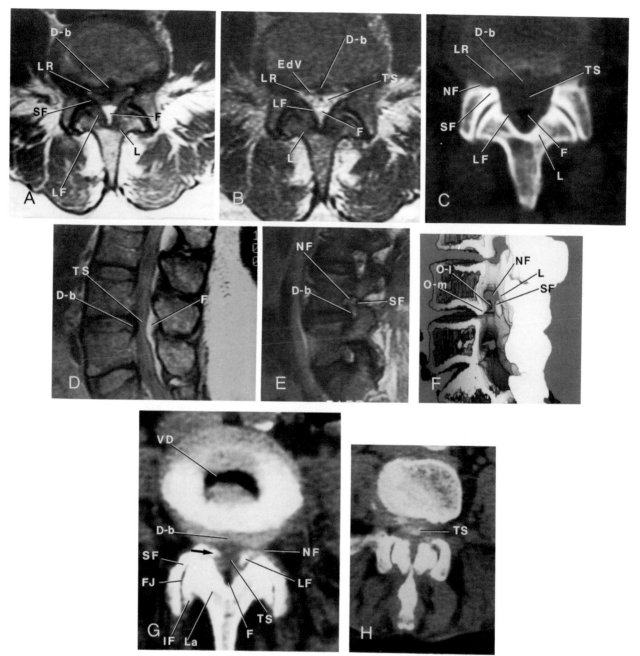

Figure 15.42.   Lumbar spondylosis and spinal stenosis. A–E, F, G, and **H** are different cases. *Axial L4–5-level presaturation technique SE 2000/30* **(A)** *and 2000/60* **(B)** *MR scans and 325/2000 CT scan* **(C)**. *Midsagittal* **(D)** *and lateral sagittal* **(E)** *SE 2000/30 flow-compensation technique MR scans. Sagittal 3-D reformation of 3-mm CT sections* **(F)**. *Axial 34/450 L3-4-level CT scan* **(G)** *and 50/500 bottom-L4 CT myelogram of another patient* **(H)**. Case 1 **(A–E):** Same case as Figure 15.30. There is a disk bulge *(D–b),* ligamentum flavum *(LF)* hypertrophy, superior facet *(SF)* hypertrophy, and thick laminae *(L)*. There is resultant stenosis of the thecal sac *(TS)* and the lateral recesses *(LR)*. The intervertebral neural foramen *(NF)* is stenosed by the combined bulging disk and superior facet hypertrophy **(E)**. The posterior epidural fat window *(F)* presents an unyielding barrier to the thecal sac causing dorsal compression **(D)**. The disk bulge displaces the epidural veins *(EdV)*. Case 2: **F.** The L4

body posterior-inferior midline osteophyte *(O–m)* and laminar hypertrophy *(L)* compromises the central spinal canal. The lateral vertebral body osteophyte *(O–l)* combined with superior facet hypertrophy *(SF)* compromises the neural foramen *(NF)*. The same process is seen at the L5–S1 neural foramen. Compare to **D** and **E.** Case 3: **G.** Neural foramen *(NF)* and thecal sac *(TS)* stenosis results from a disk bulge *(D–b),* superior facet *(SF),* ligamentum flavum *(LF),* and laminar *(La)* hypertrophy. The combined superior facet hypertrophy and ligamentum flavum calcification *(LF)* produces a right-sided spur *(arrow)* projecting into the spinal canal. There is vacuum disk phenomenon *(VD)* and inferior facet *(IF)* spurring and degenerative facet joint *(FJ)* changes. The unyielding posterior epidural fat *(F)* and the posterior disk margin define the stenotic thecal sac sagittal diameter. Case 4: **H.** The CT myelogram demonstrates marked stenosis of the thecal sac *(TS)*.

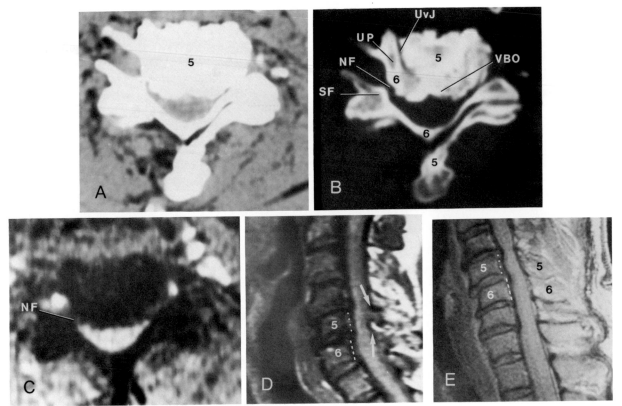

Figure 15.43. Cervical spondylosis. **A–D** and **E** are different cases. Case 1: *Axial C5–6 20/450 (A) and 327/2000 (B) CT scans and GRE 21/12 30° tip-angle MR scan (C). Midsagittal 2000/30 256 × 128 matrix without flow-compensating technique (D).* There is marked uncinate process *(UP)*, superior facet *(SF)* and vertebral body *(VBO)* hypertrophic thickening and osteophyte formation, producing neural foraminal *(NF)* and spinal canal stenosis. There is slight retrolisthesis of C5 *(dots)* over C6 *(dashes)*. Narrowing and irregularity of the uncovertebral joints *(UvJ)* is seen. *Arrows* indicate flow artifact from the pulsating CSF. Lack of detail on the sagittal section is due to flow and Gibbs artifact (256 × 128 matrix). Case 2: *Midsagittal SE 2000/30 256 × 256 matrix flow-compensation MR scan (E).* C5–6 spondylolisthesis and C4–5 and C6–7 interspace narrowing is clearly identified on this more recent MR scan **(E).**

lumbar disk disease. The cervical herniated disk may also have a typical appearance, as in Fig 15.40, establishing the imaging diagnosis.

Less commonly, severe posterior longitudinal ligament ossification ("OPLL") causes or contributes to spinal stenosis (Fig. 15.44).[74] Paget's disease may also

cause profound spinal stenosis and will be discussed later in this chapter.

Spinal cord cystic necrosis and/or myelomalacia may occur as a result of spinal cord compression.[76] MR detection of a cyst and/or abnormal spinal cord signal identifies this complication.[74] CT delayed mye-

Figure 15.44. Posterior longitudinal ligament ossification (OPLL) vs. diffuse idiopathic skeletal hyperostosis (DISH). Lateral cervical spine x-ray **(A)** and C5-level axial 371/2000 CT scan **(B).** Hypertrophic ossification of the posterior longitudinal ligament *(closed arrow)* causes stenosis of the cervical spinal canal. Marked anterior osteophyte bridging with anterior longitudinal ligament involvement is present *(open arrows).* Posteriorly, there is calcification of the ligamentum flavum. Although the predominant feature is the massive posterior longitudinal ligament ossification (OPLL), the other ligamental ossification and calcification raises the possibility of diffuse idiopathic skeletal hyperostosis (DISH).

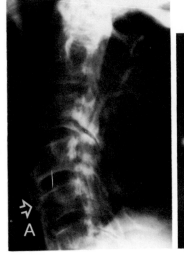
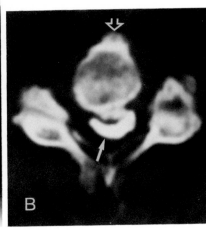

lography for contrast entrance into the cyst or area of myelomalacia is less dependable and less practical. Spinal cord cysts will be discussed later in this chapter.

At the present time, we often resort to cervical myelography for the investigation of cervical radicular pain when the MR scan is not clearly diagnostic. CT myelography for additional investigation at a particular level is often used. This method produces excellent bone and soft tissue detail (Fig. 15.40). Sagittal reformation is unnecessary due to the conventional myelogram lateral projection. The neck hyperextension used in cervical myelography exaggerates stenosis because of ligamentum flavum bulging. We expect that MR will increasingly replace the cervical myelography-CT myelography technique when recent technical MR advances become routinely employed.[30,74,75]

MR demonstrates two types of vertebral endplate changes associated with degenerative disk disease (Fig. 15.45). Abnormal vertebral body T1 and T2 water or fat signals adjacent to the apposing endplates frequently occurs in spondylotic regions.[63] Vertebral body fat deposits, some of which are remote from the endplates, have been described as age and physical stress related. These common fat deposits have a tendency to occur in the concavity of kyphotic and scoliotic spines. They range in size from 5–15 mm and should not be confused with focal pathological processes.[4] The fat-type lesions change over the course of 1–3 years and tend to convert to the water-type lesions and the water-type lesions tend to remain stable chronologically.[63] The association of the fat MR signal abnormalities with degenerative disk MR changes and their limitation to apposing surfaces helps to exclude other conditions associated with vertebral fat signal such as aging, hemangioma, osteoporosis, radiation changes, and central

focal yellow marrow. The water-type signal abnormality may require intravenous contrast injection in order to exclude an active case of osteomyelitis.[63]

A markedly destructive noninfectious form of spondyloarthropathy may occur in long-term hemodialysis patients (Fig. 15.46). Because these changes resemble septic spondylitis in a sepsis-prone population, biopsy be may necessary to exclude an infectious cause.[77]

Synovial cysts uncommonly occur adjacent to a degenerative facet joint, usually at L4-5. They probably result from synovium herniating through joint capsule tears. They appear as a CT hypodense, MR water-isointense cystic epidural mass at the facet joint often displacing the nerve root and dural sac (Fig. 15.47). They may calcify and they do not contrast enhance. Spondylosis is virtually always present. The facet joint location and cystic character differentiate these lesions from the herniated disk.[78] A continuation of the cyst and the facet joint may occasionally be identified by MR and CT may rarely document an air-filled synovial cyst continuous with a "vacuum facet" (Fig. 15.47).

Herniated nucleus pulposis is the major differential diagnostic consideration. Conjoined nerve roots should also be considered. Continuity of the lesion and the joint, cyst water-density/intensity, and joint rather than disk location should exclude all herniated disks except a rare water-density/intensity disk fragment. Conjoined roots can be excluded by lack of an enlarged asymmetrical root sleeve, normal number of root sleeve nerve roots, and a normal-size lateral recess.

CONGENITAL SPINAL STENOSIS

Patients with congenitally narrow spinal canals have short thick pedicles, thick laminae, large facets, and disproportionately vertically elongated neural

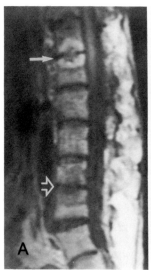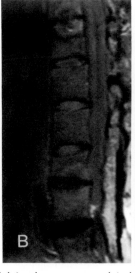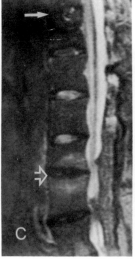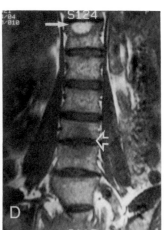

Figure 15.45. Disk and vertebral endplate changes asssociated with spondylosis. *Sagittal SE 600/25* **(A)**, *SE 2000/30* **(B)**, *and 2000/ 80* **(C)** *and coronal SE 600/25* **(D)** *MR scans.* There is T2 disk hypointensity from T11-L1 and from L3–5 with L3–5 intervertebral disk

space narrowing. There is an L3 wedge-compression deformity. Opposing T11–12 vertebral endplate and adjacent vertebral body fat signal *(closed arrows)* and L3–4 vertebral endplate and adjacent vertebral body water signal *(open arrows)* is present.

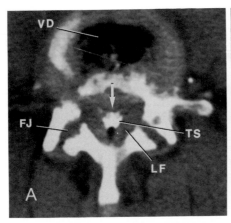
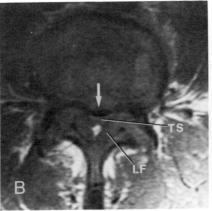
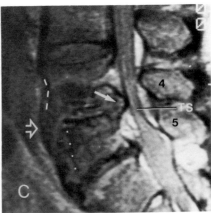

Figure 15.46. Spondyloarthropathy associated with long-term dialysis. *L4–5 axial 500/34 CT scan* **(A)** *and SE 2000/30 MR scan* **(B)**. *Midsagittal SE 2000/30 MR scan* **(C)**. The CT scan demonstrates marked vacuum disk phenomenon *(VD)* facet joint erosion *(FJ)* and ligamentum flavum hypertrophy *(LF)*. There is anterior subluxation of L4 *(dashes)* over L5 *(dots)* and profound anterior osteophyte bridging *(open arrow)*. There is a large central herniated disk *(closed arrows)* and marked stenosis of the thecal sac *(TS)*.

foramina (Fig. 15.48). The normal progressively widened lumbar interpedicular distance from L1–5 is absent. The lack of spondylotic changes in these patients differentiates the congenital from the acquired form of stenosis. These patients are highly susceptible to further canalicular or foraminal encroachment. They usually clinically present in early adulthood.[2] Abnormally small spinal canal measurements include lumbar AP diameters of less than 11.5 mm, L4–5 interpedicular diameters of less than 16 mm and cross-sectional areas less than 1.45 cm.[2] We have found that a lower lumbar thecal sac sagittal diameter of less than 10 mm can be considered stenotic. Both MR and CT accurately detect congenital spinal stenosis.

SPONDYLOLYSIS

Spondylolysis is a traumatic and/or developmental defect of the pars interarticularis. It is the most common neural arch defect. It usually involves the L5 pars interarticularis. Approximately 50% of spondylolysis patients develop spondylolisthesis. The L5-S1 level spondylolisthesis is a distinguishing feature compared to degenerative spondylolisthesis that usually occurs at L4–5. It usually begins in early adulthood and is associated with secondary degenerative changes due to the unstable articulation. The process is usually bilateral.[79]

Plain lumbar lateral oblique x-rays and complex motion tomography easily establish the diagnosis. Often the CT lateral localizer identifies the defect. CT accurately identifies the pars defect on axial scans 10–15 mm cephalad to the disk plane.[79] A contiguous CT axial series of sections is necessary in order to identify the articular facets so that the pars defect cannot be confused with degenerative facets (Fig. 15.49). An abnormal atretic pars can occasionally be identified.[79] Sagittal planar and 3-D CT reformations may be helpful for surgical planning but unnecessary for diagnosis. MR can also identify the

defect[3,75] on axial, sagittal, and coronal images. The spinal canal sagittal diameter will appear enlarged on axial views in patients with spondylolisthesis.[79]

SCOLIOSIS

Scoliosis is usually of the primary idiopathic type that commonly occurs in female adolescents. It can be associated with neurofibromatosis, Marfan's disease, neuromuscular disorders, and spinal cord tumors.[2,80] Scoliosis also occurs with congenital anomalies such as tethered cord, Chiari malformations, syringomyelia, meningomyelocele, and diastematomyelia.[80]

The MR advantages over CT for evaluation of scoliosis include direct coronal images and superior soft tissue evaluation for identification of the spinal cord and tumors. CT disadvantages include "skewed" axial sections, the need to resort to intrathecal contrast for spinal cord imaging, and lack of direct orthogonal plane imaging. We have found multiplanar reformatted CT helpful (Fig. 15.13G) but prefer MR for scoliosis evaluation. Patients with muscular dystrophy and polio may have scoliosis and will also demonstrate lower paraspinal muscle atrophy detectable by both CT and MR techniques. The presence of profound muscle group replacement by fat should differentiate these cases from idiopathic scoliosis.[81] Paraspinal masses and posterior vertebral scalloping favor the diagnosis of neurofibromatosis. Dural ectasia with aortic aneurysm favors the diagnosis of Marfan's disease. Focal fat deposits commonly occur adjacent to the vertebral endplates along the curve concavity.[4,63]

TRAUMA

The role of noncontrast CT and of CT myelography for investigation of spine trauma has been well established.[2,10] MR investigation of subacute and chronic spine injury has now gained general acceptance.[82,83] The initial difficulty of managing acutely ill patients dependent on life-support systems and electronic monitors deep within an intense magnetic field is now

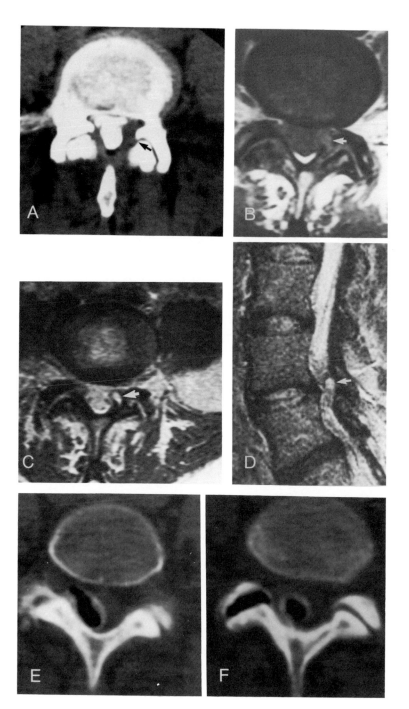

Figure 15.47. Synovial cyst. **A, B–D,** and **E–F** are different cases. Cases 1 and 2: *Axial L4–5 30/550 CT myelogram **(A)** and SE 2000/30 **(B)** and 2000/80 **(C)** MR scans. Left sagittal 2000/80 flow-compensation MR scan **(D)**.* A water-CT density/MR intensity smooth, round, small epidural mass is centered at the facet joint *(arrows)*. It indents the dural sac and displaces the left fifth lumbar root. The T1 proton density image **(B)** demonstrates continuation of the cyst and interfacet joint space. Case 3: *Axial 383/2000 CT scans at the cranial **(E)** and caudal **(F)** L4–5 level.* A "vacuum facet" is continuous with a gas-containing synovial cyst. There is marked right-sided facet degenerative change.

being overcome. The recent development of "hybrid" magnets (permanent magnets with resistive coils) markedly diminishes the fringe field and permits the use of patient supportive equipment within a mid-strength magnet. Advantages of MR in spine trauma include the orthogonal plane visualization of the spinal cord and nerves and the thecal sac without the need for intrathecal contrast injection. Early assessment of spinal cord edema and hemorrhage, cord compression, and laceration is possible. Although MR bone detail is inferior to CT, the relationships of the vertebral bodies and posterior elements and intervertebral disks are well demonstrated (Fig. 15.50).[3,82] Until an MR system becomes available at our hospital that does not interfere with life-support and monitoring equipment or until better MR-compatible equipment becomes available, we will continue to depend upon CT and, occasionally, CT myelography in acute spine trauma patients.

This section on spine trauma will discuss spinal injuries regionally. The section will therefore be divided into cervical spine injuries; thoracic, thoraco-

Figure 15.48. Congenital spinal stenosis. **A, B–C,** and **D–E** are different young adults with similar findings. *Axial L3–4 41/300 CT scan* ***(A)***. *Axial 396/2000 L4–5* ***(B)*** *and superior L5-level* ***(C)*** *CT myelogram. SE 2000/30 axial* ***(D)*** *and foraminal-level sagittal* ***(E)*** *MR scans. All cases have short pedicles (Pe), thick laminae (La), hypertrophied ligamentum flavum (LF), large superior facets (SF), and bulging disks (D–b) causing stenosis of the dural sac (DS), neural foramina (NF), and lateral recesses (LR). There is a vacuum facet phenomenon (arrow) and superior facet hypertrophy in* ***B*** *and* ***C***. *The ligamentum flavum in* ***D*** *and* ***E*** *is probably calcified, accounting for its hypointensity.* ***D*** *and* ***E*** *also demonstrate the sagittally stenotic and coronally tall neural foramina due to the short pedicles.*

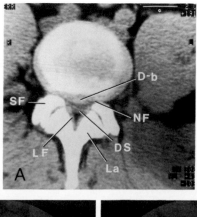

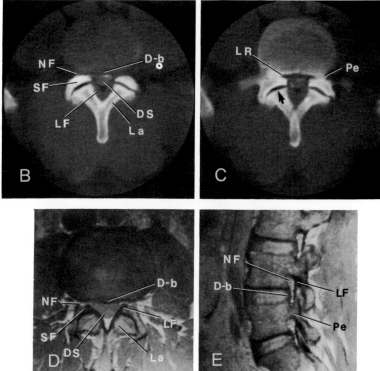

lumbar, and lumbar injuries; and penetrating injuries. A summary will conclude the spine trauma section.

Cervical Spine Injuries

One of the most important rules of spine trauma investigation (particularly cervical spine) is to analyze the total area of investigation. Following this rule, a study for cervical spine trauma includes the foramen magnum through T1.

Atlanto-occipital dislocations are usually fatal injuries. Patients with atlanto-occipital dislocations may survive, however. Hopefully, this injury will be detected on the emergency room cervical cross-table x-ray before any neck manipulation. The CT lateral localizer and the MR sagittal sequence will demonstrate a laminar line offset and an abnormal relationship of the dens to the clivus basion. Dislocation may be either anterior or posterior. Axial sections will demonstrate an abnormal occipital condylar position with respect to the atlas. Sagittal reformation of multiple thin CT sections may be helpful. Sagittal MR would be ideal. Some authors have proposed measurement of lines as a method of diagnosis. A large retropharyngeal hematoma is common.[84]

"Bursting" or "Jefferson" atlas fractures are best imaged by CT but can also be recognized by MR. The fracture is produced by vertical compression of the atlas between the occipital condyles and the axis pillars. These fractures are usually through two locations of the ring often isolating a lateral mass (Fig. 15.51).[2,10] They may be unilateral, however.[85] Those fractures involving only the posterior arch are stable.[10] Jefferson fractures occur only rarely in preadolescence but cases are referred for CT scans due to "atlas pseudospread"—the normal C1 lateral mass slight overlap of C2 on plain x-ray open-mouth views seen in children from 3 months to 4 years of age.[86] The

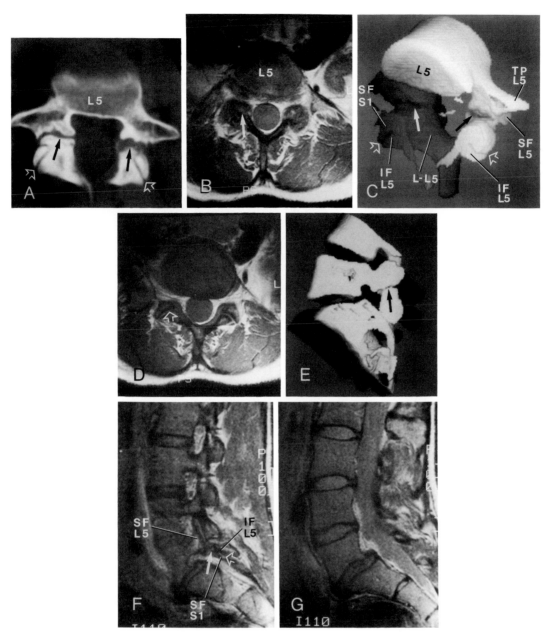

Figure 15.49. Spondylolysis and spondylolisthesis. All images are the same case. *Axial L5-level 362/2000 CT scan (A) and SE 2000/30 MR scan (B).* Three-dimensional reformation of oblique axial view from below with "removal" of the posterior half of the L5 body **(C).** *Axial L5-level SE 2000/30 MR scan caudal to B (D).* Lateral 3-D view **(E).** *Sagittal SE 2000/30 lateral (F) and midline (G) MR sections.* There are bilateral pars interarticularis defects *(closed arrows)* between the L5 superior (SF–L5) and inferior (IF–L5) facets. Identification of the L5 lamina *(L–L5)* and the S1 superior facet *(SF–S1)* excludes the possibility that the defect is a degenerative facet joint. The L5–S1 facet joint is identified *(open arrows);* TP = transverse process. There is grade I spondylolisthesis **(G)** and increased spinal canal sagittal diameter **(A).**

documentation of an intact ring excludes fracture.[86] The unfused C1 anterior and posterior ring synchondroses should not be confused with fractures (Fig. 15.16).

Atlantoaxillary rotary subluxation occasionally occurs after trauma of minimal to moderate degree or, sometimes, upper respiratory infection with resultant C1–2 rotational malalignment and persistent torticollis. Axial CT can demonstrate the rotational malalignment and, often, a characteristic increased distance between the C1 anterior arch and the dens. The nonreducible atlantoaxillary rotation is called atlantoaxillary fixation. Fixation requires treatment including collar or halo traction and occasional fusion.[87] The CT technique we use includes thick (1-cm) overlapping (5-mm) sections from the foramen magnum through C2 in neutral, head-rotated-right and head-rotated-left position angled parallel to C1 (Fig. 15.52).[2]

Cervical fractures with spinal cord injury most

Figure 15.50.   C5 fracture with spinal cord contusion and transsection-flexion injury. *Axial C5-level 300/1500 CT scan* **(A)** *and GRE 75/17 10° tip-angle MR scan* **(B).** *Midsagittal reformation of contiguous CT scans* **(C)** *and midsagittal SE 2000/80 256 × 128 4 NEX MR scan* **(D).** There is a comminuted C5 body, pedicle, and laminar fracture. A large retropulsed fragment *(closed arrow)* compresses and contuses the spinal cord *(SC) (open arrow).* Note how the spinal cord definition is obliterated and replaced with hyperintense signal. There is interspinous ligament hyperintensity **(D).** Cord transsection was found surgically. The double parallel hypointense spinal cord signal is due to Gibb's phenomenon.

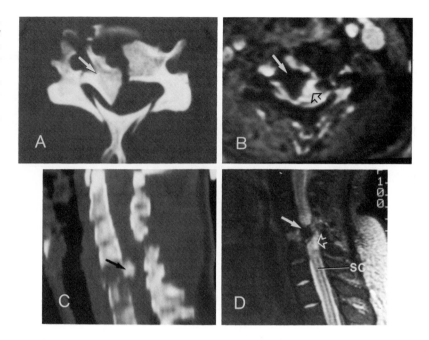

commonly occur at C4–7. Fractures at C1–2 are unlikely to be associated with spinal cord injury. Pedicle fractures are less stable than lamina fractures due to the loss of support function of the lateral mass.[2] MR is expected to be the examination of choice once the limitations for emergency use are overcome. This is because of the unique ability of the MR system to visualize spinal cord abnormalities, such as hemorrhage, edema, displacement and transsection, directly. CT may still be required for cervical fracture bone detail. Major vertebral body fractures, subluxation, and facet lock and ligamental tears are routinely recognized by MR.[35,82]

Traumatic spondylolisthesis of the axis (hangman's fracture) is usually a result of hyperextension injury. It is characterized by bilateral pedicle fractures and C2–3 spondylolisthesis. The dens and the transverse ligament are intact. This unstable fracture is usually not associated with spinal cord injury but cord injury may occur (Fig. 15.53C and D). The

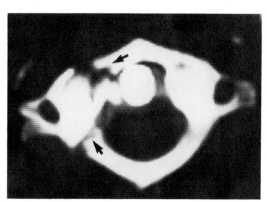

Figure 15.51.   Bursting atlas fracture, "Jefferson fracture," 82/200 CT scan. The right C1 lateral mass is isolated by two fractures *(arrows)* and rotated counterclockwise.

CT localizer film and axial sections usually suffice for diagnosis. Sagittal reformation CT may be helpful. MR has the advantage of soft tissue discrimination and direct sagittal imaging; and the disadvantage of cortical bone insensitivity.

C2 fractures have been categorized as types I, II and III. Fractures dividing the dens (type I) or at the base of the dens (type II) can be difficult to identify by CT due to the axial fracture plane. Those C2 fractures involving the C2 body (type III) are more easily recognized by CT (Fig. 15.53A and B).[82] MR, however, can identify the fracture on sagittal images. MR also identifies the spinal cord position and signal and can identify a spinal cord contusion or an epidural hematoma. Of course, review of conventional plain films or the CT or MR localizer view can identify the dens fracture.

Simple wedge compression fractures result from flexion injuries. They are easily recognized on CT lateral localizer, CT sagittal reformation, and sagittal MR images (Fig. 15.54). Axial CT may demonstrate fracture lines or simply a subtle density change.[2]

The flexion-teardrop fracture dislocation usually occurs at C4–6 and is the result of combined hyperflexion and axial compression which occurs in diving accidents, vehicular accidents, and falls. More than one body is frequently fractured. This fracture is very unstable due to pedicle involvement and ligament disruption. Vertebral body comminution results in an increased vertebral body sagittal diameter. Fragment retropulsion causes spinal canal compromise. Epidural hematoma may further compromise the spinal canal. Quadraparesis commonly occurs. Axial CT and CT myelography with sagittal, coronal, and 3-D reformation (Fig. 15.54) has proven to be accurate and useful for evaluation of spinal canal integ-

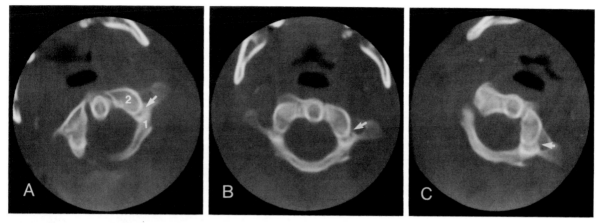

Figure 15.52.   Rotary subluxation. *Axial C1–2-level 10-mm thickness 30/3000 head rotation right **(A)**, neutral **(B)**, and left **(C)**.* There is a fixed rotation (rotary subluxation) of C1 over C2 such that the C2 and C1 lateral mass relationships *(arrows)* are unchanged with head-body positional change.

rity and spinal cord displacement, swelling, or transsection.[2,88] CT cannot reliably detect spinal cord hemorrhage. CT, however, can occasionally detect spinal epidural hematomas.[89] MR accurately assesses the spinal canal, spinal cord, ligaments, and can detect major fracture deformities and subluxation (Fig. 15.50). Spinal cord contusion and intraspinal (Fig. 15.54) and epidural hemorrhage (Fig. 15.55) are routinely recognized by MR. Spinal cord edema produces water-signal isointensity (Figs. 15.50, 15.53, 15.54, 15.56). Spinal cord hemorrhage (hematomyelia) is associated with a poor prognosis and, in this sense, MR is a good prognosticator of recovery.[35]

Ligamental injury is also well documented by MR (Fig. 15.54) and can only be inferred by CT. Axial CT is clearly superior for spine fracture detail, however, MR sagittal bone detail is usually better than CT sagittal reformation (Fig. 15.57) and MR soft tissue and vascular detail is vastly superior to CT (Fig. 15.57). At this stage of development, CT and MR are alternative and complementary methods of spine trauma investigation.[35,82,,90,91]

Facet dislocation may be either unilateral or bilateral resulting in neck rotation and/or subluxation. It is often, if not usually, associated with articular pillar fracture. Unilateral dislocations result from flex-

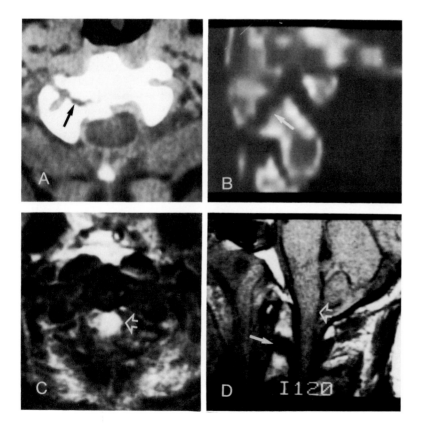

Figure 15.53.   C2 fracture dislocation—Hangman's fracture. A–B and **C–D** are different cases. *Axial C2-level 39/300 CT scan **(A)** and right paracentral sagittal reformation CT scan **(B)**. Axial C2-level SE 1500/100 **(C)** and midsagittal 700/25 **(D)** MR scans.* C2 body-pedicle fractures *(closed arrows)* are seen to better advantage by CT, however, a medullary-cervical spine contusion is identified by MR *(open arrows)*. It is characterized by spinal cord T2 hyperintensity **(C)** and T1-isointense medulla-cervical spinal cord expansion.

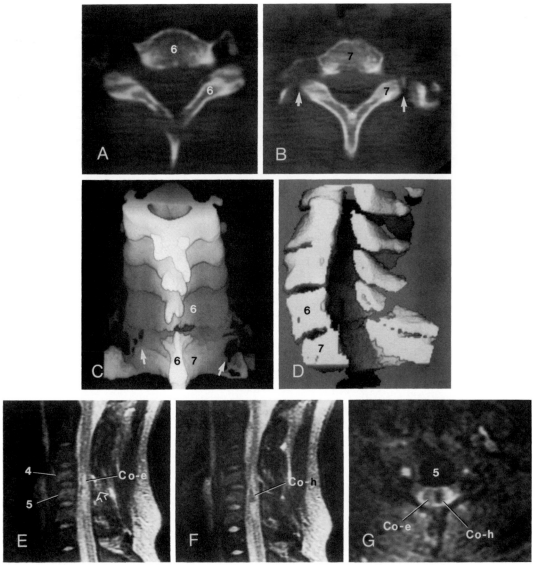

Figure 15.54. Midcervical flexion injuries. A–D and **E–G** are different cases. Case 1: Flexion C6 and C7 fracture-subluxation "teardrop fracture." *Axial C6-level (A) and C7-level (B) 449/2000 CT scans.* Three-dimensional reformation view from behind **(C)** and from a mid-sagittal perspective **(D).** There is C6–7 subluxation with comminuted C7 wedge compression, C7 pedicle fractures *(arrows),* and a C6 spinous process fracture. Case 2: C4–5 flexion fracture deformity with spinal cord contusion. *Right parasagittal (E) and left parasagittal (F) SE 2000/80 MR scans. C5 axial GRE 75/17 10· tip-angle MR scan (G).* There is a C5 slight compression fracture deformity and C4–6 slight T2-signal hyperintensity. A spinal cord contusion *(Co)* has left-sided T2-signal hypointensity *(Co-h)* probably representing deoxyhemoglobin or intracellular methemoglobin. There is right-sided T2 hyperintensity representing probable edema (Co-e). Gibb's artifact produces spinal cord parallel hypointense margins due to the 256 × 128 matrix. Note how the T2* effect of GRE imaging exaggerates deoxyhemoglobin hypointensity. Interspinous ligament T2-signal hyperintensity *(open arrow)* supports a diagnosis of ligament disruption.

ion-rotational injuries and are usually stable. Bilateral dislocations result from flexion injuries and are associated with ligament disruption and instability and cervical cord damage. Degrees of dislocation vary from facet distraction to facet perch (Fig. 15.57) and facet lock (Fig. 15.58).[2,10,92]

The CT technique for demonstration of facet dislocation is unique. Thin (3-mm or 1.5-mm) sections parallel to the facet interspace are necessary (Fig. 15.58). Sagittal reformation through the articular pillars is helpful in absence of sagittal MR scans or

sagittal complex motion tomography. CT detects most associated fractures. MR can detect the facet dislocation but posterior element fractures may be missed due to MR lack of cortical detail.[2,92]

CT of facet distraction demonstrates an abnormally increased interfacet distance. Articular pillar fractures may be misinterpreted as a facet joint (Fig. 15.54). Facet dislocation or "lock" demonstrates the flat (articular) posterior border of the superior facet posterior to the rounded posterior border of the inferior facet (Fig. 15.58). Associated articular pillar

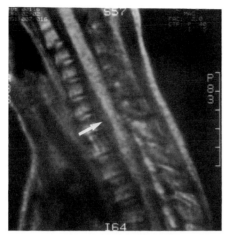

Figure 15.55.   Cervicothoracic epidural hematoma. *Midsagittal SE 1000/30 MR scan.* A CSF-isointense biconvex anterior epidural mass *(arrow)* compresses and posteriorly displaces the spinal cord.

fractures and distracted uncovertebral joints are also readily identified.[2,92]

The clay shoveler's fracture can also be recognized by the CT or MR method. It is a stable fracture of a cervical spinous process, usually C7. The spinous process fracture is commonly associated with more severe cervical injuries (Fig. 15.54).[2]

Traumatic dural tears may occur due to avulsion or a penetrating wound. A dural tear (dural laceration) may also be caused by a piercing bone fragment. The resulting tears may trap nerve roots and may also increase the risk of meningitis. The latter two sequellae to dural tears represent indications for surgical correction. Nerve root avulsion occurs due to a stretching injury, usually to an upper extremity and often produces motor and sensory paralysis ("flail-arm"). The same type of stretching injury may be unassociated with nerve avulsion but may be associated with neurological deficit due to nerve root trapping in the dural laceration.[93]

CT myelography demonstrates expanded nerve root sleeves in avulsion injuries, identifies the site of CSF extravasation into the soft tissues, and can identify pseudomeningoceles (Fig. 15.59).[2,93] MR can identify the expanded nerve root sleeves and meningomyeloceles in orthogonal views (principally axial and coronal planes) but lacks the dynamic information (flow, extravasation, communication) of the CT myelographic technique.[94]

Traumatic cervical disk herniation is an uncommon occurrence with trauma and should be included (or suspected) in the differential diagnosis of an interspace-centered anterior or anterolateral epidural mass that has CT or MR characteristics compatible with herniated disk.[95]

Post-traumatic cervical spinal sequellae include spinal cord cystic necrosis, noncystic myelomalacia, and spinal cord atrophy. A post-traumatic spinal cord cyst can be responsible for progressive myelopathy in a previously stable patient. Large cysts are responsive to shunting, thereby representing an important indication for diagnostic investigation.[96] CT myelography cannot accurately distinguish between the contrast enhancement of noncystic myelomalacia and post-traumatic spinal cord cyst (Fig. 15.60). MR distinguishes the noncystic from cystic lesion by demonstrating T1- and T2-weighted water-isointense signal.[83] Spinal cord atrophy may be quite profound on post-traumatic MR and CT myelographic studies (Fig. 15.60).

MR is superior, in general, to CT for work-up of the post-traumatic cervical spine injury patients. In addition to detection of cystic and noncystic post-traumatic myelomalacia, it can detect subluxation and facet lock, evaluate for herniated disk and spinal stenosis, and exclude various postoperative complications. If a broken fracture fixation wire-induced dural tear is suspected, CT myelography is necessary to demonstrate the site of leakage.[97]

Thoracic, Thoracolumbar, and Lumbar Spine Injuries

Fractures of the thoracic and lumbar spine are more common at the thoracolumbar junction partially because the thoracolumbar facet joint orientation approaches the sagittal plane whereas the more cranial

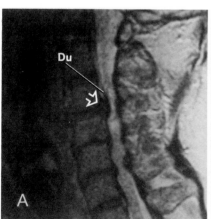

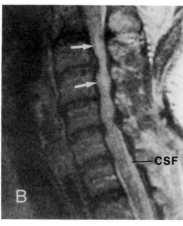

Figure 15.56.   Cervical HNP with spinal cord contusion after trauma. Sagittal SE 2000/80 flow-compensation parasagittal **(A)** and midsagittal **(B)** MR scans. There is a stenotic spinal canal and a C3–4 herniated disk with dural *(Du)* displacement *(open arrow)*. There is T2-signal hyperintensity of the compressed spinal cord *(closed arrows)*. The subarachnoid space *(CSF)* surrounding the spinal cord is obliterated from C2–6 by the stenotic spinal canal.

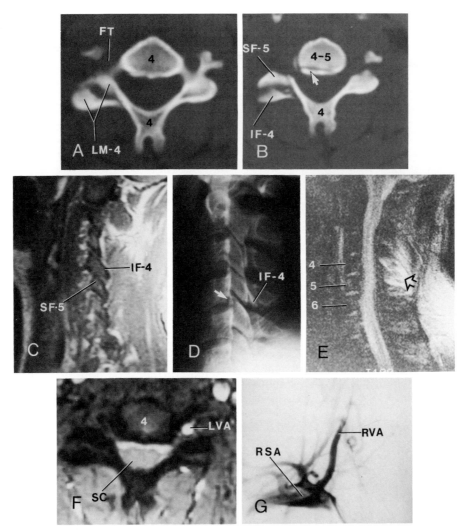

Figure 15.57. Cervical lateral mass and body fracture with perched facets, C5–6 retrolisthesis, and vertebral artery occlusion. *Axial 390/ 2000 CT scan at C4 (A) and C4–5 CT scan (B). Right sagittal SE 600/25 MR scan (C). Lateral conventional x-ray (D). Midsagittal SE 2000/100 MR scan (E). Axial GRE 50/17 30° tip-angle MR scan (F). Digital subtraction right subclavian arteriogram (G).* There are C4 lateral mass *(LM-4)* and posterior-inferior body *(closed arrow)* frac- tures. There is perching of the C4 inferior facet *(IF–4)* anteriorly over the C5 superior facet *(SF–5)*. Occlusion of the right vertebral artery *(RVA) is seen angiographically and by MR due to absent signal intensity. Compare to the left vertebral artery (LVA) on the gradient reversal axial sequence.* C5–6 retrolisthesis is present. There is interspinous ligamental edema *(open arrow)*. No definite foramen transversarium *(FT)* fracture is identified.

thoracic facet joint orientation approaches the coronal plane. The costotransverse and costovertebral articulations further protect and stabilize the thoracic spine. Fractures of the midthoracic spine do occur, however, after severe trauma. The mid-dorsal and thoracolumbar fractures are often associated with spinal cord injury.[2] CT best demonstrates bone fracture deformities in the axial plane and MR identifies neural tissue, ligaments, and gross bone abnormalities. MR is expected to become the study of choice for these injuries with CT reserved for bone-detailed examination where needed. CT myelography is necessary for detailed examination of the spinal cord when MR images cannot be obtained.

Flexion injuries of the thoracolumbar spine usually result in a simple vertebral body wedge compression fracture. Motor vehicle accidents caus- ing acute flexion injuries with lap-type seatbelt restraints may result in a horizontal neural arch-vertebral body fracture with an associated wedge compression called the Chance fracture (Fig. 15.61). Another type of acute flexion injury with seatbelt restraints disrupts the posterior longitudinal ligament, the ligamentum flavum and the interspinous ligaments with resultant facet vertical distraction. This latter type of distraction injury principally involves soft tissue disruption but may be associated with vertebral body wedge compression, posterior element fractures, and anterior subluxation of the more cranial involved vertebra. Due to the vertical distraction or dislocation, an axial CT may demonstrate unarticulated superior or inferior facets—the so-called "naked face" sign.[2,98]

Varying degrees of distraction occur. Vertical dis-

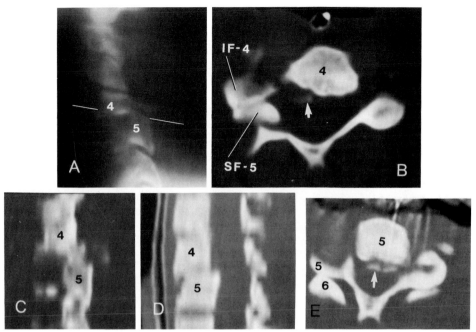

Figure 15.58.   Locked facets. A–D and **E** are different cases. Case 1: Unilateral locked facets. Right lateral mass-level sagittal conventional tomogram **(A)**. *Axial 314/1000 CT scan in the articular plane of section indicated by the line in* **A(B)**. Sagittal reformation of axial sections through the lateral mases **(C)** similar to **A**. Midsagittal reformation **(D)**. The right C4 inferior facet *(IF–4)* is subluxed anteriorly and locked in front of the C5 superior facet *(SF–5)*. The C4 body is slightly subluxed and rotated clockwise over C5. There is a small avulsion chip fragment *(arrow)*. Compare to the normal left side. Case 2: Bilateral C5–6 facet lock and vertebral body fracture. *Axial 249/2000 CT scan* **(E)**. The C6 superior facet posterior flat articular surfaces are posterior to the smooth convex posterior surfaces of the C5 inferior facets. A C5 vertebral body avulsion fracture is also present *(arrow)*. Note that the sagittal MR in Figure 15.57 is superior in bone detail to the sagittal CT reformation here.

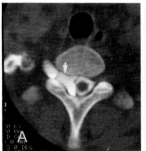
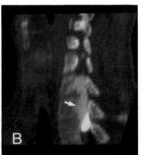
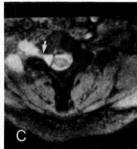

Figure 15.59.   Brachial plexus avulsion injuries. First case (A and B): *Axial T1–2 level 344/2000 CT myelogram* **(A)**. Right foraminal-level sagittal CT reformation **(B)**. The contrast-filled pseudomeningocele *(arrow)* displaces the spinal cord and involves the nerve root sleeves at three levels. Fluid/fluid levels are present. Second case **(C)**: *Axial C7-level GRE 450/12 10° flip angle MR scan.* Note the CSF-isointense pseudomeningocele having an almost identical appearance to the first case.

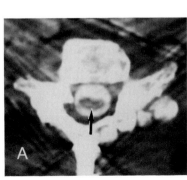
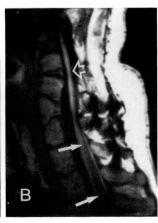

Figure 15.60.   Post-traumatic cervical myelopathy. Postcervical fracture and central spinal cord injury. Axial C7 59/1500 CT myelogram *(A)* and midsagittal SE 1500/20 MR scan without flow-compensation technique **(B).** Same case with studies 3 years apart. CT intrathecal contrast enters the central cord cystic cavity *(closed arrow)*. MR demonstrates the cavity *(closed arrows)* and the marked cervical spinal cord atrophy *(open arrow)*.

traction with a naked facet sign has already been described. The facets in this latter case may be widely separated or just barely contacting—one atop the other or "perched" (Fig. 5.57C). The facets may be anteriorly or laterally locked (Fig. 15.58). Plain films and/or AP and lateral localizer views are very helpful. The CT diagnosis of anteriorly locked thoracic facets is similar to that of cervical facet lock. The superior facet articular surface is identified posteriorly in place of the dorsal aspect of the inferior facet. Laterally locked facets are quite obvious to plain film, axial CT, and coronal CT reformations.[99] MR evaluation of spinal cord compression, contusion or hemorrhage, and ligamental rupture is important for surgical planning and prognosis.

Severe axial compressive forces and varying degrees of flexion forces sustained during rapid deceleration from a fall or motor vehicle accident can product a burst fracture.[100,101] These unstable fractures are characterized by posterior-superior-vertebral body fragment retropulsion into the spinal canal with resultant stenosis, vertebral body fracture with comminution of the superior half, bilateral laminar fractures, and increased interpedicular distance.[100,102] There is also disruption of the annulus fibrosus and posterior longitudinal ligament. Spondylolisthesis may occur. Disk material may accompany the retropulsed fragment. Nearly all burst fractures occur from T9 to L5.[100] The majority (65%) of patients in a large series presented with neurological deficits.[100] The degree of spinal canal stenosis detected by CT may not correlate with clinical neurological deficits.[100] Interfragment fracture, fragment rotation, and craniocaudal fragment migration are important characteristics to identify for surgical planning.[102]

MR demonstrates fragment retropulsion, spinal canal compromise, spinal cord injury (compression, hemorrhage, contusion), ligamental rupture, vertebral alignment, and intervertebral disk condition (Figs. 15.62 and 15.63).[35] Just as with cervical spinal cord injury, a swollen thoracic cord with edema and/or hemorrhage-MR signals can be identified. The edema signal is T1/T2 water-isointense and the hemorrhage signal depends on the degree of hemoglobin molecule oxidation and whether or not the hemorrhage RBCs have lysed. The spinal cord enlargement may be asymmetrical. The spinal cord hemorrhage usually is associated with a greater neurological deficit and has a poorer chance for recovery in an early study. The edematous spinal cord without hemorrhage has a better prognosis and abnormal findings may remit, often, within 1 week.[35]

Laminar fractures, details of superior vertebral body comminution, facet relationships, and details of a retropulsed segment (intersegment fracture and rotation) are best detected by axial CT (Figs. 15.62 and 15.63).[100,101] Sagittal reformation CT is the standard CT method. We are increasingly relying on MR bone detail which is usually superior to planar CT sagittal and coronal reformation. CT still plays a significant role as the first examination in these acutely injured patients.

Post-traumatic spinal cord sequellae, similar to that already described for cervical spine injury, occurs with thoracic spine injury. This includes spinal cord cysts, noncystic myelomalacia, and spinal cord atrophy.

Penetrating Injuries

Most spinal penetrating injuries result from gunshot wounds. Bullet fragmentation from the ricochet effect against osseous structures commonly occurs. A potential hazard with MR is the movement of a sharp fragment close to the spinal cord. Metallic artifact distorts the image on both MR and CT. Spinal cord transsection is more likely to occur with penetrating injury than with fragment retropulsion.[82]

TUMORS

This section categorizes bone tumors into vertebral bone tumors and soft tissue tumors adjacent to the vertebrae. The first category is divided into pri-

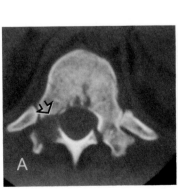
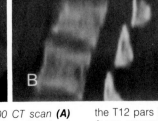
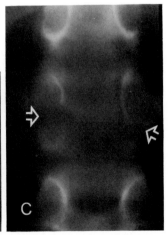

Figure 15.61. Chance fracture. *Axial T12 372/2000 CT scan* **(A)** *and facet-level CT sagittal reformation* **(B).** *Coronal pedicle-level conventional polyspiral tomogram* **(C).** *Axial fracture plane through* the T12 pars interarticularis and body *(closed arrows)* and pedicles *(open arrows). Other T12 fractures and an L1 wedge compression fracture are present.*

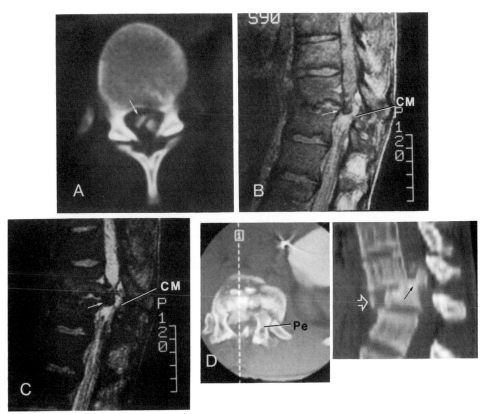

Figure 15.62.   Thoracolumbar (T12–L1) fractures with fragment retropulsion. A–C and **D** are different cases. *Axial 390/1500 CT scan* **(A)**. *Midsagittal SE 2000/30* **(B)** *and 2000/80* **(C)** *MR scans. Axial 20/ 424 CT scan with sagittal reformation* **(D)**. Retropulsed fragments in each case markedly stenose the spinal canal *(closed arrows)*. MR demonstrates contusion of the conus medullaris *(CM)*. There is an interfragment fracture in case 1 and the contused conus is MR hy-

perintense. There is T12–L1 retrolisthesis in case 1 and T12–L1 anterior subluxation in case 2. The case 2 pedicle *(Pe)* fractures explain the marked instability. In case 2, there is an anterior fragment of L1 attached to the anterior longitudinal ligament *(open arrow)*. The vertebral body is comminuted and the interpedicular distance is increased.

mary and secondary (metastatic or direct spread from other tissues). The soft tissue tumors are subcategorized as extradural, extramedullary-intradural, and intramedullary. As will be seen, CT plays a major role in the diagnosis of spine bone tumors and MR plays a dominant role in the diagnosis of soft tissue tumors of the spine.

Bone Tumors

The most common vertebral bone tumors include hemangioma, metastases, myeloma, and lymphoma. Benign tumors will be discussed first. Table 15.1 describes the differential diagnostic features of spinal bone tumors.

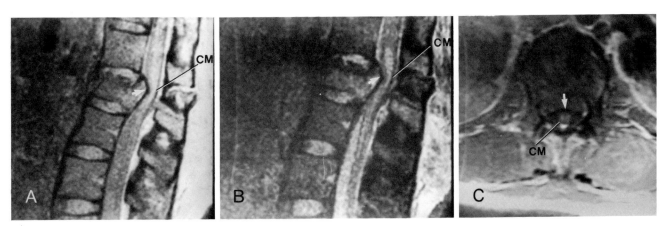

Figure 15.63.   L1 burst fracture with retropulsion and cord contusion. *Midsagittal SE 2000/30* **(A)** *and 2000/80* **(B)**, *and 2000/20 L1-level axial* **(C)** *MR scans.* A large retropulsed fragment *(arrow)* com-

presses the hyperintense contused conus medullaris *(CM)*. The intervertebral disk height and disk signal are preserved. The L1 endplates are fractured and the L1 body is compressed.

Table 15.1. Differential Diagnosis of Vertebral Bone Lesions

Lesion	CT Characteristics	MR Characteristics	Age	Sex	Differential Diagnostic Considerations	Exclusionary Factors
Hemangioma	Sharply defined low density containing "polka-dot"-thickened sparse trabeculae; single vertebra—whole or part	Characteristic mottled T1- and T2-weighted hyperintensity; single vertebra—whole or part			By CT Osteoporosis, metastasis; Paget's disease By MR Hemorrhage, bone changes adjacent to degenerative disk, vertebral fat infiltration	vs. osteoporosis—hemangioma limited to single vertebra with sparse but thickened trabeculae vs. metastasis—hemangioma has polka-dot CT and mixed T1/T2 MR hyperintensity, single vertebra vs. Paget's—Paget's is expansile, often multilevel with bizzare trabeculae vs. degenerative disk bone changes (MR)—hemangioma is usually not an endplate process vs. fat (MR)—hemangioma is usually a mixed signal intensity; cannot exclude hemorrhage by MR
Osteoid osteoma	Hypodense nidus <15 mm surrounded by sclerosis		<20	Male:female, 3.5:1	By CT Osteoblastoma, bone island	vs. osteoblastoma—osteoid osteoma has smaller nidus and occurs in younger patients vs. bone island—osteoid osteoma has a nidus; may be difficult if nidus is calcified
Bone island	Solitary small dense mass	Suspect signal-void but may vary depending on fat content			By CT Osteoid osteoma, osteoblastoma	vs. osteoid osteoma—bone island lacks a nidus vs osteoblastoma—bone island small, sharply marginated, and homogeneously hyperdense
Osteoblastoma	Expansile lytic lesion with thin sclerotic rim, may have a nidus (>20 mm)	Intraosseous expansile mass without unique intensity characteristics	20–40	Male:female, 3:1	By CT or MR Osteoid osteoma, giant cell tumor, aneurysmal bone cyst	vs. osteoid osteoma—osteoblastoma usually lacks a well-defined nidus and sclerosis; older patient vs. aneurysmal bone cyst—not aneurysmal unless coexistent vs. giant cell tumor—osteoblastoma not common in sacrum, may have a nidus, not invasive
Aneurysmal bone cyst	Lytic markedly expansile, eggshell calcification, neural arch mass, sharply marginated	Sharply marginated, markedly expansile cervical or thoracic neural arch mass	<20	Slight female preponderance	By CT or MR Giant cell tumor, osteoblastoma, myeloma	vs. giant cell tumor—aneurysmal bone cyst occurs in patients of a younger age, is more expansile with "eggshell" calcification, sharply marginated vs. osteoblastoma—may coexist, aneurysmal expansion

Table 15.1.   *(continued)*

Lesion	CT Characteristics	MR Characteristics	Age	Sex	Differential Diagnostic Considerations	Exclusionary Factors
						vs. myeloma—myeloma is destructive, in older patient
Giant cell tumor	Destructive lytic bone tumor, favors sacrum, may be expansile, possible pathological fracture	Destructive bone tumor, favors sacrum, may be expansile	20–50		By CT or MR Aneurysmal bone cyst, chordoma, myeloma, metastasis	vs. aneurysmal bone cyst—giant cell tumor occurs in older patients, lacks eggshell calcification, and is less sharply marginated

vs. chordoma—giant cell tumor usually less destructive

vs. myeloma and metastasis—giant cell tumor is singular and usually less destructive |
| Chordoma | Destructive invasive tumor favoring clivus and sacrum, vertebral lesions often involve adjacent disk, frequent calcifications | Destructive invasive tumor favors clivus and sacrum, vertebral lesions often involve adjacent disk, T2 hyperintensity with hypointense septae | 50–70 | More common in females | By CT or MR Metastasis and myeloma, giant cell tumor, osteoblastoma, sarcoma, and sacrococcygeal teratoma | vs. metastasis—chordoma is singular, usually less destructive

vs. giant cell tumor and plasmacytoma—chordoma is frequently calcified; in general, chordoma location is best clue

vs. others—chordoma cannot be excluded if lesion in the sacrum, clivus, or vertebral body |
| Myeloma | Favors vertebral body, varies from small lytic to large expansile "bubbly" lesion | Favors vertebral body, lytic destructive expansile hypointensity | Elderly | | By CT or MR Singular: giant cell tumor, chordoma, osteoblastoma, Paget's disease Multiple: metastasis | vs. giant cell tumor—difficult, myeloma tends to be more destructive

vs. chordoma—myeloma not calcified and usually more destructive

vs. osteoblastoma—myeloma occurs in elderly, lacks nidus

vs. Paget's—Paget's disease except Paget's sarcoma lacks destruction

vs. metastasis—myeloma frequently expansile |
| Osteogenic sarcomas | Invasive ossified soft tissue mass; hyperdense bone may have osteolytic areas, specific if in area of Paget's disease | Hypointense if markedly osteoblastic | 10–25 years except Paget's in elderly or post-irradiation | | By CT or MR Solitary osteoblastic or calcified metastasis, osteoblastoma, giant cell tumor, other sarcomas | vs. metastasis—marked calcium signal of bone and soft tissue mass

vs. osteoblastoma, giant cell tumor—osteogenic sarcoma in areas of Paget's or radiation, has calcification, and large soft tissue mass, more invasive

vs. other sarcomas—osteosarcoma in Paget's and radiation areas; lacks popcorn calcification not associated with osteochondroma; younger age group than chondrosarcoma |

Table 15.1. *(continued)*

Lesion	CT Characteristics	MR Characteristics	Age	Sex	Differential Diagnostic Considerations	Exclusionary Factors
Chondrosarcoma	May originate from osteochondroma, contains calcified areas		Middle-aged and elderly		By CT or MR Paraspinal—osteochondroma; intraosseous—sarcomas, metastases, osteoblastoma, giant cell tumor	vs. osteosarcoma; older age group; may arise from osteochondroma; "popcorn" calcification vs. all except osteochondroma—chondrosarcoma contains chondroid calcification vs. osteochondroma, osteoblastoma—giant cell tumor, chondrosarcoma may be very destructive
Metastasis	Destructive, usually multiple, osteolytic, and/or osteoblastic mass(es)	Destructive, usually multiple, possibly specific if melanoma			By CT or MR Tumor, osteoblastoma, plasmacytoma, lymphoma, Schmorl's nodes, degenerative vertebral endplate reactive changes, Paget's disease, hemangioma, osteomyelitis, granuloma, and osteoporotic fracture	vs. all—metastasis is usually multiple vs. Schmorl's nodes and degenerative disk disease—endplate changes—unusual metastasis location vs. Paget's—Paget's is hypertrabecular, expansile, and nondestructive vs. hemangioma—metastasis destructive, lacks CT polka-dot and MR T1/T2 mottled hyperintensity vs. infection—metastasis pedicle involvement, lesser degree prevertebral soft tissue mass Matastasis spares disk vs. osteoporosis; metastasis is destructive and not uniform

Cavernous hemangiomas are the most common local benign vertebral tumors. They usually occur in the lower thoracic or lumbar region. Vertebral involvement may be focal with characteristic abrupt margins with uninvolved bone or bone involvement may be generalized. Neurological symptoms may develop due to pathological fractures with spinal cord or nerve root compression. Bone expansion may occur but rarely causes spinal stenosis.[2,10,103]

CT demonstrates fewer than normal but thickened vertically oriented trabeculae within a clearly defined osteoporotic zone. Axial CT scans therefore demonstrate a striking polka-dot pattern. There is rarely contrast enhancement (Fig. 15.64).[2,10] CT differential diagnosis includes osteoporosis. Osteoporosis involves multiple vertebral bodies diffusely. Although there are a diminished number of trabeculae in osteoporosis, they are not thickened.

Vertebral hemangiomas cannot be definitively di-

agnosed by MR as they can by CT. MR demonstrates a characteristic mottled T1- and T2-weighted image hyperintensity. The T1 hyperintensity is caused by tumor fat content and the T2 hyperintensity is probably caused by the more cellular tumor component. Plain films or even the CT localizer film can detect the celery stalk-striations characteristic of hemangioma.

MR differential diagnosis includes vertebral body hemorrhage, bone signal changes adjacent to degenerative intervertebral disks, and vertebral body fat infiltration—all conditions that might have T1- and T2-weighted hyperintensity. The endplate T2 hyperintensity associated with degenerative disks, the focal vertebral fat infiltration of the elderly, is only slight compared to the more marked T2-weighted hyperintensity associated with the hemangioma. Vertebral hemorrhage cannot be excluded by MR.[103]

Bone islands are solitary, small, dense ossifica-

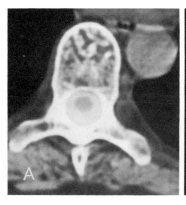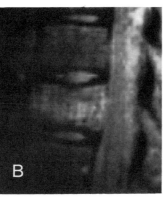

Figure 15.64. Vertebral cavernous hemangioma. **A** and **B** are different cases. *Axial T9 level CT scan (A) and midsagittal SE 2000/90 MR scan (B).* There are sparse hypertrophic cancellous bone spicules causing a CT characteristic polka-dot pattern and MR striations within the T2 hyperintense lower thoracic vertebral body. (**B** courtesy of Solomon Batnitzky, M.D., Kansas City, Kansas.)

tions that may be present in the vertebrae. They are commonly seen in the pelvic flat bones on conventional x-rays. They are seldom, if ever, symptomatic and their main importance is the potential for confusion with a neoplastic process such as an osteoid osteoma or metastasis. CT demonstrates a sharply circumscribed small homogeneously dense nonexpansile lesion that may slowly increase in size (Fig. 15.65).[104]

Osteoid osteoma is a small, benign, primary bone tumor composed of atypical bone and osteoid tissue and is characterized by an osteolytic nidus surrounded by thick bony sclerosis. The nidus measures less than 15 mm in diameter—an important diagnostic point. The nidus is initially uncalcified but may calcify with time. The nidus is surrounded by a well-defined sclerotic area. This tumor usually occurs in boys in their early teens. The male:female ratio is 3.5:1. Ten percent of osteoid osteomas occur in the spine, usually in the lumbar location and most often involving the neural arch. The patients present with gradually increasing pain, which is worse at night and promptly relieved by aspirin. Gait disturbances, radicular pain, limb atrophy, and scoliosis may occur. Nearly all osteoid osteomas have positive nuclear bone scans.[2,105]

CT findings of a smooth, round lucent nidus less than 15 mm in diameter surrounded by a well-defined sclerotic area is virtually pathognomic (Fig. 15.66). CT is the investigative method of choice following a localization estimate by clinical, nuclear medicine, or conventional x-ray methods.[105] MR can detect the lesion but is less sensitive and specific.

Osteoblastoma is a lytic benign expansile bone tumor affecting the neural arch and occasionally the vertebral body primarily in young adult males. The most common location is vertebral, usually involving the appendages. The male to female ratio is 3:1. The osteoblastoma nidus is often poorly circumscribed and is larger than that of the osteoid osteoma, usually measuring 20 mm or greater in diameter. Sclerosis is not a prominent feature.[2,106]

CT demonstrates a vertebral posterior element expansile lytic lesion with a thin sclerotic rim. Calcification may be present. Paraspinal extension and extension into the spinal canal may occur. There is usually absence of a well-defined nidus and surrounding sclerosis as is seen in osteoid osetoma and, if present, the nidus is larger. It is, therefore, a misconception to think that the typical osteoblastoma simply looks like large osteoid osteoma. MR and CT document spinal canal and neural foraminal involvement.[2,106] Aneurysmal bone cyst, giant cell tumor, and osteoid osteoma are the principal CT differential di-

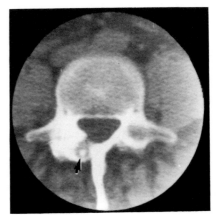

Figure 15.65. Bone island. *Sacral direct modified coronal 40/1600 CT scan.* There is a sharply defined homogeneously hyperdense right sacral ala lesion without surrounding bone abnormality.

Figure 15.66. Osteoid osteoma. *Axial L5-level 40/500 CT scan.* This case represents classic findings for an osteoid osteoma. There is a central nidus containing a small calcification *(arrow)* surrounded by sclerotic hypertrophic bone.

agnostic considerations. The differential diagnosis of these four lesions and other bone tumors of the spine is found in Table 15.1. CT is clearly not as specific for osteoblastoma as it is for osteoid osteoma.

MR of osteoblastoma demonstrates the intraosseous expansile character of the lesion and paravertebral and intracanalicular involvement.[107] Rather than resorting to a CT myelogram in particular cases where the CT suggests extension into the spinal canal, MR should be considered as the complementary exam.

Aneurysmal bone cyst is an uncommon benign markedly expansile bone lesion that often affects the vertebra and usually occurs in the cervical and thoracic neural arches. It is not a true neoplasm and may represent a reaction to a stimulus such as an osteoblastoma. Pathologically, the aneurysmal bone cyst is comprised of large, blood-filled communicating cavities. It usually affects patients under 20 years old. There is a slight preponderance toward women. The aneurysmal bone cyst may compromise the spinal canal representing an indication for MR study.

CT shows characteristic marked "aneurysmal" cortical "eggshell" expansion and thinning enclosing a noncalcified cyst. Occasionally, trabeculations are present within the cyst. Vertebral body collapse may occur (Fig. 15.67).[2,10,108] CT is probably more specific than MR for diagnosis because of improved bone detail, however, MR can demonstrate bone expansion, the spinal cord and canal, and paraspinal soft tissues in orthogonal planes. Differential diagnosis includes plasmacytoma, giant cell tumor, and osteoblastoma. The aneurysmal bone cyst is not destructive like plasmacytomas and giant cell tumors and it occurs in a younger age group. The characteristic aneurysmal pattern serves to differentiate it from osteoblastoma, however, the two lesions may coexist.

Eosinophilic granuloma is one of the three forms of histiocytosis X. It may affect the spine of young children presenting as a single vertebral body or posterior element osteolytic focus. It may extend into the spinal canal (Fig. 15.68).

Giant cell tumors are rare destructive lytic bone

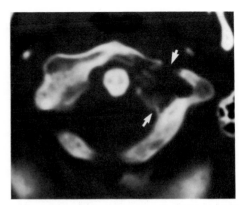

Figure 15.68. Eosinophilic granuloma. *Axial C1-level 400/1500 CT scan.* There is a left C1 lateral mass slightly expansile osteolytic mass with cortical fractures *(arrows).*

tumors that may involve the vertebral body, pedicle, or neural arch, usually in patients between 20 and 50 years old. They often behave as malignant tumors. It occurs most frequently in the sacrum.[2,108] Pathological fractures may occur and be the cause of the presenting complaint of pain. CT demonstrates a lytic noncalcified expansile mass that may have a benign appearance similar to an aneurysmal bone cyst but may also expand into surrounding soft tissues in a more aggressive fashion (Fig. 15.69).[2] As with other bone tumors, MR is less specific but it can better document the soft tissue involvement. Differential diagnosis includes osteoblastoma, aneurysmal bone cyst, plasmacytoma, and metastasis.

Chordoma is a rare invasive tumor originating from notochordal remnants which are considered to be of "low malignancy." The tumor epicenter is usually within the vertebral body or clivus (Fig. 11.22). Vertebral chordomas often involve the adjacent disk. Half (50%) of these lesions are sacrococcygeal, 35% are intracranial (usually clivus) and 15% arise from a vertebral body. Sellar and parasellar lesions also occur. Women are more frequently affected than men and chordomas usually occur in patients between 50 and 70 years of age. Approximately 10% of lesions metastasize to the lungs, liver, and other sites. The tumors are initially encapsulated but later become highly destructive and invasive and often extend into the spinal canal and the calvarium.[2,108–110]

CT of chordoma most accurately demonstrates the bone destructive process and demonstrates calcifications (Fig. 15.70). MR demonstrates T1 isointensity or hypointensity and T2 hyperintensity. The T2-hyperintense tumor often has hypointense septae.[110] In absence of MR, CT myelography with sagittal reformation is necessary for exclusion of spinal canal or cisternal involvement. Differential diagnostic considerations include metastasis and myeloma.

Myeloma is a common bone tumor of plasma cell origin that often involves the vertebral column as solitary (plasmacytoma) or multiple (multiple myeloma) lesions. The vertebral body is characteristically involved by osteolysis. It usually occurs in the

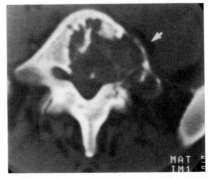

Figure 15.67. Aneurysmal bone cyst. *L5 axial 89/2000 CT scan.* There is a lytic expansile "aneurysmal cortical eggshell" slightly trabecular or compartmentalized mass of the vertebral body, left transverse process, and pedicle. The psoas muscle fat plane *(arrow)* is displaced but not invaded. The lesion expands into the spinal canal.

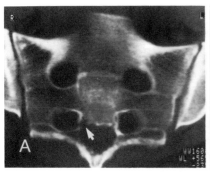
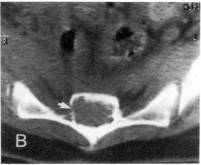

Figure 15.69.   Giant cell tumor. *S3-level modified coronal* **(A)** *and axial* **(B)** *565/1600 CT scans.* An osteolytic slightly expansile mass destroys the medial wall of the right S2–3 sacral foramen and right lateral sacral cortex *(arrows).*

elderly. Radionuclide scans are often negative or equivocal. CT characteristics vary from small lytic vertebral body lesions ("punched out") to frank expansile lytic "bubbly" lesions. Soft tissue involvement and spinal canal invasion are common (Fig. 15.71).[2,111] CT myelography for spinal canal involvement is necessary only if MR imaging cannot be performed. MR more accurately identifies extension into the soft tissues. Differential diagnostic considerations include metastasis for multiple lesions and chordoma and giant cell tumor for solitary plasmacytoma.

Otseogenic sarcoma is a rare tumor of the spine. Most cases occur between the ages of 10 and 25 years. It can result from Paget's disease degeneration and from irradiation. It can also metastasize from elsewhere to the vertebrae and/or the soft tissues.[107] Mixed osteolytic and osteoblastic pathological changes can result in a varied CT appearance (Fig. 15.72). Although CT more accurately identifies calcification, and particularly ossification within the mass, MR identifies the lesion in orthogonal planes and identifies the spinal cord.[2,107,108]

Chondrosarcomas occur predominantly in the middle-aged and elderly populations. They may arise de novo or result from degeneration of an osteochondroma, particularly in patients with hereditary multiple exostoses. CT characteristically demonstrates

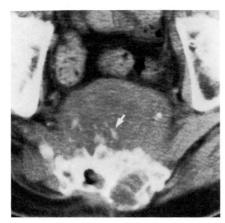

Figure 15.70.   Sacral chordoma. *Axial 125/500 midsacral CT scan.* A large presacral soft tissue mass containing calcifications *(arrow)* is continuous with a markedly destructive and partially expansile sacral bone tumor. There is also posterior soft tissue invasion.

multiple, irregularly shaped calcifications within a spine tumor or a paraspinal soft tissue mass. When the lesion is paraspinal, the chondrous calcification and destructive invasive mass strongly suggest the correct diagnosis. When the lesion is intraosseous and expansile with a sclerotic rim, the differential diagnosis includes other sarcomas, metastases, osteoblastoma and giant cell tumor.[108] MR would not be expected to be as specific as CT for diagnosis of chondrosarcoma due to the CT specificity for chondrous calcification. MR better documents tumor extent and spinal canal involvement.

Metastasis to the spine is the most common cause of vertebral tumors at our hospital. The vertebrae are the major site of bone metastases.[108] The most frequent origins of spine metastases are breast, prostate, lung, and kidney. Systemic tumors such as lymphoma,[107] leukemia,[112] and multiple myeloma[111] invade the spine. Destruction often begins at the pedicle, however, any portion of the vertebra may be involved. Both CT and MR accurately establish the diagnosis (Fig. 15.73). CT best demonstrates the lytic or blastic nature of the lesion (Figs. 15.73**A** and **B**) and MR best demonstrates tumor extent and relationship to the spinal canal, spinal cord and nerve roots (Figs. 15.73**C–F**). MR signal intensities are usually nonspecific.[3] Osteolysis is most common. Prostatic metastases and lymphoma often produce osteoblastic or mixed osteoblastic/osteolytic metastases. Breast carcinoma (particularly chemotherapy-treated) can cause osteoblastic metastasis.[108] Direct vertebral invasion with osteolysis may follow periosteal invasion of lung oat cell carcinoma and other juxtavertebral malignant tumors. Pathological fractures and tumor epidural spread commonly occur. These patients often present with focal or radicular pain and, not infrequently, with evidence of spinal cord compression. Spinal cord compression in these patients is usually caused by epidural tumor mass. Myelography with or without CT or MR are the usual means of confirming the diagnosis of epidural spinal cord compression—"block." We have recently found MR to be quite accurate for this diagnosis and feel that it will probably replace myelography for initial evaluation of epidural spinal cord compression. Cellular bone invasion results in T1 hypointensity. MR may be useful for predicting acute lymphocytic leu-

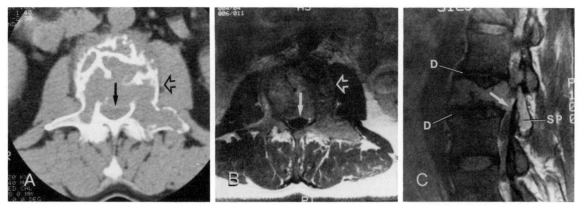

Figure 15.71. Plasmacytoma. *L3-level axial 62/550 CT scan* **(A)** *and same level SE 600/25 presaturation MR scan* **(B).** *Midsagittal 2000/30 MR scan* **(C).** CT demonstrates a lytic coarsely trabeculated "bubbly" expansile mass which is typical of plasmacytoma. MR is less specific but documents marked compression fracture deformity, spinous process involvement *(SP),* and abnormal disk *(D)* signal. Both CT and MR demonstrate mass protrusion into the spinal canal *(closed arrow)* and psoas fat plane infiltration *(open arrows).* The cause of the disk hypointense proton signal is unknown.

kemia remission or relapse on the basis of MR signal changes. T1 marrow-intensity in relapse and in the acute newly diagnosed stage is significantly lower than in remission or in healthy normal patients. Using this MR method may obviate the need for repeated bone marrow biopsy.[112] MR marrow signal within osteoporotic remote fracture cancellous bone should be expected to be normal as compared to the usually hypointense tumor cellular invasion of metastatic pathological fracture.[3]

Soft Tissue Tumors

Intraspinal tumors are categorized here by location as extradural, intradural extramedullary, or intramedullary. MR is the diagnostic procedure of choice in all three categories due to orthogonal plane imaging for longitudinal localization and soft tissue discrimination of spinal cord and nerve displacement. The full extent of the tumor mass and its relationship to the spinal cord is usually quite clear.

Figure 15.72. Osteogenic sarcoma. T9 metastasis. *T9-level 250/2000* **(A)** *and 13/400* **(B)** *CT scans with midsagittal reformation* **(C).** *Midsagittal SE 600/25 MR scan* **(D).** The markedly CT-hyperdense nonexpansile vertebral body and posterior element mass invades the paraspinal soft tissues **(A)** and the spinal canal **(B, D).** The CT sagittal reformation hyperdensity and the MR calcium signal-void *(arrows)* presents an interesting CT and MR signal comparison. The T10 MR vertebral hypointensity is due to signal dropoff at the coil periphery.

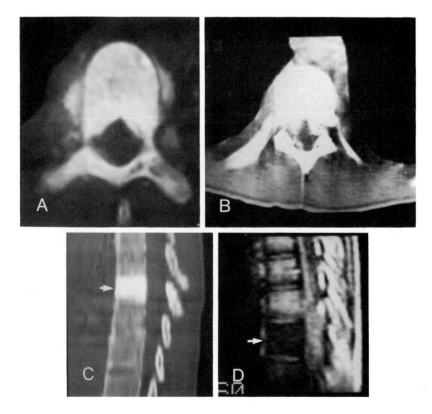

MR i.v. contrast can be used to improve definition. Without MR, CT myelography is usually necessary. An additional problem with the CT myelography technique is the necessity to determine the top level of the epidural block. This requires either a 2-hour delay exam or a lateral cervical or cisterna magna puncture and additional contrast injection.

Extradural Tumors. Most extradural intraspinal tumors are metastatic neoplasms, most commonly of breast, prostate, lung, kidney, and lymphoma.[108,113] Other tumors such as Ewing's sarcoma, reticulum cell sarcoma, leukemic chloroma, thyroid carcinoma, neuroblastoma, and melanoma produce epidural metastasis. Neurofibromas can be entirely or partly extradural but will be discussed in the "intradural extramedullary" category. The dura resists penetration by extradural masses. With metastatic lesions, there is usually bone osteolytic and/or osteoblastic involvement. The paraspinal muscles may be diffusely infiltrated (Fig. 15.73).[2,108]

The differential diagnosis of metastatic epidural tumors includes epidural tumors of primary origin, abscess, and hematoma. Primary epidural tumors are usually paraspinal soft tissue sarcomas but purely extradural neurofibromas do occur. MR may demonstrate hemoglobin signal and rarely CT can demonstrate clot density in an epidural hematoma. Epidural hematoma and, often, abscess are unassociated with destructive bone change. These latter conditions will be discussed later in this chapter. The epidural neurofibroma is usually a component of a dumbbell intradural-extradural combined mass. There is often a history of neurofibromatosis.[114] An epidural tumor such as lymphoma may have an appearance simulating a herniated disk, particularly on CT scans. Lymphoma (Fig. 15.73G—J) is often associated with epidural mass extending over several segments, with osteolytic and/or osteoblastic metastasis, and with extensive paraspinal mass component.[113] Associated metastatic bone or soft tissue involvement and absence of MR evidence for herniated disk (degenerative disk and the toothpaste sign) should establish the correct diagnosis.

Intradural Extramedullary Tumors in the Adult. The two major categories of intradural extramedullary lesions are primary tumors and intradural arachnoid implants. The most common primary intradural extramedullary neoplasms are neurofibroma, schwannoma, meningioma, and lipoma.[108] Lipomas, dermoid and epidermoid tumors associated with dysraphism have been discussed earlier in this chapter. Gd-DTPA i.v. contrast injection can improve tumor detectability and sensitivity.[115] Table 15.2 describes the differential diagnostic features of intradural extramedullary tumors.

Neurofibromas and schwannomas are tumors of spinal nerve roots and peripheral nerves. Neurofibromas take origin from perineural fibroblasts and schwannomas take origin from Schwann cells that surround axons. Since neurofibromas and schwan-

nomas cannot be reliably distinguished by CT or MR, the two lesions will be considered as neurofibromas in this text. Multiple neurofibromas characteristically occur in patients with von Recklinghausen's disease.[115]

Combined intradural extramedullary tumors (dumbbell) are the most common type of intradural neurofibroma. They commonly cause neural foraminal erosion (Fig. 15.74). They are frequently associated with plexiform neurofibromas in patients with neurofibromatosis (Fig. 15.75). Other associated abnormalities in neurofibromatosis include meningiomas, lateral meningoceles, neurofibrosarcomas and intramedullary tumors including astrocytomas, and ependymomas.[114]

MR often demonstrates neurofibroma T1-weighted slight muscle-hyperintensity and marked T2 hyperintensity commonly with a central decreased signal (Fig. 15.75).[114] Spinal cord displacement and associated epidural and paraspinal mass are well demonstrated by both MR and CT myelography. Neurofibromas are characteristically CT slightly hypodense compared to muscle and they are smoothly marginated.[108] Neural foramen erosion, although best seen by CT, is quite obviously implied by MR evidence of intraforaminal tumor. Calcification is very uncommon.[116] MR and CT i.v. contrast enhancement can be quite dramatic.[115,117]

Intraspinal meningiomas occur predominantly in the thoracic subarachnoid space in women. The female:male ratio is 4:1 and approximately 80% are thoracic. They are usually in a posterior location firmly attached to the dura. Spinal meningiomas are usually CT hyperdense compared to the spinal cord.[10] They usually CT contrast enhance. Cystic changes are unusual. Extradural extension may occur.[10,117] Spinal meningiomas are rarely multiple.[118] They have been only rarely reported to metastasize to lung.[119] There is occasional dense tumoral calcification and/or adjacent hyperostosis.[2,10,108] MR usually demonstrates T1 and T2 muscle-isointense signals typical of intracranial meningiomas with marked contrast enhancement (Fig. 15.76). Intraspinal meningiomas are occasionally of the dumbbell type.[10,108]

Lipomas account for only approximately 1% of intraspinal tumors, most of which are unassociated with dysraphism.[108] They are composed of fat and fibrous tissue. Isolated intraspinal lipomas are usually in an intradural location but may be extradural and rarely intramedullary. They can occur at any spine level but are more common in the thoracic spine.[2,108]

MR and CT demonstrates a round or slightly lobulated fat signal-intensity and CT density mass (Fig. 15.77). CT requires CT myelography to better delineate the lesion and assess spinal cord location, displacement, and compression.

Intradural extramedullary spinal teratomas are very rare tumors that may occur isolated or in association with congenital spinal anomalies.[120]

Subarachnoid tumor implantation ("seeding")

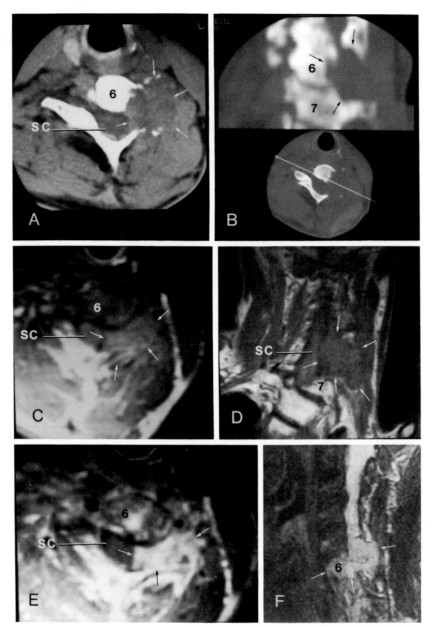

Figure 15.73. Epidural tumors. A–F, G–I, and **J** are different cases; Case 1: C6 metastatic bronchogenic carcinoma. *Axial C6-level 22/ 350 CT scan (A) and CT coronal reformation in the plane of the cursor line (B). Noncontrast axial (C) and coronal (D) SE 600/25 MR scans and same axial level gadolinium i.v. contrast MR scan (E). Sagittal 2000/80 MR scan (F).* An expansile lytic left C6 lateral elements and vertebral body mass *(arrows)* destroys and displaces the bone cortex. CT demonstrates C6 osteolysis, C7 involvement, and calcific cortical remnants surrounding the soft tissue mass. MR demonstrates a T1 muscle-isointense/T2 muscle-hyperintense contrast-enhancing mass. The spinal cord *(SC),* seen only by MR, is displaced. The C6 vertebral body T2 hyperintensity **(F)** correlates well with gadolinium contrast enhancement **(E).** Compare **E** to **C.** Para-spinal muscle infiltration is seen in **A** and **D.** Case 2: Non-Hodgkin's lymphoma thoracic spine vertebral body and epidural metastasis of the thoracic spine. *Midsagittal noncontrast (G) and Gd-DTPA i.v. contrast (H) SE 600/25 MR scans. T6-level axial i.v. contrast MR scan (I).* The T6 and T10 vertebral bodies are anteriorly markedly T1 hypointense. There is i.v. contrast enhancement of the T6 posterior isointense portion that is continuous with a circumferential epidural mass compressing the spinal cord. Case 3: Non-Hodgkin's lymphoma epidural metastasis in an AIDS patient. *T10 level axial 385/ 2000 CT myelogram (J).* An epidural mass markedly compresses the contrast-filled subarachnoid space and displaces the spinal cord. There is no detectable bone involvement.

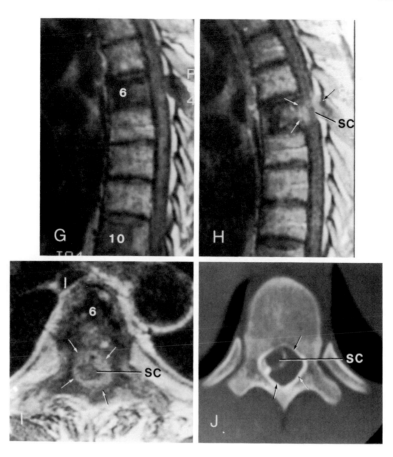

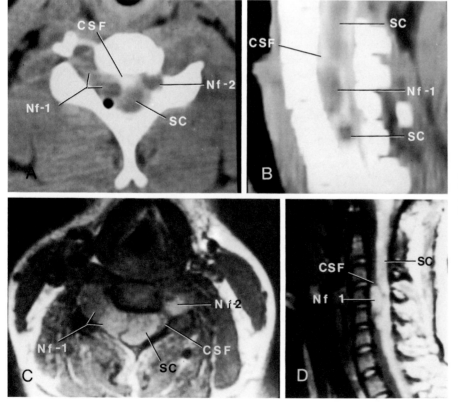

Figure 15.74. Cervical neurofibromas, von Recklinghausen's disease. *Axial top C4-level 39/450 CT myelogram **(A)** and right lateral sagittal reformation **(B)**. Axial SE 700/ 25 MR scan **(C)** at same level as **A**. Sagittal 1500/25 MR scan **(D)** at same level as **B**.* There is a sharply marginated right-sided "dumbbell" combined intradural-extramedullary and extradural intraforaminal mass *(Nf– 1)* and a left-sided extradural intraforaminal mass *(Nf–2)*. The masses are CT-slightly muscle-hypodense and MR-T1 slightly muscle-hyperintense/proton density and T2 hyperintense. The dumbbell neurofibroma erodes (widens) the neural foramen and displaces the spinal cord *(SC)*. The characteristic intradural mass ipsilateral CSF space enlargement *(CSF)* is present.

can be caused by medulloblastoma, ependymoma, and germinoma. Glioblastoma, other primary CNS malignancies and metastatic systemic carcinoma, melanoma, sarcoma, and lymphoma can also be responsible.[2,108,121]

MR and CT myelographic studies demonstrate multiple masses, usually small but often varying in size, attached to the pia arachnoid membrane producing nerve root, spinal cord, and thecal sac lesions. "Pseudowidening" of the spinal cord may result (Fig. 15.78).[108]

Intramedullary tumors. Ependymomas and astrocytomas are the most common intramedullary spinal cord tumors in order of decreasing frequency 2:1.[3] Other intramedullary tumors such as hemangioblastomas, glioblastomas, hemangiopericytomas, lipomas, and spinal cord metastasis are far less common.[2,122]

The ependymoma occurs most frequently in the conus medullaris and filum terminale although other spinal locations are common. They are most likely to occur from the third through the sixth decade and

Table 15.2. Diagnostic Considerations for Intradural Extramedullary Tumors in the Adult

Lesion	CT Characteristic	MR Characteristic	Considerations	Exclusionary Factors
Neurofibroma	Hypodense, homogeneous contrast enhancement	Slight T1 muscle-hyperintensity and T2 marked hyperintensity, may have T2 central relative hypointensity, contrast enhancement	Meningioma, liopma, arachnoid cyst, subarachnoid implantation	vs. meningioma—neurofibroma T2 hyperintensity, CT hypodensity, usual lack of calcification, multiplicity if neurofibromatosis vs. implantation—neurofibroma (in absence of neurofibromatosis), lack of multiplicity, absent evidence of primary tumor vs. lipoma—absent fat intensity/density, foraminal erosion vs. arachnoid cyst—neurofibroma lacks water signal, contrast enhances
Meningioma	Hyperdense, homogeneous contrast enhancement, calcification	T1 and T2 muscle-isointense, contrast enhancement	Neurofibroma, lipoma, subarachnoid implantation	vs. neurofibroma—meningioma has T1/T2 muscle-isointensity CT hyperdensity, adjacent hyperostosis, dense tumoral calcification, 4:1 female preponderance; 80% thoracic vs. lipoma—meningioma lacks fat signal vs. subarachnoid implantation—neurofibromas (with von Recklinghausen's disease)—meningioma is singular vs. arachnoid cyst—meningioma lacks water signal
Lipoma	Hypodensity	Fat signal intensity	Neurofibroma, meningioma, subarachnoid implantation	vs. all—lipoma has fat signal vs. subarachnoid implantation and neurofibromatosis—lipoma lacks multiplicity
Subarachnoid implantation[a]	Multiple leptomeningeal, cord, and nerve root nodular masses	Multiple T1 isointense/T2 hyperintense (compared to muscle) dural, cord, and nerve root nodular masses	Neurofibromas	vs. neurofibromatosis—subarachnoid implantation patients lack evidence for neurofibromatosis

[a]Note: Cysticercosis can present as a varied appearance, intradural extramedullary mass/masses.

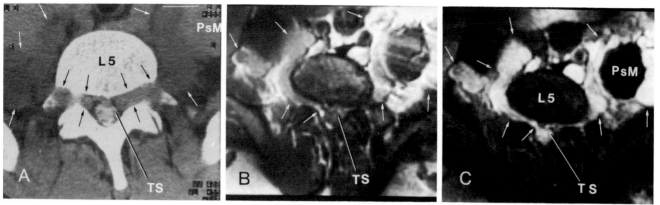

Figure 15.75. Plexiform neurofibromatosis—von Recklinghausen's disease. *L5-level axial 55/400 CT myelogram (A) and SE 1500/25 (B) and 1500/75 (C) MR scans.* There is a large bilateral paravertebral mass *(arrows)*, which is CT hypodense and MR T1 moderately hyperintense/T2 markedly hyperintense as compared to muscle. The mass enlarges and fills both intervertebral neural foramina and displaces the thecal sac *(TS)*. It displaces and surrounds the psoas muscles *(PsM)*.

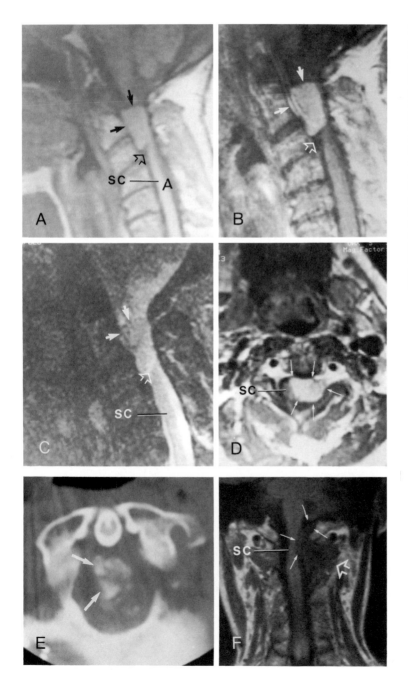

Figure 15.76. Cervical meningiomas. A–D and **E–F** are different cases. Case 1: C2–3 meningioma. *Midsagittal SE 600/25 noncontrast (A) and i.v. contrast (B), and 2000/100 (C) MR scans. Axial 600/25 i.v. contrast MR scan (D).* There is a left intradural extramedullary smoothly marginated mass *(arrows)* that compresses and deforms the spinal cord *(SC)*. It is T1/T2 spinal cord-isointense and it diffusely contrast enhances. It bulges slightly into the left neural foramen, which is seen filled with hyperintensity fat similar to the opposite side. At the tumor inferior margin there is a relatively large collection of CSF typical of intradural extramedullary masses *(open arrows)*. The tumor intensity characteristics and lack of prominent foraminal involvement favor the diagnosis of meningioma. Case 2: Calcified foramen magnum-C3 meningioma. *Axial C1-level 219/2000 CT scan (E). Coronal SE 600/25 noncontrast MR scan (F).* There is a large, partially calcified **(E)** combined intradural-extramedullary *(closed arrows)* and paraspinal *(open arrow)* mass that is T1 muscle-isointense with areas of focal greater hypointensity. The spinal cord *(SC)* (not seen by CT) is compressed and displaced. The calcification, (confirmed by CT only) supports the diagnosis of meningioma.

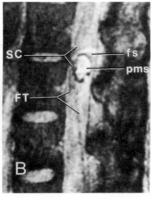
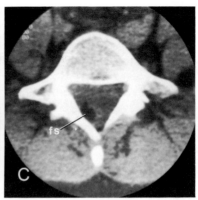

Figure 15.77. **Intradural lipomas. A–B** and **C** are different cases. Case 1: Conus medullaris-level lipoma. *Midsagittal SE 2000/20* **(A)** *and 2000/80* **(B)** MR scans. There is a sharply marginated intradural extramedullary L1–2 tumor anteriorly displacing the spinal cord *(SC)* and filum terminale *(FT)*. The tumor has two tissue types. The superior posterior portion has fat (T1 hyperintense/T2 isointense) signal *(fs)* and the larger anterior inferior portion has paramagnetic (T1/T2 hyperintense) signal *(pms)*. Chemical shift artifact at the caudal tumor margin and the inferior vertebral endplate is seen *(arrows)*. Case 2: Caudal sac lipoma. *Axial 61/550 CT scan* **(C)**. There is a sharply marginated, hypodense, small fat-signal *(fs)* mass.

are slightly more common in males. They grow slowly and may become quite large—"giant ependymoma." Above the filum, they usually are fusiform. Below the conus, they appear as sometimes lobular intradural masses. Approximately 50% of patients have some degree of cystic degeneration. Spinal canal expansion due to tumor erosion may occur and can be quite irregular in contour.[108]

Spinal intramedullary astrocytomas are most common in the thoracic and next most common in the cervical spine, occur in children, have a peak incidence in the third through fifth decades and have a slight male predominance. Like ependymomas, they usually cause a focal fusiform spinal cord enlargement. Approximately 40% of patients have tumor cystic degeneration.[3,108]

With the exception of the more frequent thoracic and cervical locations of astrocytoma and the conus and filum location of ependymomas, the CT and MR characteristics of these two tumors are indistinguishable (Fig. 15.79). They present as fusiform intramedullary masses at the spinal cord level with frequent cystic cavitation and lack of calcification.

They are usually T1 spinal cord-iso- or slightly hy-pointense and T2 hyperintense compared to normal spinal cord. Tumor cystic fluid has a higher protein content and decreased pulsatile motion compared to benign syrinx fluid and will usually not be CSF-isointense to various MR sequences. MR i.v. contrast can help define tumor margins within an edematous spinal cord but the role of i.v. MR contrast for investigation of these lesions is still unclear.[115] CT myelography with delay study is necessary in absence of MR. The delay study is necessary for detection of cystic degeneration.[2,108] CT i.v. contrast injection has not been found to be particularly useful.[117]

Spinal intramedullary hemangioblastomas are rare, usually single tumors. Approximately one-third of cases occur in patients with Hippel-Lindau disease. Spinal cord hemangioblastoma, however, occurs uncommonly (less than 5%) in patients with Hippel-Lindau disease.[108,123] These tumors usually are cystic but may be solid. The thoracic location is slightly more common than the cervical. Discovery of asymptomatic cases with MR may prove these lesions to be more common. MR demonstrates a large cyst (or cysts) associated with a small solid nodule and an abnormal vessel (or vessels) with spinal cord expan-

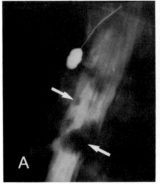
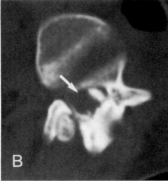
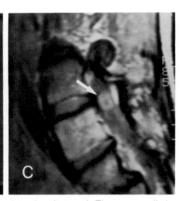

Figure 15.78. **Subarachnoid tumor deposit.** Osteosarcoma. *Conventional myelogram* **(A)** *and L3–4-level 34/450 CT myelogram* **(B)**. *Sagittal SE 1500/25 MR scan* **(C)**. There are multiple intradural tumor deposits of varying size *(arrows)*. They are well demonstrated by all three methods.

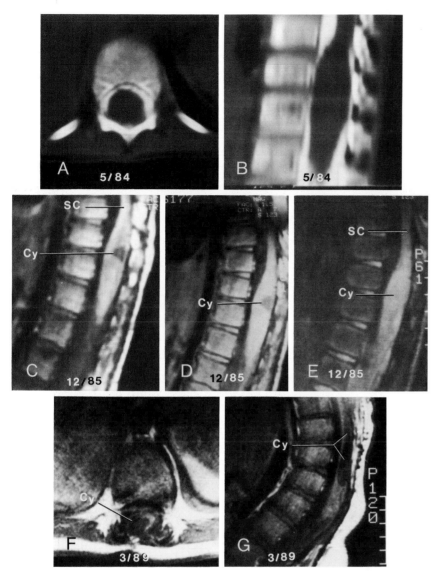

Figure 15.79. Thoracic astrocytoma. Same case with studies at different times: **A–B** at 5/84; **C–E** at 12/85; and **F–G** at 3/89. *T11-level 320/850 CT myelogram **(A)** and sagittal reformation **(B)**. Midsagittal SE 600/25 **(C)**, 1500/20 **(D)**, and 1500/80 **(E)**. Axial **(F)** and sagittal **(G)** 600/25 i.v. contrast injection MR scans.* There is a large intramedullary mass markedly expanding the spinal canal demonstrating an enlarging cystic or cavitary portion *(Cy)*. It is T1 hypointense/T2 hyperintense compared to the normal spinal cord *(SC)* with slight contrast enhancement. The cystic portion has increased over the interval.

sion (Fig. 5.36).[3,108,123,124] CT myelography demonstrates an intramedullary mass and may demonstrate abnormal draining veins.[124] Intravenous CT contrast enhancement occurs and can be a valuable clue to diagnosis.[117]

Spinal cord intramedullary metastases, previously thought to be rare occurrences, are likely to be more commonly discovered with MR examination. Primary sources of metastasis include both non-neurogenic and neurogenic tumors including lung and breast carcinoma, lymphoma, melanoma, medulloblastoma, glioma, and ependymoma. Combined leptomeningeal and spinal cord metastasis produces spinal cord widening plus surface irregularity.[122] These metastases tend to be a near-terminal event.[122]

The investigative method of choice is MR with or without i.v. contrast. As an alternative method of investigation, CT myelography can be helpful. Intravenous contrast CT scans have not been effective. By directly imaging the spinal cord, MR is very accu-

rate for intramedullary tumor detection. T1-weighted MR images demonstrate the spinal cord contour and size and T2-weighted images analyze abnormal intramedullary signals. Intramedullary metastasis has a characteristically high T2-weighted signal intensity. Spinal cord widening is usually present but may be confused with pseudowidening of subarachnoid metastasis.[122]

INFLAMMATORY DISEASES

Spinal inflammatory diseases can be caused by pyogenic, granulomatous, autoimmune, idiopathic, and iatrogenic conditions.

Infections

Direct bacterial inoculation from trauma or surgery, direct spread from paraspinal infectious processes and hemotogenous spread from primary extraspinal infections can cause septic spondylitis.[2] The most common organism is *Staphylococcus aureus*. The

Figure 15.80 Cervical epidural abscesses. A–F and **G–H** are different cases. Case 1: *Left parasagittal noncontrast SE 600/25* **(A)** *and i.v. contrast* **(B)** *preoperative MR scans. Same sagittal plane postlaminectomy 2000/100* **(C)**, *i.v. contrast 600/25* **(D)** *and C4-level axial noncontrast* **(E)**, *and i.v. contrast* **(F)** *MR scans.* There is marked contrast enhancement of a T1/T2 spinal cord-isointense left parasagittal C4–5 anterior epidural mass *(closed arrows)* that displaces and compresses the spinal cord *(SC)*. The epidural component is continuous with a paraspinal abscess *(open arrows)* and C4 and C5 septic spondylitis. All of the involved tissues contrast enhance. The postlaminectomy exam demonstrates increased contrast enhancement and T2 hyperintensity of the C4–5 disk *(4–5)* with decreased intervertebral height and erosion of adjacent cortical margins. There is marked contrast enhancement of the posterior operative site **(D and F)**. Case 2: *Axial low C2-level 18/342 i.v. contrast CT scan* **(G)**. *Axial C2–3-level SE 600/25 Gd-DTPA MR scan* **(H)**. A contrast-enhancing multilocular abscess *(open arrows)* markedly infiltrates the paraspinal and right-sided neck muscles. It is continuous with a right-sided contrast-enhancing epidural mass *(closed arrows)* that displaces the spinal cord *(SC)*. Osteomyelitis causes destruction and contrast enhancement of the C2 neural arch *(C2)*.

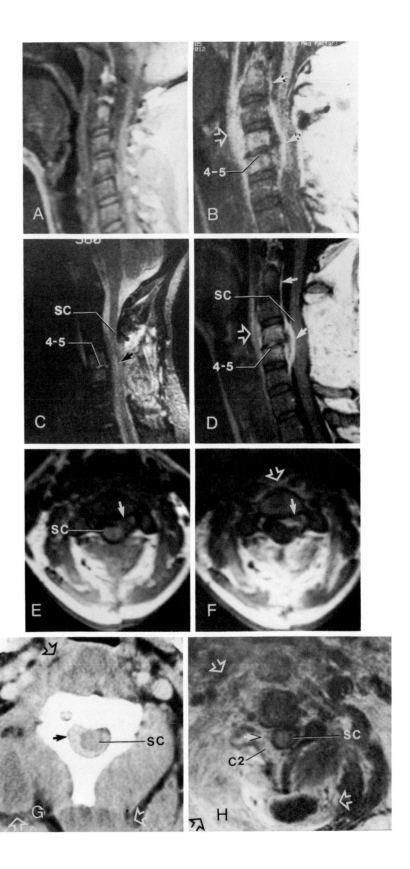

next most common is the *Enterobacter* species—a common urinary infectious organism. *Salmonella* may complicate SS and SC hemoglobinopathies.[125,126]

Osteomyelitis and Diskitis. MR is equally sensitive to radionuclide scanning for detection of osteomyelitis and diskitis. MR of septic spondylitis demonstrates vertebral body and disk T1 hypointensity and T2 hyperintensity. The inflamed disk T2 signal is characteristically very hyperintense and lacks the characteristic internuclear cleft. There is loss of the normal vertebral body-disk interface. A paraspinal mass is characteristic. Intravenous contrast injection enhances the disk, vertebral body, and paraspinal inflammatory tissue and can define epidural and other abscesses (Fig. 15.80).[125,126]

CT is also effective for diagnosis of septic spondylitis. CT demonstrates lytic fragmentation of adjacent vertebral bodies (Figs. 15.81 and 15.82), paraspinal soft tissue mass, and intervertebral disk hypodensity. The localizer view and sagittal reformation demonstrate loss of interspace height—a relatively late finding.[125,127–129] Intraosseous and paravertebral gas may be present in cases with spondylitis and paravertebral abscesses caused by gasforming organisms (Fig. 15.81). This can be confused with vacuum disk or facet and destructive change associated with paraspinal mass helps establish the diagnosis.

Spinal tuberculosis (Pott's disease) favors the thoracic and lumbar regions, most often in children and adolescents. It usually causes anterior vertebral body osteolysis and gibbus deformity. Half of patients have involvement of adjacent vertebrae with disk destruction. The posterior elements are almost never involved.[126] Paraspinal masses are common and are frequently calcified (cold abscess). Cold abscesses may involve the psoas muscles and may have epidural components.[2,126,128,130] CT demonstration of calcification of a paraspinal mass with rim contrast enhancement associated with spondylitis or anterior vertebral body osteolysis is virtually diagnostic of tuberculosis. CT will likely prove to be more specific than MR for diagnosis of tuberculous spondylitis due to calcium detection.

Vertebral osteomyelitis may be caused by *Candida* (Fig. 15.82**A** and **B**), coccidiomycosis (southwestern U.S.), and blastomycosis (central and southeastern U.S.) usually as part of a systemic illness. Coccidiodal vertebral osteomyelitis occasionally causes multilevel vertebral sclerotic-edged osteolysis and paraspinal uncalcified masses with disk preservation. Gibbus deformity is uncommon.[108]

Differential diagnosis of spondylitis and vertebral osteomyelitis includes pyogenic, granulomatous and fungal infections, and metastasis. Pyogenic and tuberculous spondylitis typically involves disk destruction. Osteolysis of posterior elements is uncommon with tuberculosis, common with pyogenic infections, and typical of metastasis. Metastasis and coccidiomycosis spare the disk. Tuberculosis favors the an-

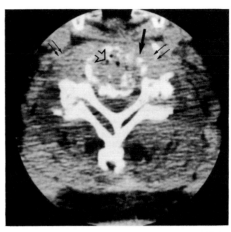

Figure 15.81.   Septic spondylitis—gas formation. *Midcervical 40/500 CT scan.* There is disk and endplate destruction *(closed arrow),* a paraspinal mass *(double arrows),* and gas formation *(open arrow).* Multiple discrete gas bubbles rather than a larger collection and the associated destructive changes and a paraspinal mass favor bacterial gas formation rather than vacuum disk.

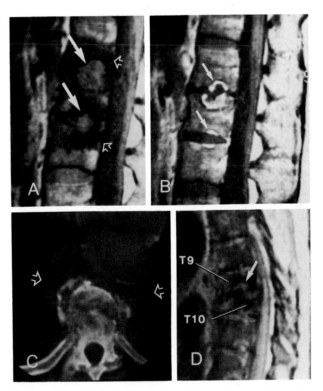

Figure 15.82.   Septic spondylitis. A–B and **C–D** are different patients. Case 1: *Candida* spondylitis L1–3 in an AIDS patient. **A** and **B** are T1-weighted pre- and post-Gd-DTPA i.v. contrast MR scans, respectively. L1–2 *(upper arrow)* and L2–3 *(lower arrow)* vertebral endplate erosion, disk and adjacent vertebral body hypointensity *(open arrows)* diminished disk height, and marked adjacent vertebral contrast enhancement is present. There is hypointense material probably containing desiccated disk within the L1–2 contrast-enhanced portion. (Courtesy of Benjamin Kuzma, M.D., Indianapolis, IN.) Case 2: *S. aureus* spondylitis. Axial T9–10 359/2000 CT scan **(C)** and sagittal SE 2000/30 MR scan **(D).** There is marked T9 and T10 endplate destruction and erosion *(closed arrow),* marked vertebral body compression deformities, and there is a large paraspinal mass *(open arrows).*

terior vertebral body producing a gibbus deformity. Calcification of paraspinal masses is typical of tuberculosis. Metastasis uniquely includes osteoblastic changes. A thin rim of marginal sclerosis is typical of nonpyogenic vertebral osteomyelitis, tends to exclude pyogenic processes but can be confused with osteoblastic changes. The metastatic paravertebral soft tissue mass usually spares or partially spares the prevertebral space whereas pyogenic processes tend to extensively involve it. Gas within the bone (not disk) and soft tissues indicates pyogenic infection.[130]

Epidural Abscess. Spinal epidural abscess most often results from hematogenous spread or, less frequently, direct extension of pyogenic infection. Immunosuppressive disorders and diabetes mellitus increase the risk of occurrence. *S. aureus* is usually responsible but Gram-negative bacilli and tuberculous spinal epidural abscesses also occur. Direct epidural infection can result from spinal puncture, spine penetrating injury, and chemonucleolysis. Early diagnosis is critical in order to begin immediate surgical and medical treatment.[131]

MR is the diagnostic method of choice due to direct visualization of the spinal cord and soft tissues in orthogonal planes (Fig. 15.80). MR demonstrates the epidural mass and associated changes of septic spondylitis. Intravenous contrast injection enhances the inflammatory epidural, disk, vertebral body, and paraspinal tissue, and defines abscesses (Fig. 15.80).[15,131]

CT demonstrates effacement of epidural fat. CT hypotensity with surrounding contrast enhancement of the abscess may be seen (Fig. 15.80). CT myelography is usually necessary in order to demonstrate the full extent of the abscess and spinal cord compression and displacement when MR is not available.[131]

Myelitis. Spinal cord pyogenic abscess can be detected by MR and CT myelography. A series of cases

is necessary to determine imaging characteristics, however, spinal cord expansion with T2 hyperintensity of the abscess would be expected. Sarcoidosis is a rare causative factor inducing myelitis. MR can demonstrate spinal cord enlargement and T2 cord hyperintensity in spinal cord sarcoidosis.[132]

Other Inflammatory Disorders

Other spinal inflammatory disorders include arachnoiditis, ankylosing spondylitis, and rheumatoid arthritis.

Arachnoiditis. Arachnoiditis is a chronic inflammatory condition which is frequently seen in patients who have had iophendylate (Pantopaque) myelography and surgery. Patients who have had both iophendylate myelography and surgery, however, often have no evidence of arachnoiditis. Arachnoiditis also occurs in patients who have had meningitis, subarachnoid hemorrhage, spinal tumors, and intrathecal medications and anesthesia.[133] Arachnoiditis is characterized by collagen arachnoid and subarachnoid deposition with subsequent adhesions affecting the theca and nerve roots with thickening, retraction and fibrosis. Postinflammatory syringomyelia may occur.[134]

MR and CT myelography demonstrate thecal sac thickening and fibrosis, and nerve root adhesions to other roots (clumping) or to the thecal sac (Fig. 15.83).[134] Iophendylate droplets may be seen by either the MR (fat-intensity) or CT (hyperdense) method but are more easily detected by CT.

Ankylosing Spondylitis. Ankylosing spondylitis is a progressive arthritic disease that primarily affects the sacroiliac joints and the apophyseal joints of the entire spine. Joint ankylosis, ligamental and annulus fibrosus ossification, vertebral endplate rim destruction, demineralization and, often, disk space narrowing occurs. Spinal canal and thecal sac dilatation is occasionally seen. Atlantoaxial subluxation

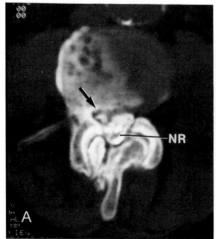 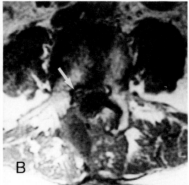 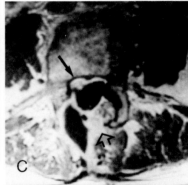

Figure 15.83.   Lumbar arachnoiditis. *L3-4 350/2000 CT myelogram **(A)**. Same level 3-month post-laminectomy noncontrast **(B)** and i.v. contrast **(C)** SE 500/20 MR Scans. There is arachnoid scarring (closed arrow) that markedly contrast enhances by MR. Note the adherent "clumped up" nerve roots (NR) demonstrated by CT myelography.

Contrast enhancement of the operative scar (open arrow) is seen adjacent to a right-sided fluid collection which communicates with the thecal sac representing a pseudomeningocele. There has been relief of the preoperative stenosis with absence of the trefoil appearance seen in A.

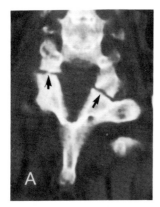
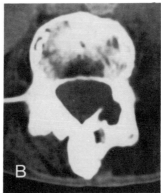
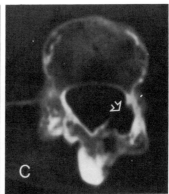

Figure 15.84. Ankylosing spondylitis. A and **B–C** are different cases. Case 1: *Modified direct coronal 336/1000 section* **(A)** *of the markedly cervical lordotic patient. There are bilateral fractures of the* C6–7 ankylosis *(arrows)*. Case 2: *Axial L5-level 67/350* **(B)** *and 370/ 2000* **(C)**. There is dural sac bulging into the smoothly marginated erosive defect *(open arrow)*. Note the ankylosed facet joints.

may occur. Fractures of the fragile fused spine tend to occur after relatively mild trauma. The resultant subluxation of the fracture fragments can produce spinal cord compression with severe clinical consequences.[2] CT more accurately identifies the bone changes characteristic of ankylosing spondylitis (Fig. 15.84). The localizer view may demonstrate syndesmophyte vertebral body ankylosis. MR can better evaluate cord compression and cord injury.

Rheumatoid Arthritis. Unlike ankylosing spondylitis, rheumatoid arthritis more severely affects the cervical spine than other levels. The thoracolumbar spine is less often affected and sacroiliac fusion is rare. Pannus formation and synovial joint erosion is associated with apophyseal joint laxity subluxation, disk bulging, and superimposed degenerative spurring (Fig. 15.85). The atlantoaxial joint is often involved with odontoid base erosion, transverse ligament laxity, and C1–2 subluxation.[2] Spinal cord compression commonly occurs at levels of subluxation and stenosis. CT and MR play complementary roles in the investigation of rheumatoid arthritis. CT best demonstrates the degree of joint and bone erosion destruction and osteophytosis, however, MR

best demonstrates spinal cord displacement, compression, and abnormal signal within the compressed cord.[135]

A mass of fibrous and granulation tissue ("pseudotumor") uncommonly occurs at the craniovertebral junction in rheumatoid arthritis cases. It also occurs in patients with other degenerative joint diseases. Because these pseudotumors are composed of fibrous tissue, they have an MR T1 and T2 low to intermediate signal intensity. This hypo- or isointensity mass, associated with subluxation, helps differentiate these lesions from craniovertebral chordomas and metastasis. Meningioma may have a similar appearance. CT is less effective demonstrating these pseudotumors due to lack of direct sagittal imaging and less sensitive tissue discrimination.[135]

EPIDURAL HEMATOMA

Spinal epidural hematoma is an uncommon lesion often associated with anticoagulant therapy and coagulopathy.[136] Less common causes include surgery, cervical or lumbar needle puncture, trauma, neoplasm, and pregnancy.[136] Symptoms of acute epidural hematoma include severe pain and rapidly de-

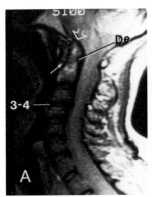
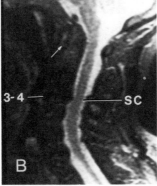
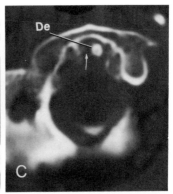

Figure 15.85. Rheumatoid arthritis. A–B and **C** are different cases. *Midsagittal flow-compensation SE 2000/30* **(A)** *and 2000/80* **(B)**. *Axial C1–2 level 468/2000 CT scan* **(C)**. Pannus *(arrows)* erodes the dens *(De)* waist. There is C1–2 subluxation and C3–4 retrolisthesis. The tip of the dens *(open arrow)* is slightly posterior and superior to its usual position immediately under the basion *(clivus tip)* indicating a slight degree of basilar invagination. The spinal cord-medullary junction is slightly angulated as a result. There is borderline C3–4 stenosis with only a thin rim of hyperintense CSF surrounding the spinal cord *(SC)*. Note the markedly small diameter of the eroded dens base **(C)**.

veloping paresis. Surgery must be immediately performed due to the rarity of spontaneous remissions.[89]

The diagnostic procedure of choice is MR scanning due to direct spinal cord visualization and tissue analysis in orthogonal planes. Acute hemorrhage signal (T1 isointense/T2 hypointense) can be identified within the epidural mass (Fig. 15.55). CT requires an initial method to determine a level of involvement accurately. For this reason, myelography is usually done first followed by CT myelography. Acute hemorrhage density may be difficult to identify in the presence of intrathecal contrast.[89]

The differential diagnosis includes epidural tumor and a rare subarachnoid hematoma.[137] Careful analysis of CT density and MR intensity should lead to the correct diagnosis.

VASCULAR MALFORMATION

These conditions include ateriovenous malformations and the very rare spinal cord cavernous hemangiomas.[138,139]

Arteriovenous malformations are fistulous communications between arteries and veins, lacking an intervening capillary network. They usually occur as intramedullary, extramedullary, or dural types with vascular supply by anterior radiculomedullary, posterior radiculomedullary, or radiculomeningeal arteries, respectively.[138]

The intramedullary and extramedullary lesions have an equal incidence in both sexes, are more common in the cervical and cervicothoracic regions, have a large shunt volume, and are present in patients younger than 50 years of age. The intramedullary nidus is deep within the anterior spinal cord and the extramedullary nidus is superficial on the dorsal cord surface.[138]

Dural (radiculomeningeal) arteriovenous malformations are present in older, predominantly male,

patients and most commonly occur in the thoracic and thoracolumbar spine. The clinical onset of dural malformation is typically a slow, progressive myelopathy as compared to the more rapid onset of the intramedullary and extramedullary types.[138]

Surface coil MR is the investigative method of choice. MR characteristically demonstrates signal-void serpentine veins, a vascular nidus, and, often, distal spinal cord hyperintensity probably representing edema (Fig. 15.86).[138] CT myelography after myelographic lesion longitudinal localization is the alternative diagnostic method. CT myelography demonstrates abnormal vessels as punctate and serpentine sharply defined structures within the contrast-enhanced subarachnoid space.[2]

SPINAL CORD INFARCTION

MR is expected to be able to detect spinal cord infarction much as it does brainstem infarcts. CT may rarely demonstrate spinal cord hemorrhagic infarcts[140] but it is not a reliable method.

MULTIPLE SCLEROSIS

Multiple sclerosis commonly affects the spinal cord. Contrast CT can occasionally demonstrate contrast enhancement of acute multiple sclerosis demyelination and CT myelography may occasionally demonstrate associated spinal cord swelling.[141] CT, nevertheless, is not a reliably sensitive method of diagnosis.[142]

MR, on the other hand, is fairly sensitive to spinal MR changes and MR i.v. paramagnetic contrast agents may improve sensitivity and specificity of the method. Multiple sclerotic spinal cord plaques preferentially occur in the dorsal and lateral segments and are characteristically elongated parallel to the cord long axis. They do not correspond to specific fiber tracts and cross gray-white matter boundaries. Acute plaques may occasionally cause focal cord expansion.[3,142]

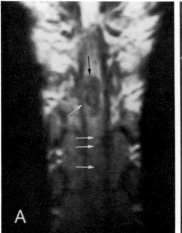
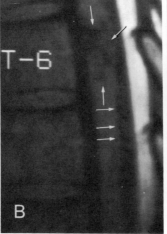
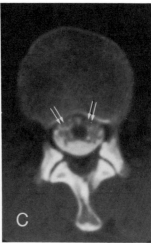

Figure 15.86. Spinal arteriovenous malformation. **A–B** and **C** are different cases. *Coronal SE 1500/30* **(A)** *and midsagittal SE 1500/20* **(B)** *T6-level nonflow-compensation MR scans. Axial 400/(conus-level) 1500 CT myelogram* **(C)**. A signal-void arterial nidus *(angular arrows)* and signal-void tortuous veins *(parallel arrows)* are seen posterolaterally below the T6 level in **A** and **B**. CT myelography demonstrates multiple abnormal dilated subarachnoid veins anterior to the conus similar in appearance to cauda equina roots in this surgically proven case **(C)**.

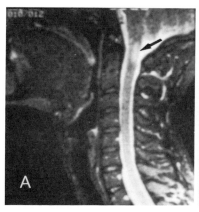
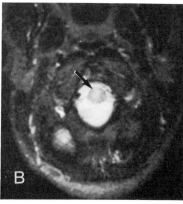

Figure 15.87. Cervical spinal cord MS plaque. *Midsagittal (A) and C1–2 axial (B) T2-weighted MR scans.* There is an abnormal hyperintense ovoid C1–2 spinal cord lesion *(arrows)*. There is no evidence of intramedullary expansion. Note how the ovoid lesion is elongated in the sagittal axis. (Courtesy of Richard D. Smith, M.D., Indianapolis, IN.)

Surface coil T2-weighted images demonstrate the characteristically hyperintense lesions (Fig. 15.87).

OTHER BONE DISEASES AND BONE ABNORMALITIES

Bone diseases and bone abnormalities that will be discussed in this section are Paget's disease, osteoporosis, and sickle cell disease.

Paget's Disease

Paget's disease of the spine causes highly vascular, coarsely trabecular, demineralized and hypertrophied vertebral bone. Spinal stenosis frequently develops due to vertebral body and neural arch hypertrophy. Malignant degeneration to osteosarcoma is uncommon. Characteristic CT changes of Paget's disease include coarsened trabeculae, zones of demineralization and of sclerosis, and bone expansile hypertrophy with spinal stenosis (Fig. 15.88).[2,10,143] MR Paget's changes are less obvious. The major differential diagnostic considerations are metastasis, myeloma, and hemangioma. The Paget's changes characteristically involve the entire vertebra, include nondestructive bone expansion with spinal stenosis, and are not accompanied by an adjacent soft tissue mass. Metastases are often focally destructive within the vertebra, are not associated with bone expansion, and are often associated with a soft tissue mass. Both Paget's disease and metastasis may involve multiple vertebrae. Osteosarcomatous degeneration of Paget's disease has typical "aggressive"

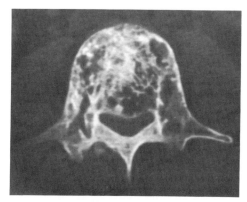

Figure 15.88. Paget's disease. *Axial L5 377/1600 CT scan.* There is thickening of bizarre trabeculae with intertrabecular irregular hypodense regions. The vertebral body and pedicle expansion has stenosed the spinal canal.

characteristics of osteosarcoma.[108,143] Myeloma and hemangioma characteristics are reviewed in Table 15.1.

Osteoporosis

Osteoporosis is a diffuse process affecting all bones throughout the body. Osteoporotic compression fractures are common and are usually of the biconcave ("fishmouth") or wedge type. Burst-type osteoporotic fractures may also occur with retropulsed fragments and neurological compromise.[144] CT demonstrates decreased numbers of thickened spongy bone trabeculae with cortical bone thinning (Fig. 15.89). These findings are sometimes confused with vertebral hemangiomas. The hemangioma, however, is limited to a single vertebra, has an abrupt transition with vertebral normal bone and lacks diffuse cortical thinning.[2] Quantitative bone density measurements can be obtained with CT technique.[145] Osteoporosis is often associated with fatty replacement of paraspinal muscles in the elderly.[81]

Sickle Cell Disease

Sickle cell disease may cause coarsened vertebral trabeculae, increased bone density, medullary space expansion, and cortical thinning. Bone infarcts, diskitis, and osteomyelitis may occur. These changes are detectable by CT. Encroachment of the intervertebral disks into the vertebral endplates produces characteristic "H-vertebral" bodies which can be detected by CT reformation and sagittal MR scanning.[2]

POSTOPERATIVE CHANGES

Postoperative changes include osseous and soft tissue changes and the presence of devices such as Harrington rods. Some postoperative changes have already been discussed, such as postdiskectomy epidural scars and arachnoiditis. Fusion mass hypertrophy may cause spinal stenosis (Fig. 15.90). Postlaminectomy bone defects, ligamentum flavum defect, and dural bulge ("pseudomeningocele") can be easily detected by CT (Fig. 15.91). Postoperative spinal epidural hematoma is most easily detected by MR. Thecal sac compression and spinal stenosis resulting from Harrington rod placement should be studied by CT and not by MR due to the metallic magnetic field distortion.

Figure 15.89. Osteoporosis. *Axial L2-level 82/400 CT scan.* **(A)** *Midsagittal reformation of 3-mm sections* **(B).** There is a generalized decreased mineralization with thickened sparce trabeculae *(closed arrows)*, L2 central compression fracture biconcave deformity, and hyperdensity is seen *(open arrow)*.

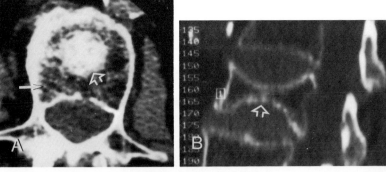

Figure 15.90. Surgical fusion evaluation. L4–S1 lateral fusion. *L5–S1 axial 305/2000 CT scan* **(A)** *and 3-D reformation scans* **(B–D).** Lateral bone grafts *(arrows)* appear solidly fused to the transverse processes *(TP)*, superior facets *(SF)*, and inferior facets *(IF)*. Fusion mass hypertrophy involves the laminae *(La)* with encroachment upon the spinal canal. The neural foramina *(NF)* are anterior to the fusion mass; spinous process *(SP)*.

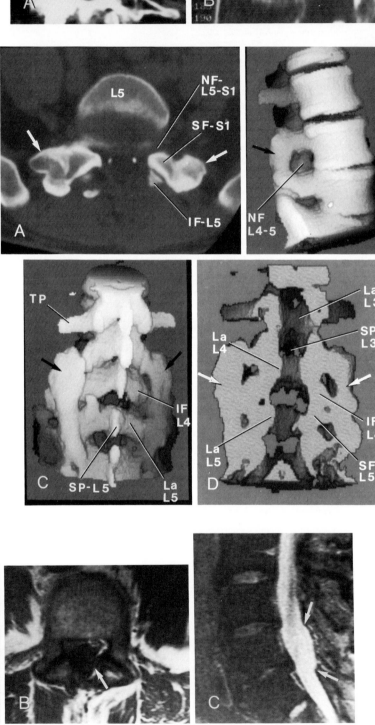

Figure 15.91. Postlaminectomy pseudomeningocele. *L4–5 349/2000 CT myelogram* **(A)** *and SE 600/25 MR scan* **(B).** *Midsagittal SE 2800/80 MR scan* **(C).** The dural sac bulges through the bilateral laminectomy defect *(arrows)*.

452

References

1. Modic MT. Normal anatomy. In Modic MT, Masaryk TJ, Ross JS (Eds). *Magnetic Resonance Imaging of the Spine.* Chicago: Year Book Medical Publishers, 1989; 35–74.
2. Grossman CB, Post JD. The adult spine. In Gonzalez CF, Grossman CB, Masdeu JM (Eds). *Head and Spine Imaging.* New York: John Wiley & Sons, 1985; 781–858.
3. Norman D. The spine. In Brant-Zawadzki M, Norman D (Eds). *Magnetic Resonance Imaging of the Central Nervous System.* New York: Raven Press, 1987; 289–328.
4. Hajek PC, Baker LI, Goobar JE. Focal fat deposition in axial bone marrow: MR characteristics. *Radiology* 1987; 162:245–249.
5. Resnick D. Degenerative diseases of the vertebral column. *Radiology* 1985; 156:3–14.
6. Grenier N, Kressel HY, Schiebler ML, et al. Normal and degenerative posterior spinal structures: MR imaging. *Radiology* 1987; 165:517–525.
7. Yu S, Sether L, Haughton VM. Facet joint menisci of the cervical spine: Correlative MR imaging and cryomicrotomy study. *Radiology* 1987; 164:79–82.
8. Goss CM. *Anatomy of the Human Body (Gray's Anatomy).* Philadelphia: Lea & Febiger, 1959.
9. Sartoris DJ, Resnick D, Guerra J Jr. Vertebral venous channels: CT appearance and differential considerations. *Radiology* 1985; 1545:745–749.
10. Haughton VM, Williams AL (eds). *Computed Tomography of the Spine.* St. Louis: CV Mosby, 1982.
11. Ullrich CG, Binet EF, Sanecki MG, et al. Quantitative assessment of the lumbar spinal canal by computed tomography. *Radiology* 1980; 134:137–143.
12. Aguila LA, Piraino DW, Modic MD, et al. The intranuclear cleft of the intervertebral disk: Magnetic resonance imaging. *Radiology* 1985; 155:8.
13. Daniels DL, Williams AL, Haughton VM. Computed tomography of the articulations and ligaments at the occipito-atlantoaxial region. *Radiology* 1983; 146:709–716.
14. Yu YL, Stevens JM, Kendall B, duBoulay GH. Cord shape and measurements in cervical spondylotic myelopathy and radiculopathy. *AJNR* 1983; 4:839–842.
15. Grogan JP, Daniels DL, Williams AL, et al. The normal conus medullaris: CT criteria for recognition. *Radiology* 1984; 151:661–664.
16. Monajati A, Wayne WS, Rauschning W, Ekholm SE. MR of the cauda equina. *AJNR* 1987; 8:893–900.
17. Kjos BO, Norman D. Strategies for efficient imaging of the lumbar spine. In Brant-Zawadzki M, Norman D (Eds). *Magnetic Resonance Imaging of the Central Nervous System.* New York: Raven Press, 1987; 279–288.
18. Flannigan BD, Lufkin RB, McGlade C. MR imaging of the cervical spine. *AJNR* 1987; 8:27–32.
19. Pech P, Daniels DL, Williams AL, Haughton VM. The cervical neural foramina: Correlation of microtomy and CT anatomy. *Radiology* 1985; 155:143–146.
20. Daniels DL, Hyde JS, Kneeland JB. The cervical nerves and foramina: Local-coil MR imaging. *AJNR* 1986; 7:129–133.
21. Osborn AG, Koehler PR. Computed tomography of the paraspinal musculature: Normal and pathological anatomy. *AJR* 1982; 138:93–98.
22. Van Dyke JA, Holley HC, Anderson SD. Review of iliopsoas anatomy and pathology. *Radiographics* 1987; 7:53–84.
23. Sze G, Abramson A, Krol G, et al. Gadolinium-DTPA in the evaluation of intradural extramedullary spinal disease. *AJNR* 1988; 9:153–163.
24. Czervionke LF, Daniels DL, Ho PSP, et al. Cervical neural foramina: Anatomic and MR imaging study. *Radiology* 1988; 169:753–759.
25. Russell EJ, D'Angelo CM, Zimmerman RD, et al. Cervical disk herniation: CT demonstration after contrast enhancement. *Radiology* 1984; 152:703–712.
26. Calvy TM, Segall HD, Gilles FH, et al. CT anatomy of the cranioverbetral junction in infants and children. *AJNR* 1987; 8:489–494.
27. Rothman SLG, Glenn WV. Spondylolysis and spondylolisthesis. In Post MJD (Ed). *Computed Tomography of the Spine.* Baltimore: Williams & Wilkins, 1985; 591–615.
28. Rosenthal DL, Stauffer AE, Davis KR, et al. Evaluation of multiplanar reconstruction in CT recognition of lumbar disk disease. *AJNR* 1984; 5:307–314.
29. Lanzieri CF, Hilal SK. Computed tomography of the sacral plexus

and sciatic nerve in the greater sciatic foramen. *AJNR* 1984; 5:315–318.
30. Haughton VM. MR imaging of the spine. *Radiology* 1988; 166:297–301.
31. Hedberg MC, Drayer BP, Flom RA, et al. Gradient echo (GRASS) MR imaging in cervical radiculopathy. *AJNR* 1988; 9:145–151.
32. Bronskill MJ, McVeigh ER, Kucharczyk W, Henkelman RM. Syrinx-like artifacts on MR images of the spinal cord. *Radiology* 1988; 166:485–488.
33. Runge VM, Schaible TF, Goldstein HA. Gd-DTPA clinical efficacy. *Radiographics* 1988; 8:147–159.
34. Runge VM, Wood ML, Kaufman D, Price AC. Gd-DTPA future applications with advanced imaging techniques. *Radiographics* 1988; 8:161–179.
35. Kulkarni MV, McArdle CB, Kopanicky D, et al. Acute spinal cord injury: MR imaging at 1.5 T. *Radiology* 1987; 164:837–843.
36. Fitz CR. The pediatric spine. In Gonzalez CF, Grossman CB, Masdeu JM (Eds). *Head and Spine Imaging.* New York: John Wiley & Sons, 1985; 759–780.
37. Naidich TP, Zimmerman RA. Common congenital malformations of the brain. In Brant-Zawadzki M, Norman D (Eds). *Magnetic Resonance Imaging of the Central Nervous System.* New York: Raven Press, 1987; 131–150.
38. Naidich TP, McLone DG, Mutluer S. A new understanding of dorsal dysraphism with lipoma (lipomyeloschisis): Radiological evaluation and surgical correction. *AJNR* 1983; 4:103–116.
39. Flannigan-Sprague BD, Modic MT. The pediatric spine, normal anatomy and spinal dysraphism. In Modic MT, Masaryk TJ, Ross JS (Eds). *Magnetic Resonance Imaging of the Spine.* Chicago: Year Book Medical Publishers, 1989; 240–256.
40. Vade A, Kennard D. Lipomeningomyelocystocele. *AJNR* 1987; 8:375–377.
41. Naidich TP, Zimmerman RA. Common congenital malformations of the brain. In Brant-Zawadzki M, Norman D (Eds). *Magnetic Resonance Imaging of the Central Nervous System.* New York: Raven Press, 1987; 131–150.
42. Scotti G, Musgrave MA, Harwood-Nash DC, et al. Diastematomyelia in children: Metrizamide and CT metrizamide myelography. *AJNR* 1980; 1:403–410.
43. Naidich TP, Harwood-Nash DC. Diastematomyelia: Hemicord and meningeal sheaths; single and double arachnoid and dural tubes. *AJNR* 1983; 4:633–636.
44. Schlesinger AE, Naidich TP, Quencer RM. Concurrent hydromyelia and diastematomyelia. *AJNR* 1986; 7:473–477.
45. Han JS, Benson JE, Kaufman B. Demonstration of diastematomyelia and associated abnormalities with MR imaging. *AJNR* 1985; 6:215–219.
46. Barkovich AJ, Raghavan N, Chuang S, Peck WW. The wedge-shaped cord terminus: a radiographic sign of caudal regression. *AJNR* 1989; 10:1223–1231.
47. Wang H, Rosenbaum AE, Reid C, et al. Pediatric patients with achondroplasia: CT evaluation of the craniocervical junction. *Radiology* 1987; 164:515–519.
48. Suss RA, Udvarhelyi GB, Wang H, et al. Myelography in achondroplasia: Value of a lateral C1-2 puncture and non-ionic, water soluble contrast material. *Radiology* 1983; 149:159–163.
49. Edwards MK, Harwood-Nash DC, Fitz CR, Chuang SH. CT metrizamide myelography of the cervical spine in Morquio syndrome. *AJNR* 1982; 3:666–669.
50. Banna M, Hollenberg R. Compressive meningeal hypertrophy in mucopolyaccharidosis. *AJNR* 1987; 8:385–386.
51. Naidich TP, McLone DG, Harwood-Nash DC. Systemic malformations. In Newton TH, Potts DG (Eds). *Modern Neuroradiology.* San Enselmo, CA: Clavadel Press, 1984; 367–382.
52. Williams AL, Haughton VM, Daniels DL, Grogan JR. Differential CT diagnosis of extruded nucleus pulposus. *Radiology* 1983; 148:141–148.
53. White JG III, Strait TA, Binkley JR, Hunter SA. Surgical treatment of 63 cases of conjoined nerve roots. *J Neurosurg* 1982; 56:114–117.
54. Hoddick WK, Helms CA. Bony spinal canal changes that differentiate conjoined nerve roots from herniated nucleus pulposis. *Radiology* 1985; 154:119–120.
55. Kieffer SA. Disk disease: Radiculopathies. In Harwood-Nash DC, Huckman MS, Lukin RR (Eds). *Syllabus: A Categorical Course in Neuroradiology.* 73rd Scientific Assembly and Annual Meeting of the Radiological Society of North America (11/29/87–12/4/87); 71–80.
56. Grenier N, Grossman RI, Scheibler ML, et al. Degenerative lumbar disk disease: Pitfalls and usefulness of MR imaging in detection of vacuum phenomenon. *Radiology* 1987; 164:861–865.
57. Maravilla KR, Lesh P, Weinreb JC, et al. Magnetic resonance im-

aging of the lumbar spine with CT correlation. *AJNR* 1985; 6:237–245.

58. Kaiser MC, Sandt G, Roilgen A, et al. Intradural disk herniation with CT appearance of gas collection. *AJNR* 1985; 6:117–118.
59. Firooznia H, Benjamin V, Kricheff II, et al. CT of lumbar spine disk herniation: correlation with surgical findings. *AJNR* 1984; 5:91–96.
60. Williams AL, Haughton VM, Daniels DL, Thornton RS. CT recognition of lateral lumbar disk herniation. *AJNR* 1982; 3:211–213.
61. Graves VB, Finney HL, Mailander. Intradural lumbar disk herniation. *AJNR* 1986; 7:495–497.
62. Eisenberg RA, Bremer AM, Northrup HM. Intradural herniated cervical disk. *AJNR* 1986; 7:492–494.
63. Modic MT, Steinberg PM, Ross JC, et al. Degenerative disk disease: Assessment of changes in vertebral body marrow with MR imaging. *Radiology* 1988; 166:193–199.
64. Ross JS, Hueftle MG. Postoperative spine. In Modic MT, Masaryk TJ, Ross JS (Eds). *Magnetic Resonance Imaging of the Spine.* Chicago: Year Book of Medical Publishers, 1989; 120–148.
65. Braun IF, Hoffman JC Jr, Davis PC. Contrast enhancement in CT differentiation between recurrent disk herniation and postoperative scar: Prospective study. *AJNR* 1985; 6:607–612.
66. Wilmink JT, Roukema JG. Effects of IV contrast administration on intraspinal and paraspinal tissues: A CT study. 1. Measurements of CT attenuation numbers. *AJNR* 1987; 8:703–709.
67. Gentry LR, Turski PA, Strother CM, et al. Chymopapain chemonucleolysis: CT changes after treatment. *AJNR* 1985; 6:321–329.
68. Huckman MS, Clark JW, McNeill TW, et al. Chemonucleation and changes observed on lumbar MR scan: preliminary report. *AJNR* 1987; 8:1–4.
69. Onik G, Maroon J, Helms C, et al. Automated percutaneous diskectomy: Initial patient experience. Work in progress. *Radiology* 1987; 162:129–132.
70. Ross JS, Perez-Reyes N, Masaryk TJ, et al. Thoracic disk herniation: MR imaging. *Radiology* 1987; 165:511–515.
71. Matsuura P, Waters RL, Adkins RH. Comparison of computerized tomography parameters of the cervical spine in normal control subjects and spinal cord injured patients. *J Bone Joint Surg* 1989; 71A:183–188.
72. Penning L, Wilmink JT, van Woerden HH, Knol E. CT myelographic findings in degenerative disorders of the cervical spine: Clinical significance. *AJNR* 1986; 7:119–127.
73. Teresi LM, Lufkin RB, Reicher MA, et al. Asymptomatic degenerative disk disease and spondylosis of the cervical spine: MR imaging. *Radiology* 1987; 164:83–88.
74. Modic MT. Degenerative disorders of the spine. In Modic MT, Masaryk TJ, Ross JS (Eds). *Magnetic Resonance Imaging of the Spine.* Chicago: Year Book of Medical Publishers, 1989; 75–119.
75. Schellinger D, Wener L, Ragsdale BD, Patronas NJ. Facet joint disorders and their role in the production of back pain and sciatica. *Radiographics* 1987; 7:923–944.
76. Jinkins JR, Bashir R, Al-Mefty O, et al. Cystic necrosis of the spinal cord in compressive cervical myelopathy: Demonstration by iopamidol CT-myelography. *AJNR* 1986; 7:693–701.
77. Kaplan P, Resnick D, Murphey M, et al. Destructive noninfectious spondyloarthropathy in hemodialysis patients: A report of four cases. *Radiology* 1987; 162:241–244.
78. Jackson DE, Atlas SW, Mani JR, Norman D. Intraspinal synovial cysts: MR imaging. *Radiology* 1989; 170:527–530.
79. Grenier N, Kressel HY, Schiebler ML, Grossman RL. Isthmic spondylolysis of the lumbar spine: MR imaging at 1.5T. *Radiology* 1989; 170:489–493.
80. Nokes SR, Murtagh FR, Jones JD III, et al. Childhood scoliosis: MR imaging. *Radiology* 1987; 164:791–797.
81. Hadar H, Gadoth N, Heifetz M. Fatty replacement of lower paraspinal muscles: Normal and neuromuscular disorders. *AJNR* 1983; 4:1087–1090.
82. Masaryk TJ. Spine trauma. In Modic MT, Masaryk TJ, Ross JS (Eds). *Magnetic Resonance Imaging of the Spine.* Chicago: Year Book of Medical Publishers, 1989; 214–239.
83. Quencer RM, Sheldon JJ, Post MJD. Magnetic resonance imaging of the chronically injured cervical spinal cord. *AJNR* 1986; 7:457–464.
84. Bools JC, Rose BS. Traumatic atlanto-occipital dislocation: Two cases with survival. *AJNR* 1986; 7:901–904.
85. Suss RA, Bundy KJ. Unilateral posterior arch fractures of the atlas. *AJNR* 1984; 5:783–786.
86. Suss RA, Zimmerman RD, Leeds NE. Pseudospread of the atlas: False sign of Jefferson fracture in young children. *AJR* 1983; 140:1079–1082.
87. Kowalski HM, Cohen WA, Cooper P, Wisoff JH. Pitfalls in the CT diagnosis of atlantoaxial rotary subluxation. *AJR* 1987; 8:697–702.

88. Pech P, Kilgore DP, Pojunas KW, Haughton VM. Cervical spinal fractures: CT detection. *Radiology* 1985; 157:117–120.
89. Laissy J-P, Milon P, Freger P, et al. Cervical epidural hematomas: CT diagnosis in two cases that resolved spontaneously. AJNR 1990; 11:394–396.
90. Hackney DB, Asato R, Joseph PM, et al. Hemorrhage and edema in acute spinal cord compression: Demonstration by MR imaging. *Radiology* 1986; 161:387–390.
91. Chakeres DW, Flickinger F, Bresnahan JC, et al. MR imaging of acute spinal cord trauma. *AJNR* 1987; 8:5–10.
92. Yetkin Z, Osborn AG, Giles DS, Haughton VM. Uncovertebral and facet joint dislocations in cervical articular pillar fractures: CT evaluation. *AJNR* 1985; 6:633–637.
93. Morris RE, Hasso AN, Thompson JR, et al. Traumatic dural tears: CT diagnosis using metrizamide. *Radiology* 1984; 152:443–446.
94. Armington WG, Harnsberger HR, Osborn AG, Seay AR. Radiographic evaluation of brachial plexopathy. *AJNR* 1987; 8:361–367.
95. Blumenkopf B, Bennett WF. Delayed presentation of post-traumatic cervical disk herniation. *AJNR* 1986; 7:722–724.
96. Gebarski SS, Maynard FW, Gabrielsen TO, et al. Post-traumatic progressive myelopathy. *Radiology* 1985; 157:379–385.
97. Dunn V, Smoker W, Menezes AH. Transdural herniation of the cervical spinal cord as a complication of a broken fracture-fixation wire. *AJNR* 1987; 8:724–726.
98. Gellad FE, Levine AM, Joslyn JN. Pure thoracolumbar facet dislocation: clinical features and CT appearance. *Radiology* 1986; 161:505–508.
99. Manaster BJ, Osborne AG. CT patterns of facet fracture dislocations in the thoracolumbar region. *AJNR* 1986; 7:1007–1012.
100. Atlas SW, Regenbogen V, Rogers LF, Kim KS. The radiographic characterization of burst fractures of the spine. *AJNR* 1986; 7:675–682.
101. Shuman WP, Rogers JV, Sickler ME, et al. Thoracolumbar burst fractures: CT dimensions of the spinal canal relative to postsurgical improvement. *AJNR* 1985; 6:337–341.
102. Guerra J Jr, Garfin SR, Resnick D. Vertebral burst fractures: CT analysis of the retropulsed fragment. *Radiology* 1984; 153:769–772.
103. Ross JS, Masaryk TJ, Modic MT, et al. Vertebral hemangiomas: MR imaging. *Radiology* 1987; 165:165–196.
104. Greenfield GB (Ed). *Radiology of Bone Diseases.* Philadelphia: JB Lippincott, 1969; 364–370.
105. Gamba JL, Martinez S, Apple J, et al. Computed tomography of axial skeletal osteoid osteomas. *AJR* 1984; 142:769–772.
106. Omojola MF, Fox AJ, Vinuela FV. Computed tomographic metrizamide myelography in the evaluation of thoracic spinal osteoblastoma. *AJNR* 1982; 3:670–673.
107. Beltran J, Noto AM, Chakeres DW, Christoforidis AJ. Tumors of the osseous spine: Staging with MR imaging versus CT. *Radiology* 1987; 162:565–569.
108. Doorwart RH, LaMasters DL, Wanatabe TJ. Tumors. In Newton TH, Potts DG (Eds). *Modern Neuroradiology Computed Tomography of the Brain and Spinal Cord,* Volume I. San Anselmo, CA: Clavadel Press, 1983; 115–147.
109. Jeyer JE, Lepke RA, Lindfors KKI et al. Chordomas: Their CT appearance in cervical, thoracic and lumbar spine. *Radiology* 1984; 153:693–696.
110. Sze G, Uichanco LS III, Brant-Zawadzki MN, et al. Chordomas: MR imaging. *Radiology* 1988; 166:187–191.
111. Schrieman J, McLeod RA, Kyle RA, Beabout JW. Multiple myeloma evaluation by CT. *Radiology* 1985; 154:483–486.
112. Moore SG, Gooding CA, Brasch RC. Bone marrow in children with acute lymphocytic leukemia: MR relaxation times. *Radiology* 1986; 160:237–240.
113. Beres J, Pech P, Berns TF, et al. Spinal epidural lymphomas: CT features in seven patients. *AJNR* 1986; 7:327–328.
114. Burk DL, Brunberg JA, Kanal E, et al. Spinal and paraspinal neurofibromatosis: Surface coil MR imaging at 1.5 T. *Radiology* 1987; 162:797–801.
115. Masaryk TJ. Spine tumors. In Modic MT, Masaryk TJ, Ross JS (Eds). *Magnetic Resonance Imaging of the Spine.* Chicago: Year Book Medical Publishers, 1989; 183–213.
116. Dross PE, Raji MR. CT myelography of calcified thoracic neurolemoma. *AJNR* 1985; 6:967–968.
117. Lapointe JS, Graeb DA, Nugent RA, Robertson WD. Value of intravenous contrast enhancement in the CT evaluation of intraspinal tumors. *AJNR* 1985; 6:939–943.
118. Puljic S, Schechter MM. Multiple spinal canal meningiomas. *AJNR* 1980; 1:325–327.
119. Dastur KJ, Raji MR, Smith WI Jr. Pulmonary metastasis from intraspinal meningioma. *AJNR* 1984; 5:483–484.

120. Smoker WRK, Biller J, Moore SA, et al. Intradural spinal teratoma: Case report and review of the literature. *AJNR* 1986; 7:905–910.
121. Kim KS, Ho SU, Weinberg PE, Lee C. Spinal leptomeningeal infiltration by systemic cancer: Myelographic features. *AJR* 1982; 139:361–365.
122. Post MJD, Quencer RM, Green BA, et al. Intramedullary spinal cord metastasis, mainly of non-neurogenic origin. *AJNR* 1987; 8:339–346.
123. Sato Y, Waziri M, Smith W, et al. Hippel-Lindau disease: MR imaging. *Radiology* 1988; 166:241–246.
124. Rebner M, Gebarski SS. Magnetic resonance imaging of spinal-cord hemangioblastoma. *AJNR* 1985; 6:287–289.
125. Modic MT, Feiglin DH, Piraino DW, et al. Vertebral osteomyelitis: Assessment using MR. *Radiology* 1985; 157:157–166.
126. Brant-Zawadzki M. Infections in computed tomography of the spine and spinal cord. In Newton TH, Potts DG (Eds). *Modern Neuroradiology CT of the Brain and Spinal Cord.* San Anselmo, CA: Clavadel Press, 1983.
127. Price AC, Allen JH, Eggers FM, et al. Intervertebral disk-space infection: CT changes. *Radiology* 1983; 149:725–729.
128. Larde D, Mathieu D, Frija J. Vertebral osteomyelitis: Disk hypodensity on CT. *AJNR* 1982; 3:657–661.
129. Golimbu, Firooznia H, Rafii M. CT of osteomyelitis of the spine. *AJNR* 1983; 4:1207–1211.
130. Van Lom KJ, Kellerhouse LE, Pathria MN. Infection versus tumor in the spine: Criteria for distinction with CT. *Radiology* 1988; 166:851–855.
131. Angtuaco EJC, McConnell JR, Chadduck WM, Flanigan S. MR imaging of spinal epidural sepsis. *AJNR* 1987; 8:879–883.
132. Kelly RB, Mahoney PD, Cawley KM. MR demonstration of spinal cord sarcoidosis: Report of a case. *AJNR* 1988; 9:197–199.
133. Simmons JD, Newton THH. Arachnoiditis. In Newton TH, Potts DG (Eds). *Computed Tomography of the Spine and Spinal Cord.* San Anselmo, CA: Clavadel Press, 1983; 223–230.
134. Ross JS, Masaryk TJ, Modic MT, et al. MR imaging of lumbar arachnoiditis. *AJNR* 1987; 8:885–892.
135. Sze G, Brant-Zawadzki MN, Wilson CR, et al. Pseudotumor of the craniovertebral junction associated with chronic subluxation: MR imaging studies. *Radiology* 1986; 161:391–394.
136. Zilkha A, Irwin GAL, Fagelman D. Computed tomography of spinal epidural hematoma. *AJNR* 1983; 4:1073–1076.
137. Abla A, Rothfus WE, Maroon JC, Deeb ZL. Delayed spinal subarachnoid hematoma: A rare complication of C1-C2 cervical myelography. *AJNR* 1986; 7:526–528.
138. Masaryk TJ, Ross JS, Modic MT, et al. Radiculomeningeal vascular malformations of the spine: MR imaging. *Radiology* 1987; 164:845–849.
139. Fontaine S, Melanson D, Cosgrove R, Bertrand G. Cavernous hemangiomas of the spinal cord: MR imaging. *Radiology* 1988; 166:839–841.
140. Post MJD. CT update: The impact of time, metrizamide and high resolution on the diagnosis of spinal pathology. In Post MJD (Ed). *Radiographic Evaluation of the Spine.* New York: Masson, 1980; 259–294.
141. Latack JT, Gabrielsen TO, Knake JE, et al. Computed tomography of spinal cord necrosis from multiple sclerosis. *AJNR* 1984; 5:485–487.
142. Larsson E-M, Holtås S, Nilsson O. Gd-DTPA-enhanced MR of suspected spinal multiple sclerosis. AJNR 1989; 10:1071–1076.
143. Zatkin MB, Lander PH, Hadjipavlau AG, Levine JS. Paget disease of the spine: CT with clinical correlation. *Radiology* 1986; 160:155–159.
144. Kaplan PA, Orton DF, Asleson RJ. Osteoporosis with vertebral compression fractures, retropulsed fragments and neurological compromise. *Radiology* 1987; 165:533–535.
145. Gilsanz V, Gibbens DT, Roe TF, et al. Vertebral bone density in children: Effect of puberty. *Radiology* 1988; 166:847–850.

INDEX

Page numbers in *italics* denote figures; those followed by "t" denote tables.